Clinico Radiological Series

TEMPORAL BONE IMAGING

Clinico Radiological Series
TEMPORAL BONE IMAGING

Second Edition

Editors

Ashu Seith Bhalla MD MAMS FICR
Professor
Department of Radiodiagnosis
All India Institute of Medical Sciences
New Delhi, India

Manisha Jana MD DNB FRCR
Additional Professor
Department of Radiodiagnosis
All India Institute of Medical Sciences
New Delhi, India

Co-editor

Smita Manchanda MD DNB MNAMS
Associate Professor
Department of Radiodiagnosis
All India Institute of Medical Sciences
New Delhi, India

Surgical Content Editors

Suresh C Sharma MS
Professor
Formerly Head
Department of Otorhinolaryngology and
Head and Neck Surgery
All India Institute of Medical Sciences
New Delhi, India

Alok Thakar MS DNB FRCS
Professor and Head
Department of Otorhinolaryngology and
Head and Neck Surgery
All India Institute of Medical Sciences
New Delhi, India

JAYPEE

JAYPEE BROTHERS MEDICAL PUBLISHERS

The Health Sciences Publisher

New Delhi | London

Jaypee Brothers Medical Publishers (P) Ltd

Headquarters

Jaypee Brothers Medical Publishers (P) Ltd
4838/24, Ansari Road, Daryaganj
New Delhi 110 002, India
Phone: +91-11-43574357
Fax: +91-11-43574314
Email: jaypee@jaypeebrothers.com

Overseas Office

J.P. Medical Ltd
83 Victoria Street, London
SW1H 0HW (UK)
Phone: +44-20 317 08910
Email: info@jpmedpub.com

EU GPSR Authorised Representative

Logos Europe, 9 rue Nicolas Poussin
17000, La Rochelle, France
Phone: +33 (0) 6 67 93 73 78
E-mail: Contact@logoseurope.eu

Website: www.jaypeebrothers.com
Website: www.jaypeedigital.com

Clinico Radiological Series: Temporal Bone Imaging

First Edition: 2016
Second Edition: **2021**
ISBN: 978-93-90020-73-7

Dedicated To

Surgeons whose never ending questions compel us to push the boundaries

Contributors

Aanchal Kakkar MD
Assistant Professor
Department of Pathology
All India Institute of Medical Sciences
New Delhi, India

Adarsh Ghosh MD
Research Fellow
Department of Radiology
Children's Hospital of Philadelphia
PA, USA

Ajay Garg MD DM
Professor, Department of Neuro
Radiology
All India Institute of Medical Sciences
New Delhi, India

Alok Thakar MS DNB FRCS
Professor and Head
Department of Otorhinolaryngology and
Head and Neck Surgery
All India Institute of Medical Sciences
New Delhi, India

Ankur Goyal MD DNB MNAMS
Assistant Professor
Department of Radiodiagnosis
All India Institute of Medical Sciences
New Delhi, India

Anuradha Singh MD DNB
Assistant Professor
Sanjay Gandhi Postgraduate Institute of
Medical Sciences
Lucknow, Uttar Pradesh, India

Aparna Irodi MD FRCR
Professor
Department of Radiodiagnosis
Christian Medical College
Vellore, Tamil Nadu, India

Arvind Kumar Kairo MS
Associate Professor
Department of Otorhinolaryngology and
Head and Neck Surgery
All India Institute of Medical Sciences
New Delhi, India

Ashu Seith Bhalla MD MAMS FICR
Professor
Department of Radiodiagnosis
All India Institute of Medical Sciences
New Delhi, India

Atin Kumar MD MNAMS FICR
Professor
Department of Radiodiagnosis
All India Institute of Medical Sciences
New Delhi, India

Chandrashekhara SH MD DNB MNAMS
Additional Professor
Department of Radiodiagnosis
All India Institute of Medical Sciences
New Delhi, India

Chirom Amit Singh MS
Additional Professor
Department of Otorhinolaryngology and
Head and Neck Surgery
All India Institute of Medical Sciences
New Delhi, India

Devasenathipathy Kandasamy MD
DNB FRCR
Additional Professor
Department of Radiodiagnosis
All India Institute of Medical Sciences
New Delhi, India

Gh Mohammad Wani MD
Former Fellow in Thoracic Radiology
Department of Radiodiagnosis
All India Institute of Medical Sciences
New Delhi, India

Hitesh Verma MD DNB MNAMS
Associate Professor
Department of Otorhinolaryngology and Head and Neck Surgery
All India Institute of Medical Sciences
New Delhi, India

Jyoti Kumar MD DNB MNAMS
Professor
Department of Radiology and Imaging
Maulana Azad Medical College
New Delhi, India

Kapil Sikka MD DNB MNAMS
Additional Professor
Department of Otorhinolaryngology and Head and Neck Surgery
All India Institute of Medical Sciences
New Delhi, India

Madhavi K DNB
Assistant Professor
Christian Medical College
Vellore, Tamil Nadu, India

Manisha Jana MD DNB FRCR
Additional Professor
Department of Radiodiagnosis
All India Institute of Medical Sciences
New Delhi, India

Priyanka Naranje MD DNB MNAMS
Associate Professor
Department of Radiodiagnosis
All India Institute of Medical Sciences
New Delhi, India

Shivanand Gamanagatti MD DNB
Professor
Department of Radiodiagnosis
All India Institute of Medical Sciences
New Delhi, India

Shuchita Singh MS DNB MNAMS
Associate Professor
Department of Otorhinolaryngology and Head and Neck Surgery
All India Institute of Medical Sciences
New Delhi, India

Smita Manchanda MD DNB MNAMS
Associate Professor
Department of Radiodiagnosis
All India Institute of Medical Sciences
New Delhi, India

Surabhi Vyas MD DNB MNAMS
Additional Professor
Department of Radiodiagnosis
All India Institute of Medical Sciences
New Delhi, India

Suresh C Sharma MS
Professor, Formerly Head
Department of Otorhinolaryngology and Head and Neck Surgery
All India Institute of Medical Sciences
New Delhi, India

Vinit Baliyan MBBS MD
Clinical Fellow
Emergency Radiology
Massachusetts General Hospital
Boston, MA, USA

Foreword to the First Edition

The sentiment that "Temporal Bone Imaging" is a complex topic is echoed by most radiologists—both neophytes and experts. The advances in surgical technique and the growing number of cochlear implant surgeries over the last decade mandate accurate delineation of the anatomy of this region. The advent of multidetector computed tomography (MDCT) has revolutionized the understanding of pathology of this region but has also made the reporting of temporal bone pathology more complex. Using postprocessing tools on MDCT, it is now possible to trace even minute structures in multiple planes. "Temporal Bone Imaging" is a dynamic field requiring constant effort on the part of managing clinicians to keep abreast with recent advances.

This book is the first volume of a series titled "*Clinico Radiological Series*" and the authors have chosen a team of experts mostly from the All India Institute of Medical Sciences (AIIMS), New Delhi, India. They have attempted to simplify this rather complex topic and give a "management" context to the radiologists while reporting. The book also has invaluable contributions from Head and Neck surgeons, presented in lucid chapters.

There is detailed coverage of anatomy in a user-friendly compact, bulleted text complemented by high-quality illustrations throughout the book. There is no compromise on detail and the book should prove useful to the surgeons as well. A unique feature is the formulation of structured reporting format for various disease groups which is enhanced by illustrative cases.

The topic and format of this should make it a "trusted guide" for postgraduates and residents of Radiology as well as Otorhinolaryngology. It will be an asset to practicing radiologists and surgeons as well and reminds me of the adage "less is more"!

Raju Sharma
Professor
Department of Radiodiagnosis
All India Institute of Medical Sciences (AIIMS)
New Delhi, India

Preface to the Second Edition

"Change is the only constant"
— Heraclitus

The *"Clinico Radiological Series"* started its journey in 2016; and *"Temporal Bone Imaging"* was the first book in this series. The whole concept of a combined handbook having both clinical and imaging inputs was much like walking on a road less traveled. To our satisfaction, the overwhelming response to the first edition of this book encouraged us to explore this path again.

As with any other field in medicine, the understanding of temporal bone diseases and surgical techniques have undergone significant change in the past few years. Cochlear implant, e.g., is one such front. It is hence the need of the hour that we keep abreast with the recent advances in this field. In this Second Edition of the book, we have incorporated new imaging as well as relevant surgical advances. We hope this will be beneficial to both the radiologists as well as ENT surgeons alike.

Keeping in mind the need of the radiologists and surgeons-in-training, this edition has been further enhanced by addition of more number of high-quality illustrations, flowcharts, and tables, wherever required. Another addition is the self-assessment module, containing examination-oriented long questions and MCQs with elaborate explanations. It also contains 50 interesting spotters, which we hope the postgraduates will find extremely useful.

We thank our readers for their faith and support in us, and welcome feedback and suggestions for further improvement.

Ashu Seith Bhalla
Manisha Jana

Preface to the First Edition

"What the mind does not know; the eyes do not see"; and Head and Neck radiology, especially temporal bone essays the phrase better than any other radiologic subspecialty. Head and Neck anatomy is complex; and so is the radiology of Head and Neck diseases. The range of diseases involving head and neck is wide and varies according to the anatomic region involved. Amongst them all, temporal bone probably harbors the most complex anatomic intricacies and hence the most difficult area to interpret the abnormalities of. Vital to hearing and equilibrium; temporal bone is the seat of various disease processes which are unique to it. A thorough knowledge of the regional anatomy and the normal variations is crucial in order to identify the imaging abnormalities, which can be quite subtle at times. And even a trained eye may miss significant yet subtle findings unless a systematic approach is adopted for reporting.

Otorhinolaryngology and Head and Neck surgery is a rapidly expanding medical specialty which relies heavily on imaging. Practicing surgeons need to be aware of the basics of imaging involving their area of interest, as the same holds true for temporal bone surgeries. Similarly, radiologists practicing Head and Neck radiology need to be aware of the details of temporal bone anatomy and provide a structured and comprehensive report to the surgeon. Cochlear implant surgery is being performed quite frequently now; and the radiologists need to be aware of the imaging requirements for the procedure. For the purpose, this book contains a separate dedicated section on cochlear implant imaging. This book is not intended to be a detailed text on temporal bone imaging but we hope that it will help the busy radiologists and surgeons in interpreting images of the temporal bone. The structured reporting format and illustrative cases at the end of each section are aimed at this.

We welcome any feedback on enhancing the content of the book, which can be incorporated in the subsequent editions.

Ashu Seith Bhalla
Manisha Jana

Acknowledgments

We wish to thank all the contributors, for their efforts in compiling this text. We sincerely thank Professor Suresh C Sharma and Professor Alok Thakar for guiding us in this new endeavor. We are also grateful to Dr Kapil Sikka for compilation of the surgical contents of the book, and Dr Aanchal Kakkar for her contribution in elucidating the concepts in temporal bone pathology.

We would also like to extend our appreciation to our sincere and grateful thanks to Shri Jitendar P Vij (Group Chairman), Mr Ankit Vij (Managing Director), Mr MS Mani (Group President), Dr Richa Saxena (Associate Director-Professional Publishing), Ms Nedup Denka Bhutia (Development Editor), and other staffs of M/s Jaypee Brothers Medical Publishers (P) Ltd, New Delhi, India, for their efforts and input enabling timely publication of the book.

Contents

Section 1: Normal Anatomy and Imaging Technique

Section 2: Congenital Anomalies of External and Middle Ear

Section 9: Examination Section

1

SECTION

Normal Anatomy and Imaging Technique

1

Imaging Techniques in Temporal Bone Evaluation

Ankur Goyal

- Radiographs
  - Frontal Views
  - Lateral Views
  - Oblique View
- Computed Tomography
  - High-resolution Computed Tomography
  - Cone-beam Computed Tomography
- Magnetic Resonance Imaging
- Advanced Imaging Techniques
  - Postprocessing Tools
  - Three-dimensional Variable Flip-angle FLAIR MRI Sequence
  - Facial Nerve Visualization
  - Contrast Magnetic Resonance Angiography
  - Diffusion-weighted MRI
  - MR Spectroscopy and Perfusion MR
  - Diffusion-tensor Imaging

- Temporal bone constitutes the lateral skull base and contributes to middle and posterior fossa and the lateral calvarium. It is situated lateral to the temporal lobe of brain.
- It comprises of five portions: (1) Squamous; (2) Mastoid; (3) Tympanic; and (4) Petrous parts; and (5) Styloid process (**Fig. 1**).
- The small tympanic part houses the tympanic cavity (middle ear), which communicates with the mastoid.
- Petrous portion houses the otic capsule (inner ear) at its base.
- Lower six cranial nerves and major vessels (internal carotid artery and jugular vein) pass in relation to the temporal bone.

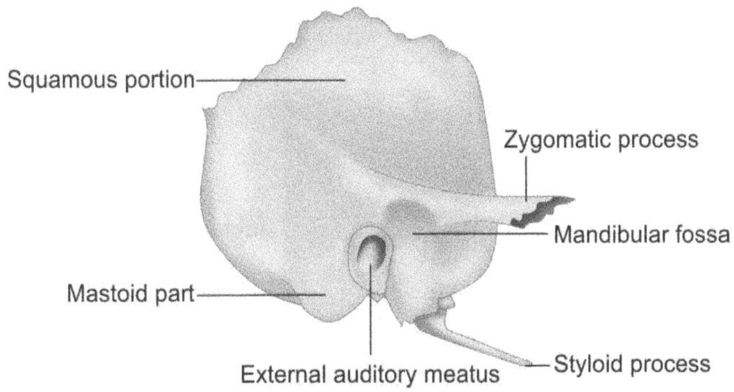

FIG. 1: Diagram showing the parts of temporal bones (view from outside) (petrous part is hidden from view).

- This book focusses on the imaging of ear and related structures, including the petrous apex and lateral skull base.
- The role and techniques of various imaging modalities are discussed in this chapter.
- Always compare with the opposite side on cross-sectional imaging modalities and look for symmetry while reporting.

RADIOGRAPHS

- Radiographs give an overview of the entire temporal bone and indicate the status of pneumatization of the mastoids and petrous pyramids.
- Opacification/sclerosis of air cells indicates otomastoiditis and large lesions can produce osseous lytic destruction, evident on the radiographs.
- Radiographs are also useful to evaluate the position and integrity of cochlear implants, demonstrating the continuity of the wires.
- In addition to intraoperative use, pre- and postoperative radiographs are also very useful.
- Serial radiographs serve to assess the clinical course and disease progression/response.
- Commonly performed projections include frontal view, lateral view, and oblique view.

Frontal Radiographs

Transorbital view:

- It is obtained with orbitomeatal line of the patient perpendicular to the detector and radiation beam going anteroposteriorly or posteroanteriorly, directed at the center of the orbit.
- It provides a frontal projection of the mastoid and petrous pyramid.
- Petrous apex is foreshortened because of its obliquity and internal auditory canal (IAC) is seen as lucent canal extending through it. Vestibule, semicircular canals, and cochlea are also discernible.

Towne's view: This is an anteroposterior radiograph of the skull with a 30° fronto-occipital tilt (**Fig. 2**). This radiographic view enables visualization of the temporal

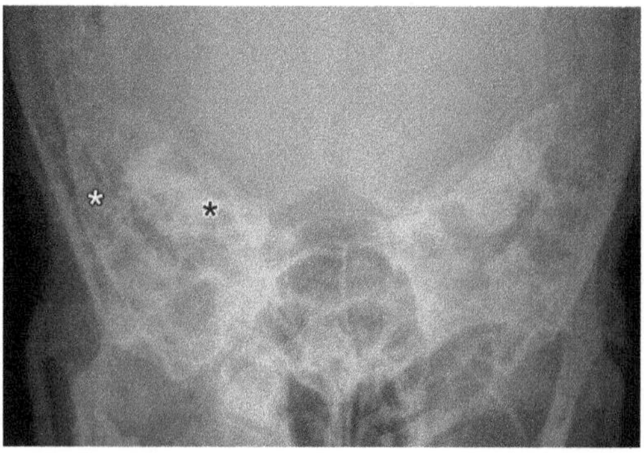

FIG. 2: Towne's view of skull including both mastoid areas: White asterisk marks the region of pneumatized mastoid part of temporal bone while black asterisk indicates the petrous part of temporal bone.

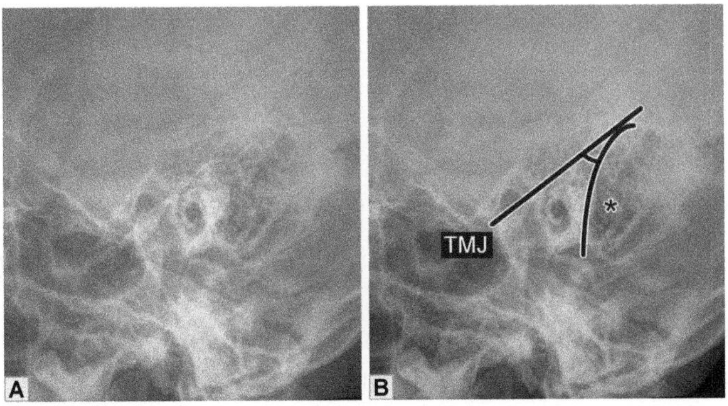

FIGS. 3A AND B: Schuller's view of mastoid: (A) and (B) depict radiographs without and with graphical annotations. Curved vertical line indicates sinus plate while the straight line depicts dural plate. The angle formed between the two is the sinodural angle (shown). Asterisk marks the area of pneumatized mastoid.

bones, mastoid antrum, superior semicircular canal (SSC), internal auditory meatus, cochlea, petrous apex, and external auditory meatus.

Lateral Radiographs

Schuller's projection (**Figs. 3A** and **B**):

- This is a lateral view of the mastoid with the sagittal plane of the patient's skull parallel to the table and X-ray beam directed 30° caudally to separate the two mastoids.
- It gives accurate depiction of degree, extent, and distribution of aeration of mastoid with superimposition of IAC and external auditory canal (EAC).
- The sinus plate is seen as a dense vertical line posterior to the EAC and merges posterosuperiorly with similar dense line (dural plate).
- The sharp angle at the junction of these plates is called as the sinodural angle of Citelli, which becomes obtuse in secondary sclerosis [chronic suppurative otitis media (CSOM)].
- More anteriorly is the superior petrous ridge, which crosses the radiolucency of the EAC and extends to the mandibular condyle.

Law's projection: This employs a 15° caudal tilt instead of 30°.

Oblique (Stenver's) View

- In this view, the patient's head faces the film with slight flexion and 45° rotation to the opposite side, so that ipsilateral orbit touches the image receptor. The X-ray beam is directed 12° cranially.
- The entire petrous apex is visualized in full length while the porus acusticus is seen enface (**Figs. 4A** and **B**). Vestibule, semicircular canals, and mastoid are also seen.

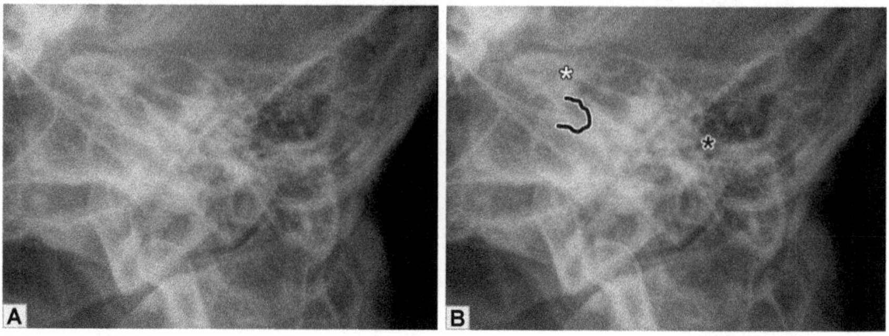

FIGS. 4A AND B: Stenver' view: (A) and (B) depict radiographs without and with graphical annotations. White asterisk marks the petrous apex while black asterisk denotes the pneumatized mastoid. The region of internal auditory canal is also marked (curved line).

COMPUTED TOMOGRAPHY

High-resolution Computed Tomography

- High-resolution multidetector CT is the most frequently employed imaging modality for evaluation of temporal bone.
- Widespread availability, relatively low cost, high spatial resolution, and quick acquisition make it a robust investigation.
- Indications of temporal bone CT include:
    - Congenital/acquired hearing loss (both in conductive and sensorineural)
    - Trauma
    - Neoplasms
    - Infections
    - Preoperative evaluation (for cochlear implant and mastoidectomy)
- *Technique*:
    - Noncontrast thin collimation volumetric CT of both temporal bones is routinely done.
    - Patient lies supine on the CT table and no gantry tilt is employed.
    - Axial acquisition is performed from top of petrous apex to inferior tip of mastoid with acquisition plane parallel to infraorbitomeatal line (**Figs. 5A** and **B**).
    - Small field of view (FOV) (15–20 cm) and high matrix resolution (512 × 512).
    - Data is reconstructed into 0.6 mm thickness overlapping axial and coronal sections. High spatial resolution bone algorithm is used. Large window width (4,000 HU) and low window level (e.g., 0–200 HU) is used.
    - About 2 mm thickness soft tissue window is also reconstructed.
    - Axial images are reconstructed from the top of the petrous apex to the inferior tip of mastoid, parallel to the lateral semicircular canal (LSC).
    - Coronal reformation is done from the anterior margin of the petrous apex to the posterior margin of mastoid.
    - Three-dimensional (3D) multiplanar reformats in different planes are increasingly used to better depict the complex anatomy.

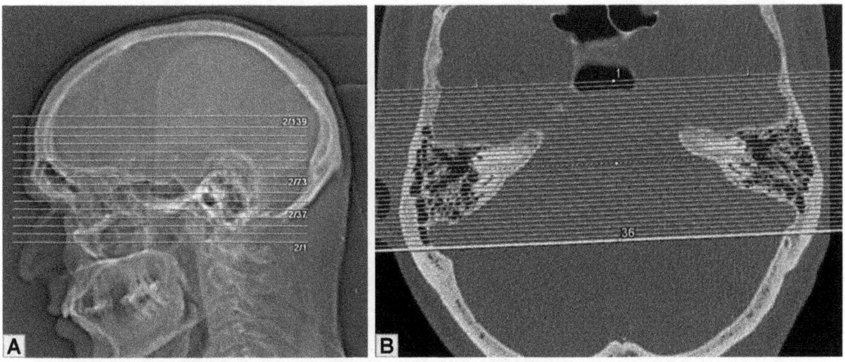

FIGS. 5A AND B: CT planning: (A) Scout CT image showing planning of acquisition for HRCT temporal bone; (B) Coronal multiplanar reformats are then generated from the axial images (plane of reformation shown).

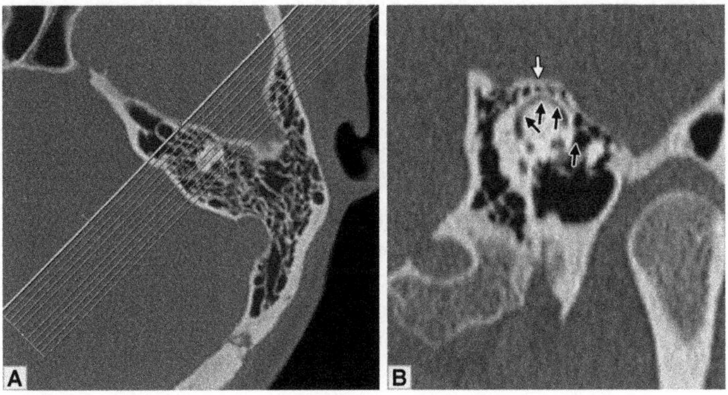

FIGS. 6A AND B: Pöschl plane: (A) Axial CT image depicts section orientation in Pöschl plane (perpendicular to petrous); (B) The resultant CT image at the level of superior semicircular canal shows the canal in its entire extent (small black arrows) with air cells cranial to it (white arrow).

- *Indications of contrast administration* include suspected tumor, abscess formation, vascular involvement, and complications (like sigmoid sinus thrombosis or intracranial spread of disease).
- *Special planes of reconstruction* for each temporal bone (reconstructed in 0.6 mm thickness bone window):
  - *Pöschl plane* (**Figs. 6A** and **B**):
    - Sections are oriented parallel to the SSC and perpendicular to long axis of temporal bone.
    - This is the best plane to detect dehiscence of the roof of SSC.
  - *Stenver's plane* (**Figs. 7A** to **D**):
    - Sections are oriented perpendicular to the SSC and parallel to the long axis of petrous bone.

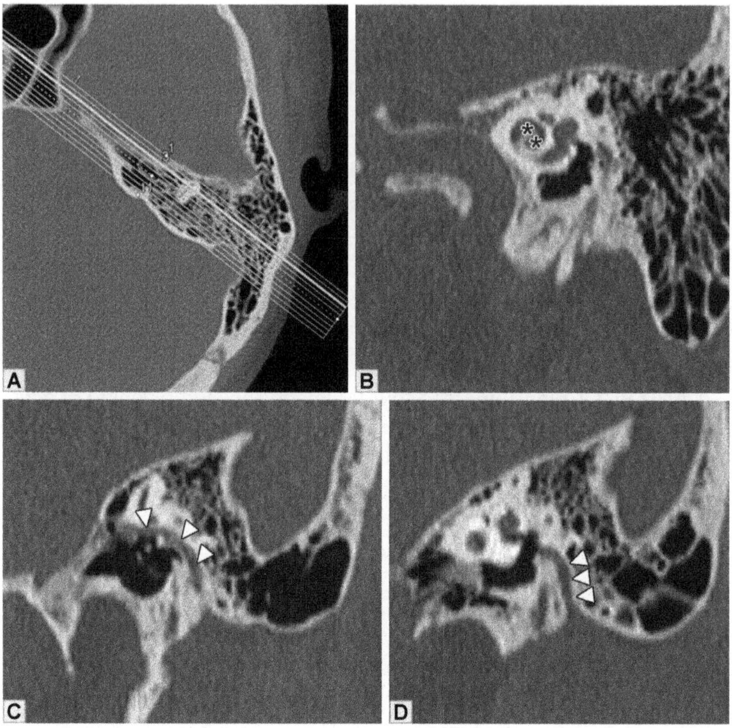

FIGS. 7A TO D: Stenver's plane: (A) Axial CT image depicts orientation of Stenver's plane (parallel to petrous); (B) The resultant plane provides enface depiction of cochlear turns (asterisks); (C) A slight modification of Stenver's plane results in depiction of entire tympanic and proximal mastoid portions of the bony canal of facial nerve (arrowheads); (D) Adjacent section shows distal mastoid portion of the bony canal of facial nerve (arrowheads).

- The result is an oblique coronal short-axis plane of cochlea with enface depiction of all three cochlear turns.
- This is useful for evaluation of temporal bone fractures.
- A slight modification results in depiction of entire tympanic and mastoid segment of facial nerve canal (**Figs. 7C** and **D**).

◦ *Unconventional planes*: Various single and double oblique planes have been described for optimal depiction of ossicles and inner ear structures.[1]
- Double-oblique coronal plane is best for depiction of malleus and incus. The primary reference plane is axial, where line is drawn at 150° to the left vector of the horizontal axis.
- The secondary reference plane is sagittal where line is drawn at 85° for malleus (**Figs. 8A** to **C**) and 60° for incus (**Figs. 9A** and **B**).
- There are separate planes for stapes-oval window complex both in long (double oblique axial) and short axes (double oblique sagittal).

- Three-dimensional volume-rendering postprocessing tools enable easy understanding of the normal structures and pathologies (discussed later).

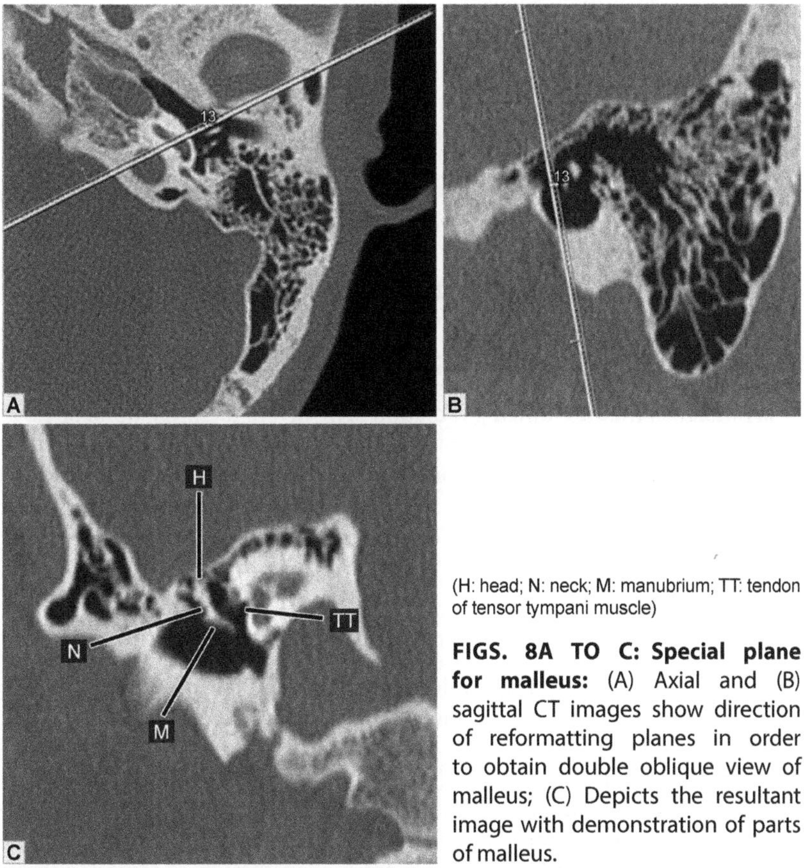

(H: head; N: neck; M: manubrium; TT: tendon of tensor tympani muscle)

FIGS. 8A TO C: Special plane for malleus: (A) Axial and (B) sagittal CT images show direction of reformatting planes in order to obtain double oblique view of malleus; (C) Depicts the resultant image with demonstration of parts of malleus.

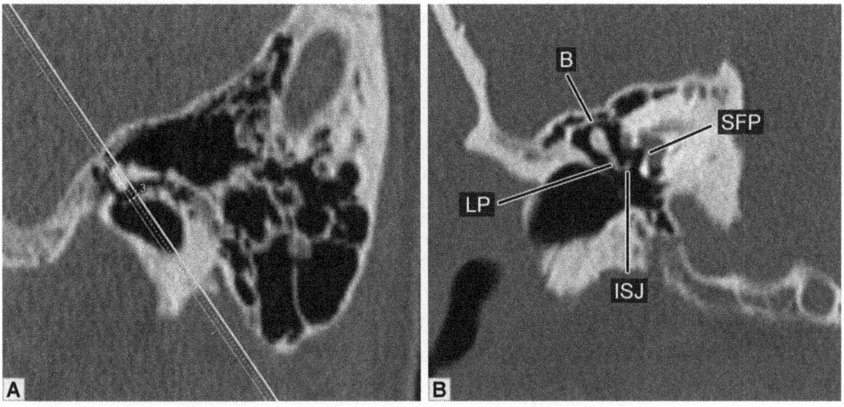

(B: body; ISJ: incudostapedial joint; LP: long process; SFP: stapedial foot plate)

FIGS. 9A AND B: Special plane for incus: (A) Sagittal CT image shows direction of reformatting plane in order to obtain double oblique view of incus. Orientation on axial CT image is same as in **Figure 7A;** (B) Demonstrates the parts of incus on resultant image.

Cone Beam Computed Tomography

- Cone beam CT (CBCT) employs a cone-shaped X-ray beam, directed toward the temporal bone onto a two-dimensional (2D) detector. Since it uses the entire FOV of the 2D X-ray detector, only a single gantry rotation is required to acquire a 3D-volumetric dataset.
- Advantages over multidetector computed tomography (MDCT) include low radiation dose despite high spatial resolution and less metallic and beam hardening artifacts.
- However, acquisition time is long and thus it is prone to motion artifacts.

MAGNETIC RESONANCE IMAGING

- Advantage is that no ionizing radiation is involved. It can be done at 1.5–3T. Sedation is required for children.
- *Indications*: For evaluation of brainstem, cerebellopontine angle, IAC, 7th to 8th nerve complex and signal intensity of cochlea-vestibular apparatus (modality of choice for inner ear evaluation).

Basic Sequences

These include:

- Three-dimensional axial isotropic thin-section (0.3–0.6 mm) cisternography-type sequences of bilateral inner ear and IAC regions. Two types of MR sequences may be done:
    - Steady-state free precession (SSFP) gradient-echo sequences (FIESTA or TrueFISP or balanced SSFP) highlight structures with high T2/T1 ratios [constructive interference in steady state (CISS) on Siemens, FIESTA+C on GE, bSSFP on Philips]; enabling optimal evaluation of cerebellopontine angles and inner ears.
    - An alternative is heavily T2-weighted (T2W) fast/turbo spin-echo sequence (RESTORE on Siemens, FRFSE on GE, DRIVE on Philips) (**Figs. 10A** to **C**). Susceptibility artifacts are lesser compared to balanced SSFP sequences.
    - Sagittal oblique reformatted images are then generated perpendicular to the 7th to 8th nerve complex in the IAC and cerebellopontine angle. The fluid-filled spaces of membranous labyrinth and semicircular canals are well seen.
- Thin section (1.25–2 mm) axial and coronal T2W.
- Thin section (2–3 mm) axial and coronal T1W.
- Thin section axial and coronal (or 3D) postcontrast T1W (fat-suppressed).
- A multiphasic scan may also be done to evaluate the contrast kinetics as well as for perfusion studies in case of mass lesions. Detection of delayed enhancement may help in differentiating postoperative granulation tissue from residual cholesteatomas.
- Screening fluid-attenuated inversion recovery (FLAIR) (axial or 3D) and diffusion-weighted imaging (DWI) of entire brain with postcontrast scans.

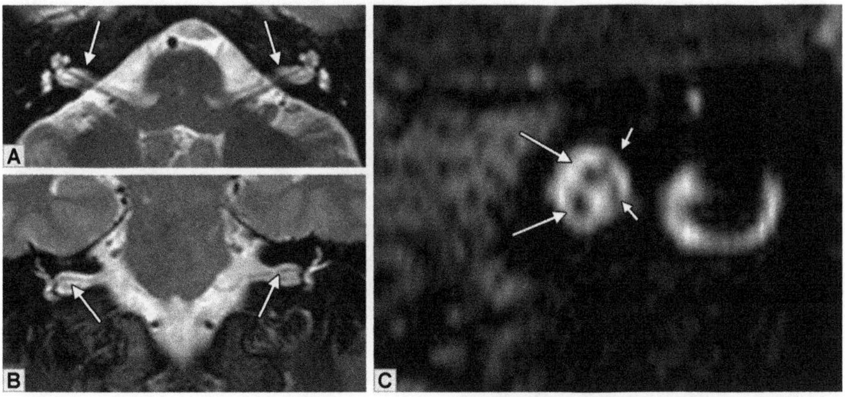

FIGS. 10A TO C: MRI for depiction of nerves in internal auditory canal (IAC): (A) Axial T-2 weighted (T2W) MR image at the level of 7th to 8th nerve complexes shows both IACs (white arrows) with cochlea and vestibule; (B) Coronal T2W MR image, at the level of IAC, showing 7th to 8th nerves (arrows) with bilateral semicircular canals; (C) Sagittal oblique image of constructive interference steady state (CISS) sequence shows anterosuperiorly facial nerve (superior long arrow), anteroinferiorly cochlear nerve (inferior long arrow), superior and inferior vestibular nerves posteriorly (short arrows).

ADVANCED IMAGING TECHNIQUES

Postprocessing Tools

- These include 3D surface reconstructions (**Figs. 11A** to **C**) [surface-shaded display (SSD)] and volume rendering technique (VRT) to have an overview of fluid-filled cochlea-vestibular apparatus [in magnetic resonance imaging (MRI)] and/or associated auricle anomalies (in CT).
- Image segmentation can be done and various structures (like ossicles) can be seen in isolation in three dimensions after clipping out surrounding regions.
- Virtual endoscopy of the middle ear structures is also possible because of high contrast between the bony structures and air spaces in CT. These structures can be rotated in space and dissected in different planes, enabling understanding of the complex anatomy of ossicles and inner ear structures.
- Other postprocessing tools include maximal intensity projection (MIP) and minimal intensity projections (MinIP).

Three-dimensional Variable Flip-angle FLAIR MRI Sequence

- These include SPACE FLAIR on Siemens, cube FLAIR on GE, and FLAIR VISTA on Philips (please see Chapter 20).[2]
- Fluid signal is suppressed and brain signal is accentuated.
- This is useful in evaluation of Ménière's disease because it permits distinct visualization of endolymphatic and perilymphatic components.[3]
- It is also useful to detect labyrinthine hemorrhage and to monitor the degree of functional impairment in case of vestibular schwannoma.

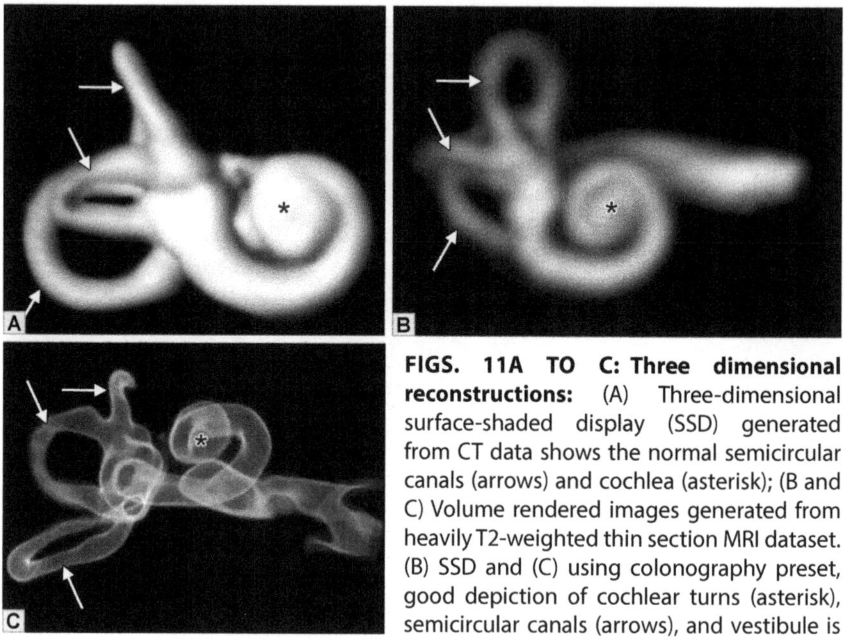

FIGS. 11A TO C: Three dimensional reconstructions: (A) Three-dimensional surface-shaded display (SSD) generated from CT data shows the normal semicircular canals (arrows) and cochlea (asterisk); (B and C) Volume rendered images generated from heavily T2-weighted thin section MRI dataset. (B) SSD and (C) using colonography preset, good depiction of cochlear turns (asterisk), semicircular canals (arrows), and vestibule is possible.

- This sequence has also been found to be helpful after contrast administration, for the evaluation of Ménière's disease.
- Endolymphatic hydrops may be detected on 3D heavily T2W sequences where saccular dilatation may be seen as enlarged hypointense structure.
- However, postcontrast 3D FLAIR imaging is better validated for this purpose. Contrast may be administered intratympanically or more commonly intravenously followed by delayed phase imaging.
- Usually, double dose of contrast is administered intravenously and acquisition is done at 4 hours after contrast injection. 3T acquisition is better to accentuate the contrast opacification of perilymph and better assess the nonenhancing cochlear duct. Also, the perilymph enhancement has been found to be more dramatic in the ears affected by Ménière's disease.
- Recently, constant high flip-angle technique has been sound to have higher intensity ratio compared to heavily-T2 variable flip-angle method.[4]

Facial Nerve Visualization

- Cisternal and intracanalicular parts of facial nerve are well seen on 3D cisternography sequences mentioned above. However, it is difficult to visualize the labyrinthine, tympanic, and mastoid segments. Parotid part can be seen by 3D double-echo steady state (DESS) sequence with water excitation (**Figs. 12A** and **B**).

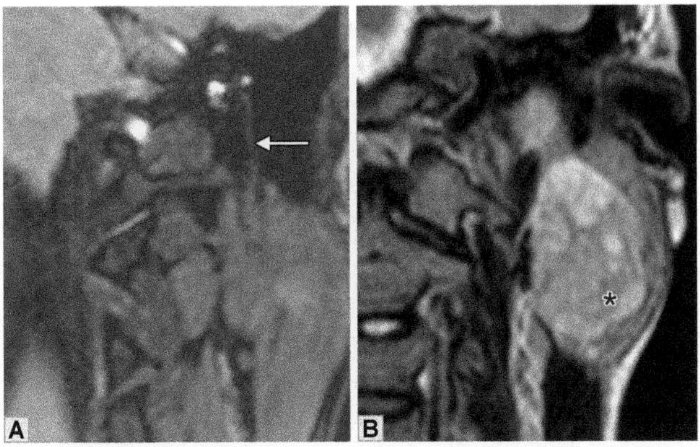

FIGS. 12A AND B: Facial nerve: (A) Coronal double-echo steady state image shows the facial nerve in mastoid and parotid segments (arrow); (B) Corresponding coronal T2-weighted magnetic resonance image depicts pleomorphic adenoma in left parotid gland (asterisk).

- *Postcontrast T1W 2D sequence*: Facial nerve faintly enhances in the region of geniculate ganglion, tympanic and mastoid segments after contrast administration. However, rest of the segments does not enhance and thus any enhancement in these regions may suggest inflammation/neoplastic pathology.
- *Postcontrast T1W 3D*: Spoiled gradient acquisition in the steady state [spoiled gradient recalled (SPGR) in GE, VIBE in Siemens and FFE in Philips].
- *Three-dimensional inversion recovery fast spoiled gradient recalled (IR-FSPGR) sequence:* Compared to SPGR, facial nerve shows significantly higher signal on this sequence in majority of the segments on both unenhanced and contrast-enhanced images.
- *Pointwise encoding time reduction with radial acquisition (PETRA) ultra-short echo time sequence*: Usually done at 3T, this MR sequence enables visualization of facial nerve from its origin, through the temporal bone, to the stylomastoid foramen.[5]

Contrast Magnetic Resonance Angiography

- Magnetic resonance arteriography and venography can be employed to assess the vascular structures in the jugular foramen and carotid canal, especially in case of large mass lesions.
- Time-of-flight (ToF) sequence enables this evaluation without the need of contrast, but the method of choice is contrast-enhanced angiography.
- Three-dimensional MR angiography provides excellent demonstration of both intracranial and extracranial vessels and arteries and veins can be separately imaged (**Figs. 13A** to **D**).

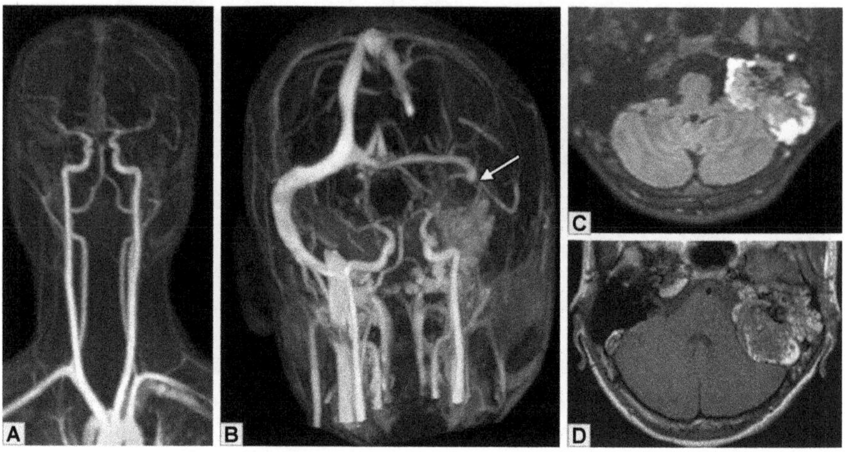

FIGS. 13A TO D: MR angiogram: MR angiogram arterial phase postcontrast MIP image provides excellent depiction of arteries of head and neck. (A) No tumor feeder arteries seen; (B) MR angiogram venous phase postcontrast MIP image (seen from anterior) depicts nonvisualization of left-sided sigmoid sinus (compressed due to mass effect). Arrow shows abrupt termination of left transverse sinus; (C) Axial 3D FLAIR image of the same patient demonstrates heterogeneously hyperintense mass lesion in left retrocochlear region; (D) Axial T1W image shows peripheral hyperintensity, suggesting hemorrhage within. Histopathology revealed endolymphatic sac tumor.

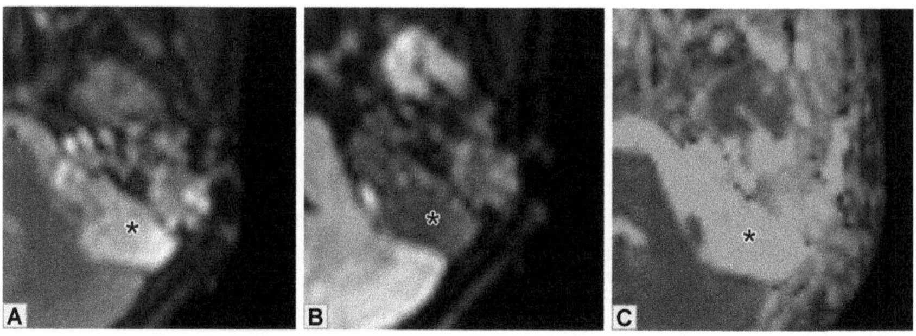

FIGS. 14A TO C: Diffusion-weighted MR imaging in tumors: (Same patient as in Figure 13). (A) Axial diffusion-weighted image at low b-value (0 s/mm^2); (B) High b-value (800 s/mm^2), and (C) Apparent diffusion coefficient) map shows that there is no restriction of diffusion within the mass lesion, suggested by low signal intensity on (B) and high signal on (C) (asterisks).

Diffusion-weighted MRI

- It detects the Brownian motion of water molecules, which is facilitated or restricted based on tissue characteristics (**Figs. 14A** to **C**).
- *Single-shot echo planar imaging (EPI) based sequence* is prone to susceptibility artifacts and geometric distortion.
- Thus, multishot or segmented EPI sequences are used.

- These include MUSE in GE, RESOLVE in Siemens, and multishot EPI in Philips.
- Reduced FOV technique can be employed to generate high resolution images in EPI-based diffusion (FOCUS in GE, ZOOMit in Siemens, and ZOOM Diffusion in Philips).

- *Non-EPI sequences*:
  - These include fast spin-echo sequences like PROPELLER in GE, BLADE AND HASTE in Siemens, and MULTIVANE in Philips.
  - There is higher spatial resolution, thinner sections can be acquired (for smaller lesions) and less susceptibility artefacts using this technique.
- b-values of 0 and 800–100 s/mm^2 are often used.
- Restricted diffusion is the hallmark of congenital cholesteatomas with smooth bony remodeling.
- Residual/recurrent cholesteatomas can also be detected with high accuracy along with delayed postcontrast imaging.
- Tumors and abscesses also show restricted diffusion.
- Magnetic resonance spectroscopy (MRS) and perfusion MRI may be employed for characterization of mass lesions, especially in retrocochlear region. Elevated choline on MRS indicates increased cell turnover, suggesting a neoplastic lesion (**Figs. 15A** and **B**).
- Diffusion tensor imaging may be helpful in detection of disruptions of the brainstem auditory pathway (**Fig. 16**).
- Digital subtraction angiography (DSA) is primarily reserved for preoperative embolizations and demonstration of cross circulation.

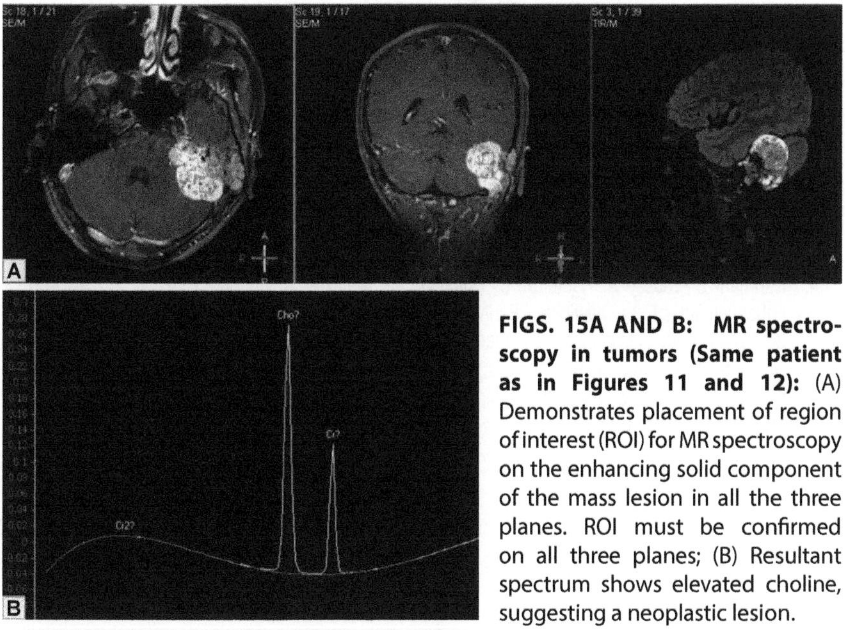

FIGS. 15A AND B: MR spectroscopy in tumors (Same patient as in Figures 11 and 12): (A) Demonstrates placement of region of interest (ROI) for MR spectroscopy on the enhancing solid component of the mass lesion in all the three planes. ROI must be confirmed on all three planes; (B) Resultant spectrum shows elevated choline, suggesting a neoplastic lesion.

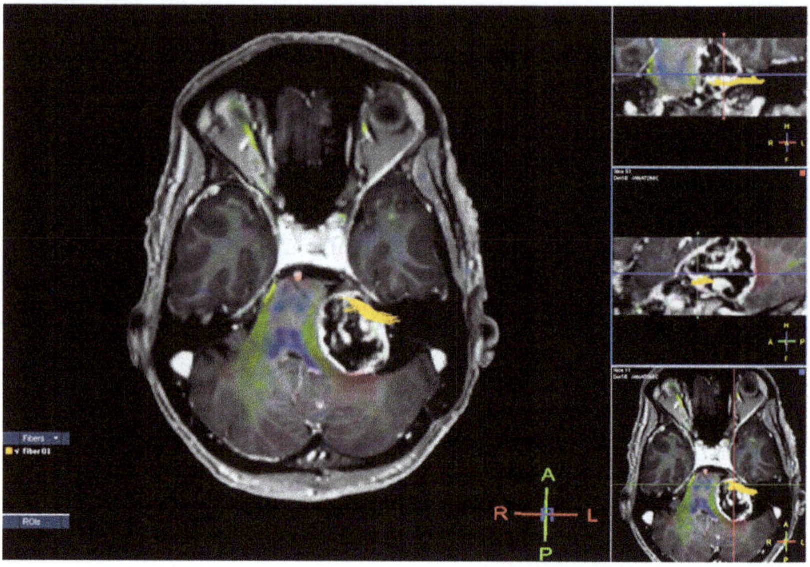

FIG. 16: Diffusion-tensor imaging. Axial image generated from three-dimensional tractography with color-coded fractional anisotropy map depicts mass effect on the 7th to 8th nerves in the cisternal and canalicular portion by cystic schwannoma.

Courtesy: Professor Ajay Garg.

CONCLUSION

Knowledge of basic imaging techniques and indications is important to optimally utilize different modalities. Imaging advancements have enabled increased role of imaging in taking patient management decisions.

REFERENCES

1. Lane JI, Lindell EP, Witte RJ, DeLone DR, Driscoll CLW. Middle and Inner Ear: Improved Depiction with Multiplanar Reconstruction of Volumetric CT Data. Radiographics. 2006;26(1):115-24.
2. Jambawalikar S, Liu MZ, Moonis G. Advanced MR Imaging of the Temporal Bone. Neuroimaging Clin N Am. 2019;29(1):197-202.
3. Bernaerts A. MRI in Menière's Disease. J Belgian Soc Radiol. 2018;102(S1):13.
4. Nahmani S, Vaussy A, Hautefort C, Guichard JP, Guillonet A, Houdart E, et al. Comparison of Enhancement of the Vestibular Perilymph between Variable and Constant Flip Angle–Delayed 3D-FLAIR Sequences in Menière Disease. Am J Neuroradiol. 2020;41(4):706-11.
5. Guenette JP, Seethamraju RT, Jayender j, Corrales CE, Lee TC. MR Imaging of the Facial Nerve through the Temporal Bone at 3T with a Noncontrast Ultrashort Echo Time Sequence. Am J Neuroradiol. 2018;39(10):1903-6.

2 Three Dimensional Printing and Its Applications in the Temporal Bone

Adarsh Ghosh, Ashu Seith Bhalla

- Acquisition of subcentimetric isovoxel images using high-resolution computed tomography (HRCT) and three-dimensional (3D) magnetic resonance imaging (MRI) provides exquisite anatomical details. Radiologists are trained in the visualization of such volumetric data on two-dimensional (2D) screens. However, sharing this valuable information with clinical counterpart becomes challenging.
- 3D printing, with its roots in the manufacturing industry, enables translation of such volumetric data into models enabling better visualization of anatomy and pathology by surgeons.
- 3D printing allows patient-specific preoperative surgical planning and training, designing of a patient-specific prosthesis, and enables the creation of teaching tools.
- Radiologists occupy a pivotal role in any 3D printing service. We cover the basics of 3D printing, hoping to give our readers a basic preview of the various nuances involved in 3D printing of the temporal bone.

FILE FORMATS

- Also known as additive manufacturing, the process of 3D printing creates a 3D object from a digital file. The digital file contains pertinent information specifying how the individual layers of materials are successively laid down to create the object.
- 3D printers do not recognize digital imaging and communications in medicine (DICOM) images, and the first step in 3D printing involves the conversion of DICOM images to a format compatible with a 3D printer.
- Any object for 3D printing needs to be defined in space by several non-overlapping surfaces. *Standard Tessellation Language (STL)* is the most commonly used standardized format. In STL, each surface is defined as multiple sets of triangles or "facets" fitting together like a jigsaw puzzle (**Figs. 1A** and **B**).

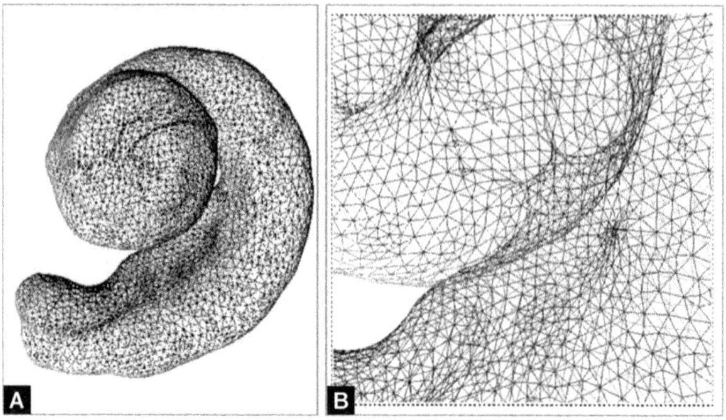

FIGS. 1A AND B: 3D printer specific file formats: The 3D model is defined as being enclosed by multiple surfaces for its conversion into the Standard Tessellation Language (STL) format. In STL file format each surface is defined as multiple sets of triangles or "facets" fitting together like a jigsaw puzzle (A) and each surface is reconstructed using a specified number of triangular facets (B).

- The *Additive Manufacturing File Format (AMF)* is sometimes used as an alternative. AMF allows additional descriptors (e.g., tactile texture of the surface being printed, and materials used for printing of different surfaces) to be incorporated into the final 3D printed model.

3D MODELS VERSUS VOLUME RENDERING TECHNIQUES

- 3D printing may be considered an extension of volume rendering techniques (VRTs) available on several commercial radiology workstations.
- Volume rendering technique allows 2D display on the console of a discrete 3D rendering of a DICOM data.
- These renditions may be rotated in space, cropped, and sectioned in any plane; however, they do not provide the functionality of a dedicated 3D image-based engineering software.
- A targeted 3D printing compatible software (**Table 1**) provides a much more extensive range of image editing options, such as automated and advanced segmentation; 3D cropping and image manipulation; preoperative fracture reconstruction; and operative implant planning which helps in better visualization of data. Further, these software allow the conversion of the DICOM images into specific 3D printing compatible file formats.

TABLE 1 Software platforms available for three-dimensional (3D) image post-processing.

3D Slicer	https://www.slicer.org	Free
CRAFTWARE	https://craftbot.com/craftware	Free
CURA	https://ultimaker.com/software/ultimaker-cura	Free
MATERIALISE MIMICS	https://www.materialise.com/en/medical/mimics-innovation-suite/mimics	Paid
REPETIER	https://www.repetier.com	Free
3D TOOL	https://www.3d-tool.com	Free
BLENDER	https://www.blender.org	Free
MESHFIX	http://meshrepair.org	Free
HOROS	https://horosproject.org	Free
OSIRIX	https://www.osirix-viewer.com	Free ± Paid

STEPS OF 3D PRINTING

- *Image acquisition*: Three-dimensional printing needs a volumetric data set (usually <1.25 mm voxel size). Most commonly, HRCT temporal bone is used—however, isovolumetric MRI datasets or fusion of imaging modalities may also be used (**Figs. 2A** and **B**).[1,2]
- *Segmentation*: This refers to the accurate delineation of anatomy to be printed using regions of interest (ROIs) (**Fig. 2 C**), which label the various structures on the DICOM images for conversion into the STL format.
  - Radiologists are indispensable for the segmentation task, and manual segmentation by a radiologist is taken to be the gold standard.
  - While a detailed discussion of the various segmentation methods available is beyond the scope of this text, the threshold method often suffices for bone segmentation and is commonly used in temporal bone 3D printing.
  - In the *threshold method*, all voxels above a particular value are segmented to represent one specific anatomical structure (e.g., pixels above 700 HU are taken to represent bone) (**Fig. 2 C**).
  - The segmented voxels in the ROI are rendered in 3D (**Fig. 2D**) and are then enclosed in a 3D surface allowing this surface to be reconstructed using a specified number of triangular facets, thus enabling conversion to an STL format. The size and the number of the triangles used in recreating the surface determine the anatomical fidelity and the smoothness of the model thus generated.

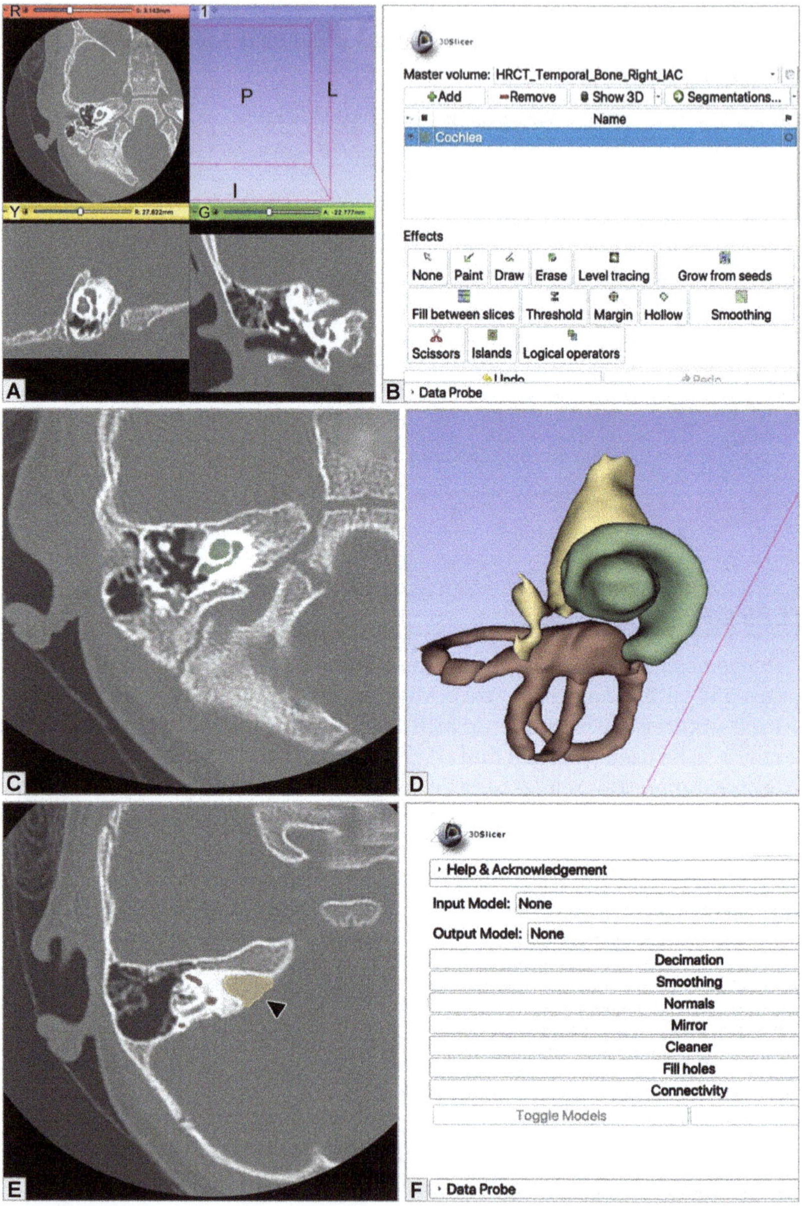

FIGS. 2A TO F: Steps of three-dimensional (3D) printing: (A) A HRCT or isotropic 3D MRI sequence is used; (B) The images are imported in digital imaging and communications in medicine (DICOM) format into a dedicated processing software; (C) The anatomy of interest is segmented using various tools including thresholding; (D) A 3D model is generated; (E and F) Several postprocessing steps including closing of open-ended structures such as internal auditory meatus (E; black arrowhead) and automated filling of holes (F) are carried out on the 3D model generated before the model is exported in the Standard Tessellation Language (STL) format. Scaffolds and supports may be added in this stage or later finally before passing on the model to a 3D printer.

- Additional postprocessing steps include:
    - Evaluating the mesh of triangles created for inadvertent holes or intersecting facets using automated software-driven mesh smoothening and hole filling.
    - Connecting unconnected surfaces to be printed.
    - Closing ends of the open-ended structures and filling various gaps (**Fig. 2E**).
    - Filling internal spaces with honeycomb grids to decrease the amount of raw material used for printing (**Fig. 2F**).
    - Adding supports and scaffolds to the 3D model to be printed so that the model does not collapse during printing.
    - Inscribing a patient identifier allowing easy identification at a later date
- *Printing*: A wide variety of printers, printing methodology, and print materials are available for 3D printing. While cost remains an important determinant, availability, color of materials, autoclavability, and malleability of the printing material determine the method and materials selected for printing (**Table 2**).

TABLE 2 **Different three dimensionally (3D) available methods by which generated files are 3D printed.**

Stereolithography	A 3D object is printed using a liquid plastic source which is laid down one layer at a time. The resin is placed on a transparent vat, and a ultraviolet light traces the pattern of interest—solidifying (curing) the resin. The solidified structure is progressively removed from the container of resin by a lifting platform while the laser creates a new layer—resulting in a 3D shape
Material jetting	May be considered a 3D inkjet printer. Material is jetted onto a build platform where it solidifies, and the model is built layer by layer
Binder Jetting	A liquid bonding agent is selectively deposited to join powder particles. Layers of material are then bonded to form an object
Material extrusion	A 3D object is constructed using a thermoplastic filament. The model is built layer by layer after extruding the heated thermoplastic material through a heated nozzle
Powder bed fusion	May use either a laser or electron beam to melt and fuse the material powder

APPLICATIONS IN TEMPORAL BONE

While 3D printing has been used extensively in various surgical and medical applications, it has a very niche role in temporal bone surgeries as discussed.

Surgical Planning

- 3D printing effectively communicates to surgeons the information contained in 2D images.

- It allows visuospatial and tactile reorientation essential for surgeons enabling a better understanding of patient-specific pathology required for detailed preoperative planning, especially in complex reconstructive surgeries.
- Drilling can be practiced on pathological anatomy before actually working on the patient; improving surgical precision, reducing complications, and enabling the development of a mental road-map for the procedure. This is especially important in the temporal bone where small anatomical space and complex anatomy makes visualization of 3D pathology on computer screens difficult.
- Surgical planning may be more precise in cases where previous surgery has significantly altered the normal anatomy and determination of residual bone thickness, and surrounding structures becomes essential for surgical success.
- Demonstration of the surgical procedure to the patient on the 3D model enables a better explanation of the method and greater patient confidence, enabling delivery of patient-specific care.[3]
- One of the specific presurgical applications has been its use in bone-anchored hearing aids (BAHA) and cochlear implant (CI) planning.

BAHA Planning

- Bone-anchored hearing aids is used for patients with moderate to severe conduction or mixed hearing loss *(see Chapter 6).*
- The implantation requires placement of the transducer into the temporal bone, and placing this bulky structure requires precise preoperative planning ensuring adequate bone thickness and evaluation of relation with critical anatomical structures like the sigmoid sinus and the dura.
- While preoperative planning with 3D reconstruction on a computer console provides adequate information—3D printing allows the surgeon to plan the BAHA implantation on the patient's anatomy accurately in real time.
- As compared to 3D rendered imaging, 3D printing provides the surgeon with the essential visuospatial and tactile cues which allow them to evaluate the feasibility of implanting BAHA versus other methods and utilize surface anatomy to optimize the location of the implant.
- In a study by Mukherjee et al.[4] superiority of 3D printing over computer-based preoperative planning was demonstrated by the fact that surgeons choose a site different from the one suggested on computerized planning after using 3D printed models.

Cochlear Implant Planning

- Inner ear malformations result in profound sensorineural hearing loss and are treated using CI surgery.
- Cochlear implant surgery is complicated in these cases because of altered surgical landmarks (lateral semicircular canal, promontory, and facial nerve)
- 3D visualization of the malformation using segmented 3D models or directly 3D printing these models can provide the operating surgeon more significant insights into the operative anatomy (**Figs. 3** and **4**).[5]

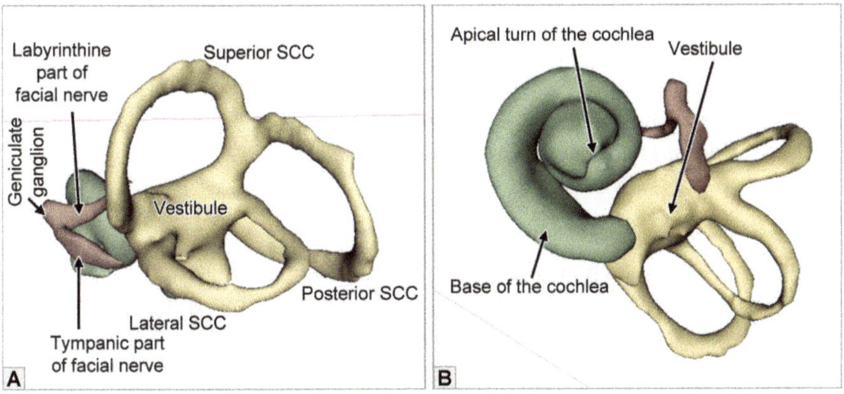

FIGS. 3A AND B: Cochlear implant planning: (A and B) The surgeon can visualise the course of the facial nerve in relation to the cochlea and this greatly aids cochlear implant planning.

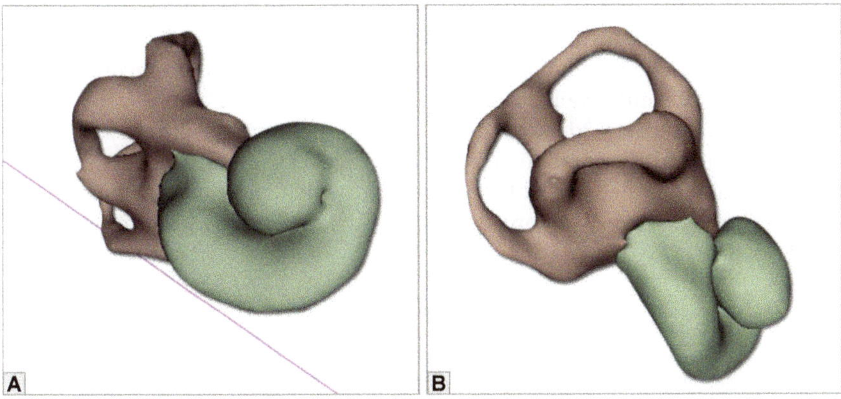

FIGS. 4A AND B: Cochlear malformation: (A and B) Surgeons can directly visualise the cochlear malformation enabling better cochlear implant planning further augmenting the findings reported in the radiologist report (type 2 incomplete partition with cystic apex).

Surgical Training

- Cadaveric temporal bones are classically used for resident training.
- Its use, however, is limited by cadaver availability, cadaver preparation, handling, and post-training clean-up.
- 3D printed temporal bones have been explored as a viable alternative.
- Besides decreasing dependence on cadaveric bone, 3D printed models can mimic various pathologies allowing better hands-on training for residents. This may translate into better resident confidence in dealing with rarer pathologies.

- However, the material used for 3D printing temporal bone needs to closely resemble human bone mechanically, especially while drilling.
- Further difficulties include recreating the middle ear ossicles and retained printing powder in the mastoid air cells.
- Inhalation of the powdered print material generated as a result of drilling may have additional unknown adverse health effects.

3D Printed Biocompatible Grafts and Prostheses

- Preliminary research in animal models has shown promise.
- Biocompatible grafts using 3D printed biocompatible (polycaprolactone) scaffolds have been created to culture human cells, which can then be implanted.
- May find use in plastic surgeries for pinna reconstruction; tympanic membrane grafting and ossicular prosthesis.

Ossicular Prosthesis

- Ossicular chain disruption due to a variety of causes is treated with ossicular reconstruction using a prosthesis. Currently manufactured prosthesis does not capture the mechanical advantages of normal ossicles. Poor size fitting, positioning, and angulation are assumed to result in poorer outcomes while using the currently available prosthesis.
- A study by Hirsch et al.[6] demonstrated that 3D printed ossicular prosthesis could be used for reconstructing the ossicular chain using CT imaging-detected anatomy. This enables proper sizing of the prosthesis, which may translate to improved prosthesis fit, decreased operative times, and improved surgical outcomes (**Figs. 5A** to **D**).

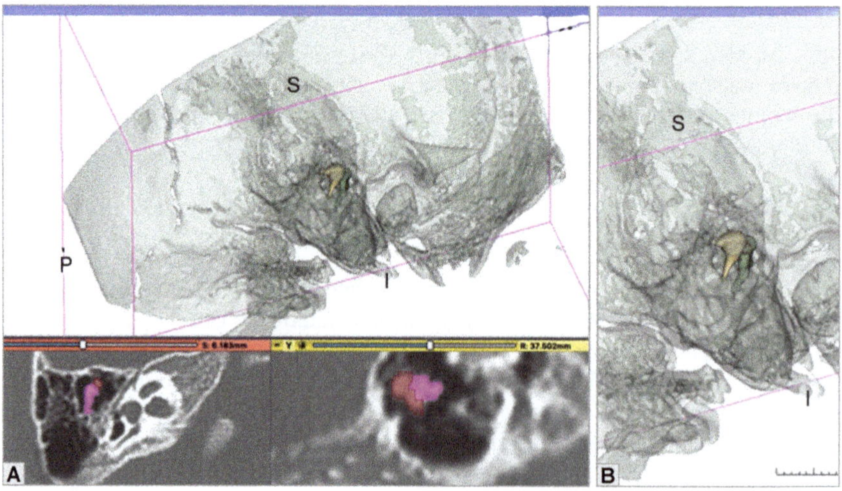

FIGS. 5A TO D: *Continued*

Continued

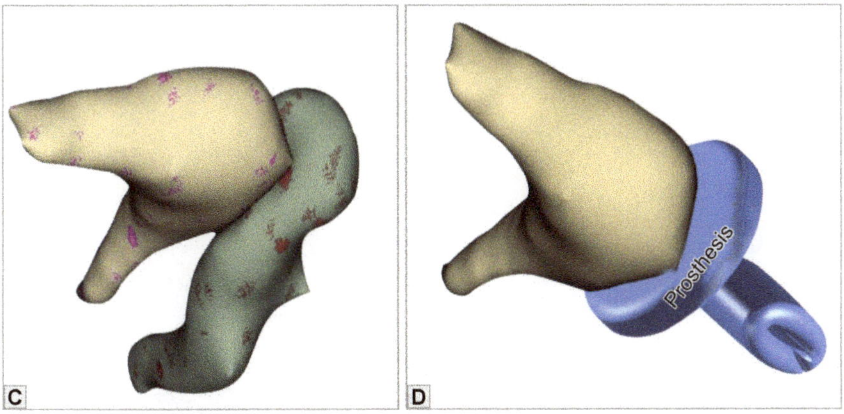

FIGS. 5A TO D: 3D printing of ossicular prosthesis: (A and B) Ossicles on routine clinical HRCT images (A) are segmented, separate from the temporal bone. (A and B) The segmented surface models of the ossicles (C) are then used to design the prosthesis (D) 3D printing allows the trough of the prosthesis to be modelled such that it exclusively fits and aligns with the manubrium of the malleus. This ensures development of an accurate prosthesis which can be tailored for use in a particular patient.

Microtia Rehabilitation

- Microtia and anotia pose significant rehabilitative challenges.
- Reconstruction of the pinna usually requires the use of autogenous cartilage, temporoparietal fascial flaps, and skin flaps.
- Recent case reports demonstrate the use of computer-aided design and 3D printing of bilateral magnetically retained custom silicone ear prosthesis (**Figs. 6A** to **D**).
- BAHA is also commonly used in patients with microtia, and 3D printing, as described previously has a definitive role in preoperative BAHA implantation planning.

LIMITATIONS

- All studies utilizing 3D printing are proof of concept, and more extensive clinically-validated studies are needed to evaluate the applicability of 3D printing in routine clinical practice.
- The financial costs of starting 3D printing services are prohibitively high. Regulatory approval for software, printing machines, and materials add to the cost of 3D printing services.
- 3D printing is time-consuming, and it may take an upward of 14 hours to print half a skull (this includes both pre- and postprocessing).
- 3D printing is technologically intensive, and clinicians or radiologists are required to acquire newer skill sets involving computer-aided design and image processing to set up 3D printing services.
- Medical 3D printing services is predominantly underorganized in India.

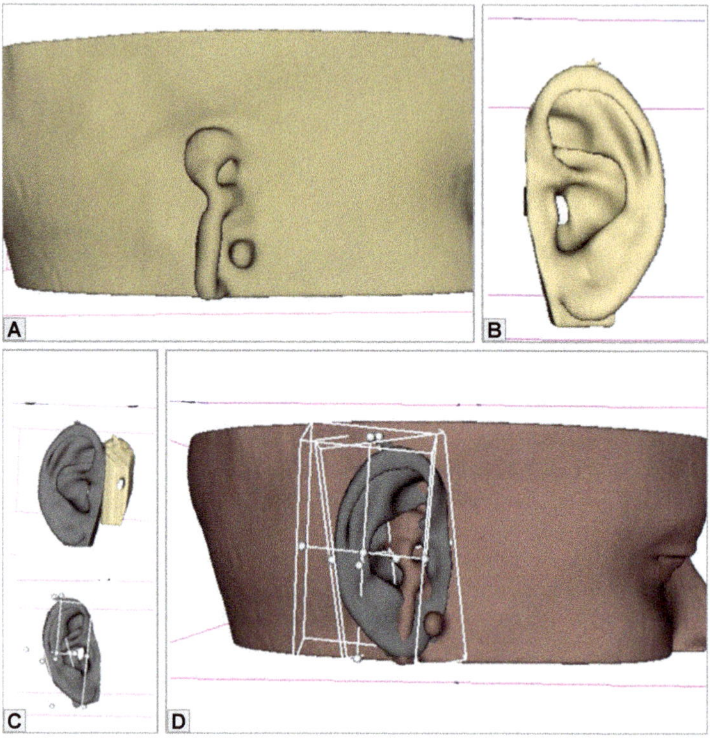

FIGS. 6A TO D: 3D printing finds a unique role in auricular reconstruction of microtia. (A) A case with right-sided microtia; (B) The normal left ear is segmented and it is flipped (C) to create a mirror image model of a normal right ear (C and D). The final positioning of this model is evaluated (D) before the model is taken for 3D printing. The 3D printed model can be used for auricular reconstruction.

REFERENCES

1. Mitsouras D, Liacouras P, Imanzadeh A, Giannopoulos AA, Cai T, Kumamaru KK, et al. Medical 3D Printing for the Radiologist. Radiographics. 2015;35(7):1965-88.
2. Crafts TD, Ellsperman SE, Wannemuehler TJ, Bellicchi TD, Shipchandler TZ, Mantravadi AV. Three-Dimensional Printing and Its Applications in Otorhinolaryngology–Head and Neck Surgery. Otolaryngol Neck Surg. 2017;156(6):999-1010.
3. Ospina JC, Fandiño A, Hernández S, Uriza LF, Aragonéz D, Mondragón IF, et al. 3D-printed pediatric temporal bone models for surgical training: a patient-specific and low-cost alternative. J 3D Print Med. 2019;3(3):135-43.
4. Mukherjee P, Cheng K, Flanagan S, Greenberg S. Utility of 3D printed temporal bones in pre-surgical planning for complex BoneBridge cases. Eur Arch Otorhinolaryngol. 2017;274(8):3021-8.
5. Dhanasingh A, Dietz A, Jolly C, Rolland P. Human Inner-ear Malformation Types Captured in 3D. J Int Adv Otol. 2019;15(1):77-82.
6. Hirsch JD, Vincent RL, Eisenman DJ. Surgical reconstruction of the ossicular chain with custom 3D printed ossicular prosthesis. [online]. Available from https://threedmedprint.biomedcentral.com/articles/10.1186/s41205-017-0015-2 [Last accessed September, 2020].

3

Temporal Bone Anatomy: Structure-wise

Jyoti Kumar

This chapter discusses the basic foundation of normal anatomy of temporal bone under the headings of external, middle, and inner ear. Detailed relevant anatomies have also been covered in specific chapters. Structure-wise pathologies are discussed in Section 6.

EXTERNAL EAR

External ear comprises of pinna and external auditory canal (EAC) and is separated from the middle ear by tympanic membrane (TM).

Pinna

- The pinna or the *auricle* is a cartilaginous structure except its lobule.
- The outer curvature is called the *helix* and inner curve, the *antihelix*, that divide superiorly into inferoanterior and superoposterior crura (**Fig. 1**).
- *Concha* is the central depression which leads to the EAC.
- An elevation of cartilaginous tissue just anterior to the beginning of EAC is the *tragus* and opposite to it is the *antitragus*.

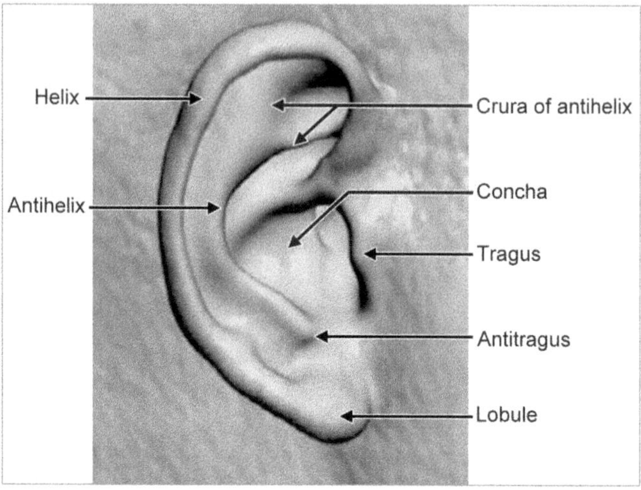

FIG. 1: Pinna: Volume rendering technique (VRT) image showing various parts of pinna.

External Auditory Canal

- External auditory canal is an air-filled canal extending from *external auditory meatus* to TM in S-shaped course (**Figs. 2A** and **B**).
- It is formed by squamous part of temporal bone superiorly, mastoid part posteriorly, and by tympanic portion of temporal bone anteriorly and inferiorly.
- It is approximately 25 mm in length.
- Its outer one-third is the *fibrocartilaginous part* which is lined by thick skin, hair follicles along with ceruminous glands. Its medial two-thirds is the *osseous portion* which is lined by thin skin which is devoid of both hair follicles as well as ceruminous glands.
- Defects that are present in the cartilaginous part are called *fissures of Santorini*. These can act as conduits of infection and malignancy to and from the EAC.

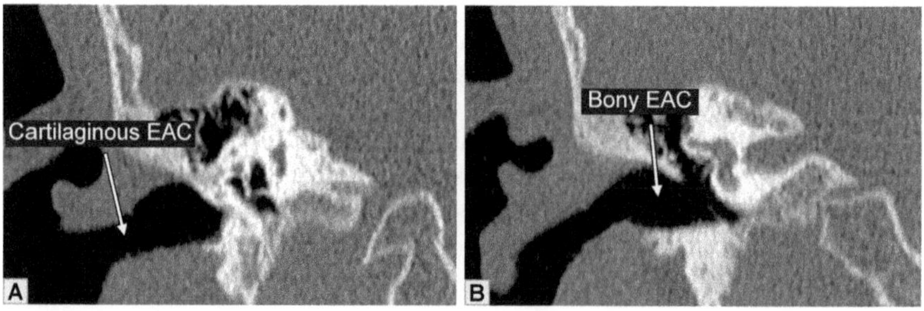

FIGS. 2A AND B: External auditory canal: Coronal CT images showing the outer cartilaginous (A) and inner bony part (B) of external auditory canal.

- A defect in the anteroinferior osseous part that communicates with the temporomandibular joint is called *foramen tympanicum (foramen of Huschke).*

Tympanic Membrane

- Tympanic membrane separates the EAC from middle ear.
- It is 9–10 mm in diameter and 1 mm thick. It is angulated ~140° along posterosuperior to anteroinferior orientation with respect to the superior border of EAC (**Figs. 3A** to **C**).
- It has a peripheral fibrocartilaginous annulus which has a superior defect called the *notch of Rivinus.* It is divided into two porions—superior pars flaccida and inferior pars tensa.
- *Pars flaccida* is the smaller, lax but thicker part, extending superiorly from the lateral process of malleus to the scutum.
- *Pars tensa* is the larger, taut and more fibrous inferior part. The handle of the malleus pulls it medially leading to a depression called the umbo.

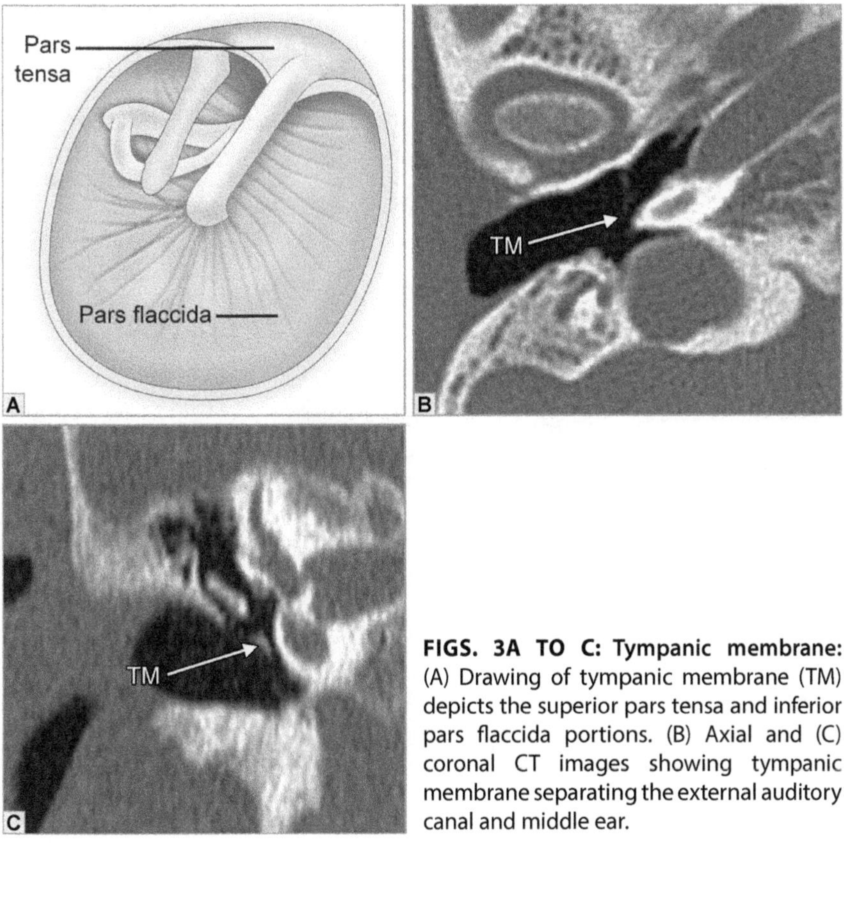

FIGS. 3A TO C: Tympanic membrane: (A) Drawing of tympanic membrane (TM) depicts the superior pars tensa and inferior pars flaccida portions. (B) Axial and (C) coronal CT images showing tympanic membrane separating the external auditory canal and middle ear.

MIDDLE EAR

- The lateral border of the middle ear is the TM and medial is the inner ear.
- The middle ear is divided into *mesotympanum* (the region of the cavity immediately opposite the pars tensa) separated from *epitympanum* above and *hypotympanum* below by tangential lines through superior and inferior margins of EAC (**Fig. 4**).[1-3]
- The major part of the ossicles resides in the epitympanum, with the handle of the malleus and long process of incus seen in the mesotympanum. The hypotympanum is empty and nearly featureless.
- Epitympanum communicates with the mastoid antrum via the *aditus* (**Fig. 5**).

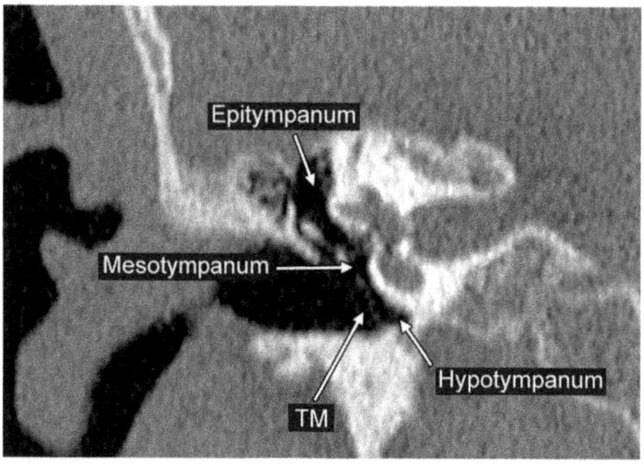

FIG. 4: Middle ear cavity: Coronal CT image depicts the division of middle ear into epitympanum superiorly, mesotympanum [opposite the tympanic membrane (TM)], and hypotympanum inferiorly.

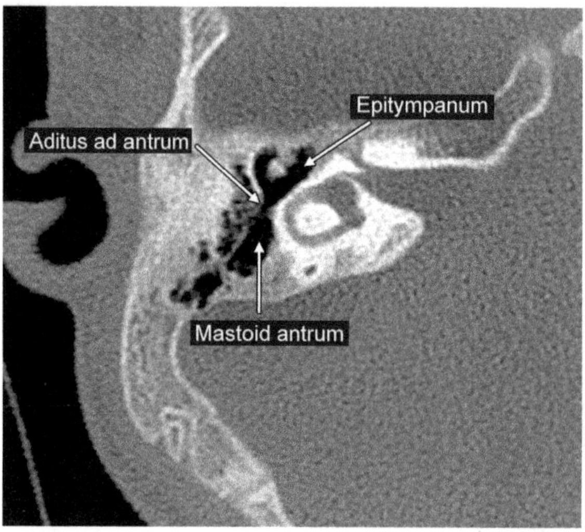

FIG. 5: Aditus ad antrum: Axial CT image depicts the communication of the epitympanum with mastoid antrum via aditus ad antrum.

Anterior Wall

- The anterior wall has two openings (**Fig. 6**)—*eustachian tube* and *semicanal for tensor tympani,* the latter running parallel and lateral to the Eustachian tube.
- Bony eustachian tube is air filled (posteriorly located) while cartilaginous extension is collapsible and not air filled, and anteriorly located.
- Carotid canal is the most medial structure.

Medial Wall

- The *promontory* covering the basal turn of cochlea occupies the anteromedial wall.
- Extends posteriorly up to *oval and round windows* and then diverges into two ridges of bone—ponticulus superiorly and subiculum inferiorly (**Fig. 7**).
- Round window niche is beneath the subiculum and oval window is superior to ponticulus.[4,5]

Posterior Wall

- The *pyramidal eminence* is the most prominent ridge in the posterior wall—stapedius tendon originates from this eminence (**Fig. 8**).
- Medial to pyramidal eminence is the *sinus tympani,* a recess of variable depth.
- Subiculum separates the sinus tympani from the *round window niche.*
- Lateral to the pyramidal eminence is the *facial recess.* The facial nerve (2nd genu) lies medial to the facial recess and chorda tympani nerve lies lateral to it.
- Facial recess is used by surgeons to place cochlear implant electrodes via the round window.[4,5]

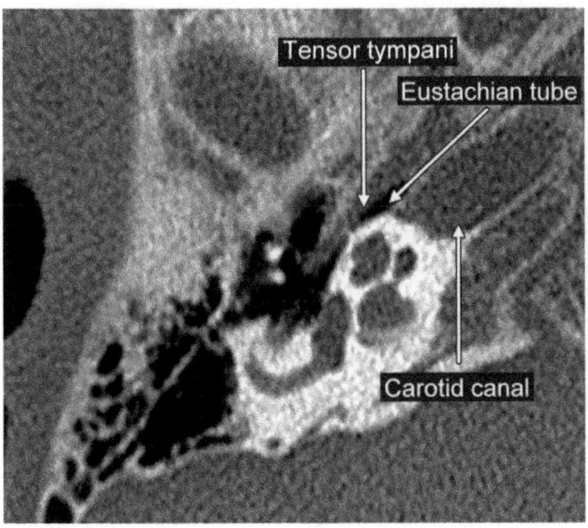

FIG. 6: Anterior wall of middle ear: Axial CT image showing the structures in the anterior wall of the middle ear.

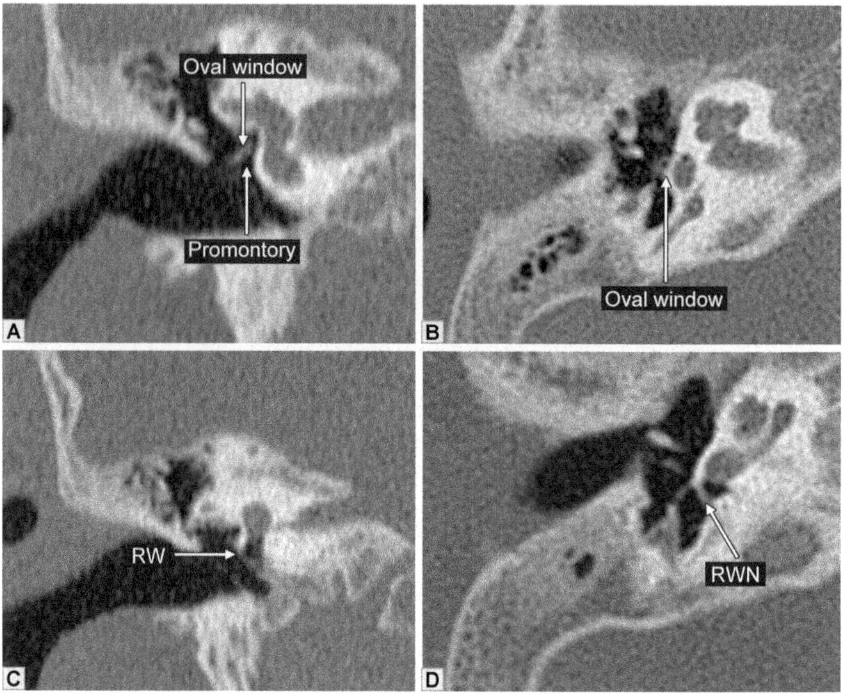

FIGS. 7A TO D: Oval window and round window niche (RWN) in medial wall of middle ear: (A) Coronal and (B) axial CT images show the oval window at the foot plate of stapes. Promontory is seen covering the basal turn of cochlea; (C) Coronal and (D) axial CT images depict the air filled RW and its opening (RWN) in the medial wall of the middle ear.

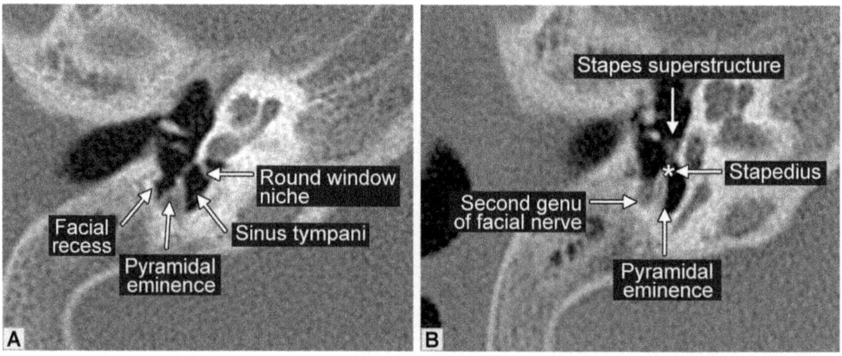

FIGS. 8A AND B: Posterior wall of middle ear: Axial CT image reveals the posterior wall of the middle ear showing the most prominent ridge (pyramidal eminence) and facial recess and sinus tympani on either side of this ridge (A). The second genu of facial nerve lies medial to the facial recess. The stapedius tendon originates from the pyramidal eminence (origin shown with asterisk) and attaches to stapes (B).

Roof

- *Tegmen tympani* is the thin bony roof that separates the epitympanum from temporal lobe (**Fig. 9**).
- It continues as tegmen mastoideum posteriorly that covers the aditus and mastoid antrum.

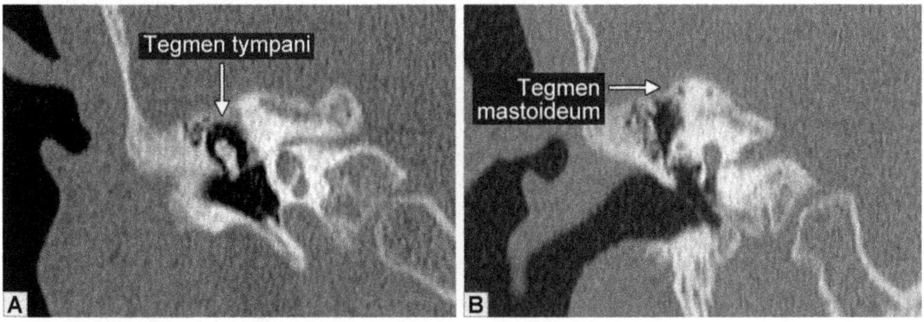

FIGS. 9A AND B: Tegmen tympani and tegmen mastoideum: (A) Coronal CT image showing tegmen tympani; (B) A more posterior image showing tegmen mastoideum forming the roof of the middle ear and mastoid, respectively.

Floor

- Thin bony shell separates the middle ear cavity from carotid artery and jugular vein
- *Jugulocarotid crest* separates the carotid artery from jugular vein.[1-3]
- Jugular fossa divided into two parts by a thin bony or fibrous septum (*jugular spine*): Pars nervosa anteriorly and pars vascularis posteriorly (**Fig. 10**).
- Pars nervosa contains the inferior petrosal sinus and glossopharyngeal nerve [cranial nerve (CN 9)].
- Pars vascularis contains the jugular bulb, vagus (CN 10), and spinal accessory nerves (CN 11)

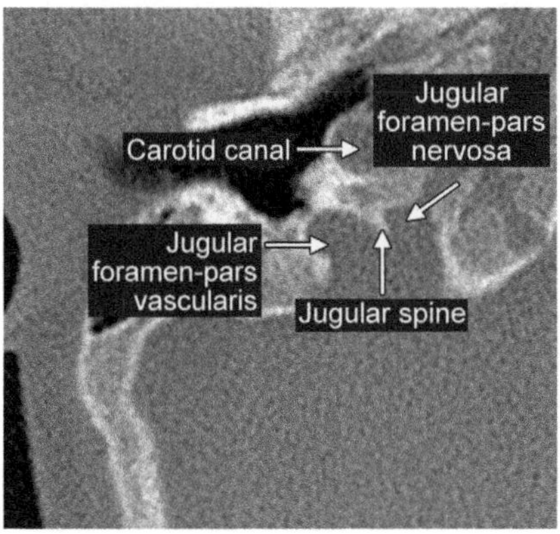

FIG. 10: Floor of middle ear: Axial CT image depicting the level of the carotid canal and jugular foramen and its parts just beneath the floor of the middle ear.

Ossicles

The ossicular chain comprises of malleus, incus, and stapes (**Figs. 11** and **12**).

- *Malleus*: It has the following parts—head, neck, lateral (short) process, anterior process, and handle (manubrium).
    - Lateral process and manubrium are embedded within TM.
    - Head of malleus articulates with body of incus (malleoincudal articulation in the attic).

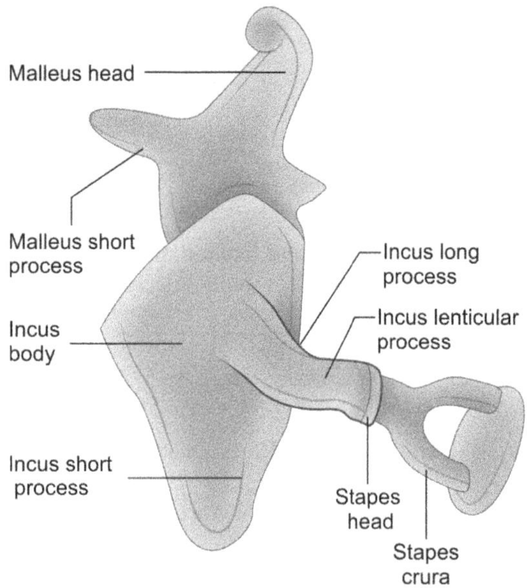

FIG. 11: Ossicular chain: Diagram of ossicular chain showing all the parts.

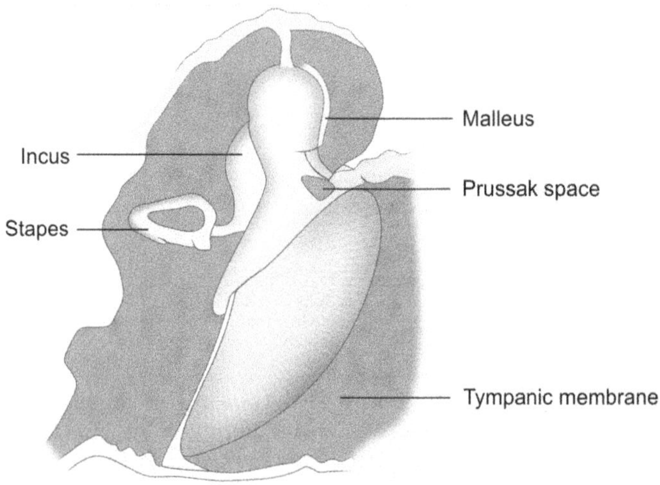

FIG. 12: Middle ear contents: Diagram of the ossicular chain, tympanic membrane, and Prussak space in the middle ear.

- *Incus*: It has the following parts—body (major bulk), short, long, and lenticular processes.
    - Short process of incus is housed in fossa incudis immediately below aditus. It acts as a fulcrum on which incus rotates and bears a close relationship with 2nd genu of facial nerve.
    - Long process of incus has lenticular process at the terminal end which articulates with head of stapes (synovial joint).
    - Long and lenticular processes are commonly eroded in inflammatory disease of the middle ear.
- *Stapes*: Suprastructure includes capitulum (head), anterior and posterior crura, tympanic portion of foot plate, and is a 2nd branchial arch derivative; vestibular portion of footplate and annular ligament are derived from otic capsule (neuroectoderm).
- *Appearance on imaging*: Axial CT depicts the following parts of the ossicles from superior to inferior (**Figs. 13A** to **C**):
    - Epitympanum: Head of malleus and body of incus articulate forming the malleoincudial articulation, giving an "*ice-cream cone*" appearance.
    - Mesotympanum: The following structures are seen in the mesotympanum:
        - Neck of malleus anteriorly, and long process of incus posteriorly; forming "*two dots*" appearance.
        - Manubrium of malleus anteriorly and long process of incus posteriorly; seen as *two parallel lines*.
        - Incus lenticular process and stapes head forming incudostapedial joint, anterior and posterior crus of stapes, and the footplate resting on the oval window.

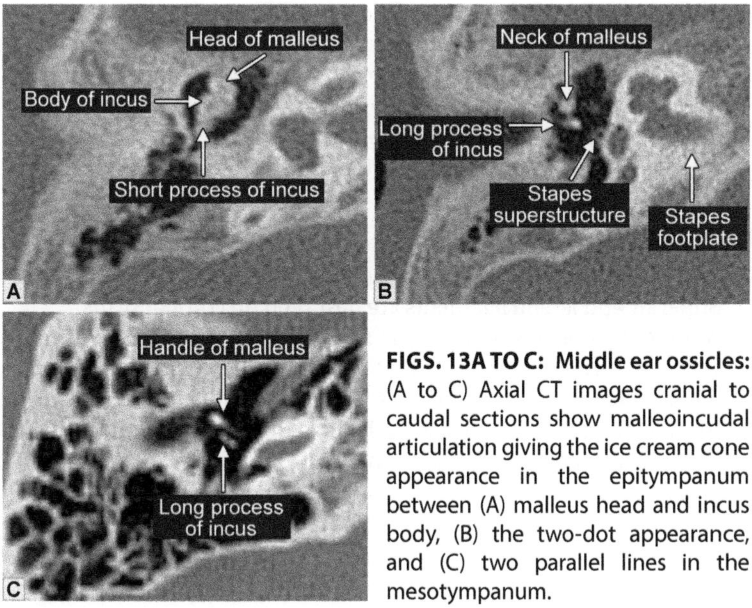

FIGS. 13A TO C: Middle ear ossicles: (A to C) Axial CT images cranial to caudal sections show malleoincudal articulation giving the ice cream cone appearance in the epitympanum between (A) malleus head and incus body, (B) the two-dot appearance, and (C) two parallel lines in the mesotympanum.

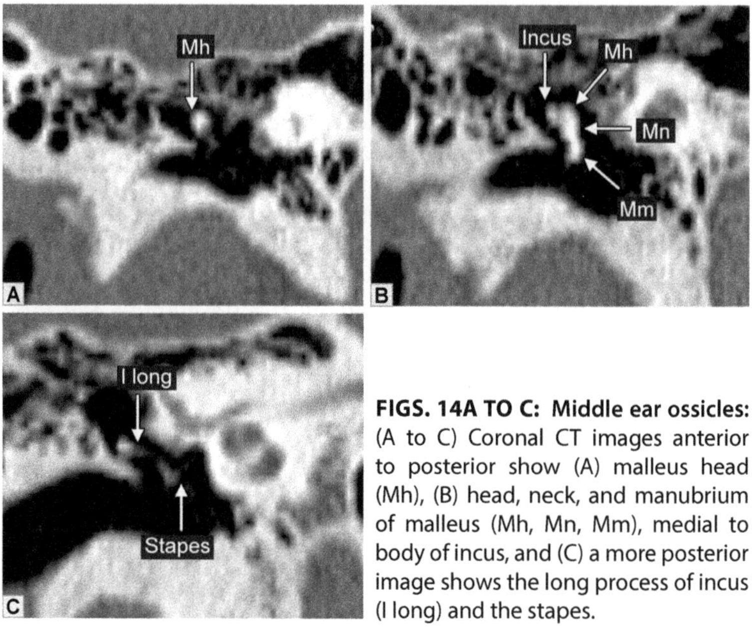

FIGS. 14A TO C: Middle ear ossicles: (A to C) Coronal CT images anterior to posterior show (A) malleus head (Mh), (B) head, neck, and manubrium of malleus (Mh, Mn, Mm), medial to body of incus, and (C) a more posterior image shows the long process of incus (I long) and the stapes.

- *Appearance on imaging*: Coronal CT depicts the following parts of ossicles from anterior to posterior (**Figs. 14A** to **C**).
  - *Anterior*: Head of malleus is seen most anteriorly.
  - More posterior images reveal head of malleus medial to the body of incus; and the handle of malleus.
  - Further posteriorly, malleoincudial articulation and tensor tympani tendon attachment to malleus is seen.
  - Sequentially posterior images show long and short processes of incus in a line vertically oriented, and stapes at a right angle to it. Incus is posterior to malleus and appears parallel to scutum.
  - More posterior image shows short process of incus as a dot.

Suspensory Ligaments

- Malleus is supported by superior, anterior, and lateral malleal ligament.[1-3]
  - Superior and lateral ligaments are best seen on coronal scans.
  - Anterior ligament is best seen on axial sections (**Fig. 15**).
- Incus is supported by superior and posterior ligaments. Posterior incudal ligament attaches the short process of incus to the fossa incudis. Superior incudal ligament is thin, attaches the head of the incus to the roof of tympanic cavity and is usually not visualized on CT.

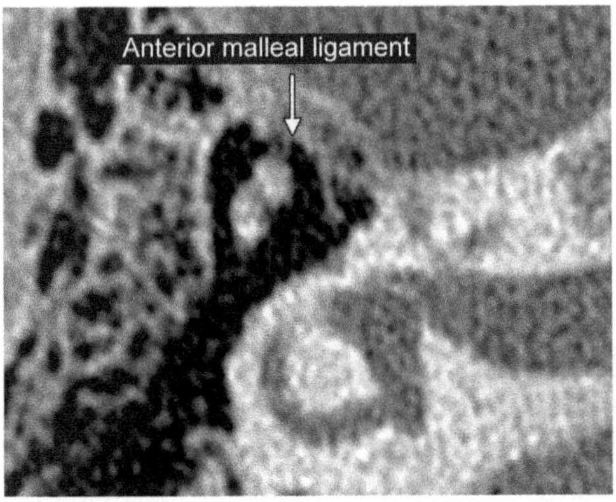

FIG. 15: Anterior malleal ligament: Axial CT image showing anterior malleal ligament.

Muscles

Tensor tympani and *stapedius* muscles tighten the TM and annular ligament of stapes, respectively, hence protecting the cochlea from intense acoustic stimulation.

- *Tensor tympani* (**Figs. 16A** and **B**):[1-3]
  - It is a first branchial arch derivative.
  - The muscle lies in a narrow canal parallel and medial to Eustachian tube
  - Cochleariform process (depression adjacent to cochlea and slightly anterior to oval window; also a surgical landmark indicating proximity to facial nerve canal) houses the tendon for tensor tympani which then courses laterally and attaches to malleus neck.
- *Stapedius muscle* (**Figs. 17A** and **B**):
  - It emerges from pyramidal eminence.
  - It courses medial to second genu of facial nerve canal to attach to stapes.

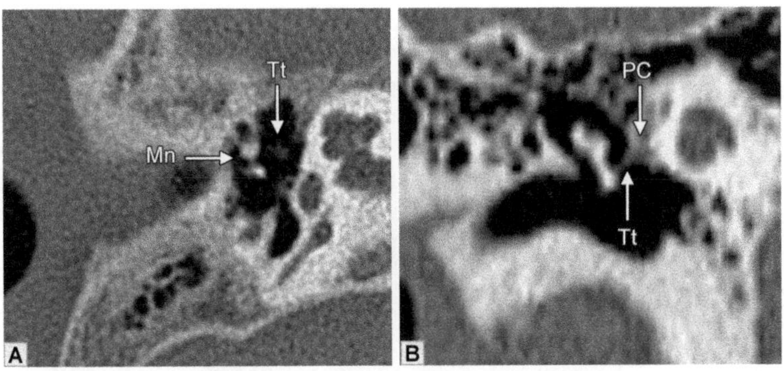

FIGS. 16A AND B: Tensor tympani (Tt) tendon: Axial (A) and coronal (B) CT images showing Tt tendon from processus cochleariformis (PC) to malleus neck (Mn).

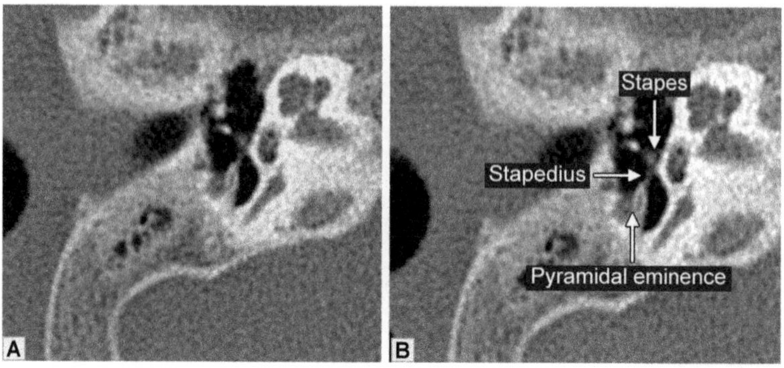

FIGS. 17A AND B: Stapedius muscle: Axial CT image (A) shows the stapedius muscle originating from the pyramidal eminence and attaching to stapes (labelled in B).

Recesses

- *Prussak space*—superior recess of TM (**Figs. 18A** and **B**):
  - It is bounded laterally by pars flaccida, medially by malleal neck, superiorly by lateral malleal ligament, and inferiorly by malleus short process.
  - It is the common site of origin for acquired attic cholesteatoma.
- *Anterior epitympanic recess (AER) (supratubal recess)* (**Fig. 19**):
  - It is anterior to attic, superior to eustachian tube, and anteromedial to head of malleus.
  - It is bounded posteriorly by thin transverse septum called the cog.
  - Proximal tympanic segment of the facial nerve canal lies immediately medial to AER.
- *Sinus tympani*:
  - It lies medial to pyramidal eminence, and of variable depth, which may not be directly visualized by the surgeon.[4,5]

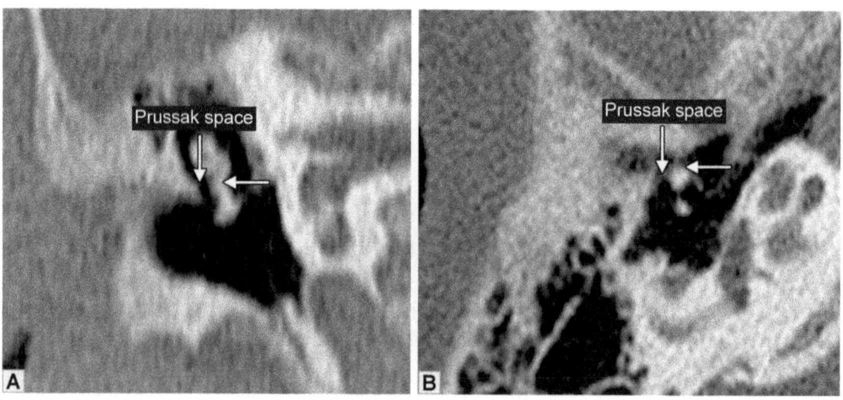

FIGS. 18A AND B: Prussak space: (A) Coronal and (B) axial CT images show the Prussak space lateral to the neck of malleus (short arrow).

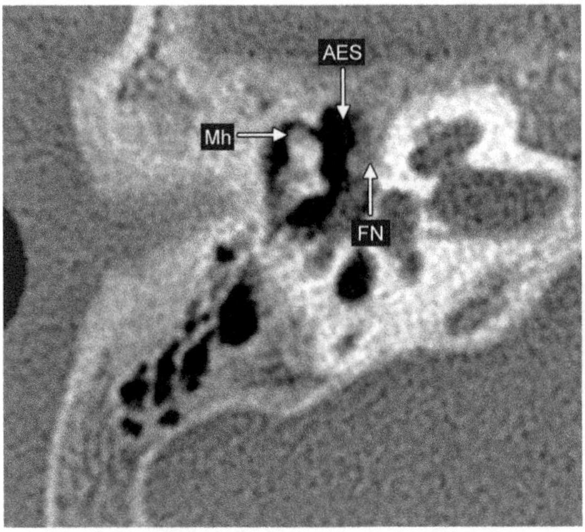

FIG. 19: Anterior epitympanic recess (AER): Axial CT image shows the AES anterior to the malleus head (Mh) in the attic with proximal tympanic segment of the facial nerve (FN) lying immediately medial to it.

- Surgeon should be cautioned against an extremely deep sinus tympani if present.
- Extensive involvement of sinus tympani by granulation tissue warrants a retrofacial (nerve) approach to disease.

- *Facial recess*:
  - This recess lies directly lateral to the pyramidal eminence. It is often much shallower than sinus tympani.
  - Lateral to facial recess is chordal eminence through which chorda tympani nerve enters middle ear.[4,5]

INNER EAR

- The inner ear consists of inner membranous labyrinth that contains the functional sensory epithelium. This is surrounded by the bony labyrinth. Between the osseous and membranous labyrinth is the perilymph fluid.
- *Perilymph* cushions the membranous labyrinth and has an ionic composition similar to that of extracellular fluid with high sodium and low potassium concentration.
- *Membranous labyrinth* consists of utricle, saccule, semicircular ducts, cochlear duct, and endolymphatic duct and sac. These structures contain endolymph.[1-3]
- *Endolymph* nourishes the sensory epithelium. It has an ionic composition similar to that of intracellular fluid with low sodium and high potassium concentration.
- *Osseous labyrinth* surrounds the membranous labyrinth and comprises of the vestibule (that contains utricle and saccule), semicircular canals (SCCs) (that contains semicircular ducts), and the vestibular aqueduct (containing endolymphatic duct).

Vestibule and Semicircular Canals

- Vestibule is the largest component of the osseous labyrinth (**Figs. 20** and **21**).
- It is perforated posterolaterally by the oval window.

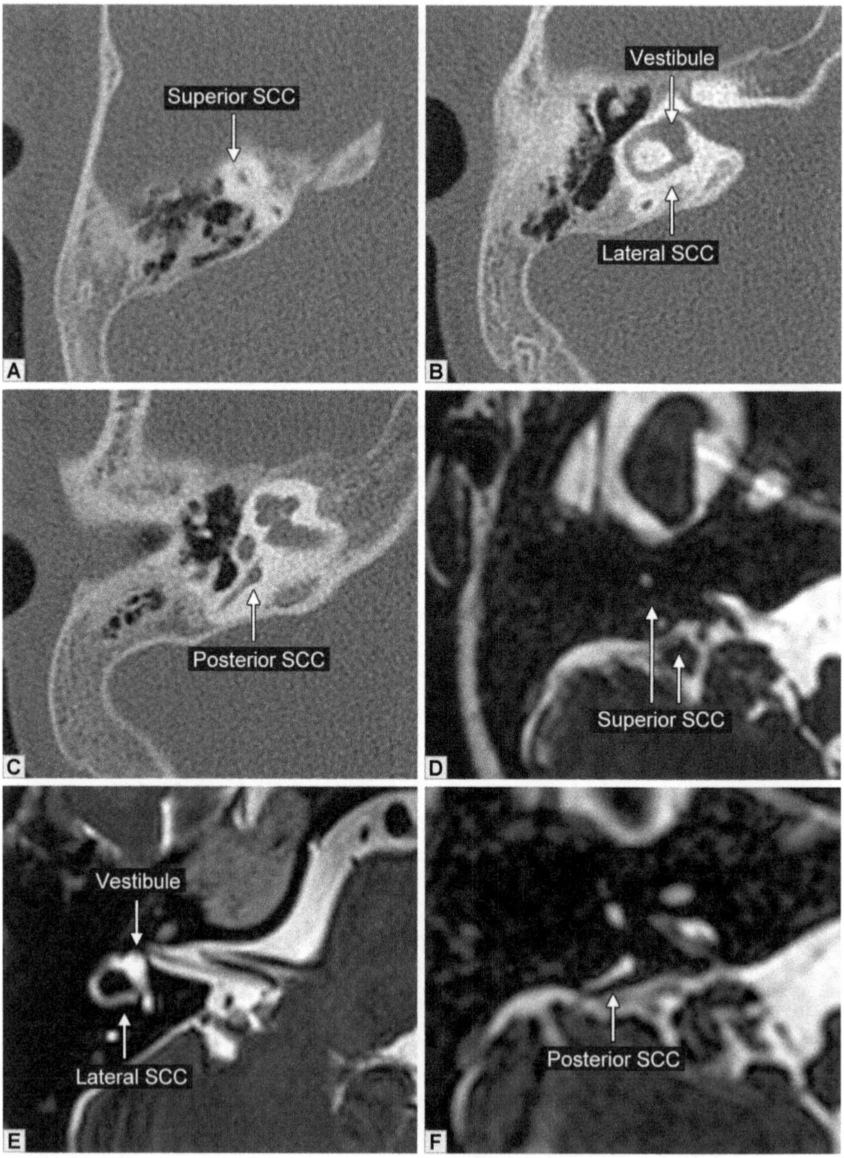

FIGS. 20A TO F: Vestibule and semicircular canals (SCCs): (A to C) Axial CT images cranial to caudal sections and (D to F) axial constructive interference in steady state (CISS) MR images cranial to caudal showing the vestibule and SCCs.

- The SCCs (superior, lateral, and posterior) are attached to the vestibule in a series of arches oriented along three orthogonal planes. There are five openings of SCCs into the utricle, as the medial arms of posterior and superior SCC form a common crus (**Figs. 20** and **21**).

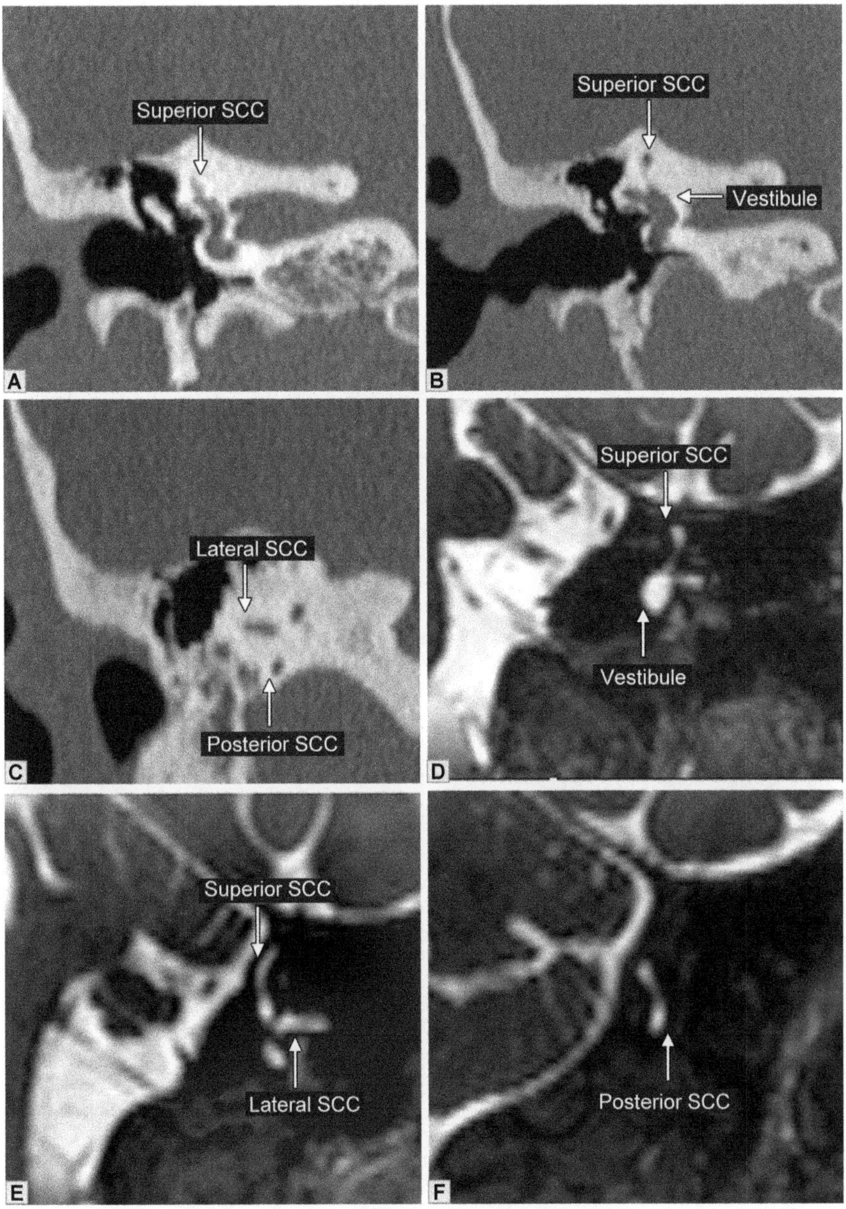

FIGS. 21A TO F: Vestibule and semicircular canals (SCCs): (A to C) Coronal CT images anterior to posterior sections of the right ear and (D to F) coronal CISS MR images anterior to posterior of the left ear showing the vestibule and SCCs.

Cochlea

- Cochlea consists of 2 1/2 to 2 3/4 turns—*apical, middle, and basal.*
- The rounded basal turn of the cochlea is separated from the middle ear by the promontory (**Figs. 22** to **24**).
- *Modiolus* is the central bony axis of cochlea, composed of spongy bone. Cochlear nerve runs centrally within the modiolus.
- *Osseous spiral lamina* projects outward from the modiolus and contains the cochlear duct (scala media). It separates the outer anterior scala vestibuli from inner posterior scala tympani (perilymph-containing structures within bony cochlea).

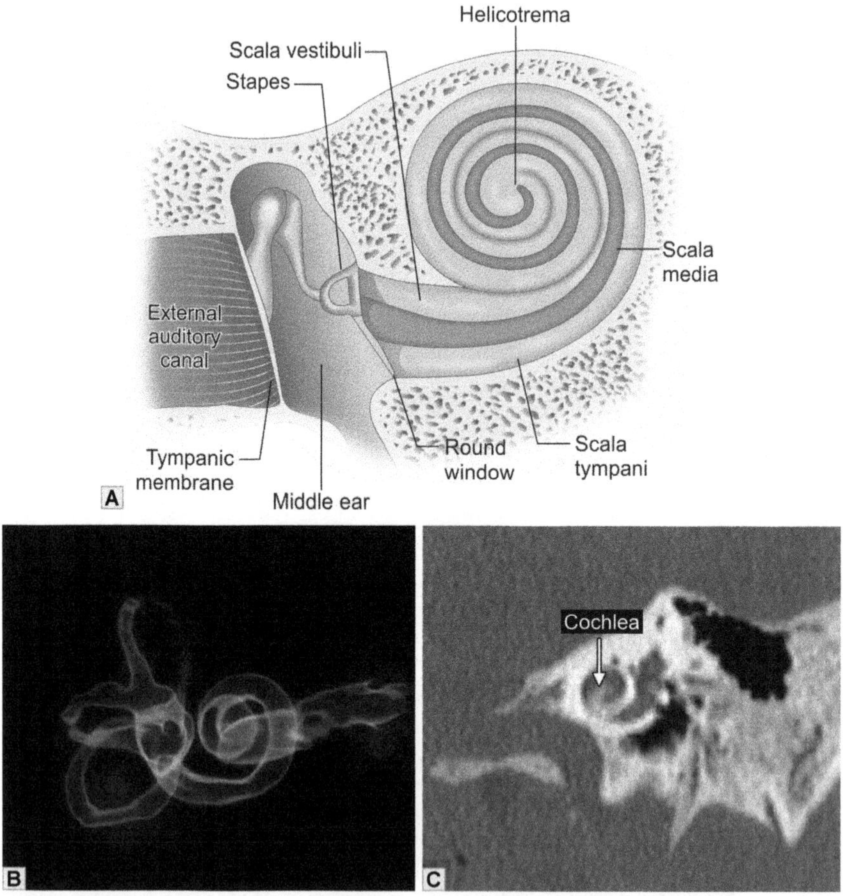

FIGS. 22A TO C: Cochlea: (A) Line diagram of the cochlear duct and perilymph containing scala vestibuli and scala tympani; (B) Volume rendering technique (VRT) of MR; (C) Maximum intensity projection (MIP) of CT images showing the cochlea.

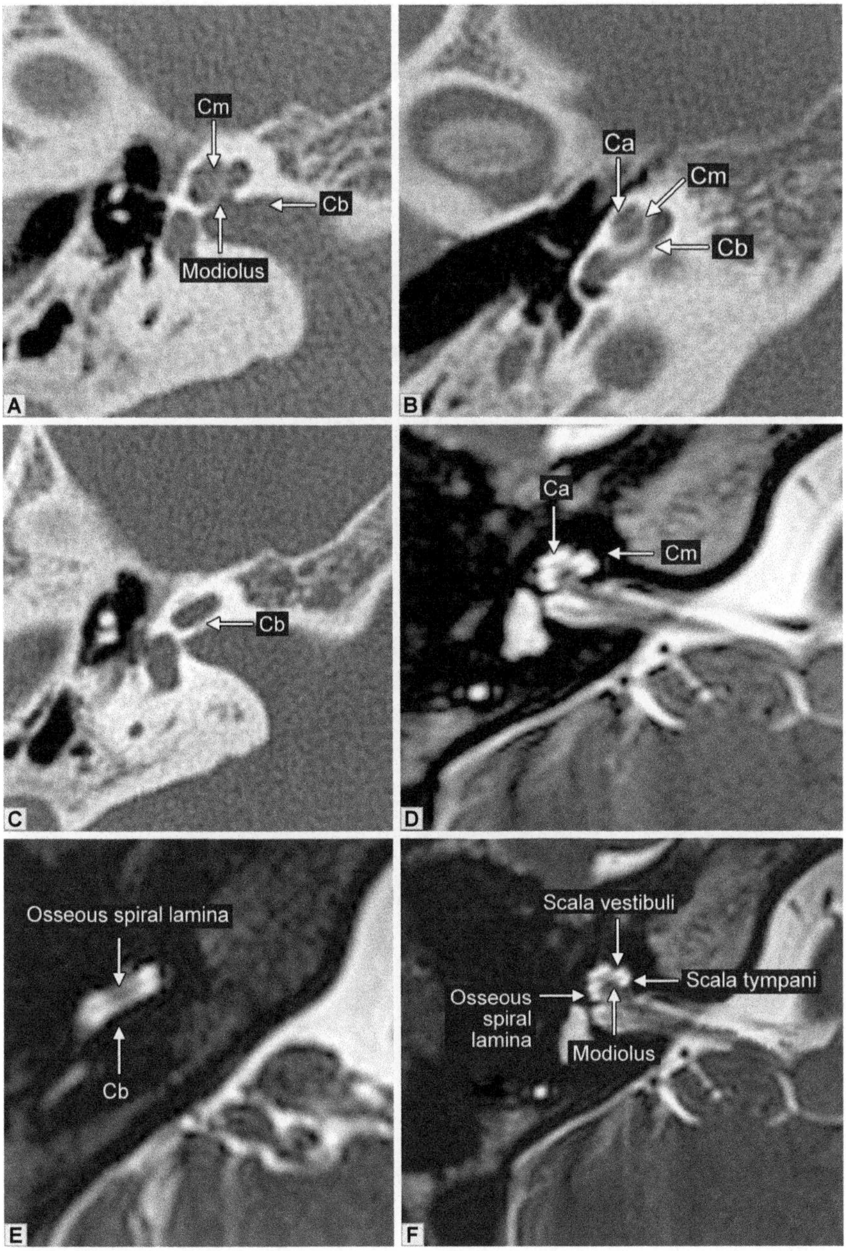

(Ca: apical turn; Cb: basal turn; Cm: middle turn)

FIGS. 23A TO F: Cochlea: (A to C) Axial CT images cranial to caudal and (D to F) axial high-resolution constructive interference in steady state (CISS) images showing the cochlear turns and osseous spiral lamina within the cochlea. Scala tympani and scala vestibuli are seen separated by the osseous spiral lamina within the cochlea.

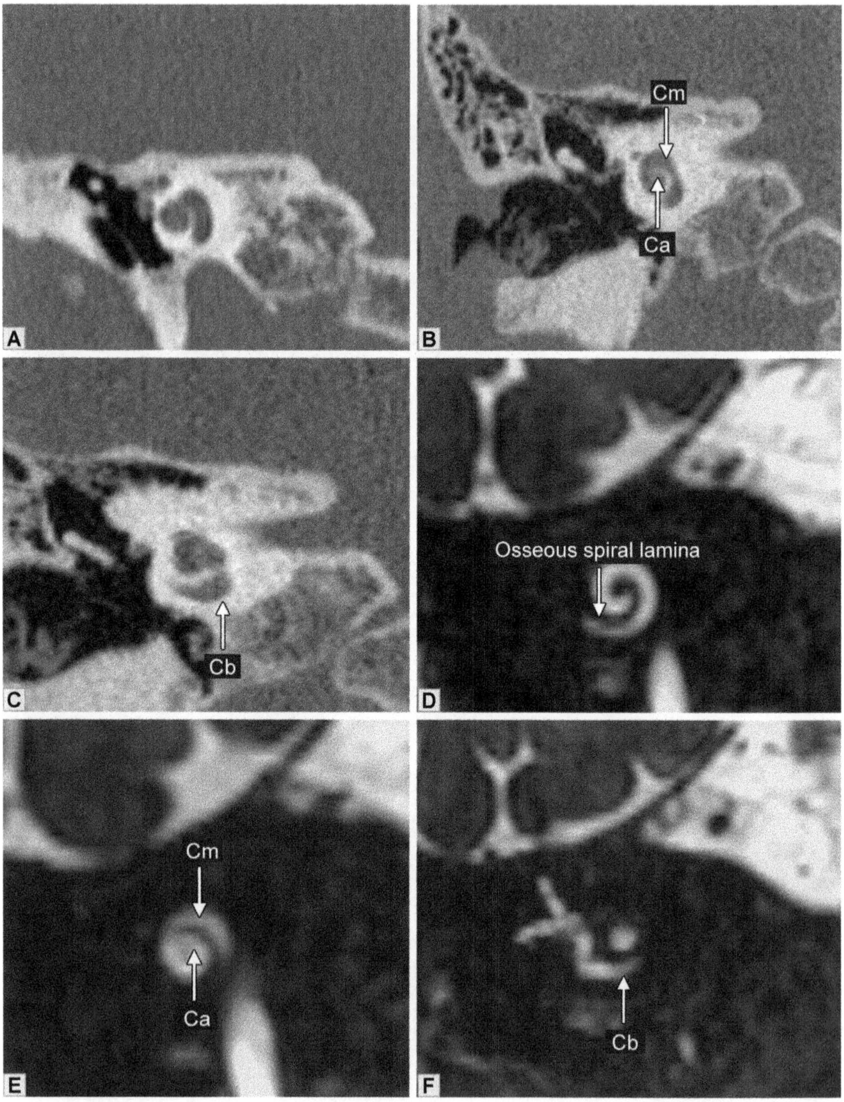

(Ca: apical turn; Cb: basal turn; Cm: middle turn)

FIGS. 24A TO F: Cochlea: (A to C) Coronal CT images anterior to posterior sections of the right ear and (D to F) coronal CISS MR images anterior to posterior showing the cochlear turns and the osseous spiral lamina.

- The *interscalar septum* also projects outward from the modiolus and separates the apical from middle turn of the cochlea. It is much thicker than osseous spiral lamina.
- Sound waves travel from oval window through the vestibule to perilymph within scala tympani and reach up to helicotrema (cochlear apex). These fluid wave stimulate the organ of Corti in the cochlear duct and converted into electrical impulses through the cochlear nerve fibers. The perilymphatic waves then pass via scala tympani to be eventually dissipated at round window.

Vestibular Aqueduct

- This is a bony channel originating from the vestibule near the common crus and drains the endolymph.

  It courses posteriorly, laterally, and inferiorly along the posterior petrous surface (**Fig. 25**).
- It is considered large if it measures more than 1.5 mm in width at its midpoint between the common crus and the external aperture.
- It houses the endolymphatic duct system—*endolymphatic duct and sac.*
- The endolymphatic sac lies within the terminal part of the aqueduct which widens to accommodate the sac. This widening along the posterior surface of temporal bone forms a small impression called the *foveate impression.*

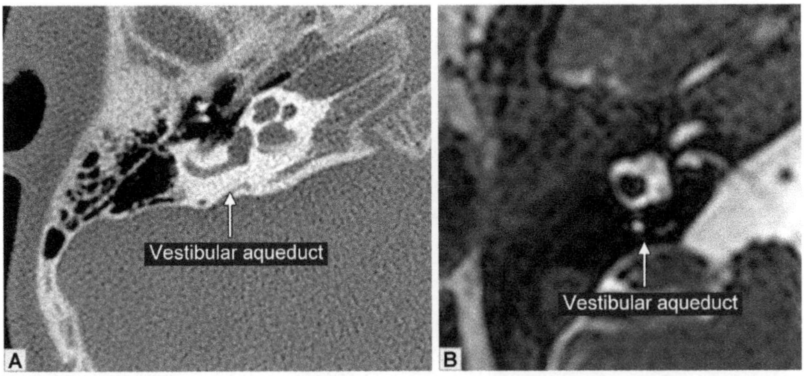

FIGS. 25A AND B: Vestibular aqueduct: (A) Axial CT and (B) CISS MR image showing the vestibular aqueduct.

Cochlear Aqueduct

- It is a narrow bony canal containing perilymph and loose connective tissue.
- It is a potential communication between the scala tympani (near round window niche) and subarachnoid apace (**Fig. 26**).
- It runs roughly parallel and immediately inferior to the internal auditory canal (IAC).

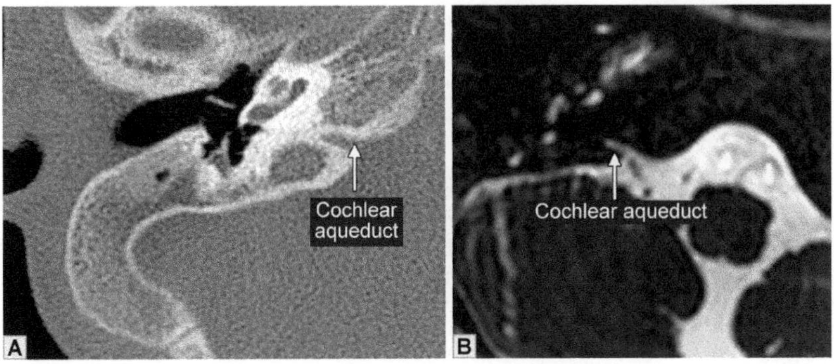

FIGS. 26A AND B: Cochlear aqueduct: (A) Axial CT and (B) CISS MR image showing the cochlear aqueduct in a direction parallel to the internal auditory canal.

Internal Auditory Canal

- It is a bony channel communicating with the subarachnoid space medially through which the vestibulocochlear and facial nerves travel to reach the petrous temporal bone (**Fig. 27**).
- The normal dimensions of the canal range between 2 mm and 8 mm, measured at its midpoint between the porus acousticus (medial end) and fundus (lateral end).[1-3]
- It is directed along the coronal plane and is divided by horizontal bone called *crista falciformis* into superior and inferior parts.
- The facial nerve and superior vestibular nerve lie in the superior compartment and cochlear nerve and inferior division of the vestibular nerve lien in the inferior compartment (**Fig. 28**).
- The superior compartment is also divided by the vertical Bill's bar. This separates the facial nerve from the superior vestibular nerve within the superior compartment.
- At the *fundus* (most lateral part of the IAC) of the IAC are the exit foramina where the canal forks in a Y shape—the ventral arms are the exit foramina of cochlear and facial nerves and dorsal for the vestibular nerves.

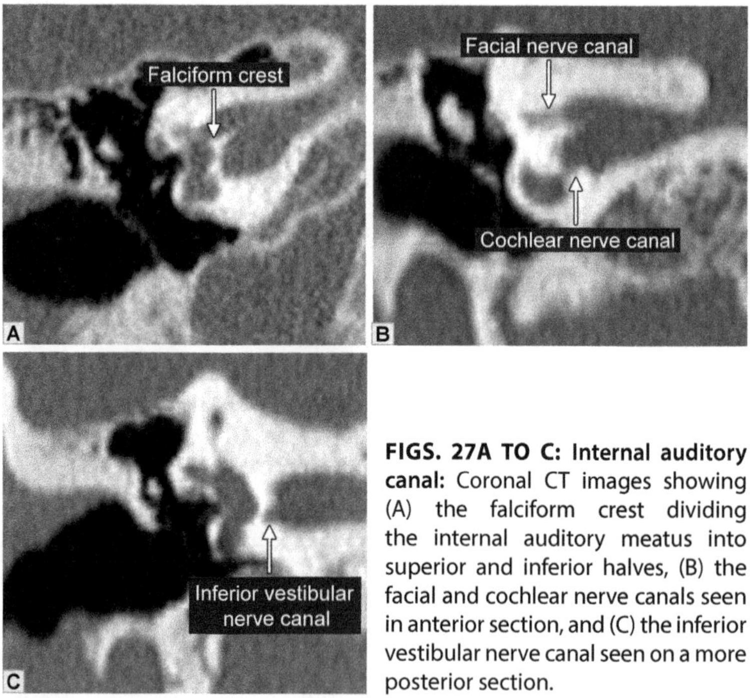

FIGS. 27A TO C: Internal auditory canal: Coronal CT images showing (A) the falciform crest dividing the internal auditory meatus into superior and inferior halves, (B) the facial and cochlear nerve canals seen in anterior section, and (C) the inferior vestibular nerve canal seen on a more posterior section.

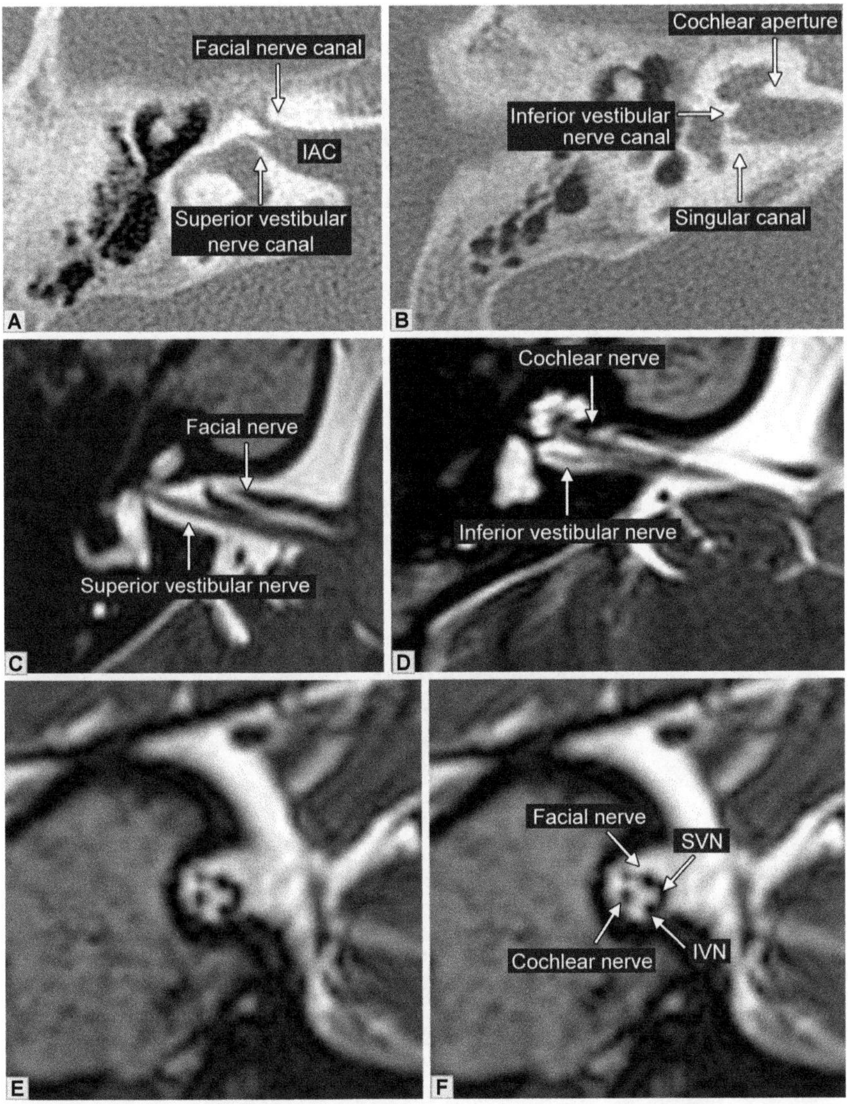

FIGS. 28A TO F: Facial and vestibulocochlear nerves: Axial CT scans (A) through the internal auditory canal (IAC) through its superior aspect shows the canal for the facial nerve and superior vestibular nerve and (B) through the mid IAC level shows the cochlear aperture and inferior vestibular nerve. Singular canal reaching the posterior semicircular canal (SCC) is also seen at this level. Axial high-resolution T2-weighted MR images (C) through the IAC through its superior aspect shows the facial nerve and superior vestibular nerve and (D) through the mid IAC level shows the cochlear nerve entering the cochlea and inferior vestibular nerve. Sagittal oblique high-resolution T2-weighted MR image through the IAC shows (E, F) the facial nerve and superior vestibular nerve (SVN) in its superior part and the cochlear nerve and inferior vestibular nerve (IVN) in its inferior part.

Facial Canal

- The facial canal, also called the fallopian canal, is the bony canal containing the facial nerve within petrous temporal bone.

  It is divided into three segments—the labyrinthine segment, tympanic segment, and mastoid segment (**Figs. 29** and **30**).

  i. *Labyrinthine segment*: It begins at the fundus of IAC and courses anteriorly ending at the geniculate ganglion. It runs between the vestibule and the cochlea.
     - *First genu*: At its first genu, it takes a hairpin turn and extends posteriorly as the tympanic segment. Here, it gives off its first branch which is the greater superficial petrosal nerve.

  ii. *Tympanic segment*: It runs along the medial wall of the tympanic cavity to the pyramidal eminence. This lies lateral to the ampulla of the lateral SCC in its anterior portion and just below the level of lateral SCC posteriorly. It runs above the level of oval window and below the level of lateral SCC.
     - *Second genu*: Posterior tympanic segment runs inferior to the short process of incus and turns at the posterior genu where it becomes the mastoid segment. The second genu lies between the facial recess laterally and pyramidal eminence medially.[4,5]

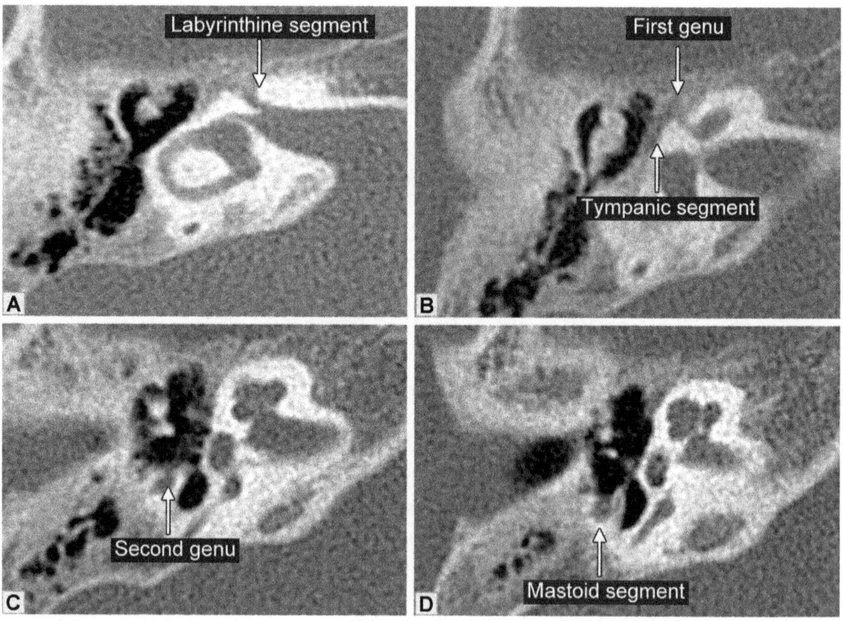

FIGS. 29A TO D: Facial nerve canal: Axial CT images (A–D) tracing the course of the facial nerve.

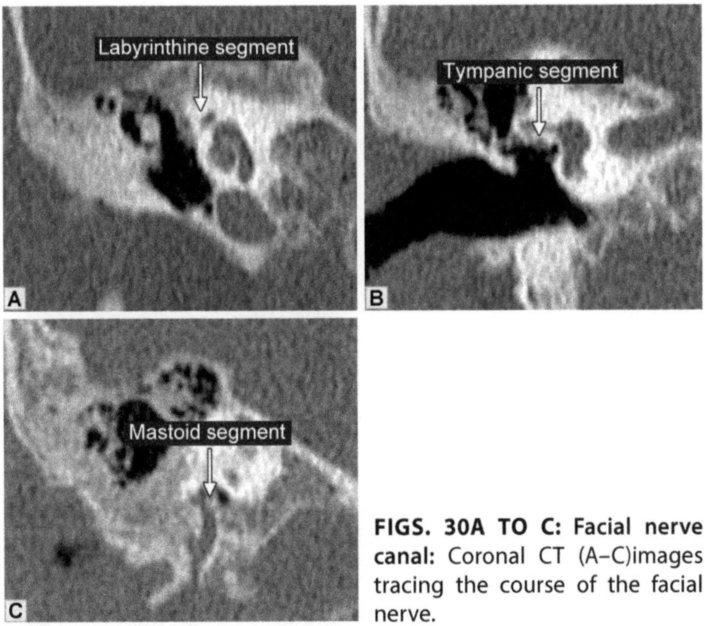

FIGS. 30A TO C: Facial nerve canal: Coronal CT (A–C)images tracing the course of the facial nerve.

iii. *Mastoid segment*: The mastoid segment courses vertically to exit through the stylomastoid foramen. Medial to the mastoid segment is the jugular bulb. The mastoid segment gives off two branches—stapedius nerve and chorda tympani nerve.
   – *Singular nerve*: It supplies the ampulla of the posterior SCC.

MASTOID

- The mastoid region is divided into mastoid antrum, central mastoid tract, and peripheral mastoid air cells. The antrum communicates with the epitympanum via the aditus.
- *Mastoid antrum* lies superiorly at the level of epitympanic recess and IAC.
- The *central mastoid tract* is direct inferior extension of the antrum seen at the level of EAC. *Peripheral mastoid area* are additional cells that arise from the antrum. These are tabulated in **Table 1**. The mastoid antrum is pneumatized at birth. Further peripheral pneumatization is seen to occur through early childhood (**Figs. 31** and **32**).
- Accessory regions of pneumatization of temporal bone (apart from middle ear, mastoid, perilabyrinthine, and petrous apex) include squamous, zygomatico-occipital, and styloid region.
- Pneumatization of mastoid is called pneumatic when it is complete, diploic when it has a diploic texture, and sclerotic when density is increased.

TABLE 1 **Types of peripheral mastoid air cells.**

Location	Name
Immediately surrounding mastoid antrum	Periantral cells
In tegmen above mastoid antrum	Tegmental cells
Posteromedial to mastoid antrum	Sinodural cells
Lateral to mastoid antrum	Squamosal cells
Ventral to central tract	Facial cells
Dorsal to central tract	Spinal cells
In the mastoid process and tip	Tip cells

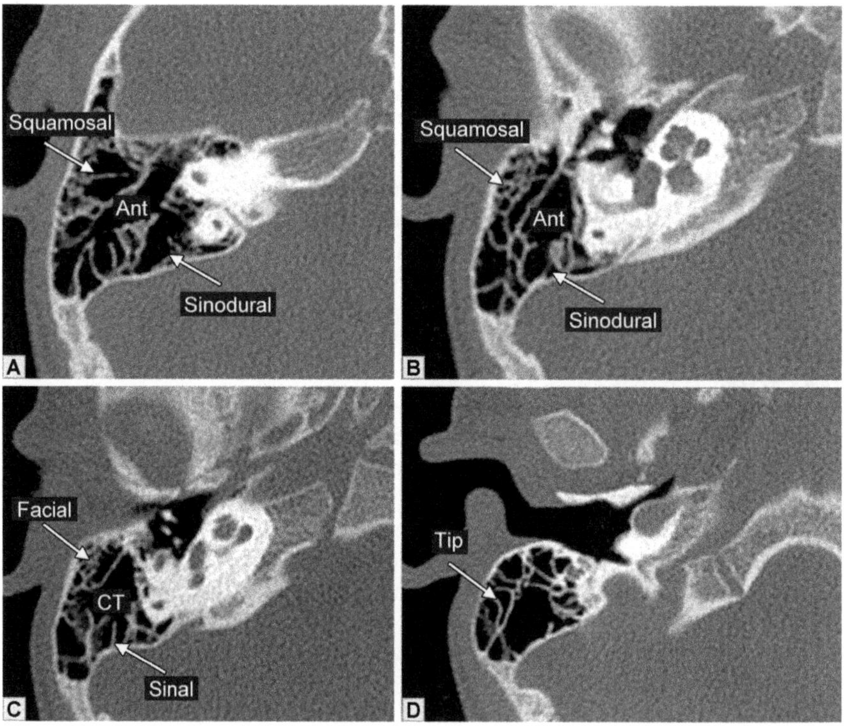

(Ant: antrum; CT: central tract)

FIGS. 31A TO D: Mastoid air cells: Axial CT images from superior to inferior (A–D) showing the mastoid air cells.

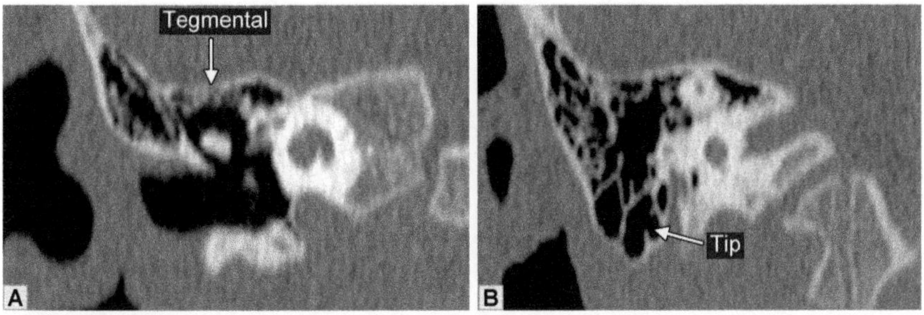

FIGS. 32A AND B: Mastoid air cells: Coronal CT images from anterior to posterior showing tegmental (A) and tip (B) mastoid air cells.

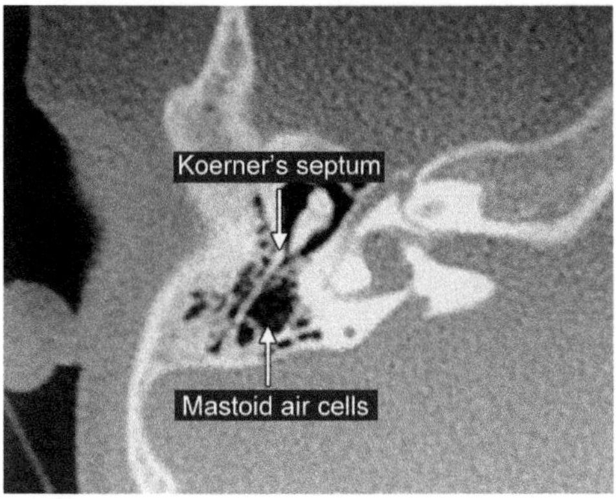

FIG. 33: Koerner's septum: Coronal CT images depicting the Koerner's septum in the lateral portion of the mastoid antrum. This is the plane of fusion between petrous and mastoid parts of temporal bone.

- *Koerner's septum* (**Fig. 33**): It is a thin osseous partition in the mastoid antrum oriented in the sagittal plane lateral to the facial nerve canal, and is a continuation of the petrosquamosal fissure. It courses from the glenoid fossa extending inferiorly toward the mastoid tip and coursing lateral to the facial nerve canal. It is variably sized and may be confused with medial wall of the antrum by the otologic surgeon, especially when it is thick.
- *The petromastoid canal (PMC)* (**Fig. 34**): It is an anteriorly convex channel that passes between superior and lateral SCC connecting the cranial cavity to the mastoid antrum. It usually measures 0.5–1 mm. PMC contains the subarcuate artery and is a potential channel for spread of infection to and from the mastoid antrum. It should not be mistaken for a fracture line in the setting of trauma.

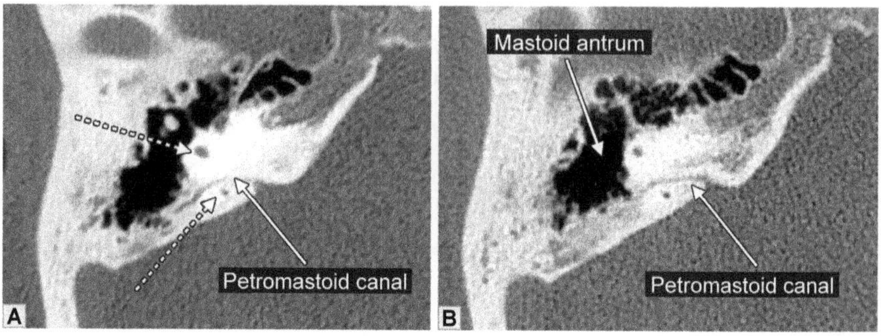

FIGS. 34A AND B: Petromastoid canal: Axial CT images (A and B) tracing the petromastoid canal coursing through the crura of the superior semicircular canal (dashed arrows) connecting the mastoid antrum with the cranial cavity.

- *Mastoid emissary vein* is a valveless vein connecting sigmoid sinus and posterior auricular/occipital vein (craniocerebral anastomosis). It is usually seen at the posterior margin of the mastoid (**Fig. 35**).
- Inadvertent injury to mastoid emissary vein can lead to brisk bleeding and even sinus thromboembolism. Preoperative mention of the same is important on imaging especially if prominent.

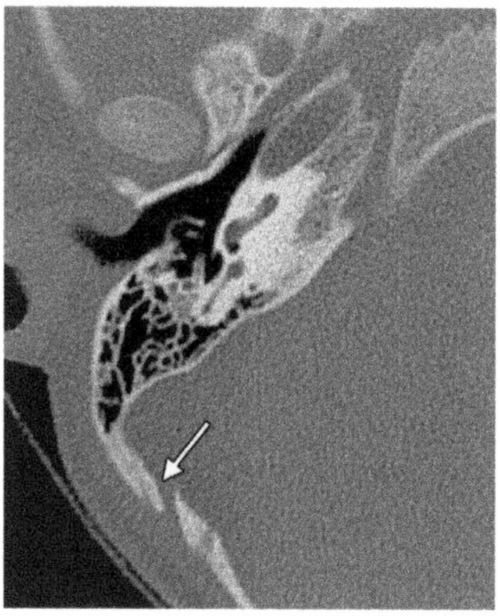

FIG. 35: Mastoid emissary vein: Axial CT image showing the mastoid emissary vein (arrow).

In conclusion, meticulous survey of the HRCT in multiple planes allows for delineation of most structures. The CT should be viewed both 'section wise' and 'structure wise' to avoid missing findings.

REFERENCES

1. Juliano AF. Cross Sectional Imaging of the Ear and Temporal Bone. Head Neck Pathol. 2018;12(3): 302-20.
2. Yamashita K, Hiwatashi A, Togao O, Kikuchi K, Matsumoto N, Momosaka D, et al. Ultrahigh-resolution CT scan of the temporal bone. Eur Arch Otorhinolaryngol. 2018;275(11):2797-803.
3. Virapongse C, Rothman SL, Kier EL, Sarwar M. Computed tomographic anatomy of the temporal bone. Am J Neuroradiol. 1982;139:739-49.
4. Bartling SH, Shukla V, Becker H, Brady TJ, Hayman A, Gupta R. High-resolution flat-panel volume-CT of temporal bone—part 1: axial preoperative anatomy. J Comput Assist Tomogr. 2005;29:420-3.
5. Gleeson TG, Lacy PD, Bresnihan M, Gaffney R, Brennan P, Viani L. High resolution computed tomography and magnetic resonance imaging in the pre-operative assessment of cochlear implant patients. J Laryngol Otol. 2003;117:692-5.

4

Temporal Bone Anatomy: Section-wise

Jyoti Kumar

- Consecutive Axial CT Sections
- Consecutive Coronal CT Sections
- Consecutive Axial MRI Sections
- Consecutive Coronal MRI Sections
- Consecutive Sagittal Oblique MRI Sections

CONSECUTIVE AXIAL CT SECTIONS (CRANIAL TO CAUDAL) (FIGS. 1A TO F, E1)

- Axial scans very well depict the structures on the anterior and posterior wall of the middle ear, the aditus, and the antrum.
- The superior semicircular canal (SCC) is seen at the most superior sections (A and B).
- The internal auditory canal (IAC) appears on successive caudal section (D). The normal diameter of IAC ranges 4-6 mm.
- The first part of the facial nerve canal is seen on the anterolateral part of the outermost part of the IAC.
- The first part of the facial nerve canal leads to an acute bend, the first genu of the facial nerve canal, which then continues to the second part of the canal (E, E1: magnified view of E).
- The cochlea appears as a spiral structure with 2.5 turns; and the basal turn in located in relation to the IAC, separated by a thin bony partition.
- The cochlear middle turn, vestibule, aditus, head of malleus, and short process of incus are seen at the same axial level (ice-cream cone appearance of the ossicles) (F).
- The common crus of the superior and posterior SCC is seen to communicate with the vestibule at the same level.

Key

A—antrum	AAA—aditus ad antrum
C—cochlea	Ca—cochlea (apical turn)
CCs—common crus of superior and posterior semicircular canal	FN—facial nerve
FN1—labyrinthine part of facial nerve	FN2—tympanic part of facial nerve
IAC—internal auditory canal	SSCC—superior semicircular canal
MAC—mastoid air cells	

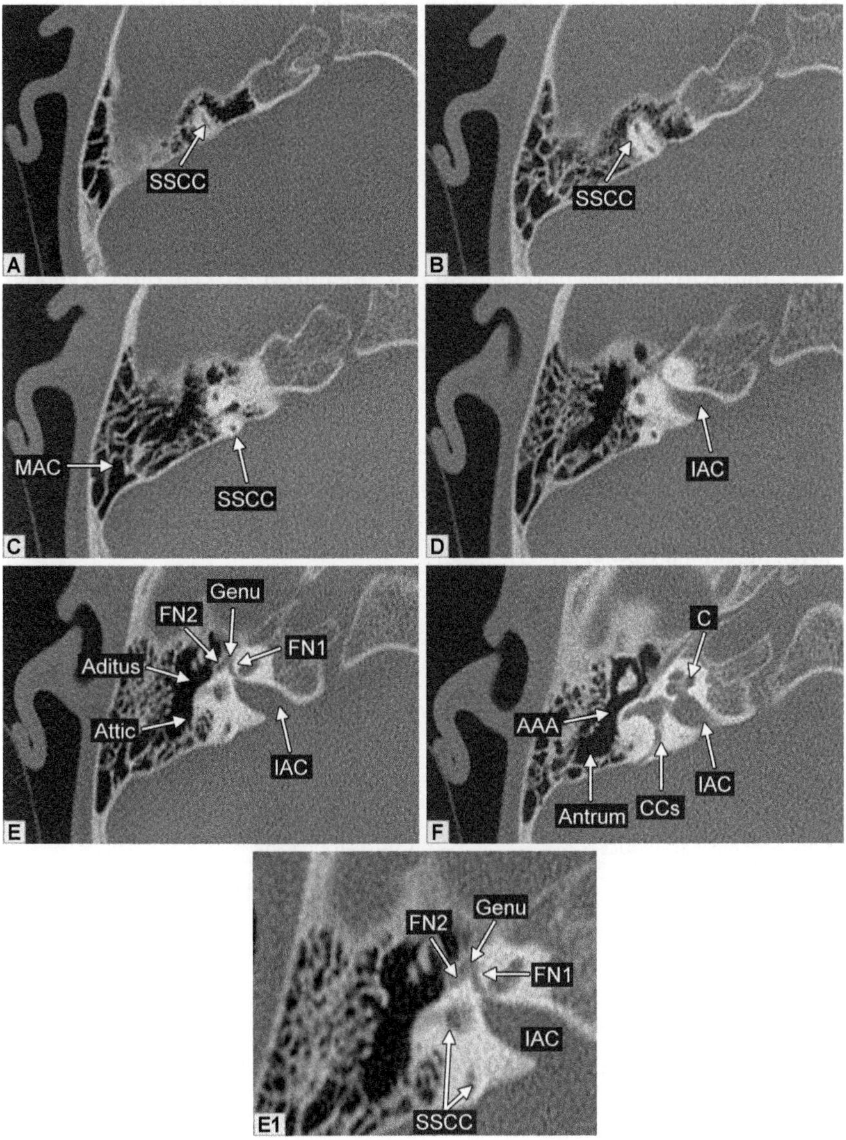

FIGS. 1A TO F, E1

SUBSEQUENT AXIAL CT SECTIONS (CRANIAL TO CAUDAL) (FIGS. 1G TO L, G1)

- These sections show the middle ear ossicles in the mesotympanum, the entire cochlea and vestibule.
- The bony modiolus is seen best in these sections.
- The posterior SCC and the vestibular aqueduct are seen at the same level.
    - The diameter of the vestibular aqueduct should be measured at the mid-part between the common crus and the external aperture. It should not be >1.5 mm or larger than the adjacent posterior SCC.
- The cochlear aqueduct is seen parallel to the IAC, at more caudal sections.
- The basal turn of cochlea is seen at the caudal sections; and posterior to it lies the round window niche.
- The middle ear ossicles show three different patterns; the ice-cream cone appearance at cranial sections (G), two dot appearance on subsequent caudal sections (H) and finally two parallel lines at the most caudal sections (I). Magnified view of G (G1).
- The footplate of stapes is seen to be attached to the oval window.
- The jugular bulb appears at the most caudal section.

Key

CAq—cochlear aqueduct	CC—carotid canal
Et—Eustachian tube	FN3—third part of facial nerve canal
FR—facial recess	I—incus
IMJ—incudomalleal joint	JB—jugular bulb
LSCC—lateral semicircular canal	M—malleus
PE—pyramidal eminence	OW—oval window
PSCC—posterior semicircular canal	RW—round window
ST—sinus tympani	TM—tympanic membrane
Tt—tensor tympani	VAq—vestibular aqueduct

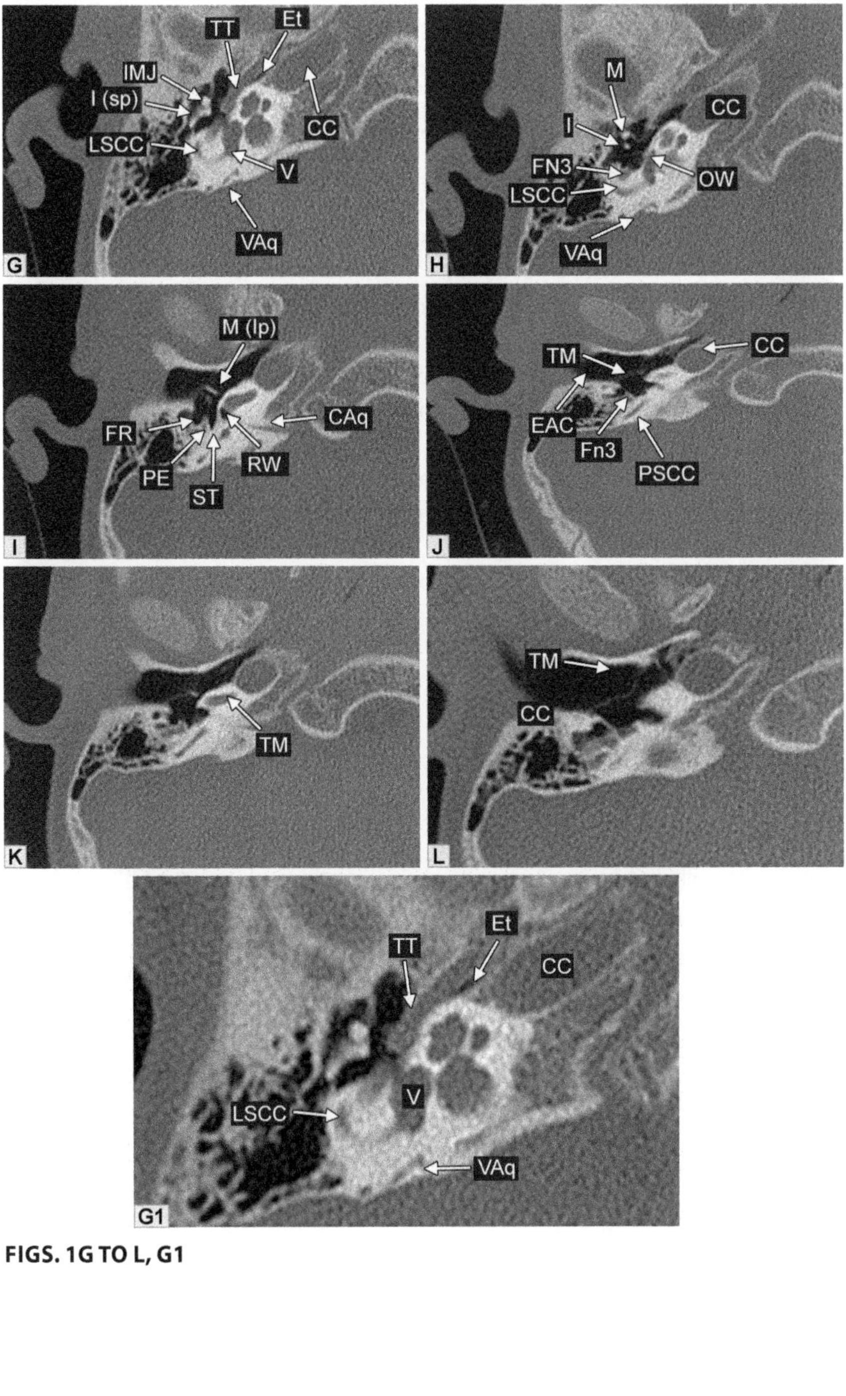

FIGS. 1G TO L, G1

CONSECUTIVE CORONAL MPR CT IMAGES (ANTERIOR TO POSTERIOR) (FIGS. 2A TO F, C1)

- While making the reformats, symmetry should be maintained.
- The head and handle of malleus appears on the most anterior sections (B), followed by the malleoincudal joint more posteriorly; the long process of incus and incudostapedial joint on even more posterior sections (D to F), and the short process of incus at extreme posterior sections.
- The apical turn of cochlea appears first (B), followed by the middle and basal turn (C and D).
- The tympanic membrane with the superior pars flaccida and inferior pars tensa, and attachment of handle of malleus is seen at the same level as the promontory (caused by basal turn of cochlea) (D).
- The epitympanum, mesotympanum and the hypotympanum, the tegmen tympani, and tegmen mastoideum are shown best on coronal images (C). Magnified view of C (C1).
- Prussak space is seen on anterior coronal images (B); located lateral to head of malleus.

Key

C—cochlea	Cb—cochlea basal turn
Cm—cochlea middle turn	CC—carotid canal
ET—epitympanum	FN—facial nerve canal
FN2—second part of facial nerve canal	HT—hypotympanum
I—incus	IMJ—incudomalleolar joint
MT—mesotympanum	OW—oval window
PS—Prussak space	S—stapes
Sc—scutum	TM—tympanic membrane
Tt—tegmen tympani	

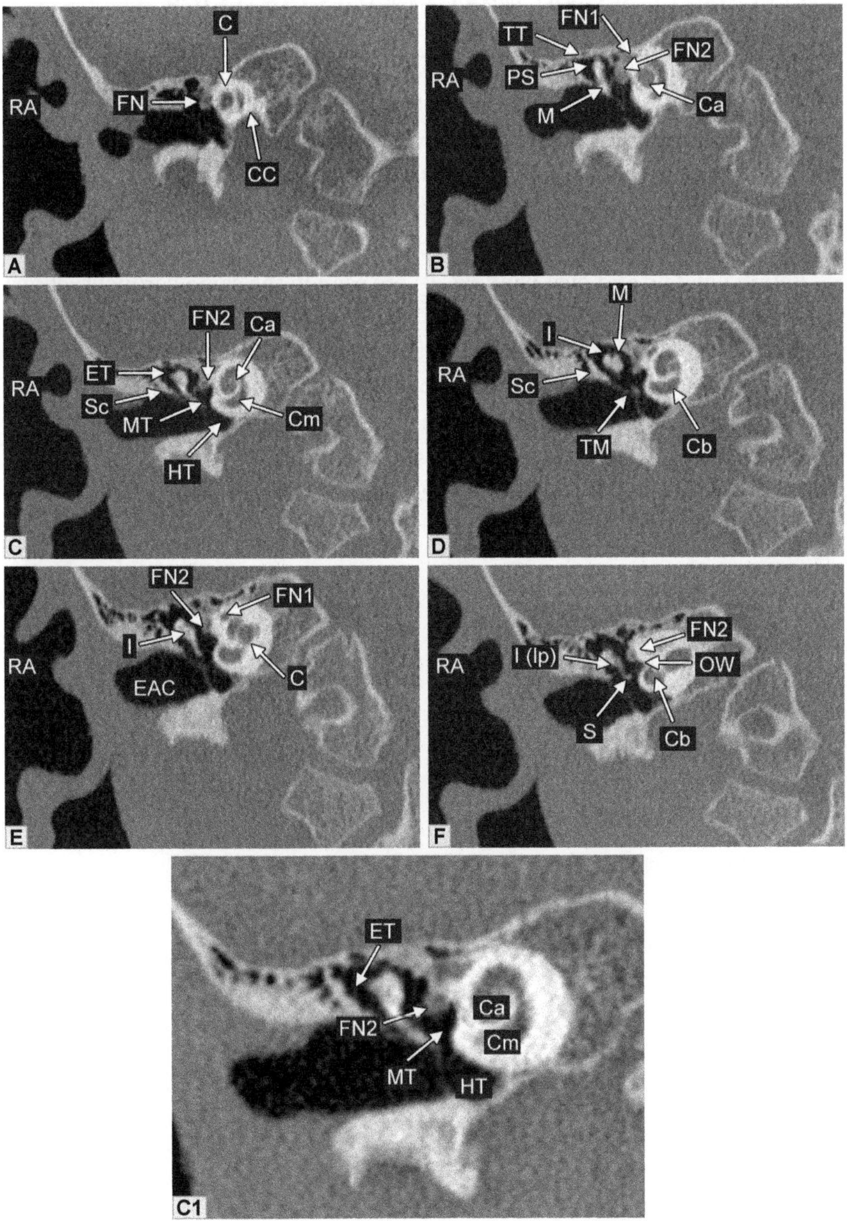

FIGS. 2A TO F, C1

SUBSEQUENT CORONAL MPR CT IMAGES (ANTERIOR TO POSTERIOR) (FIGS. 2G TO L, B1)

- These sections show the IAC, the vestibule, and the SCCs:
  - The medial part of the IAC is known as porus acousticus.
  - The lateral part is known as fundus.
  - Falciform crest (A) is a bony projection within the IAC at the lateral part, which divides it into superior and inferior part.
- Round window and oval window (B) are seen in the same coronal sections where IAC is completely seen. Round window is located inferiorly in relation to oval window. Magnified view of B (B1).
- In more posterior sections, the vestibule and SCCs are seen.
- The superior SCC and lateral SCC are seen on a relatively anterior section (C).
- Posterior SCC are seen on a more posterior section (F).
- In the posterior sections, the vertical part of the facial nerve canal (E) is visualized.

Key

FC—falciform crest	FN3—descending part of facial nerve canal
IAC—internal auditory canal	JB—jugular bulb
LSSCC—lateral superior semicircular canal	OW—oval window
PSCC—posterior semicircular canal	RW—round window
SSCC—superior semicircular canal	V—vestibule

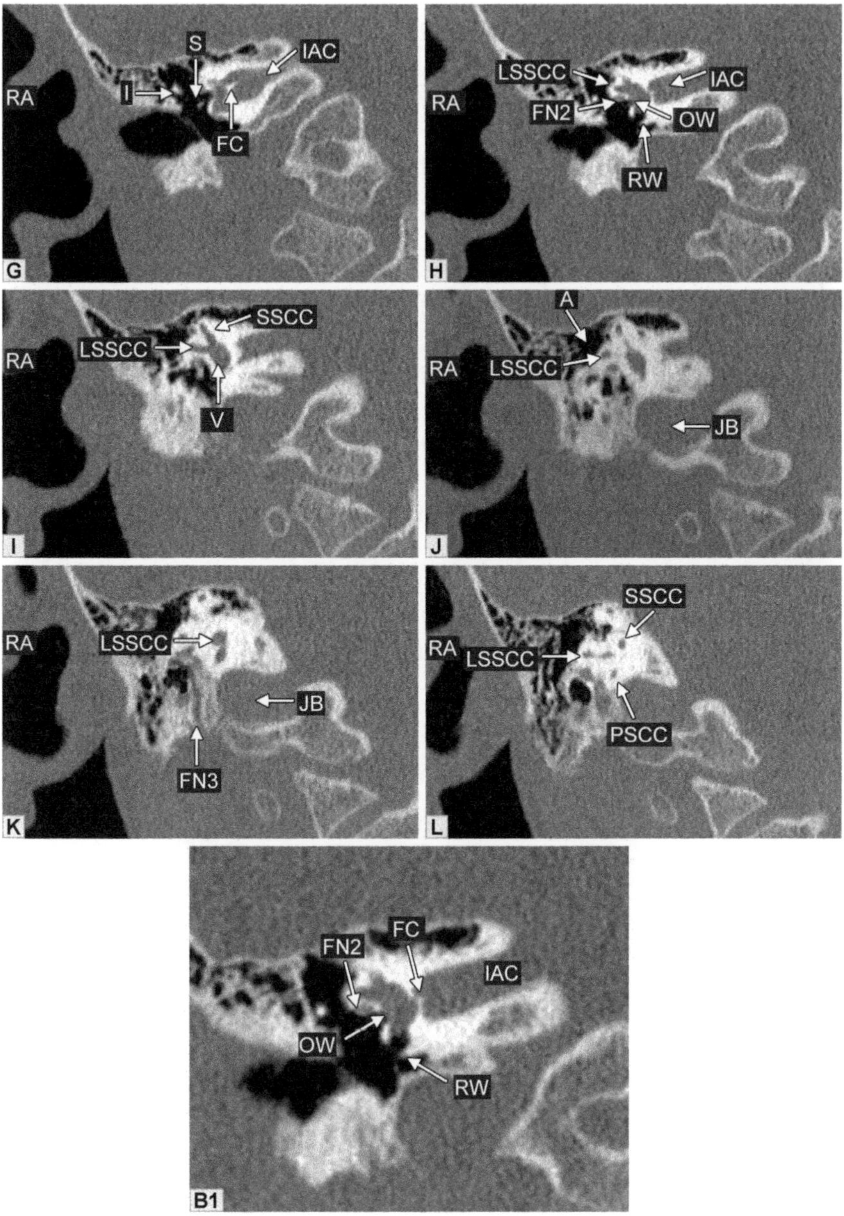

FIGS. 2G TO L, B1

CONSECUTIVE AXIAL HEAVILY T2W MR IMAGES (CISS SEQUENCE) (CRANIAL TO CAUDAL) (FIGS. 3A TO F, E1)

- On heavily T2-weighted (T2W) MR images, the fluid-containing structures [cerebrospinal fluid (CSF), perilymph, and endolymph] appear as bright.
- The superior SCC is seen as a bright linear structure at the most cranial section (A).
- The nerves on the IAC are visualized in great detail on MRI (C to E).
  - On the cranial sections, the facial and superior vestibular nerves are seen as hypointense structures (C). Relationship of facial nerve: Anterior; superior vestibular nerve: Posterior.
  - On a more caudal section (D and E), the inferior vestibular nerve and cochlear nerve are seen. The cochlear nerve is located anterior to inferior vestibular nerve.
- The internal architecture of cochlea is well visualized on MRI. The modiolus and osseous spiral lamina are seen as linear hypointense structures within the bright signal of cochlea (E, E1). Osseous spiral lamina is better seen on axial magnified image of basal turn of cochlea (F). Magnified view of E (E1).
- Lateral SCC, common crus, and the IAC are seen in the same axial level (B and C).

Key

Cn—cochlear nerve	FN—facial nerve
LSSCC—lateral superior semicircular canal	Mod—modiolus
OSL—osseous spiral lamina	PSCC—posterior semicircular canal
St—scala tympani	Sv—scala vestibule
VnI—inferior vestibular nerve	VnS—superior vestibular nerve

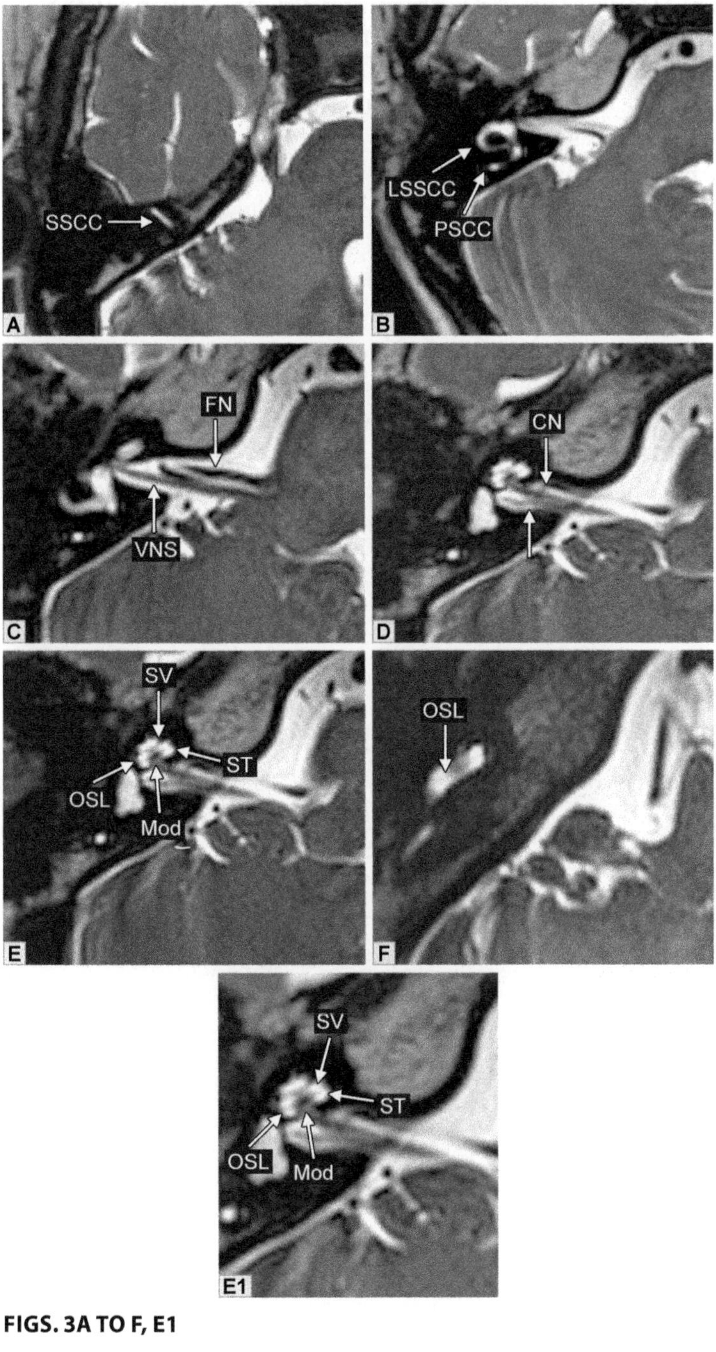

FIGS. 3A TO F, E1

CONSECUTIVE CORONAL HEAVILY T2W MR IMAGES (CISS SEQUENCE) (ANTERIOR TO POSTERIOR) (FIGS. 4A TO F)

- The middle ear structures and mastoid air cells are not visualized (as the air within produces a signal void).
- The middle ear ossicles also are not visualized.
- The labyrinthine anatomy and IAC can be evaluated in detail.
- The apical and middle turn of cochlea (A) are seen on more anterior sections. The basal turn of cochlea (B) is seen more posteriorly.
- The vestibule and the IAC is seen in the same coronal level (C).
- The superior SCC and lateral SCC are seen on a relatively anterior section (C). Posterior SCC is seen on a more posterior section (D to F).
- Superior and inferior vestibular nerves are seen in the same section where all three SCCs are first seen (D).
- Presence of high signal intensity within the middle ear or mastoid indicates pathology (otitis media or mastoiditis).

Key

Ca—apical turn of cochlea	Cb—basal turn of cochlea
Cm—middle turn of cochlea	LSSCC—lateral superior semicircular canal
PSCC—posterior semicircular canal	SSCC—superior semicircular canal
V—vestibule	VnI—inferior vestibular nerve
VnS—superior vestibular nerve	

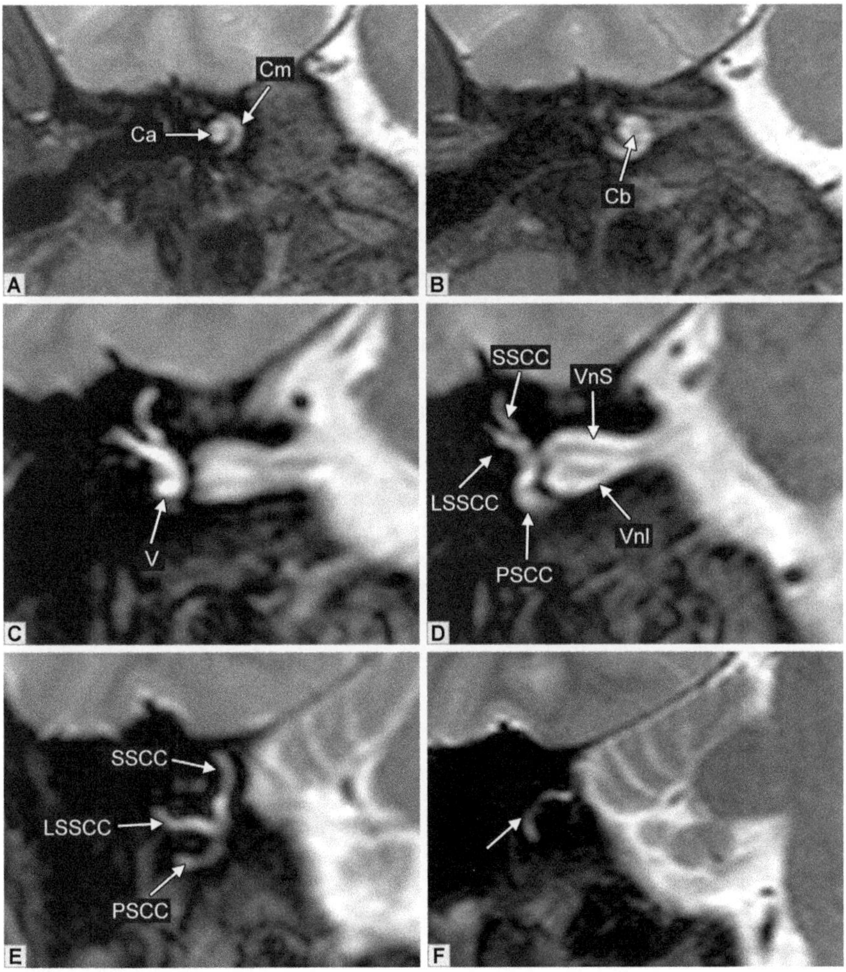

FIGS. 4A TO F

CONSECUTIVE SAGITTAL OBLIQUE HEAVILY T2W MR IMAGES (CISS SEQUENCE) (MEDIAL TO LATERAL) (FIGS. 5A TO F, C1)

- The 7th and 8th cranial nerves leave the brainstem at anterolateral upper medulla, travel across the cerebellopontine angle cistern (A and B).
- On a more lateral section, they are seen to enter the porus acousticus of IAC (C).
- The 8th nerve divides within IAC into superior vestibular, inferior vestibular, and cochlear divisions (C and D).
- Sagittal oblique images perpendicular to the nerves in the IAC enable visualization of these nerves in cross-section.
- These appear as four dots in the IAC (C, magnified view of C: C1)
  1. Anterosuperior: Facial nerve
  2. Anteroinferior: Cochlear nerve
  3. Posterosuperior: Superior vestibular nerve
  4. Posteroinferior: Inferior vestibular nerve

Key

Cn—cochlear nerve	CPA—cerebellopontine angle cistern
FN—facial nerve	IAC—internal auditory canal
VnI—inferior vestibular nerve	VnS—superior vestibular nerve

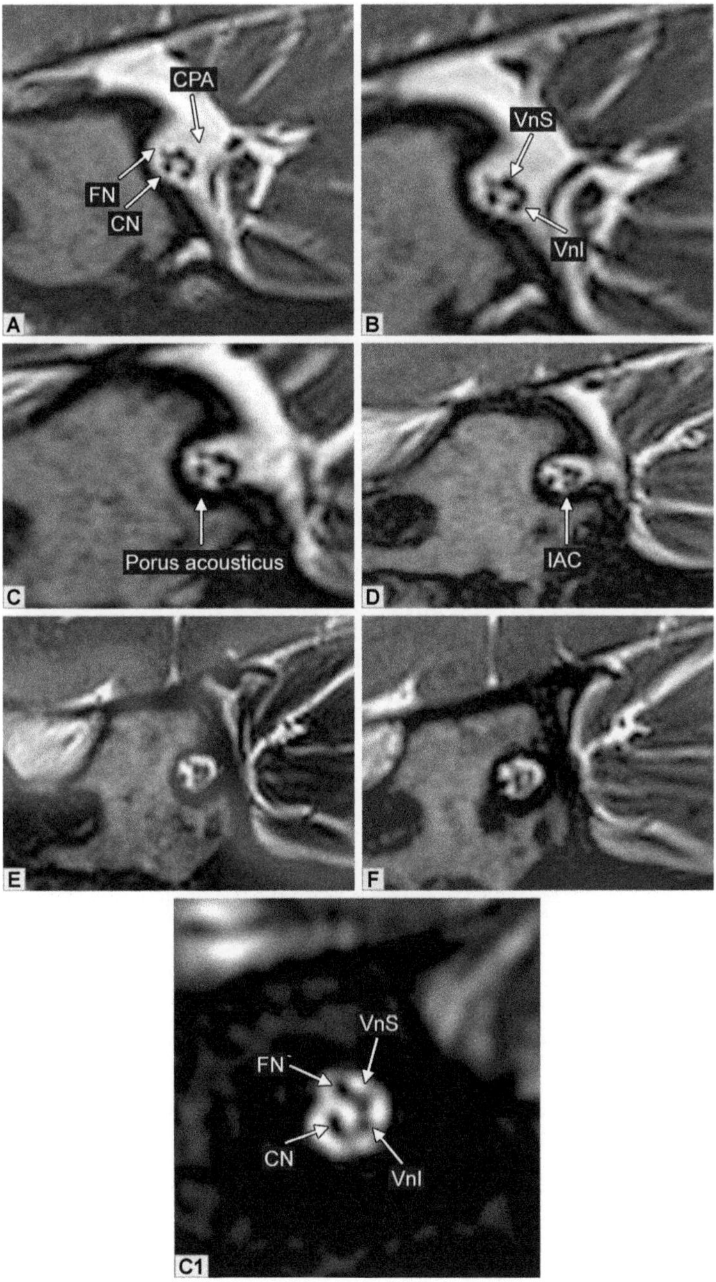

FIGS. 5A TO F, C1

2
SECTION

Congenital Anomalies of External and Middle Ear

5

Congenital Anomalies of External and Middle Ear

Ashu Seith Bhalla, Priyanka Naranje

- Congenital anomalies of external and middle ear result from aberrations during embryogenesis. These are also synonymous with congenital aural atresia, microtia (small ear), and microtia-anotia.
- *Incidence:* 1 in 10,000–15,000 births, more common in males, right side is affected more as compared left; and bilateral involvement is seen in 15% of the cases.[1] Common embryological development leads to various combinations of external and middle ear malformations. Concomitant involvement of inner ear anomalies is unusual because of its independent development pathway.
- *Clinical presentation:* Patients present with deformed pinna, conductive hearing loss, facial nerve palsy, and associated facial deformities in the syndromic forms.

EMBRYOLOGY

- External and middle ear develop from first and second branchial/pharyngeal arches during the 7th to 8th week of gestation.
- First branchial arch, also referred to as the mandibular arch, gives rise to mandible, maxilla, palate, and muscles of mastication. First branchial arch derivatives in the ear are incus, malleus, and tensor tympani muscle.
- Second branchial arch also referred to as the hyoid arch contributes to structures in the front and side of the neck. Second branchial arch derivatives in the temporal bone are stapes, facial nerve canal, stapedius, and styloid process.

IMAGING MODALITY

- High-resolution computed tomography (HRCT) temporal bone is the imaging modality of choice to delineate detailed external and middle ear anatomy, as well as for evaluation of associated anomalies of the inner ear and surrounding structures. HRCT by assessing the severity of involvement helps to prognosticate and triage patients into surgical and nonsurgical candidates.

STRUCTURES INVOLVED

The various anomalies are discussed structure-wise: Pinna, external auditory canal (EAC), middle ear structures, mastoid pneumatization, facial canal, associated inner ear anomalies, associated vascular anomalies and the temporomandibular joints (TMJ).

Pinna/Auricle Deformity

- Most patients present with varying severity of pinna deformity which is graded clinically (also see Chapter 6).
- Many classification/grading systems exist for grading of the pinna deformity, with number of grades ranging from 3 to even 10. The classifications are designed from point of view of planning of reconstruction of the pinna.
- A commonly used clinical classification is the *Weerda classification* which divides the dysplasia into three grades.[2] Grade 1: Most structures of the pinna are recognizable; Grade II: Moderate dysplasia with some structures of the auricle being recognized while in the Grade III or severe form the normal structures of the pinna are not recognizable (anotia) (**Fig. 1**).

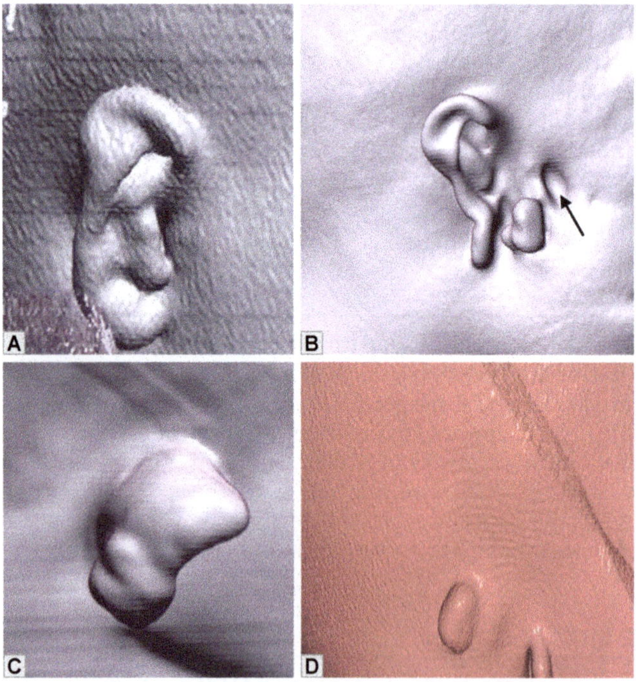

FIGS. 1A TO D: Clinical grading of microtia: Volume-rendered reconstructions showing various grades of pinna deformities in different patients: (A) Grade I, (B) Grade I with preauricular tag and pit (black arrow), (C) Grade II, and (D) Grade III.

- Another commonly used classification system is by *Marx* which has four grades.[3] Grades I and II being similar to *Weerda*. Grade III refers to a very small auricular tag and Grade IV as anotia.
- The severity of the microtia does not necessarily correlate with the severity of associated external or middle ear anomalies.[4]
- In addition, the pinna can be abnormal in position, mostly low lying.
- Preauricular or less commonly postauricular tags/cysts or pits may also be seen.

External Auditory Canal

External auditory canal abnormalities range from complete atresia to mild stenosis. Presence of EAC even if narrowed facilitates surgical reconstruction of the canal and ossicular chain, proving a landmark which aids the surgeon in reaching the tympanic cavity safely. Various EAC abnormalities are enumerated below:

- Combined cartilaginous and bony atresia (most common form) (**Fig. 2**)
- Isolated cartilaginous atresia
- Isolated bony canal atresia
- Stenotic cartilaginous EAC (**Fig. 3**)

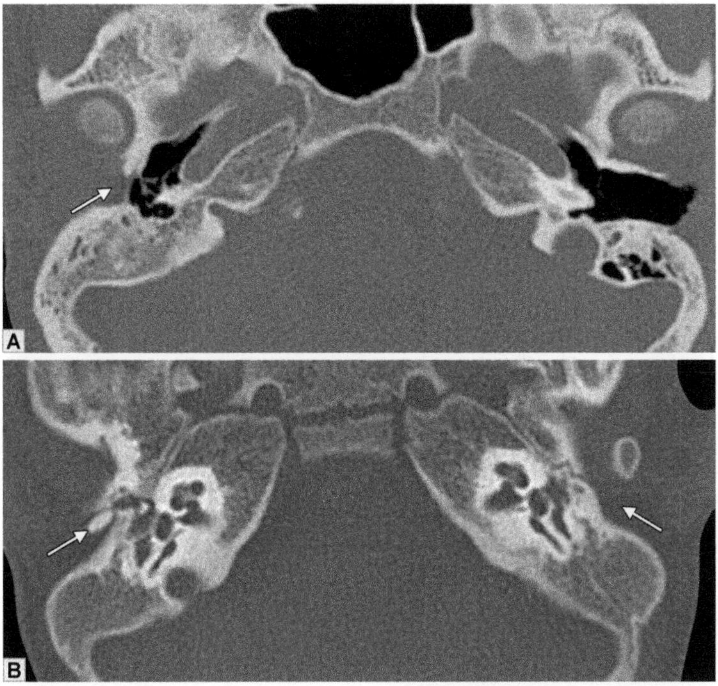

FIGS. 2A AND B: External auditory canal (EAC) atresia: (A) Patient 1 showing combined cartilaginous and bony atresia (arrow) on right side, with a normal left side; (B) Patient 2 with bilateral ear atresia (arrows). The associated middle (ME) ear anomalies are detailed subsequently.

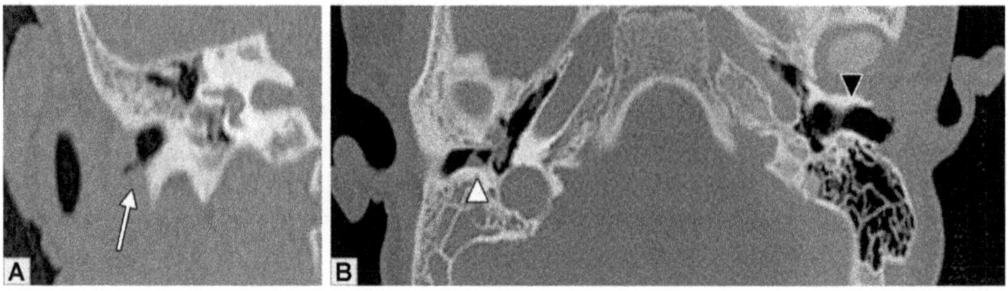

FIGS. 3A AND B: External auditory canal (EAC) stenosis: A 7-year-old boy with Grade I right microtia showing narrowing of the cartilaginous (white arrow) and bony parts (white arrowhead) of the right EAC. The left EAC is normal in its cartilaginous and bony parts (black arrowhead). Associated reduced volume of right middle ear with otomastoiditis is present.

The types of EAC anomalies are classified into three types according to *Weerda*:[2]

1. External auditory canal stenosis type A—marked narrowing of the EAC with an intact skin layer.
2. External auditory canal stenosis type B—partial development of the EAC with an atresia plate at the medial part.
3. Type C—complete bony EAC atresia.

Tympanic membrane may be dysplastic or even absent in cases of microtia and otoscopic evaluation is required for surgical planning.

Middle Ear Anomalies

Middle ear abnormalities can affect the size of tympanic cavity, ossicles, oval window, and rarely, the round window.

- The middle ear size can be assessed quantitatively. The middle ear width is measured as the distance between promontory and atretic plate (as measured in the coronal plane). If it is <3 mm, then surgical reconstruction is difficult (**Fig. 4**).
- Middle ear (tympanic cavity) space is often reduced in size in these cases. The mesotympanum and hypotympanum are affected more often than the epitympanum (**Fig. 5**).[5]

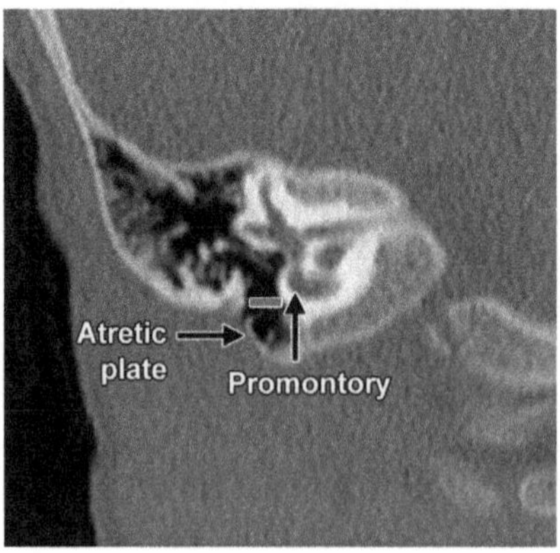

FIG. 4: The width of the middle ear is measured on a coronal section as the distance between the atretic plate and promontory.

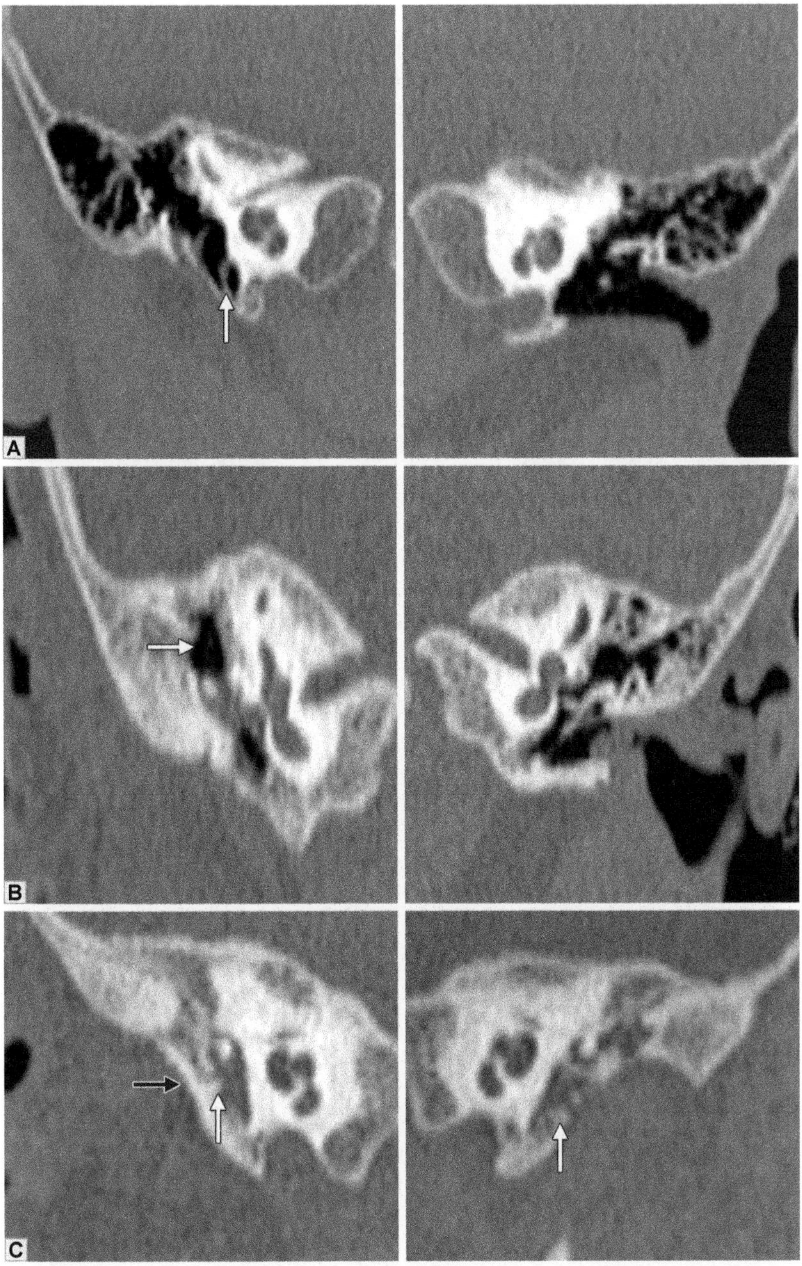

FIGS. 5A TO C: Reduced middle ear (ME) capacity: Coronal HRCT scans of *different patients* showing varying degrees of reduced middle ear capacity with contralateral side shown for comparison. (A) Preserved ME width with only mild reduction in the hypotympanum size (arrow); (B) Moderate reduction in capacity of meso- and hypotympanum with relatively larger epitympanum (arrow); (C) Marked decrease in size of entire ME cavity bilaterally (white arrows). Also note thick atretic plate on right side (black arrow).

Ossicular Anomalies

- Variable ossicular dysplasias are seen; and the ossicles are often adherent to the atretic plate. Single or all three ossicles may be hypoplastic in entirety or in parts. In the more severe forms, the ossicles may even be absent. There may be separation of ossicles or malleoincudal fusion (**Fig. 6**) in some cases. In severe cases, stapes may be absent (**Fig. 7**). An intact stapes is critical to surgery.

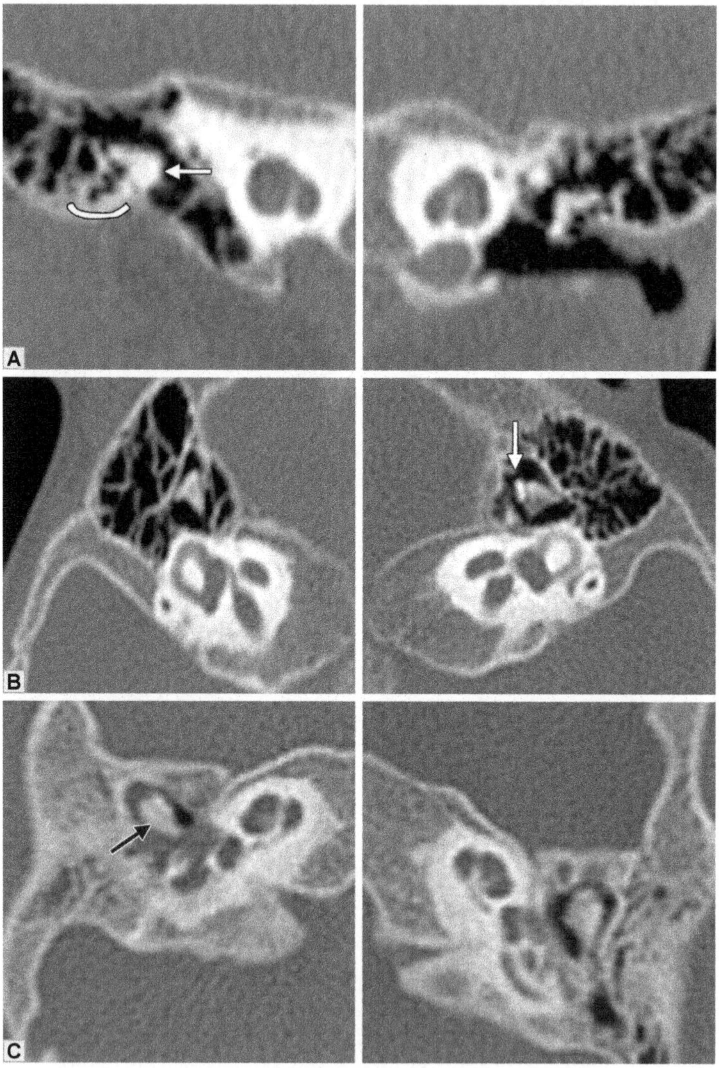

FIGS. 6A TO C: Incudomalleal dysplasias: *Patient 1*—(A) Right side malleus is dysplastic (arrow) and adherent to the atretic plate (block arrow); left side is normal; (B) Axial sections reveal missing handle of malleus on the right side, which is normal on left side (arrow); (C) *Patient 2* with bilateral microtia showing a dysplastic incus (black arrow).

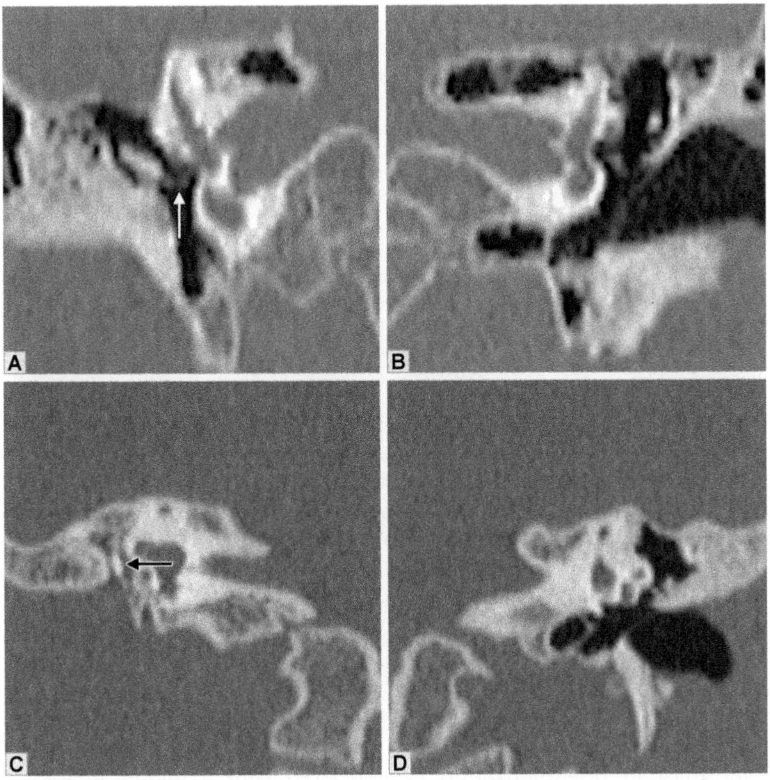

FIGS. 7A TO D: Stapes and oval window involvement: *Patient 1* (A and B)—right side (A) EAC atresia with normal incudostapedial articulation, stapes (arrow) and oval window. Left side ear (B) is normal. *Patient 2* (C and D)—right side (C) EAC atresia with flat oval window (black arrow) and nonvisualization of stapes. Left side (D) is normal.

- There may be isolated abnormality of ossicles without other anomalies (**Fig. 8**). These are classified as a type of "minor middle ear anomalies." Teunissen classification (1993) of congenital middle ear anomalies had classified these ossicular abnormalities into four forms:[6] (1) Congenital stapes ankylosis as type I; (2) Stapes ankylosis associated with another congenital ossicular chain anomaly as type II; (3) Ossicular anomalies without stapedial ankylosis as type III; and (4) Aplasia or severe dysplasia of oval window or round window as type IV. (also see Chapter 21)

Round Window and Oval Window

- Abnormality of windows can be absence or closure by a bony plate. The oval window is more often affected than round window. An atretic oval or round window is a poor surgical risk. A minimum height of 1 mm (as measured on a coronal scan) is deemed necessary for surgery.
- Oval window atresia can be seen in isolation and is classified as a "minor middle ear anomaly." (also see Chapter 21)

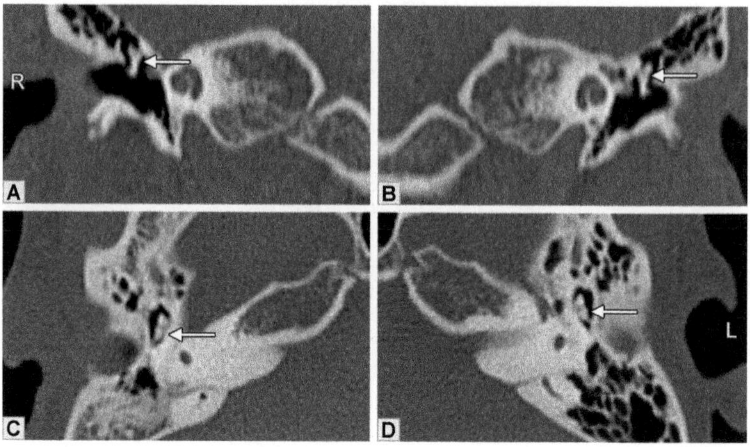

FIGS. 8A TO D: Isolated ossicular dysplasia: 19 years old female, presenting with bilateral conductive hearing loss. HRCT shows bilateral dysplastic incus and malleus with partial malleoincudal fusion (arrows). No other external ear or inner ear abnormality was seen.

Cholesteatoma

- Microtia is a cause of congenital cholesteatoma and otitis media.
- Soft tissue in the middle ear is present with other imaging features of a cholesteatoma (**Fig. 9**) as detailed in Chapter 16.
- Poor mastoid pneumatization is associated with a higher incidence of congenital cholesteatoma.

Mastoid Pneumatization

- The mastoid air cells show variable pneumatization which often correlates with mesotympanum volume, although it is not always so (**Fig. 10**).
- Also, the thickness of the atretic plate generally correlates with pneumatization of the mastoid, with thicker plates seen in sclerotic mastoids (**Fig. 11**).
- Delineating these in the report is important as anterior approach involves drilling of the atretic plate while mastoid thickness is important if transmastoid (TM) approach is planned.

Facial Canal Anomalies

- The vertical part of the facial nerve canal tends to be more anterior in location and a shortened course and is thus more prone to injury during mastoid drilling (**Fig. 12**).
- Complete dehiscence of the tympanic segment, location closer to the round or oval window, and duplication of mastoid segments are other reported anomalies. Canal dilatation is less commonly seen (**Fig. 13**).
- Due to these abnormal locations, facial nerve injury is a feared complication of microtia surgery and hence delineating its course preoperatively is critical.

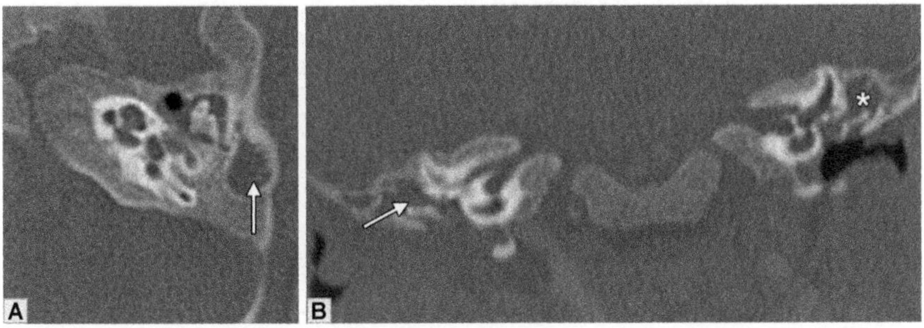

FIGS. 9A AND B: Congenital cholesteatoma: (A) 1-year old child with bilateral microtia, EAC atresia, poor mastoid pneumatization and soft tissue in the middle ear and mastoids (arrows); (B) Different patient with right EAC atresia with soft tissue filling the middle ear (arrow). Left EAC is normal but cholesteatoma present in the epitympanum (asterisk).

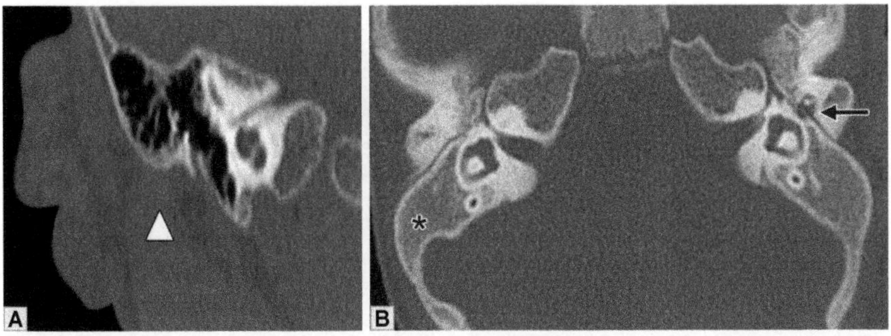

FIGS. 10A AND B: Variable mastoid pneumatization: (A) Good mastoid air cell pneumatization in a patient with isolated external auditory canal atresia (arrowhead); (B) Bilateral markedly reduced middle ear size (black arrow) with nonpneumatization of mastoid air cells (asterisk).

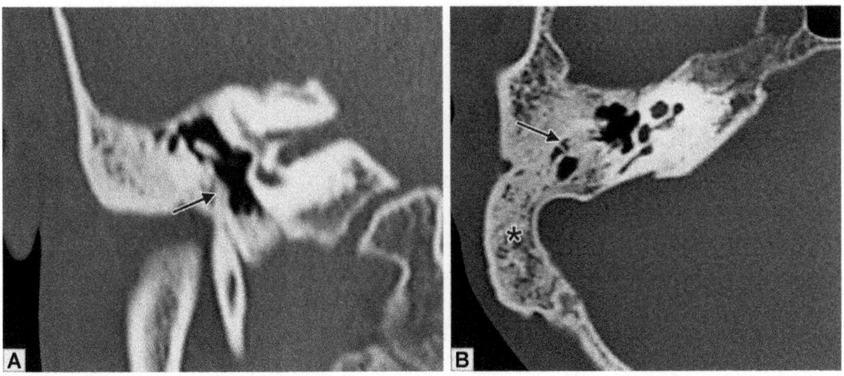

FIGS. 11A AND B: Atretic plate: 24 years old male with Grade II microtia shows mild reduction of the mesotympanum volume, and poor pneumatization of the mastoid air cells (star), as well as the atretic plate (arrow). Contralateral side is normal.

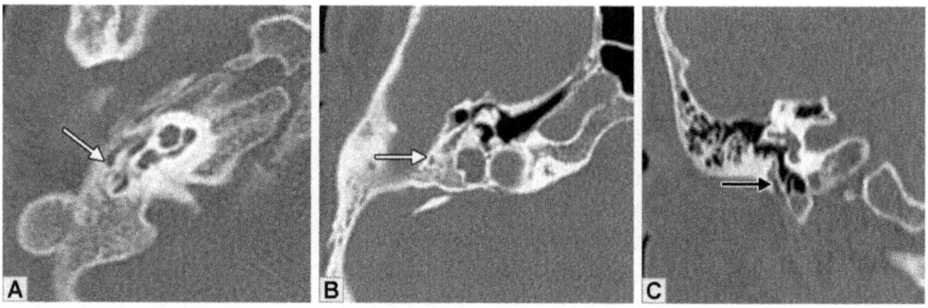

FIGS. 12A TO C: Facial canal anomalies: *Different patients.* Patient with bilateral microtia and reduced ME size showing anterolateral displacement of the facial nerve canals (FNC) (arrow) on (A) axial scan; (B) Reduced middle ear volume, the tympanic segment of the FNC is severely narrowed (arrow) and not delineated; (C) Anterior displacement of the vertical part of the FNC (black arrow). The vertical part of the FNC is normally seen in a more posterior section.

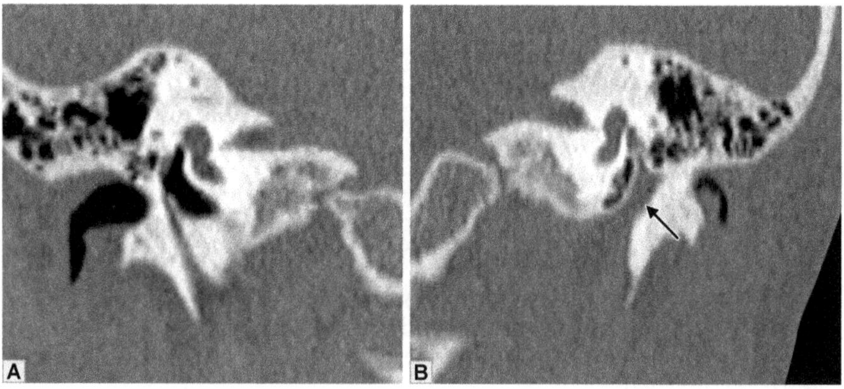

FIGS. 13A AND B: Facial canal dilatation: Patient with left external auditory canal atresia. The vertical part of the FNC is dilated on the left side (black arrow). The normal right side is shown for comparison (A).

Inner Ear/IAM Anomalies

- As inner ear has a different embryological origin, their occurrence in microtia patients is uncommon. The reported incidence is variable across various studies.
- *The spectrum includes:* Cochlear dysplasias and other inner ear anomalies (Refer to Chapter 11) (**Fig. 14**). Narrowing of internal acoustic meatus (IAM) and canal may also be seen. (**Fig. 15**). Delineating these anomalies is critical in view of increasing trend of use of cochlear implant in these patients (Chapter 11 and 14).

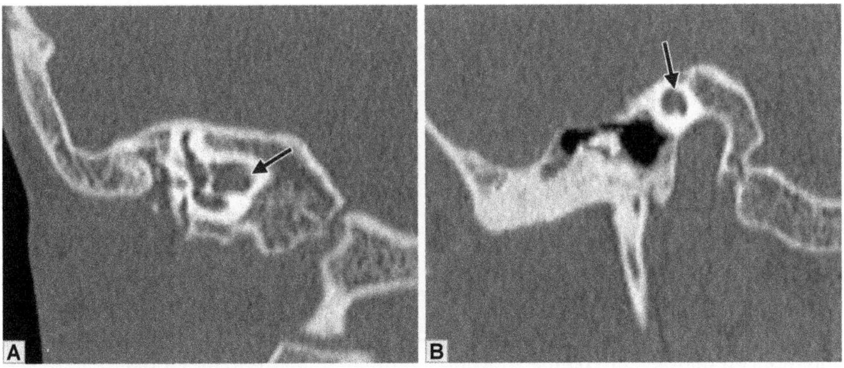

FIGS. 14A AND B: Associated inner ear anomalies: (A) Patient with external auditory canal atresia and reduced middle ear volume showing vestibule—lateral semicircular canal dysplasia (black arrow); (B) *Different patient* with microtia showing incomplete partition of cochlea (black arrow).

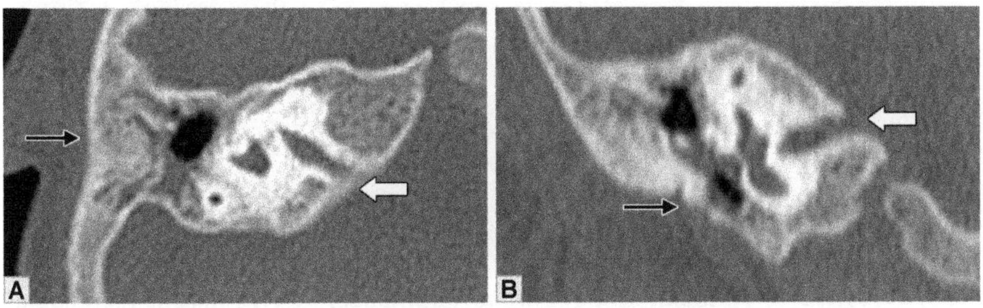

FIGS. 15A AND B: Internal acoustic meatus (IAM) anomalies: External auditory canal atresia (black arrow), reduced middle ear size, and narrow IAM (block arrow).

Vascular Anomalies

- Presence of associated vascular anomalies presents a surgical risk, and hence, reporting these becomes imperative. Reduced middle ear size results in distortion of course of the adjoining vessels. These include:
  - Aberrant course of internal carotid artery in the middle ear
  - High riding jugular bulb (**Fig. 16**)
- Absence of the carotid canal may also be seen.

Temporomandibular Joints

- Mandibular condylar abnormalities such as hypoplastic or bifid condyles (**Fig. 17**) may be seen associated with microtia. Altered TMJ structural relationship with no functional joints may also be associated.[8]

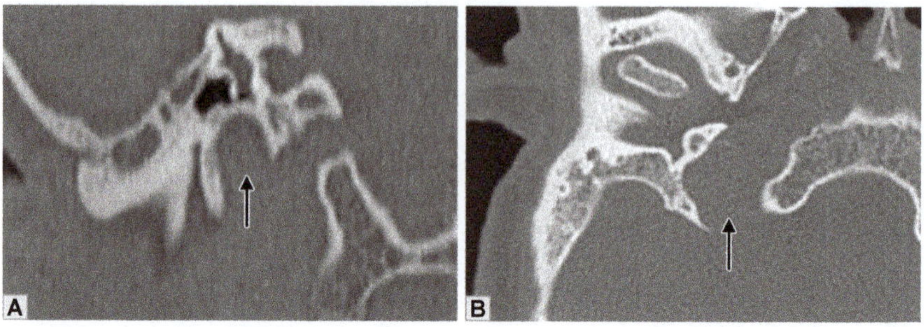

FIGS. 16A AND B: High-riding jugular bulb: Patient with right-sided aural atresia and reduced middle ear volume showing a prominent, high-riding jugular bulb (black arrow).

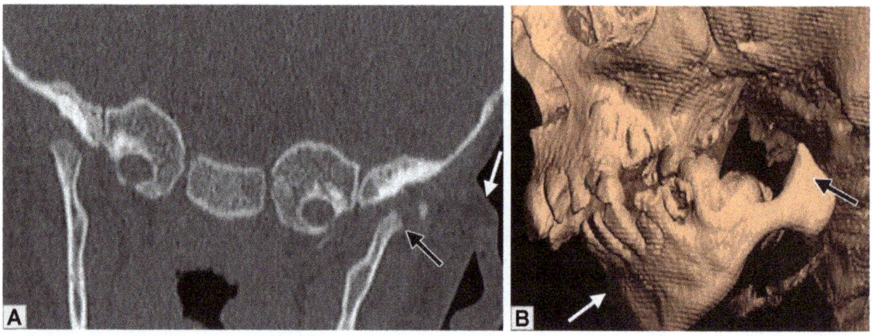

FIGS. 17A AND B: Associated mandibular anomalies: (A) Hypoplastic mandibular condyle and ramus (black arrow) with low placed pinna (white arrow). Right mandibular condyle is also hypoplastic with a shallow glenoid fossa. (B) VRT image of a different patient showing mandibular ramus and condylar hypoplasia (black arrow) resulting in retrognathia (white arrow).

SYNDROMES

- Microtia may be associated with other craniofacial syndromes. This association being due to common embryological origin from first and second branchial arches.
- Craniofacial syndromes associated with external and middle ear anomalies include:
  - *Goldenhar syndrome (**Fig. 18**)*: Also called Oculo-Auriculo-Vertebral (OAV) syndrome or hemifacial microsmia. It is characterized by anomalies involving the ear, nose, soft palate, lip, and mandible; usually on one side. Spine is also involved.

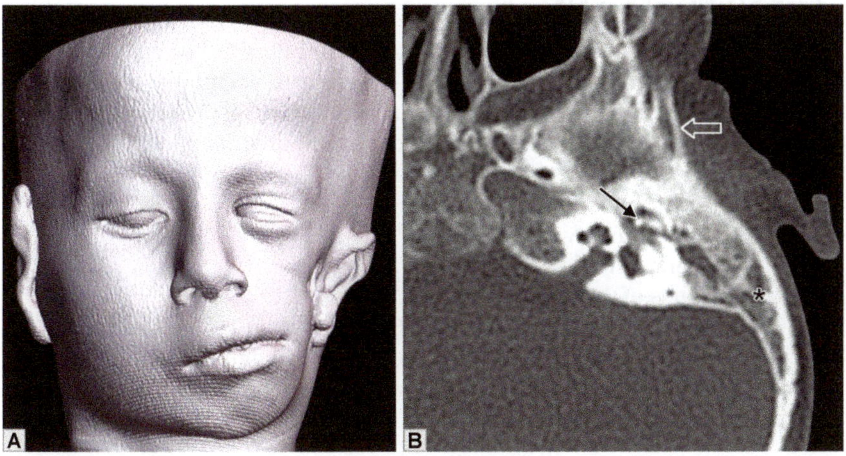

FIGS. 18A AND B: Goldenhar syndrome: (A) Volume rendering technique (VRT) image showing left-sided facial anomalies (hemifacial microsmia); (B) External auditory canal atresia (white arrow), hypoplastic middle ear with dysplastic ossicles (black arrow), dysplastic squamous part of the temporal bone (open arrow), and sclerosed mastoids (asterisk). Inner ear structures are normal.

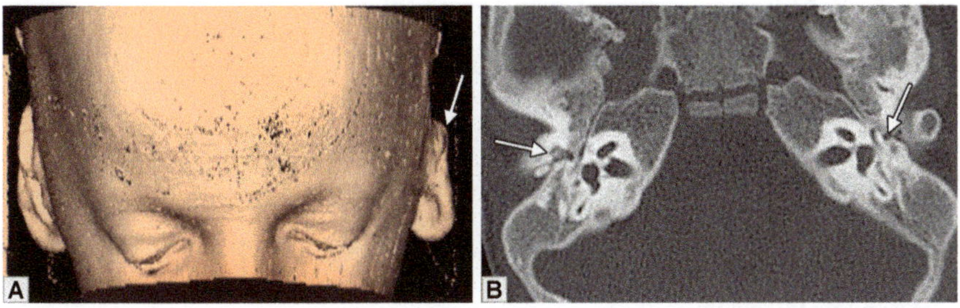

FIGS. 19A AND B: Treacher Collins syndrome: (A) Volume rendering technique (VRT) image showing downward-slanting eyes and deformed left pinna (white arrow); (B) Bilateral external auditory canal atresia, markedly reduced middle ear volume (arrows) with dysplastic ossicles.

  - *Treacher Collins syndrome (**Fig. 19**)*: Also called mandibulofacial dysostosis or midfacial syndrome. It is characterized by downward-slanting eyes with drooping eyelids, micrognathia (mandibular hypoplasia), external and middle ear anomalies, as well as anomalous maxilla. The involvement is mostly bilateral, and patients also have airway narrowing.
  - *Pierre Robin syndrome:* Microtia may be seen as association along with micrognathia, cleft palate, and glossoptosis.
- More severe grades of external and middle ear anomalies seen in these cases, with the involvement often being bilateral.

CT GRADING SYSTEMS

Based on clinical appearances and HRCT, surgical rating scales have been developed by various authors.[4,8] These CT-based scales include scores based on the configuration of structures deeming crucial to success of operative middle ear reconstructions. Some of the critical structures required for successful surgery include:

- Regular stapes
- Regular round window
- Sufficient aerated middle ear space
- Regular course of the facial nerve

Different grading systems are used on CT as shown in **Tables 1** and **2**.

While classification systems mentioned in **Tables 1** and **2** aid in deciding the surgical options, a newer treatment modality is bonebridge (BB) which needs evaluation of special measurements.

TABLE 1 Yeakley and Jahrsdoerfer's CT-based prognostic system.

Parameters	Points
Stapes present	2
Oval window open	1
Middle ear space	1
Facial nerve	1
Malleus/ Incus complex	1
Mastoid pneumatized	1
Incus-stapes connection	1
Round window	1
Appearance of external ear	1

- Maximum of 10 points
- Of major importance is an existing stapes
- Reasonable prognosis if minimum of 7 points
- Below 5, surgery is not undertaken

TABLE 2 Siegert's prognostic indices.

Structure	Findings	Points
External meatus	• Normal • Soft tissue atresia • Bony atresia	2 1 0
Aeration of mastoid	• Excellent • Fair • Missing	2 1 0

Continued

Continued

Structure	Findings	Points
Middle ear space	• Large • Medium • Missing	2 1 0
Aeration of middle ear	• Major • Minor • Missing	2 1 0
Facial nerve	• Normal • Minor dislocation • Major dislocation	4 2 0
Vessels	• Normal • Minor dislocation • Major dislocation	2 1 0
Malleus + incus	• Normal • Dysplastic • Missing	2 1 0
Stapes	• Normal • Dysplastic • Missing	4 2 0
Oval window	• Open • Obliterated	4 0
Round window	• Open • Obliterated	4 0
Summation		0–28

- It is a more diversified system.
- It assigns maximum of 28 points.
- High numbers (4 each) assigned to an open oval or round window.
- Minimum of 15 points for bilateral atresia, and 20 points for unilateral atresia are required for surgical option.

BONEBRIDGE CT MEASUREMENT

- The floating mass transducer (FMT) of the BB can be placed TM or retrosigmoid. The site of implantation is chosen based on the mastoid pneumatization, volume, and thickness of the underlying bone (**Fig. 20**).
- The FMT is basically cylindrical in shape with two flanges on the side. Part of this cylinder needs to be implanted (at least 4 mm) into well corticated bone, that is healthy; while avoiding critical structures.
- Critical structures that need to be avoided while implanting BB are:
  - External auditory canal
  - Large air cells (avoid penetration)
  - Inner table of skull
  - Sutures
  - Emissary veins/sigmoid sinus

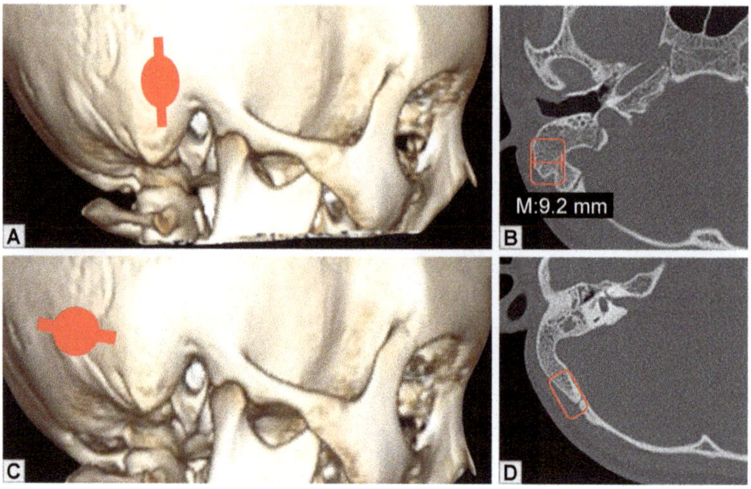

FIGS. 20A TO D: (A and B) Transmastoid FMT. VRT and axial CT showing the site for the placement of TM FMT. The measurement of >8.7 mm depth provides ample mastoid bone to accommodate FMT entirely. (C and D) Retrosigmoid FMT. VRT and axial CT showing the site for the placement of RS FMT. Lifts will be required to elevate FMT from skull surface in this case.

MANAGEMENT ISSUES (DISCUSSED IN DETAIL IN CHAPTER 6)

- It is difficult to assess the severity of hearing impairment, since most of the patients are infants.
- Brainstem audiometry is useful in this regard.
- While assessing the benefits of surgery, potential complication of facial nerve paresis should be kept in mind.
- High-resolution computed tomography-grading systems are used in triage of candidates for surgery.
- In cases with unfavorable anatomy—hearing aids are preferred.
- The goals of management are:
  - Reconstruction of pinna
  - Reconstruction of EAC
  - Restoration of hearing
- Since the reconstruction is a difficult surgery with complications; hence, traditional thinking is that further intervention is not necessary in unilateral microtia, if there is normal hearing in the other ear.
- Restoration of hearing is imperative in those with bilateral conductive hearing loss.
- The preferable site of placement of FMT is TM (between EAC anteriorly and sigmoid sinus posterolaterally). However, when mastoid cells are sclerosed [chronic suppurative otits media (CSOM)] or hypoplastic or poorly pneumatized (microtia), the mastoid volume may not be enough to accommodate the FMT, and the rectosigmoid position may be employed.[7]

REFERENCES

1. Kösling S, Omenzetter M, Bartel-Friedrich S. Congenital malformations of the external and middle ear. Eur J Radiol. 2009;69(2):269-79.
2. Weerda H. Classification of congenital deformities of the auricle. Facial Plast Surg. 1988;5(5):385-8.
3. Baluch N, Nagata S, Park C, Wilkes GH, Reinisch J, Kasrai L, et al. Auricular reconstruction for microtia: A review of available methods. Plast Surg (Oakv). 2014 Spring;22(1):39-43.
4. Jahrsdoerfer RA, Yeakley JW, Aguilar EA, Cole RR, Gray LC. Grading system for the selection of patients with congenital aural atresia. Am J Otol. 1992;13(1):6-12.
5. Patil AR, Bhalla A, Gupta P, Goyal D, Vishnubhatla S, Ramavat A, et al. HRCT evaluation of microtia: A retrospective study. Indian J Radiol Imaging. 2012;22(3):188-94.
6. Teunissen EB, Cremers WR. Classification of congenital middle ear anomalies. Report on 144 ears. Ann Otol Rhinol Laryngol. 1993;102(8 Pt 1):606-12.
7. Wang Y, Xing W, Liu T, Zhou X, Qian J, Wang B, et al. Simultaneous auricular reconstruction combined with bone bridge implantation-optimal surgical techniques in bilateral microtia with severe hearing impairment. Int J Pediatr Otorhinolaryngol. 2018;113:82-7.

6

Congenital External and Middle Ear Anomalies: Surgical Perspectives

Chirom Amit Singh, Suresh C Sharma

TERMINOLOGY

- *Microtia*: Small ear refers to the deformities of pinna.
- *Auricle*: It refers to external ear/pinna.
- *Aural*: More inclusive term implying related to ear as a whole.

CONGENITAL DEFORMITIES OF PINNA/AURICLE

Classification

Classification by Aguilar and Jahrsdoerfer is described in **Table 1**. Weerda[1] also divides the congenital auricular anomalies into similar three grades (see Chapter 5).[1]

Aims of Treatment

The aim of surgery is cosmetic correction and restoration of hearing. Usually, Grade I microtia does not require any correction. Grade II and III microtia can be treated with a variety of surgeries to improve cosmesis.

TABLE 1 **Clinical classification of congenital auricular anomalies (Aguilar and Jahrsdoerfer classification).[2]**

Grade	Description
Grade I	Pinna smaller in size in any dimension
Grade II	External ear with structural deficiencies: Absence of scapha, lobule; broadened helical rim; missing helix, missing conchal bowl or missing antihelical fold (**Figs. 1A** and **B**)
Grade III	• Ear having the classic "peanut" deformity • No recognizable structures present, anotia (**Fig. 1C**)

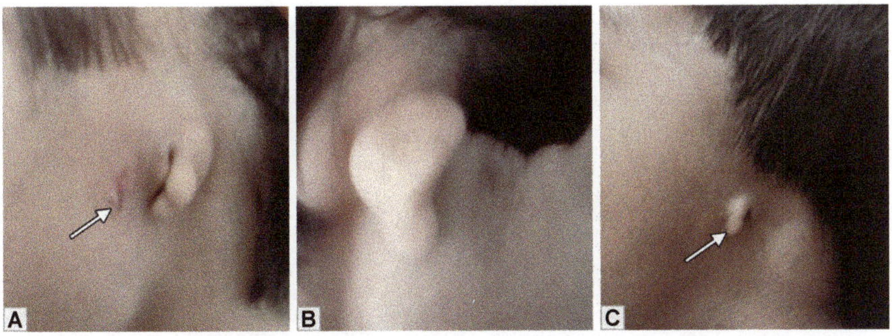

FIGS. 1A TO C: Clinical grading of microtia: (A and B) Grade II microtia and (C) Grade III microtia. Note the preauricular tag (arrow).

Treatment Options

Current widely accepted treatment options for higher grade of microtia are:

- Autogenous reconstruction (Gold standard)
- Implant-retained prosthesis

Autogenous Reconstruction

- This surgery is usually performed when the child reaches 6–10 years of age.
- By this time, the chance of harvesting adequate amount of chest cartilage is good to create a good cartilage framework. Additionally, the risk of postharvest chest deformity is less at this age. Also, by 6 years, the child has attained 95% of size of adult pinna.
- It involves complex multiple-staged surgeries which include construction of a three-dimensional (3D) cartilage framework and placement beneath the non-hair-bearing mastoid skin; lobule rotation, conchal excavation, tragus formation; and elevation of the pinna. This cartilage framework is carved from 6–8 costal cartilages.
- There is literature showing some role of preoperative 3D computed tomography (CT) scan of the rib cage to determine the length of costal cartilages from which the cartilage framework are planned to be made (see Chapter 2).

Implant-retained Prosthesis

- This is a prosthetic rehabilitation in which an auricular prothesis is fixed to the desired location of lateral face using two percutaneous osseointegrated fixtures/abutments (**Figs. 2A** and **B**).
- For optimal position of the abutments, ideally there should be around 3 mm of cortical bone.
- Preoperative high-resolution computed tomography (HRCT) provides the following information for the surgery:
    - Bone thickness of the cortical bone where the abutments are to be placed. The superior abutment is placed in the suprameatal crest. This place is chosen because there is a triangle of dense bone between the middle cranial fossa and middle ear (ME) cleft here. The inferior one is placed at least 2 cm from the superior fixture.
    - Preoperative determination of the implant location.

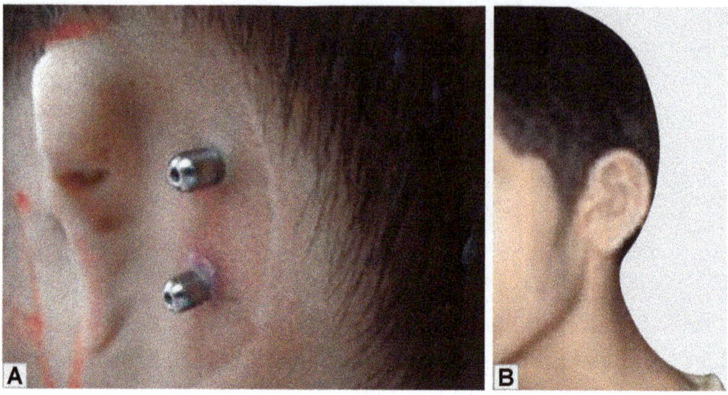

FIGS. 2A AND B: Implant-retained prosthesis: (A) Two osseointegrated fixtures; (B) Postprosthesis photograph with good cosmetic result.

Courtesy: Dr Rakesh Kumar and Dr Veena Jain, AIIMS, New Delhi.

CONGENITAL AURAL ATRESIA

This mainly refers to congenital combined abnormalities of external auditory canal (EAC) and ME as they are closely related.

Classification

- *Altman's classification of aural atresia (**Table 2**)*: It is one of the widely used classifications of congenital aural atresia (CAA) which was developed in 1955.
- CT-based classification of aural atresia is described in Chapter 4.

Management

Goal of reconstructive surgery:

- *Main goal:* To restore sufficient hearing so that amplification is no longer needed (postoperative air-bone gap within 20–30 dB)
- Create a patent and skin-lined EAC
- Stable long-term hearing result

TABLE 2 Altman's classification of aural atresia.[3]

Group	Description
Grade I	• Tympanic membrane hypoplastic • Various types of ossicular malformations • Stapes is usually mobile
Grade II	• Atretic plate present • Tympanic bone hypoplastic; or may even be absent • Facial nerve course may be abnormal • Tympanic cavity within normal limits
Grade III	• Above-mentioned abnormalities, with severely hypoplastic tympanic cavity

Source: Modified from Altmann F. Congenital aural atresia of the ear in men and animals. Ann Otol Rhinol Laryngol. 1955;64:824-58.

Timing of surgery:
- Child with unilateral canal atresia may not require any intervention as the contralateral ear is normal and the parents can be reassured that the language and intellectual development will be normal.
- Child with bilateral canal atresia needs some intervention from early age as his hearing is impaired.
- Atresia repair surgery should be performed after the pinna reconstruction surgery (usually after 6 years of age).
- Before the surgery, child should be kept on bone conduction hearing aid.
- Bone-anchored hearing aids (BAHA) may be considered in children older than 5 years of age.

Preoperative evaluation: The preoperative imaging study is HRCT of the temporal bone in both axial and coronal planes to look for:
- The status of the inner ear
- The size and status of the ME cavity
- The extent of pneumatization in temporal bone
- The facial nerve course, with emphasis on the relationship of the horizontal portion to the footplate of stapes; and the location of the mastoid segment
- The presence of the oval window and stapes footplate
- Delineation of the thickness and form of the atretic bone
- Soft tissue contribution to the atresia
- The presence or absence of congenital cholesteatoma
- Temporomandibular joint

Treatment Options

- Atresiaplasty/Canalplasty
- Implantable hearing devices

Atresiaplasty/Canalplasty

- This surgery includes creation of skin-lined EAC, tympanic membrane with or without ossicular reconstruction (ossiculoplasty).
- Different surgical approaches have been described; namely anterior, transmastoid, and modified anterior approaches (**Fig. 3**).
- Long-term hearing result (air-bone gap <30 dB) with atresiaplasty ranges from 47.8 to 84.4%.[4,5]

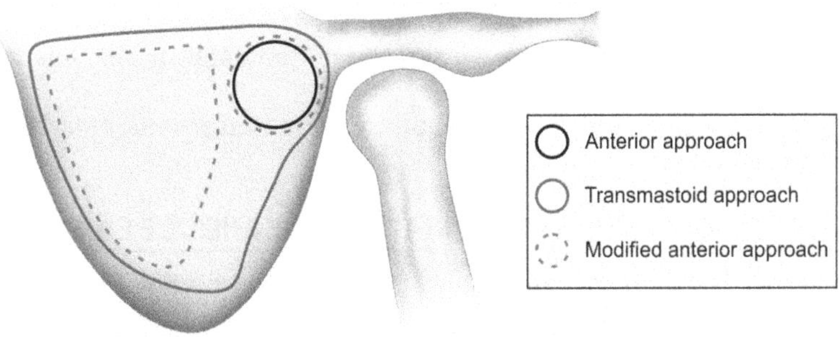

FIG. 3: Surgical approaches of atresiaplasty.

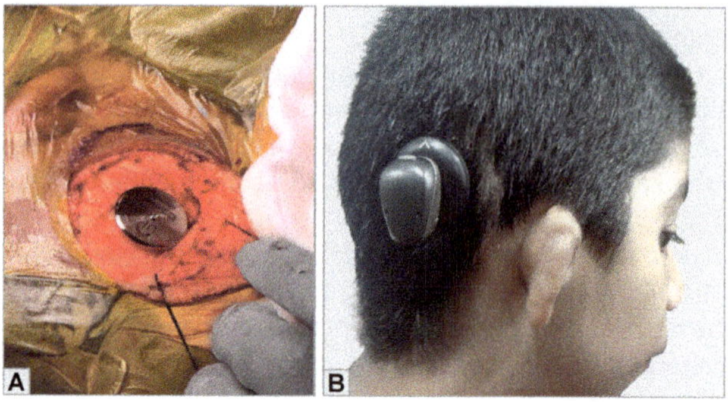

FIGS. 4A AND B: (A) BAHA titanium and abutment placed below the skin and periosteum; (B) Patient with BAHA sound processor worn over the implant.

Implantable Hearing Devices

Implantable hearing devices used in CAA are:

- Bone-anchored hearing aid (BAHA)
- Bonebridge (BB)
- Vibrant sound bridge (VSB)

Bone-anchored Hearing Aid

- Works with the concept of bone conduction hearing mechanism and osseointegration.
- Bone-anchored hearing aid fixture is usually implanted around 50–55 mm posterosuperior to ear canal.
- Preoperative 3D CT can be done to determine the optimal implant site.
- Skull thickness of 3–4 mm is required for successful BAHA surgery.
- *BAHA has two types*: (1) BAHA connect which uses transcutaneous titanium abutment; and (2) BAHA attract which uses implant magnet there by leaving the overlying skin intact (**Figs. 4A** and **B**).
- BAHA gives a consistently hearing gain when compared to atresiaplasty.[6]

Bonebridge

- This also works with the principle of bone conduction but does not require osseointegration.
- Skull thickness of >8.7 mm is required as the transducer part of the implant is thicker. Thus, the patient must be 5 years or older.

Vibrant Sound Bridge

- Unlike BAHA and BB, VSB is implanted in ME; either attached to stapes or placed over round window depending on the status of ME. This in turn stimulates the inner ear.
- This is more technically demanding surgery and carries risk of facial nerve and inner ear injury.

MINOR CONGENITAL MALFORMATIONS OF MIDDLE EAR

Though HRCT of temporal bone is the imaging modality of choice for congenital malformations of ME, definitive diagnosis of the minor malformations is often made by findings on exploratory tympanotomy only (**Table 3**).

TABLE 3 Teunissen and Cremer's classification of minor congenital malformations.[7]

Class	Malformations	Percentage
1	Ankylosis or isolated congenital stapes fixation: • Superstructure fixation • Footplate fixation	30.6%
2	Stapes ankylosis associated with other ossicle malformations: • Deformities of the incus and/or malleus, or aplasia of the long process of the incus • Bone fixation of malleus and/or incus	38.1%
3	Congenital anomalies of the ossicular chain with mobile stapes footplate: • Disruption of the ossicular chain • Tympanic fixation • Epitympanic fixation	21.6%
4	Congenital aplasia or severe dysplasia of the oval and round windows (see Chapter 4): • Aplasia • Dysplasia • Prolapse of the facial nerve • Persistent stapedial artery	9.7%

Source: Modified from Teunissen EB, Cremers WR. Classification of congenital middle ear anomalies. report on 144 ears. Ann Otol Rhinol Laryngol. 1993;102:606-12.

Other nonossicular congenital ME anomalies which should be looked for are:
- Congenital perilymphatic fistula (mainly intraoperative diagnosis)
- High jugular bulb
- Aberrant internal carotid artery

REFERENCES

1. Weerda H. Classification of congenital deformities of the auricle. Fac Plast Surg. 1988;5:385-8.
2. Aguilar EA, Jahrsdoerfer RA. Surgical repair of microtia and atresia. Otaolaryngol Head Neck Surg. 1988;98:600-6.
3. Altmann F. Congenital aural atresia of the ear in men and animals. Ann Otol Rhinol Laryngol. 1955;64:824-58.
4. De la Cruz A, Teufert KB. Congenital aural atresia surgery: long-term results. Otolaryngol Head Neck Surg. 2003;129:121-7.
5. Patel N, Shelton C. The surgical learning curve in aural atresia surgery. Laryngoscope. 2007;117:67-73.
6. Farnoosh S, Mitsinikos FT, Maceri D, Don DM. Bone-Anchored Hearing Aid vs. Reconstruction of the External Auditory Canal in Children and Adolescents with Congenital Aural Atresia: A Comparison Study of Outcomes. Front Pediatr. 2014;2:5.
7. Teunissen EB, Cremers WR. Classification of congenital middle ear anomalies. report on 144 ears. Ann Otol Rhinol Laryngol. 1993;102:606-12.

7

Reporting Templates and Illustrative Cases: Microtia

Smita Manchanda, Ashu Seith Bhalla

- This section on reporting templates attempts to provide structured reporting formats for commonly encountered situations while reporting temporal bone CT/MRI scans.
- There are a few points which should be borne in mind before interpreting these images.
- It is critical to always ensure symmetry.
- Most CT scans today are performed on multidetector computed tomography (MDCT) scanners today. Hence axial images are acquired and subsequently the coronal and sagittal planes are reconstructed from the initial data set.
- Often the primary imaging (axial) maybe obliquely oriented, especially so in children. Hence, manipulate the axial and coronal scans cross checking against each other the main landmarks to ensure symmetry.
- Also the other major leap in interpreting temporal bone images is the reporting of these scans on workstations rather than on films. Hence the focus on section-wise interpretation has shifted to structure-wise interpretation. The normal anatomy in Chapters 3 and 4 has hence been provided both ways.
- It is advisable to report structure-wise tracking the structure in its entire extent while scrolling through the images.
- Optimal special planes should also be reconstructed as detailed in Chapter 1.
- In MRI, the 3D image sets such as heavily T2-weighted constructive interference in steady state (CISS)/fast imaging employing steady-state acquisition (FIESTA) cycled phases sequences (depending on the scanner) should also be manipulated accordingly.
- Volume rendering technique (VRT) and the other 3D representatives are useful to the surgeon but do not form the primary reporting image sets for the radiologist.
- As the reader may notice through the book, several classification/staging systems exist in most disease entities. In the reporting templates we have adopted the most frequently used/quoted systems.
- However, the preference may vary in different institutions.

The classification system adopted should always preferably be in consultation with the surgeons.

Reporting Templates and Illustrative Cases: Microtia

Right Left

EXTERNAL EAR

1. Bony EAC (Normal/Stenosis/Atresia)
2. Cartilaginous EAC (Normal/Stenosis/Atresia)

MIDDLE EAR

1. Size of middle ear cavity (Normal/Small)
2. Middle ear width
3. Soft tissue density/cholesteatoma (Present/Absent)
4. Ear ossicles (Normal/Dysplastic/Eroded):
    a. Malleus
    b. Incus
    c. Stapes
5. Incudostapedial articulation
6. Incudomalleal articulation
7. Facial nerve canal tympanic part:
    a. Size (Normal/Stenosis/Dilatation)
    b. Course (Normal/Displaced)
8. Facial nerve canal mastoid part:
    a. Size (Normal/Stenosis/Dilatation)
    b. Course (Normal/Displaced)

INNER EAR

1. Internal auditory canal (Normal/Stenosis/Dilatation)
2. Cochlea and vestibule (Normal/Dysplastic)

Mastoid air cells (Pneumatized/Opacified/Sclerotic)
Any Other Abnormality

N: Normal; S: Stenosis; A: Atresia; Dil: Dilatation; Sm: Small; D: Dysplastic; E: Eroded; P: Present; Ab: Absent; Dis: Displaced; Pn: Pneumatized; Op: Opacified; Sc: Sclerotic

IMPRESSION

(In accordance with Yeakley and Jahrsdoerfer Grading—see Chapter 5)

CASE 1 (FIGS. 1A TO F)

A 13-year-old female presenting with right Grade I microtia (**Fig. 1A**).

	Right	Left
EXTERNAL EAR		
1. Bony EAC (Normal/Stenosis/Atresia) (arrow in **Fig. 1B**)	***A***	N
2. Cartilaginous EAC (Normal/Stenosis/Atresia) (**Fig. 1B**)	***A***	N
MIDDLE EAR		
1. Size of middle ear cavity (Normal/Small)	N	N
2. Middle ear width (measured in **Fig. 1E**)	4.5 mm	5 mm
3. Soft tissue density/cholesteatoma (Present/Absent)	Ab	Ab
4. Ear ossicles (Normal/Dysplastic/Eroded):		
a. Malleus	N	N
b. Incus	N	N
c. Stapes	N	N
5. Incudostapedial articulation	N	N
6. Incudomalleal articulation	N	N
7. Facial nerve canal tympanic part:		
a. Size (Normal/Stenosis/Dilatation)	N	N
b. Course (Normal/Displaced)	N	N
8. Facial nerve canal mastoid part:		
a. Size (Normal/Stenosis/Dilatation)	N	N
b. Course (Normal/Displaced)	N	N
INNER EAR		
1. Internal auditory canal (Normal/Stenosis/Dilatation)	N	N
2. Cochlea and vestibule (Normal/Dysplastic)	N	N
Mastoid air cells (Pneumatized/Opacified/Sclerotic) (**Fig. 1F**)	***Sc***	Pn
Any Other Abnormality	None	

N: Normal; S: Stenosis; A: Atresia; Dil: Dilatation; Sm: Small; D: Dysplastic; E: Eroded; P: Present; Ab: Absent; Dis: Displaced; Pn: Pneumatized; Op: Opacified; Sc: Sclerotic

IMPRESSION: Right microtia (Yeakley and Jahrsdoerfer Grading 8) with:
- **Bony and cartilaginous EAC atresia**

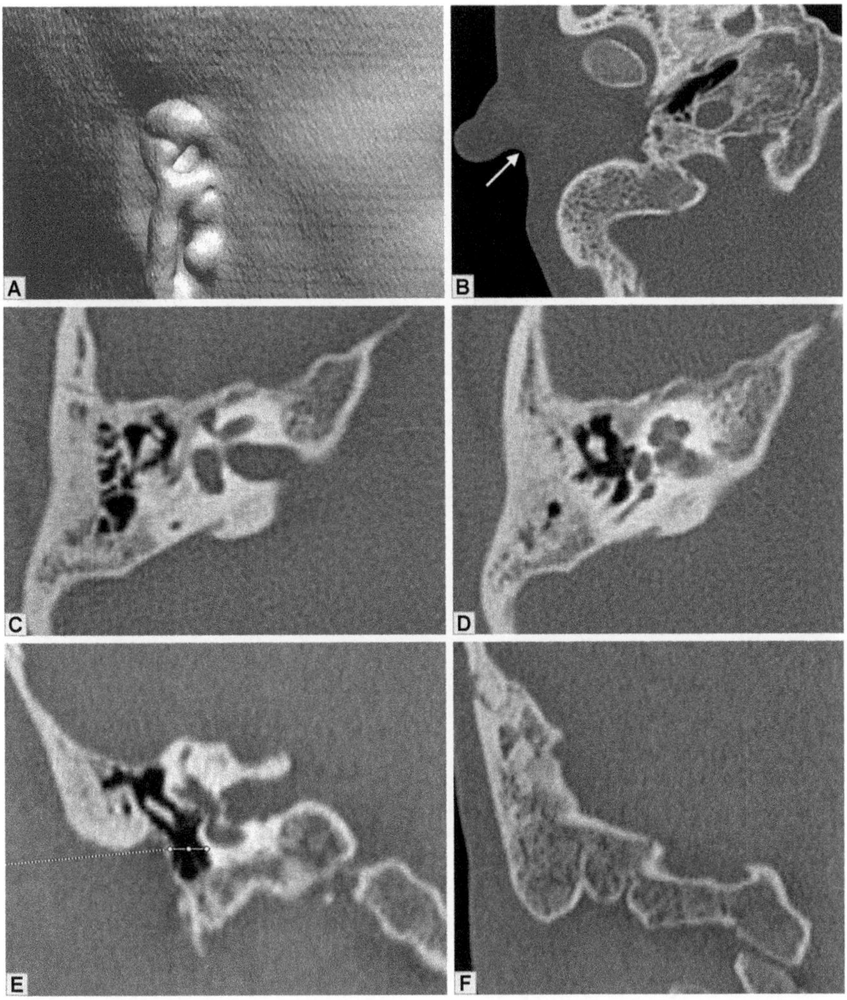

FIGS. 1A TO F: Right microtia (Yeakley and Jahrsdoerfer Grading 8) with bony and cartilaginous EAC atresia: (A) VRT. Right grade 1 microtia; (B to D) Axial HRCT superior to inferior. Bony and cartilaginous atresia (arrow in B); (E and F) Coronal HRCT anterior to posterior. Middle ear width measured in E (4.5 mm).

CASE 2 (FIGS. 2A TO F)

A 14-year-old boy with right microtia (**Fig. 2A**), mixed hearing loss and LMN Grade II facial palsy.

	Right	Left
EXTERNAL EAR		
1. Bony EAC (Normal/Stenosis/Atresia) (**Fig. 2B**)	**S**	N
2. Cartilaginous EAC (Normal/Stenosis/Atresia) (arrow in **Fig. 2B**)	***S***	N
MIDDLE EAR		
1. Size of middle ear cavity (Normal/Small)	N	N
2. Middle ear width (**Fig. 2E**)	5.0 mm	5.2 mm
3. Soft tissue density/cholesteatoma (Present/Absent)	P	Ab
4. Ear ossicles (Normal/Dysplastic/Eroded):		
a. Malleus (**Fig. 2E**)	***D***	N
b. Incus (**Fig. 2E**)	***D***	N
c. Stapes	***D***	N
5. Incudostapedial articulation	***D***	N
6. Incudomalleal articulation (arrow in **Fig. 2E**)	***D***	N
7. Facial nerve canal tympanic part (arrow in **Fig. 2C**):		
a. Size (Normal/Stenosis/Dilatation)	***S***	N
b. Course (Normal/Displaced)	N	N
8. Facial nerve canal mastoid part:		
a. Size (Normal/Stenosis/Dilatation)	**S**	N
b. Course (Normal/Displaced)	N	N
INNER EAR		
1. Internal auditory canal (Normal/Stenosis/Dilatation)	N	N
2. Cochlea and vestibule (Normal/Dysplastic) (arrows in **Figs. 2D** and **F**)	***D***	N
Mastoid air cells (Pneumatized/Opacified/Sclerotic)	***Sc***	Pn

Any Other Abnormality (**Fig. 2E**) ***Erosion of scutum and tegmen tympani***

N: Normal; S: Stenosis; A: Atresia; Dil: Dilatation; Sm: Small; D: Dysplastic; E: Eroded; P: Present; Ab: Absent; Dis: Displaced; Pn: Pneumatized; Op: Opacified; Sc: Sclerotic

IMPRESSION: Right microtia (Yeakley and Jahrsdoerfer Grading 1) with:
- **Cholesteatomatous CSOM**
- **Dysplastic ossicles**
- **Markedly narrow facial canal**
- **Incomplete partition type I deformity**

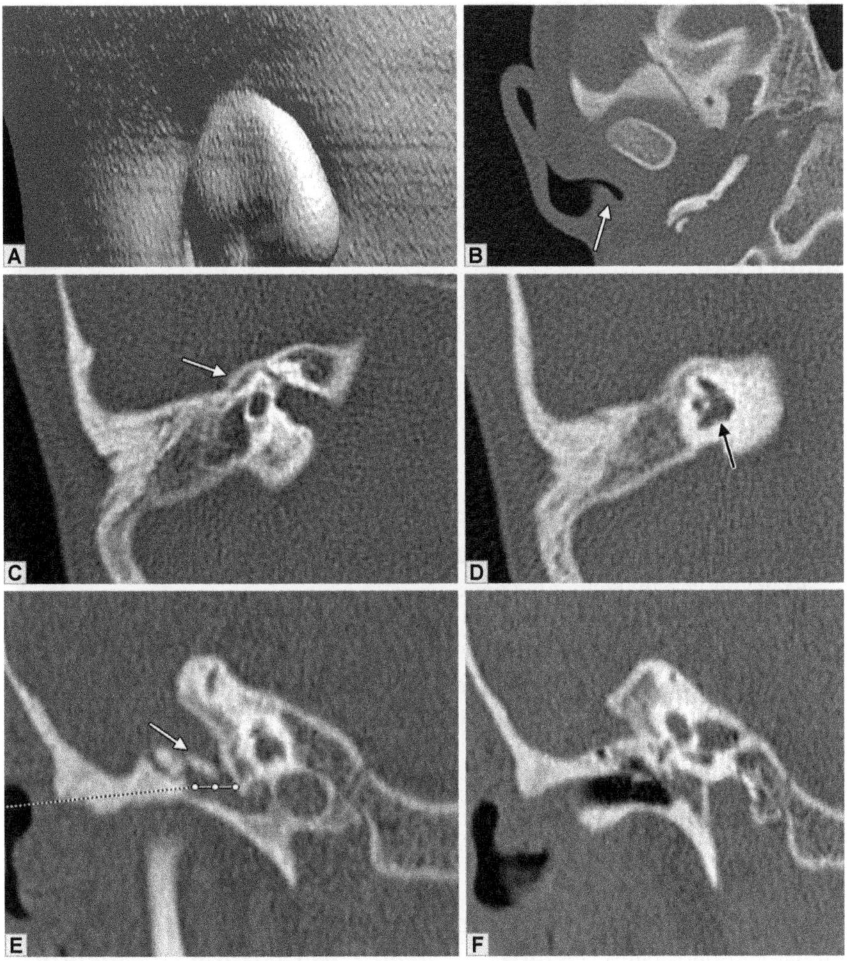

FIGS. 2A TO F: Right microtia (Yeakley and Jahrsdoerfer Grading 1) with cholesteatomatous CSOM, dysplastic ossicles, markedly narrow facial canal, incomplete partition type I deformity: (A) VRT; (B to D) Axial HRCT superior to inferior. Stenosis of bony and cartilaginous EAC (arrow in B), stenotic tympanic facial canal (arrow in C), dysplastic vestibule (arrow in D); (E and F) Coronal HRCT anterior to posterior. Dysplastic ossicles (arrow in E).

CASE 3 (FIGS. 3A TO F)

A 17-year-old male presenting with right Grade I microtia (**Fig. 3A**).

	Right	Left
EXTERNAL EAR		
1. Bony EAC (Normal/Stenosis/Atresia)	***A***	N
2. Cartilaginous EAC (Normal/Stenosis/Atresia)	***A***	N
MIDDLE EAR		
1. Size of middle ear cavity (Normal/Small)	N	N
2. Middle ear width (arrow in **Fig. 3E**)	5.8 mm	5.7 mm
3. Soft tissue density/cholesteatoma (Present/Absent)	Ab	Ab
4. Ear ossicles (Normal/Dysplastic/Eroded):		
a. Malleus (**Fig. 3B**)	***D***	N
b. Incus (**Fig. 3B**)	***D***	N
c. Stapes (arrow in **Fig. 3C**)	N	N
5. Incudostapedial articulation	N	N
6. Incudomalleal articulation (arrow in **Fig. 3B**)	***D***	N
7. Facial nerve canal tympanic part:		
a. Size (Normal/Stenosis/Dilatation)	***S***	N
b. Course (Normal/Displaced)	N	N
8. Facial nerve canal mastoid part (arrow in **Fig. 3F**):		
a. Size (Normal/Stenosis/Dilatation)	***S***	N
b. Course (Normal/Displaced)	***Dis***	N
INNER EAR		
1. Internal auditory canal (Normal/Stenosis/Dilatation) (black arrow in **Fig. 3D**)	***Dil***	N
2. Cochlea and vestibule (Normal/Dysplastic)	N	N
Mastoid air cells (Pneumatized/Opacified/Sclerotic)	***Sc***	Pn
Any Other Abnormality (**Fig. 3D**)	***Dilated right lateral SCC (white arrow)***	

N: Normal; S: Stenosis; A: Atresia; Dil: Dilatation; Sm: Small; D: Dysplastic; E: Eroded; P: Present; Ab: Absent; Dis: Displaced; Pn: Pneumatized; Op: Opacified; Sc: Sclerotic

IMPRESSION: Right microtia (Yeakley and Jahrsdoerfer Grading 6) with:
- **Bony and cartilaginous EAC atresia**
- **Dysplastic ossicles**
- **Narrow facial canal with anteriorly displaced mastoid segment**
- **Dilated IAC and lateral SCC**

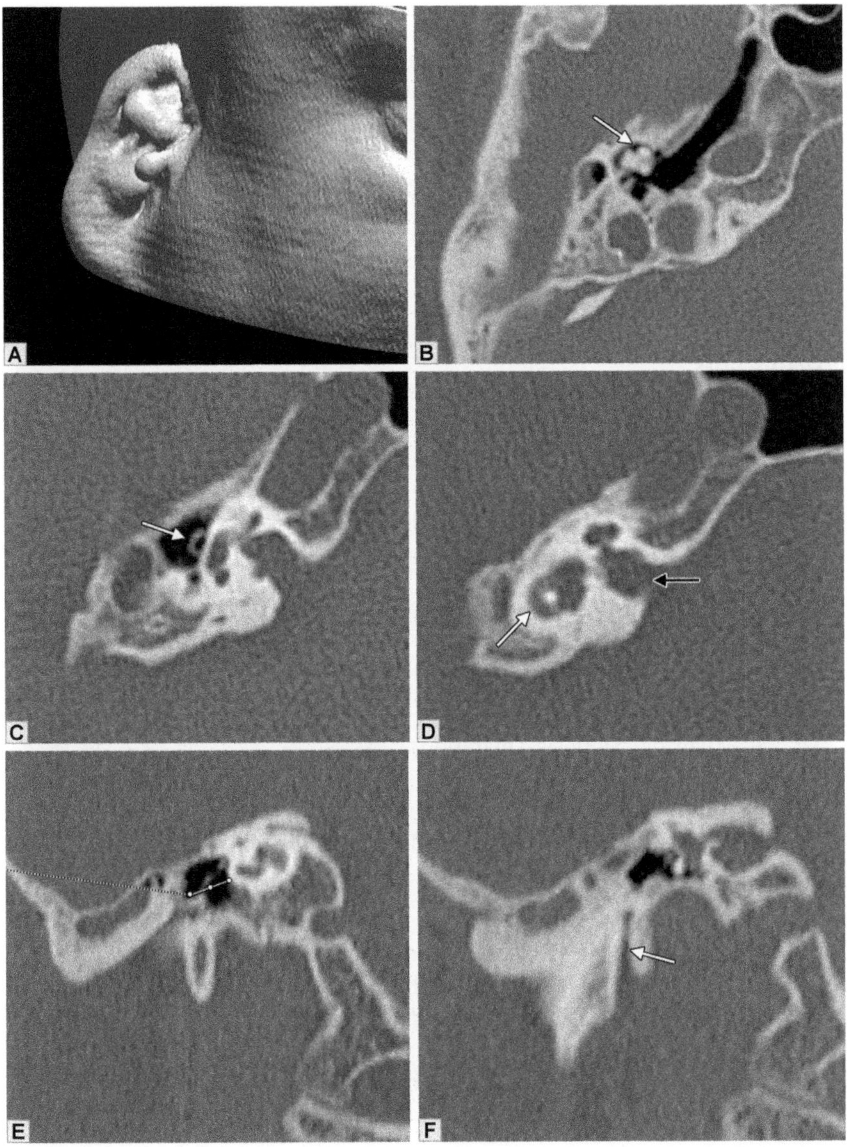

FIGS. 3A TO F: Right microtia (Yeakley and Jahrsdoerfer Grading 6) with bony and cartilaginous EAC atresia, dysplastic ossicles, narrow facial canal with anteriorly displaced mastoid segment, dilated IAC and lateral SCC: (A) VRT; (B to D) Axial HRCT superior to inferior. Dysplastic malleus and incus (arrow in B), normal stapes (arrow in C), dysplastic LSCC (white arrow in D) and dilated IAC (black arrow in D); (E and F) Coronal HRCT anterior to posterior. Middle ear width measured in E (5.8 mm), stenotic mastoid segment of facial canal (arrow in F).

CASE 4 (FIGS. 4A TO F)

An 11-year-old female presenting with right Grade II microtia (**Fig. 4A**) and hearing loss.

	Right	Left
EXTERNAL EAR		
1. Bony EAC (Normal/Stenosis/Atresia) (**Fig. 4B**)	***A***	N
2. Cartilaginous EAC (Normal/Stenosis/Atresia) (arrow in **Fig. 4B**)	***S***	N
MIDDLE EAR		
1. Size of middle ear cavity (Normal/Small)	N	N
2. Middle ear width	4.3 mm	4.5 mm
3. Soft tissue density/cholesteatoma (Present/Absent) (arrow in **Fig. 4D**)	***P***	Ab
4. Ear ossicles (Normal/Dysplastic/Eroded):		
a. Malleus (**Fig. 4D**)	***D***	N
b. Incus (**Fig. 4D**)	***D***	N
c. Stapes	***D***	N
5. Incudostapedial articulation	***D***	N
6. Incudomalleal articulation (**Fig. 4D**)	***D***	N
7. Facial nerve canal tympanic part:		
a. Size (Normal/Stenosis/Dilatation)	N	N
b. Course (Normal/Displaced)	N	N
8. Facial nerve canal mastoid part:		
a. Size (Normal/Stenosis/Dilatation)	N	N
b. Course (Normal/Displaced)	N	N
INNER EAR		
1. Internal auditory canal (Normal/Stenosis/Dilatation)	N	N
2. Cochlea and vestibule (Normal/Dysplastic)	N	N
Mastoid air cells (Pneumatized/Opacified/Sclerotic) (arrow in **Fig. 4E**)	***Sc***	Pn
Any Other Abnormality	***Lateral SCC hypoplasia (arrow in Fig. 4C)*** ***Atretic plate thin and eroded (arrow in Fig. 4F)***	

N: Normal; S: Stenosis; A: Atresia; Dil: Dilatation; Sm: Small; D: Dysplastic; E: Eroded; P: Present; Ab: Absent; Dis: Displaced; Pn: Pneumatized; Op: Opacified; Sc: Sclerotic

IMPRESSION: Right microtia (Yeakley and Jahrsdoerfer Grading 3) with:

- **Bony and cartilaginous atresia**
- **Dysplastic ossicles**
- **Thin and eroded atretic plate**
- **Lateral SCC hypoplasia**

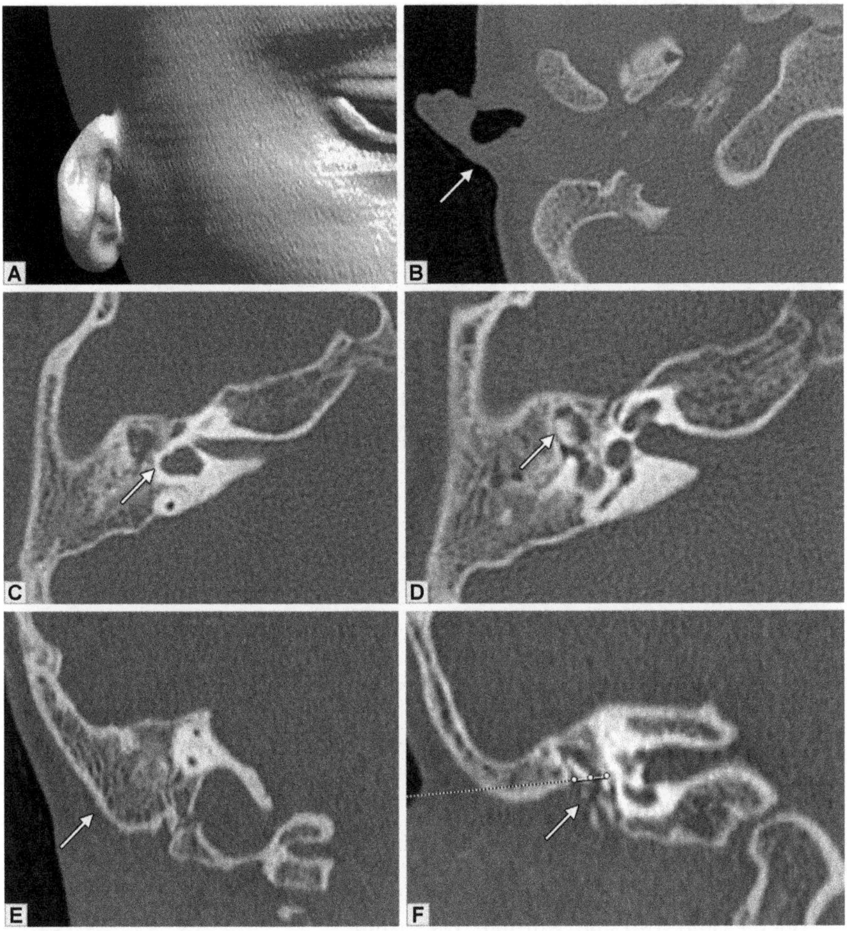

FIGS. 4A TO F: Right microtia (Yeakley and Jahrsdoerfer Grading 3) with bony and cartilaginous atresia, dysplastic ossicles, thin and eroded atretic plate, lateral SCC hypoplasia: (A) VRT; (B to D) Axial HRCT superior to inferior. Stenotic cartilaginous EAC (arrow in B), lateral SCC hypoplasia (arrow in C), dysplastic ossicles (arrow in D); (E and F) Coronal HRCT anterior to posterior. Sclerotic mastoiditis (arrow in E), thin and eroded atretic plate (arrow in F).

CASE 5 (FIGS. 5A TO E)

A 4-year-old male presenting with facial and ear (**Fig. 5A**) deformity.

	Right	Left
EXTERNAL EAR		
1. Bony EAC (Normal/Stenosis/Atresia) (**Fig. 5C**)	***A***	***A***
2. Cartilaginous EAC (Normal/Stenosis/Atresia) (arrow in **Fig. 5C**)	***S***	***A***
MIDDLE EAR		
1. Size of middle ear cavity (Normal/Small) (arrow in **Fig. 5D**)	***Sm***	***Sm***
2. Middle ear width (measured in **Fig. 5D**)	2.7 mm	2.7 mm
3. Soft tissue density/cholesteatoma (Present/Absent)	***P***	***P***
4. Ear ossicles (Normal/Dysplastic/Eroded):		
a. Malleus (**Fig. 5D**)	***D***	***D***
b. Incus (**Fig. 5D**)	***D***	***D***
c. Stapes	***D***	***D***
5. Incudostapedial articulation	***D***	***D***
6. Incudomalleal articulation (**Fig. 5D**)	***D***	***D***
7. Facial nerve canal tympanic part:		
a. Size (Normal/Stenosis/Dilatation)	***S***	***S***
b. Course (Normal/Displaced)	N	N
8. Facial nerve canal mastoid part:		
a. Size (Normal/Stenosis/Dilatation)	***S***	***S***
b. Course (Normal/Displaced)	N	N
INNER EAR		
1. Internal auditory canal (Normal/Stenosis/Dilatation)	N	N
2. Cochlea and vestibule (Normal/Dysplastic)	N	N
Mastoid air cells (Pneumatized/Opacified/Sclerotic)	***Sc***	***Sc***
Any Other Abnormality	***Hypoplastic mandible*** (**Fig. 5B**)	

N: Normal; S: Stenosis; A: Atresia; Dil: Dilatation; Sm: Small; D: Dysplastic; E: Eroded; P: Present; Ab: Absent; Dis: Displaced; Pn: Pneumatized; Op: Opacified; Sc: Sclerotic

IMPRESSION: Treacher Collins syndrome with:

- **B/L microtia (Yeakley and Jahrsdoerfer Grading Right—1; Left—1)**
- **Mandibular hypoplasia**
- **B/L dysplastic ossicles**
- **B/L stenotic middle ear cavity and facial canal**

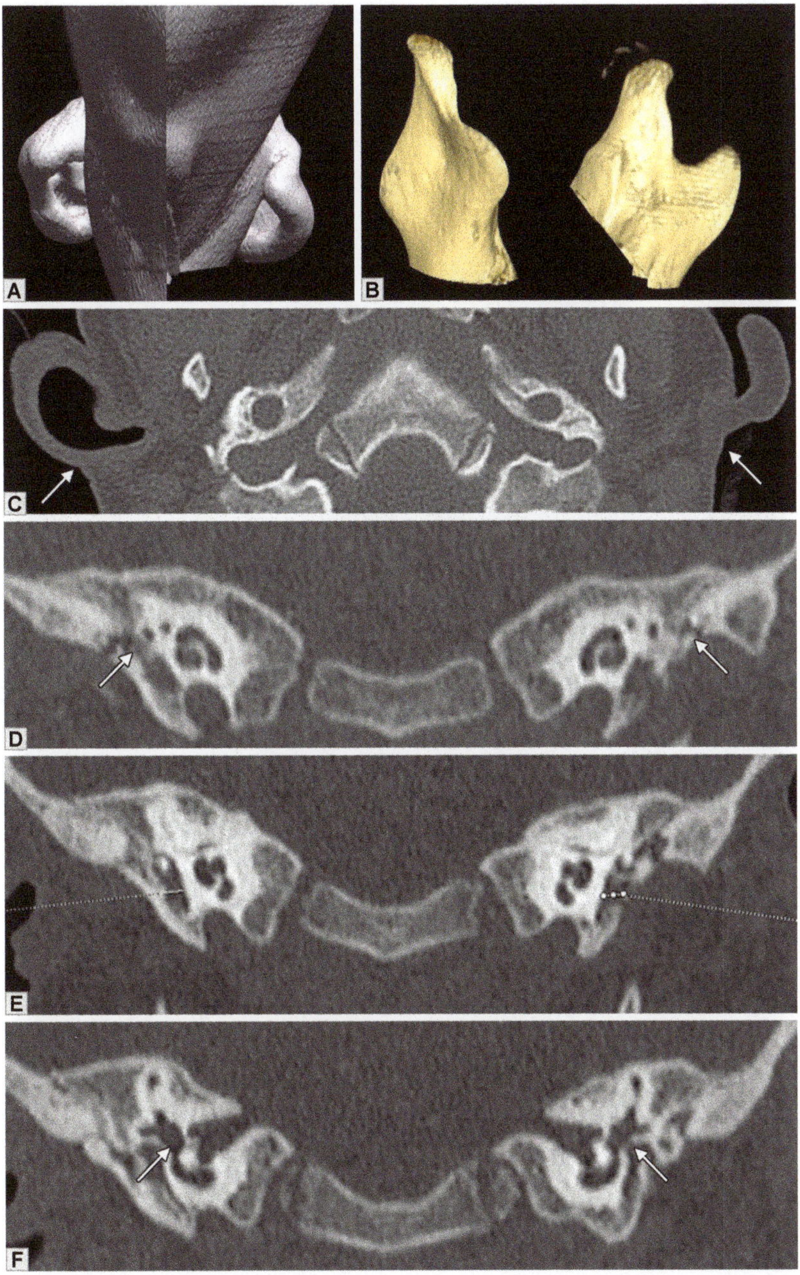

FIGS. 5A TO F: Treacher Collins syndrome with B/L microtia (Yeakley and Jahrsdoerfer Grading Right—1; Left—1), mandibular hypoplasia, B/L dysplastic ossicles and B/L stenotic middle ear cavity: (A) VRT pinna; (B) VRT mandible showing mandibular hypoplasia; (C) Axial HRCT. Cartilaginous atresia (arrow in C); (D to F) Coronal HRCT anterior to posterior. Dysplastic ossicles (arrows in D), middle ear width measured in E (narrow-2.7 mm bilaterally), normal vestibule (arrow in F).

3
SECTION

Infections of External and Middle Ear

8

Infections of External and Middle Ear: Imaging

Madhavi K, Aparna Irodi

- Infectious diseases of the ear are common indications for imaging. Imaging is performed to evaluate the extent and nature of the disease, and to resolve specific diagnostic challenges. Computed tomography (CT) is ideal to depict bone erosion, but, is less optimal than magnetic resonance imaging (MRI) for depicting the changes in soft tissues of the neck and intracranial extension and also marrow changes.
- For a systematic approach this topic can been divided into four sections, viz. external ear, middle ear and mastoid, inner ear; and petrous apex and skull base. This chapter will focus on otomastoid and external ear. Infections of petrous apex and skull base will be discussed in other chapters.

EXTERNAL EAR

Acute Otitis Externa

- Otitis externa (OE) refers to infection/inflammation of the external ear. It may involve the pinna and external auditory canal (EAC), either in combination or alone. It is primarily of bacterial origin, (viral infection may be caused by herpes zoster).
- Otitis externa is related to high humidity and warm temperature, swimming and self-inflicted trauma.
- Clinical findings include diffuse infection of the entire EAC or a localized furuncle, or isolated pinna involvement.
- Diagnosis is in most of the cases easily established clinically and no imaging performed.

Necrotizing External Otitis

- It is also known as "malignant otitis externa" (MOE).
- It is a frequent cause of otogenic skull base osteomyelitis (SBO).
- A life-threatening complication of OE when infection fails to resolve with topical antibiotics and aural toileting and instead, infection becomes invasive and extends to involve surrounding soft tissues and bones.
- Seen in elderly diabetics or immunocompromised patients.
- *Pseudomonas aeruginosa* is the most common pathogen. Other bacteria such as *Staphylococcus aureus, Proteus,* and *Klebsiella* have also been reported. Fungi (e.g., *Aspergillus fumigatus*) may also be the causative agent.

Clinical Findings

There is severe otitis with visible granulation tissue, neurologic symptoms, and/or cranial nerve deficits.

Spread of Infection

After colonizing the ear canal, *Pseudomonas* causes infection of the soft tissues; slowly progressing to cellulitis, chondritis, and osteomyelitis. It has a tendency to spread along soft tissues and vessels rather than pneumatized spaces. The routes of spread are as follows (**Flowchart 1**).

Anteriorly

- Via the fissures of Santorini (gaps in the cartilaginous and at osteocartilaginous junction in EAC) to involve the subtemporal tissues including stylomastoid foramen, parotid gland, masticator space, infratemporal fossa, jugular foramen, foramen lacerum, and retrocondylar fat.
- It can also spread along the petrotympanic fissure or patent foramen of Huschke to the temporomandibular joint.

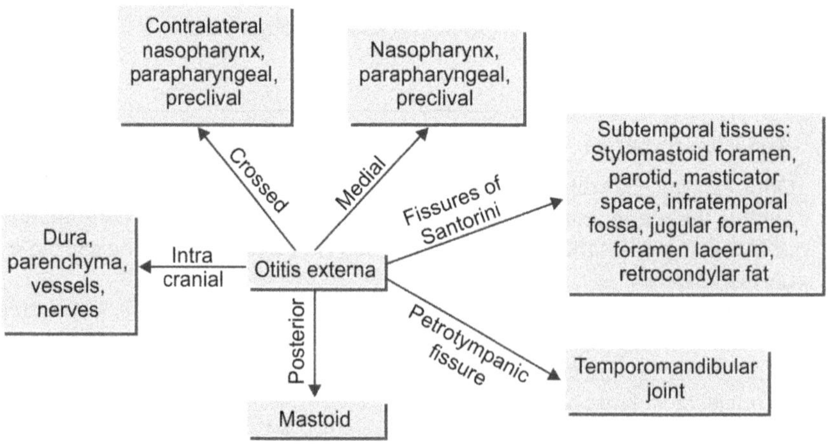

FLOWCHART 1: Routes of spread of malignant otitis externa.

Medially

- Commonly via the Eustachian tube to involve ipsilateral nasopharyngeal wall, parapharyngeal space (PPS) with or without involvement of preclival soft tissues.
- Crossed extension to involve contralateral nasopharyngeal wall and contralateral preclival soft tissues.
- Intracranial extension with involvement of dura with our without involving brain parenchyma, dural venous sinuses, arteries, and nerves.

Posteriorly

Into mastoid air cells.

Imaging Findings

Computed tomography and MRI may be complimentary. Contrast-enhanced examinations should be performed in suspected cases.

Computed Tomography

- Involvement can be seen on CT as demineralization or erosion or destruction of bone, obliteration of fat planes, and soft tissue thickening with enhancement. Occasionally, collections can also be seen with peripheral enhancement. Therefore images should be reconstructed and evaluated in both bone [high-resolution CT (HRCT)] as well as soft tissue kernels (**Fig. 1**).
- In the early stages, nonspecific soft tissue swelling and erosion at the petrotympanic fissure, and obliteration of the retrocondylar fat pad can be seen (**Fig. 1**).
- Different extensions as described above can have different imaging appearances; like fat stranding and soft tissue thickening in the PPS, nasopharynx, masticator space, around the stylomastoid foramen; widening of the temporomandibular joints space with bone erosions (**Figs. 1** and **2**).
- Osteomyelitis causes erosion, expansion, and bone destruction of the skull base, which may involve the walls of the EAC, petrotympanic fissure, petrous bone, jugular fossa, stylomandibular foramen, foramen lacerum, and clivus.

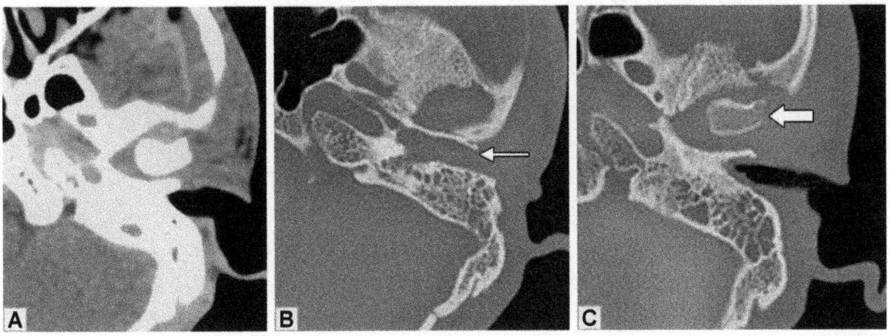

FIGS. 1A TO C: CT appearance of malignant otitis externa: *Soft tissue window (A)*: Nonspecific soft tissue thickening involving left external auditory canal (EAC) (A), parotid and masticator spaces. *Bone window (B and C)*: Soft tissue within bony EAC (arrow in B); and erosion of left mandibular condyle (block arrow in C).

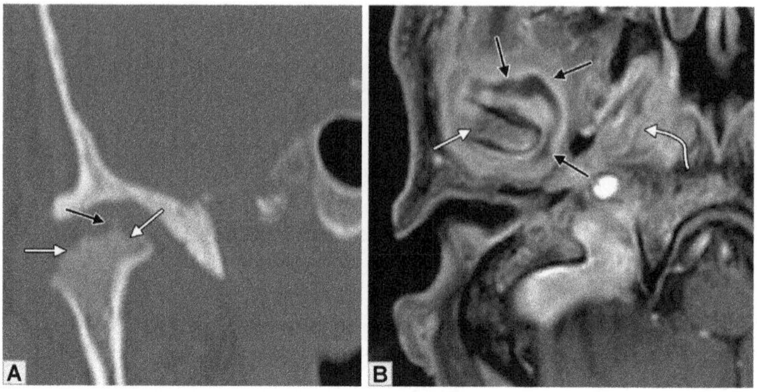

FIGS. 2A AND B: Temporomandibular (TM) joint involvement by malignant otitis externa: (A) Coronal CT: Widening of the TM joint space (black long arrow) with erosions in the mandibular condyle (white arrows). (B) Axial T1-weighted (T1W) fat-saturated postgadolinium MRI: Synovial and capsular thickening and enhancement of right TM joint (black arrows), erosion and marrow enhancement in mandibular condyle (white arrow). Note the involvement of right parapharyngeal space (curved arrow in B) as well.

- Cortical bone erosion, best seen on CT, is a crucial factor to establish the diagnosis, but, may not always be seen, especially in early disease.

MRI

- Soft tissue changes can be seen as thickening of tissues and loss of the normal high signal intensity of the fat on T1-weighted (T1W) images; in the subtemporal regions including the stylomastoid foramen, masticator space, PPS, and around other skull base foraminae (**Fig. 3**).
- Involvement of temporomandibular joint can be seen as joint effusion, synovial thickening and enhancement, marrow signal alteration, and erosions in the mandibular condyle (**Fig. 2**).

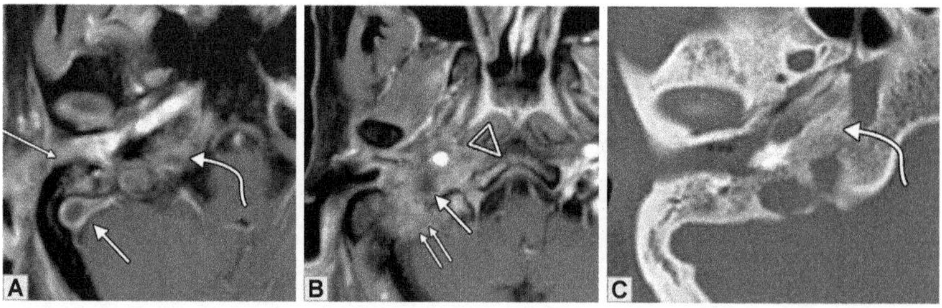

FIGS. 3A TO C: Malignant otitis externa with skull base osteomyelitis and intracranial complications: (A and B) Axial T1W fat-suppressed MR: Enhancing soft tissue in right external auditory canal (long thin arrow), marrow enhancement in the right petrous apex (curved arrow), mastoid (double arrows) and clivus (open arrow head). Note associated thrombosis of the right sigmoid sinus and internal jugular vein (thick short arrows). (C) HRCT: Subtle rarefactions and sclerosis in the right petrous apex (curved arrow).

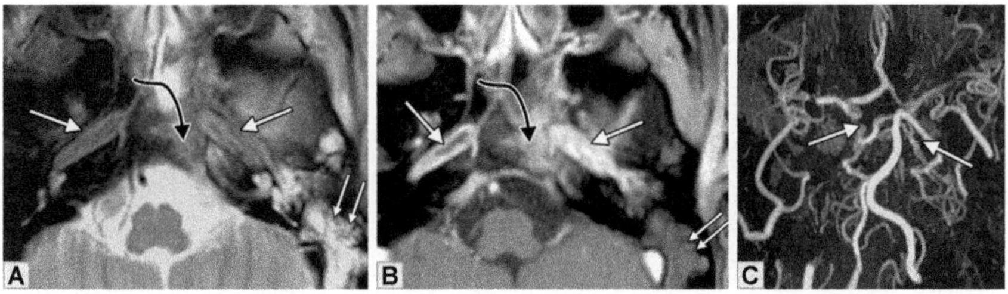

FIGS. 4A TO C: Malignant otitis externa with skull base osteomyelitis and intracranial complications (ICA thrombosis): (A) Axial T2-weighted (T2W), (B) T1W fat-saturated axial postgadolinium, and (C) MRA images. Abnormal marrow signal and enhancement in left half of clivus (curved arrow in A and B). *ICA thrombosis* loss of signal void in bilateral ICAs (white arrows in A); and filling defects in right ICA, wall enhancement along left ICA (white arrows in B), and loss of flow in the ICAs on the MRA (white arrows in C). *Left mastoid effusion* (double arrows in A and B). This was related to subtemporal inflammatory tissue narrowing the Eustachian tube (not shown).

- Unlike other inflammatory changes, these areas will usually be hypointense on T2W images as well, which is hypothesized to be related to the reduced vascularity in the diabetic patients, which results in reduced inflammatory response, and also due to presence of associated fibrosis.
- Flow voids of the carotid artery, jugular vein, and sigmoid sinus should be carefully scrutinized to ensure patency of the vessels. Filling defects should be looked for in postgadolinium images (**Fig. 3**). If the flow void is lost or if there is suspicion of thrombosis, MR angiography and MR venography could also be performed (**Fig. 4**).
- Bone involvement is seen on MRI as marrow edema with loss of the normal high signal intensity of the marrow in the temporal bones, and other bones of the skull base, on nonfat-suppressed T1W images, with enhancement on postgadolinium images (**Fig. 3**).
- Intracranial extension (**Figs. 3** and **4**) manifests as dural sinus thrombosis, signs of meningitis, or cerebral abscesses. More extensive the disease involvement, worse is the prognosis; with more mortality and more relapses despite treatment.

Nuclear Imaging

Various tracers can be used for imaging in MOE, whose role is discussed in **Table 1**. Positron emission tomography (PET)-CT and PET-MRI combine anatomical and functional imaging giving accurate information on the disease status (**Figs. 5** and **6**).

Differential Diagnoses

- Differentials to consider would include:
  - Squamous cell carcinoma of EAC (**Fig. 7**) or nasopharyngeal carcinoma (depending on which sites are more involved)
  - Lymphoma
  - Metastatic processes or myeloma (when there is predominant bone involvement)

TABLE 1 **Different radioisotopes and nuclear scans that can be performed in malignant otitis externa.**

Tracer/Scan	Mechanism	Advantages	Disadvantages	Additional comments
Technetium-99m methylene diphosphonate bone scan (**Fig. 5**)	Shows increased osteoblastic activity (even 10% increase can be detected)	• Cheap • Easily available	• Nonspecific • Increased uptake can be seen in tumors, postoperative conditions, etc. • Findings lag behind improvement and so cannot be used for monitoring therapy	Has to be used with SPECT as regular planar images of bone scan lack anatomic detail
Technetium-labeled leucocytes	Detect infectious process	More specific	• Expensive and more laborious • Difficult to detect low level infections	Cost is a limiting factor
Gallium-67-citrate (**Fig. 6**)	Binds to actively dividing cells like white blood cells	• Accumulates in bones and soft tissues with inflammation or infection • Correlates well with disease activity • Can be used for therapy monitoring	• Expensive • High radiation dose	Has to be used with SPECT
2-fluor-2-deoxy-glucose (FDG)	Detects increased metabolism as it is a glucose analog	• Good spatial resolution • Less radiation as compared to Gallium	• Not specific for infection. FDG avidity seen in malignancies as well	Good for therapy monitoring

(SPECT: single-photon emission computed tomography)

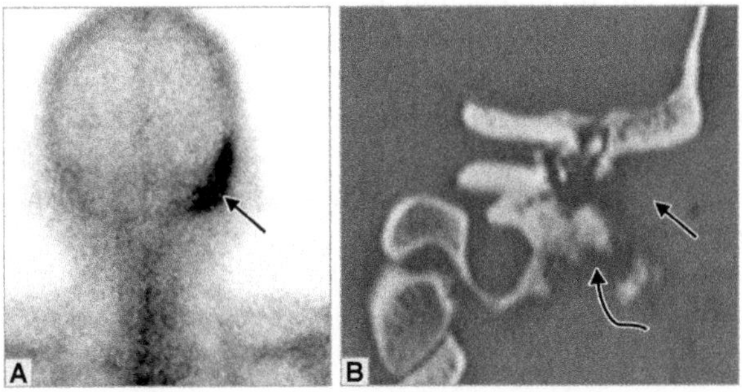

FIGS. 5A AND B: Scintigraphy in left malignant otitis externa: (A) Technetium-*99m methylene diphosphonate* bone scan: Nonspecific tracer uptake in left ear region (arrow). (B) Coronal HRCT Erosions of the floor and posterior wall of external auditory canal (EAC) (curved arrows), and soft tissue thickening left EAC (arrow). Biopsy showed inflammatory tissue and *Pseudomonas aeruginosa* grew in culture.

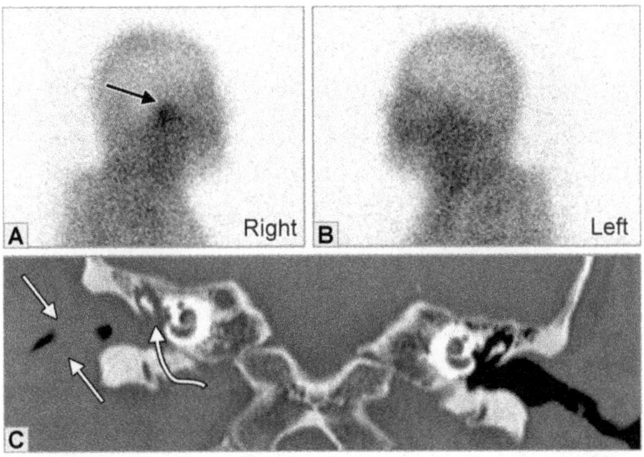

FIGS. 6A TO C: Right malignant otitis externa with middle ear extension: (A and B) *Gallium-67-citrate scintigraphy*: Abnormal concentration of tracer in right ear region (arrow in A). (C) Coronal HRCT Sheet like soft tissue thickening in external auditory canal (arrows), extending to involve the middle ear cleft as well (curved arrow).

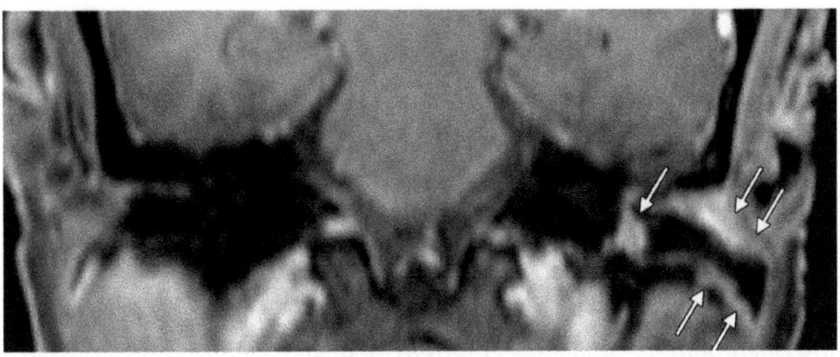

FIG. 7: Biopsy proven left external auditory canal (EAC) squamous cell carcinoma: Coronal T1W fat-suppressed postgadolinium MR image shows nodular circumferential soft tissue thickening and enhancement along the left EAC (arrows) which was initially suspected to be otitis externa.

- Although reliable differentiation of infection from neoplastic causes is difficult on imaging; infection tends to respect fascial planes and shows less restricted diffusion [higher apparent diffusion coefficient (ADC) values] than lymphoma or nasopharyngeal carcinoma. However, abscess formation could result in significant restricted diffusion.
- Peripheral enhancement on postgadolinium images would help in this regard to help establish the abscess formation as cause for restricted diffusion.
- Often biopsy for histopathology as well as culture maybe required to establish a definite diagnosis.

Treatment

- Prolonged course of high-dose antipseudomonal antibiotics and control of diabetes or immunocompromised state is advocated.
- There is no consensus regarding the timing/role of aggressive surgical debridement.
- Infection can frequently relapse and so patients have to be on continued surveillance.

Assessment of Response to Therapy and to Look for Relapse

- Computed tomography alone is less reliable to assess response to treatment as bone remineralization lags behind disease resolution.
- Resolution of the soft tissue changes as well as marrow edema on MR imaging also lags behind disease resolution.
- Gallium-67-citrate scans/18-FDG PET-CT or PET-MRI would be ideal for follow up as FDG avidity reduces promptly with reduction in the infection and neutrophil activity.

MIDDLE EAR AND MASTOID

Otitis media (OM) refers to infective or inflammatory process affecting the middle ear.

Types of Otitis Media

- Several terms have been used to classify OM, of which most commonly used are acute and chronic OM (**Table 2**).
- Acute infectious processes develop in a well-pneumatized mastoid of a child, while chronic infectious processes develop in a more sclerotic otomastoid with a Eustachian tube dysfunction.

Acute Otitis Media

- Acute OM is more common in children, who present with fever, painful ear, and show hyperemic tympanic membrane (TM).
- It is most commonly caused by *Streptococcus pneumoniae.* Other pathogens include *Haemophilus influenzae, S. aureus,* or mixed bacterial and viral pathogens.
- Most often, appropriate therapy with analgesia, evacuation of exudates or aural toileting and antibiotics as required, and leads to healing. If the patient responds to treatment, imaging is not indicated.

TABLE 2 **Different methods of classifying otitis media (OM).**

Basis of classification	Terms
Duration of symptoms	• Acute OM (**Fig. 8**) • Chronic OM (**Fig. 9**)
Whether fluid is present or not	• OM with effusion (**Fig. 4**) • Aero-OM (without effusion)
Nature of fluid	• Suppurative OM • Nonsuppurative OM (These terms are not encouraged as they may be different stages of same pathological process) • Terms like active, inactive, or healed may also be used
Cause	• Bacterial • Tubercular (**Fig. 10**) • Syphilitic • Autoimmune

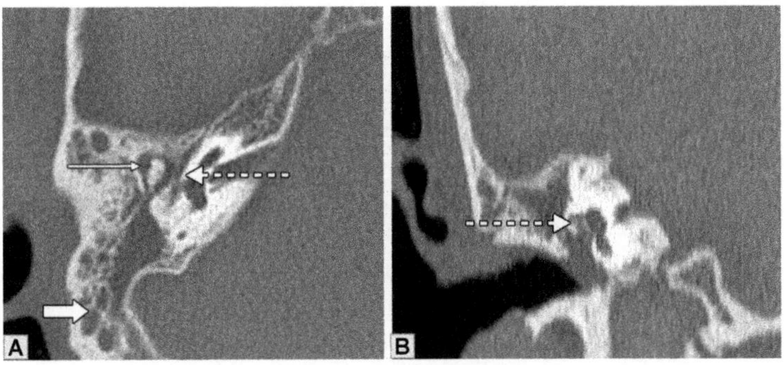

FIGS. 8A AND B: Acute otomastoiditis in a patient with acute leukemia: (A) Axial and (B) Coronal HRCT Soft tissue opacification of right middle ear (thin arrow) and mastoid (block arrow) causing erosion of the tympanic portion of the bony facial nerve canal (dotted arrow).

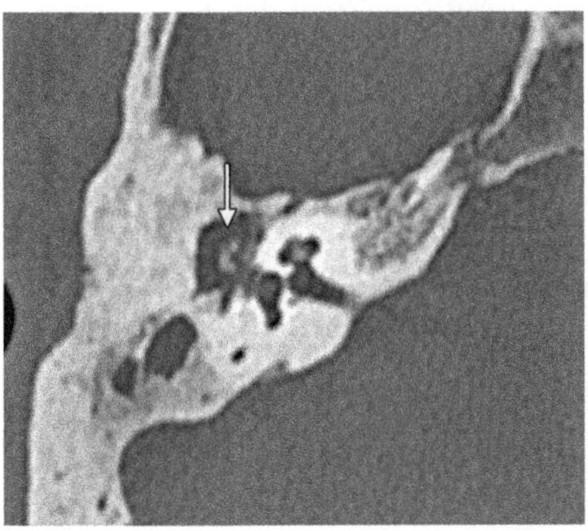

FIG. 9: Chronic right otomastoiditis with ossicular erosion: Axial HRCT image reveals soft tissue opacification of right middle ear and mastoid region with erosion of the ossicular chain (arrow).

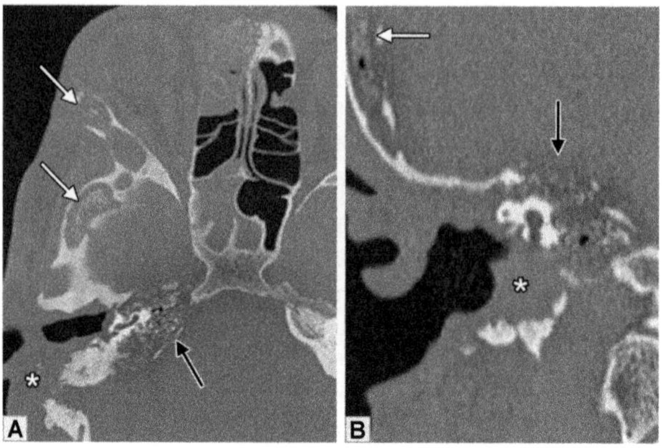

FIGS. 10 A AND B: Tubercular otomastoiditis in a patient with chronic otorrhea for several years: (A) Axial and (C) Coronal HRCT Soft tissue opacification of right middle ear cavity and mastoid (*) with mastoid erosion.
- Destruction of petrous apex and skull base (black arrows) with evidence of "button" sequestrum (arrows).

- If the infection persists, more serious extracranial or intracranial complications may occur (**Table 3**), when imaging may be indicated.
- In acute labyrinthitis, CT may be normal. MRI can show enhancement in the membranous labyrinth.

Spread to Adjacent Structures

- Extension of suppuration in the adjacent structures may largely depend on the status of mastoid cell pneumatization.
- Petrositis or petrous apicitis refers to extension of infection into pneumatized petrous apex.

TABLE 3 Different outcomes and complications of acute otitis media (OM).

Fate of acute OM	Possibilities	Imaging
Healing with treatment	Resolution of signs and symptoms	Not indicated
Extracranial complications	Acute mastoiditis	• CT—opacified mastoid air cells (**Fig. 9**) • MRI—opacified mastoid air cells with variable T1 and T2 SI and with diffusion restriction
	Coalescent mastoiditis (extends beyond the mucoperiosteum and involves the bony septae of mastoid air cells)	Mastoid is opacified and bony septae of mastoid air cells are resorbed

Continued

Continued

Fate of acute OM	Possibilities	Imaging
	Subperiosteal abscess	Rim enhancing collections around the mastoid
	Facial nerve (FN) paralysis	Erosion of bony FN canal (**Fig. 8**) or collections along course of FN canal or stylomastoid foramen
	Labyrinthitis	See Table 6 on labyrinthitis
	Petrositis or petrous apicitis, Gradenigo's syndrome—triad of petrous apicitis, VI nerve palsy, and trigeminal neuralgia	• CT—opacified petrous apex cells initially and later bone erosion (**Fig. 10**) • MRI—opacified petrous apex cells with restricted diffusion and rim enhancement (**Fig. 11**). Can extend to adjacent Meckel's cave and meninges
	Bezold's abscess	Collection related to the mastoid attachment of the sterno-cleidomastoid muscle (**Fig. 12**)
	Citelli's abscess	Collection tracking along the posterior belly of digastric muscle
Intracranial complications	Meningitis	Abnormal pachymeningeal and leptomeningeal enhancement, more in the posterior and middle cranial fossa (**Fig. 13**)
	Extradural abscesses	Biconvex-shaped extra-axial collection; bone erosion better demonstrated on CT
	Subdural abscess	Crescentic extra-axial collection with peripheral enhancement
	Otogenic brain abscesses	• CT—peripherally enhancing intracerebral lesion • MRI—peripherally enhancing lesion with central restricted diffusion (**Fig. 13**)
	Lateral sinus thrombosis	• CT—hyperdense TS/SS on plain • CT, with filling defect on contrast-enhanced CT (CECT) which may even extend to the IJV • MRI—loss of flow void in TS or SS on SE images, filling defects on CEMRI (**Fig. 14**). MRV will also help
	Otitic hydrocephalus	

(IJV: internal jugular vein; MRV: magnetic resonance venogram; SE: spin echo; SI: signal intensity; SS: sigmoid sinus; TS: transverse sinus)

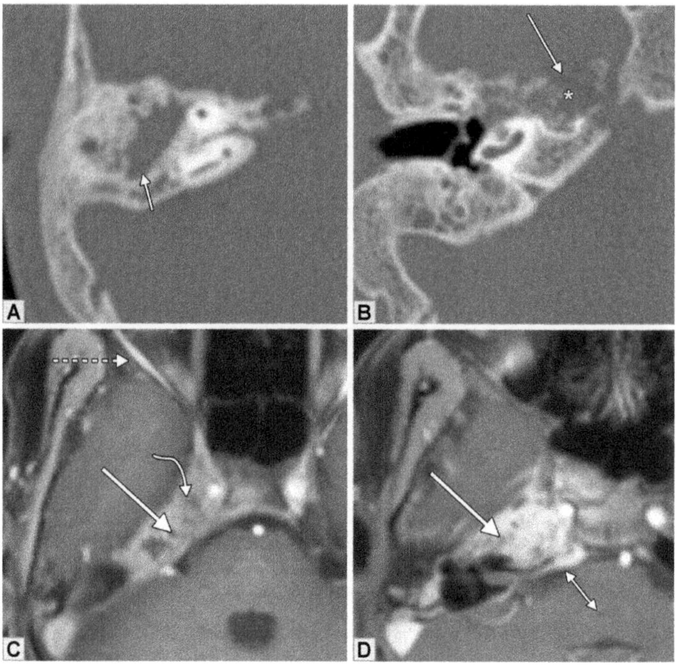

FIGS. 11A TO D: Gradenigo syndrome: Patient presented with right facial pain and lateral rectus palsy. (A and B) Axial HRCT: Soft tissue opacification of the right mastoid (arrow in A) and pneumatized right petrous apex cells (asterisk); with erosion of petrous apex (long white arrow in B). (C and D) Postgadolinium MR images: Enhancing soft tissue in the petrous apex (thick white arrows) extending to the cavernous sinus with dural thickening and enhancement along the Meckel's cave (curved arrow), middle cranial fossa, and Dorello's canal (double headed white arrow). Thinning of right lateral rectus muscle (dotted arrow).

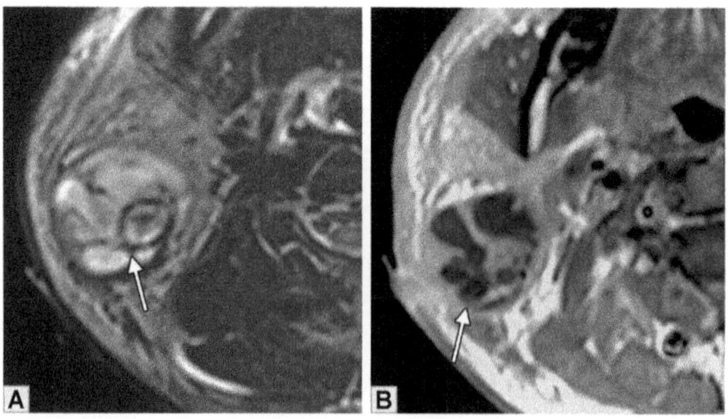

FIGS. 12A AND B: Bezold's abscess in a patient with otitis media: (A) STIR axial MRI: A multiloculated heterogeneously hyperintense collection within the right sternocleidomastoid (white arrow). (B) Axial T1W postgadolinium images: Thick enhancing wall with enhancing septae (arrow in B).

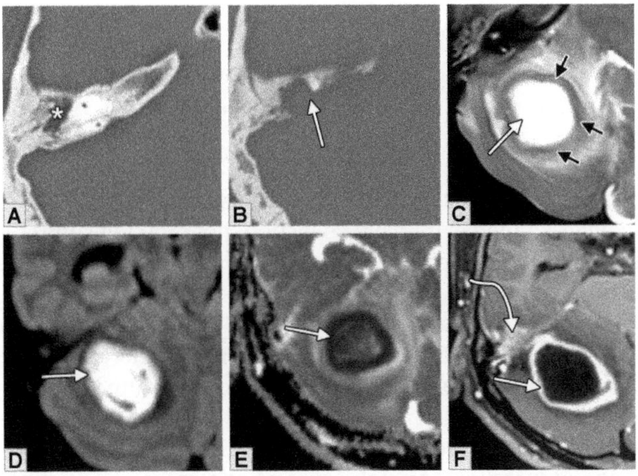

FIGS. 13A TO F: Acute otomastoiditis with cerebellar abscess and meningitis: (A and B) Axial HRCT: Soft tissue opacification of the middle ear (asterisk) and mastoid, with defect in the tegmen (arrow). (C) Axial T2-weighted (T2W), (D) diffusion weighted (DW), (E) apparent diffusion coefficient (ADC), (F) postgadolinium axial MR images show an abscess in right cerebellar hemisphere. Center of the abscess (arrow in C to E) is hyperintense on T2W and DW images (C and D) and hypointense on ADC map (E). Thick peripheral rim of the lesion shows T2W hypointensity (small black arrows in C) and contrast enhancement (arrow in F). Note the thickening and enhancement of tentorium cerebelli and dura (curved arrow in F).

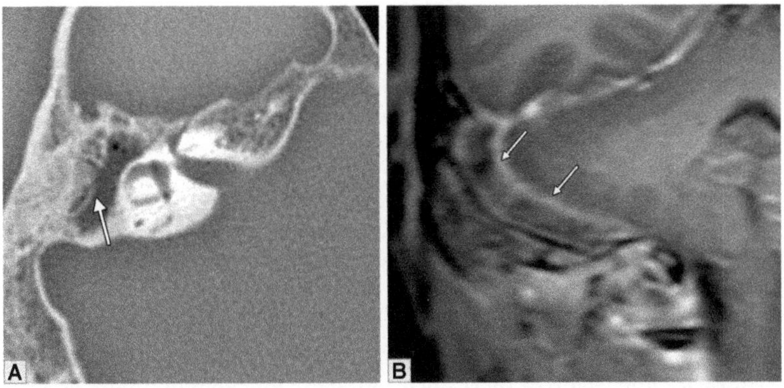

FIGS. 14A AND B: Acute otomastoiditis with sigmoid sinus thrombosis: (A) Axial HRCT: Soft tissue opacification of the right middle ear (arrow); (B) Postcontrast coronal MR: Right sigmoid sinus thrombosis (double arrows).

- Petrous apex osteomyelitis can occur in nonpneumatized petrous apex, and is part of SBO due to extension from OE.
- Bezold's abscess is more common in pneumatized mastoid tip cells in adults, and uncommon in children due to nonpneumatization.

Intracranial Complications

Intracranial complications may manifest as meningitis, intracranial abscesses (extradural, subdural, or intraparenchymal), venous sinus thrombosis, or otitic hydrocephalus.

- Extradural abscesses are a result of bone erosion and direct extension of infection. They can occur in middle or posterior cranial fossa. They appear as biconvex-shaped extra-axial collection, not crossing sutures and showing peripheral enhancement. Central content may show diffusion restriction on diffusion-weighted imaging (DWI).
- Subdural abscess can occur due to spread of infection via veins and venules. It is seen as crescentic extra-axial collection with peripheral enhancement. Otitic subdural abscess is more common along the tentorium and interhemispheric fissure.
- Intraparenchymal abscesses (otogenic brain abscess) can be due to direct extension of infection; through osteitic bone or via pre-existing foramina or via hemotagenous route. They are most commonly seen in temporal lobe or in cerebellum.
- Transverse sinus thrombosis can be secondary to epidural abscess or secondary to thrombophlebitis (intact bone plate).

Otitis Media with Effusion

- *Synonyms*: Glue ear/mucoid or secretory or serous OM.
  This refers to acute or chronic accumulation of serous or mucoid (nonpurulent) fluid in the middle ear cleft.
- In children, OM with effusion could be related to Eustachian tube dysfunction due to adenoid enlargement or hyperactivity of middle ear glands. Imaging is generally not indicated in children.
- In adults, any lesions obstructing the Eustachian tube (like nasopharyngeal carcinoma) need to be excluded by clinical examination and CT or MRI (**Fig. 4**).

Imaging

- High-resolution CT shows complete opacification of the middle ear cleft without ossicular or bone erosion.
- The noninfected serous fluid appears bright on T2W images, hypointense on T1W images, with no restricted diffusion and no enhancement. In adults, close scrutiny for any lesion or mass obstructing the Eustachian tube is essential.

Chronic Otitis Media

- *Classification/Terminology*: As is OM overall, several bases are employed to classify chronic OM. It can be classified as active, inactive, or healed. Chronic OM can also be classified as chronic suppurative and chronic nonsuppurative OM.
- The term chronic suppurative otitis media (CSOM) is used when there is TM perforation with chronic persistent ear discharge. It can also be called

as "chronic active mucosal otitis media"/"chronic tympanomastoiditis or otomastoiditis."

- If the TM is intact and there is chronic middle ear effusion without discharge, then it can be termed nonsuppurative or non-CSOM which includes chronic OM with effusion, chronic serous/mucinous/seromucinous OM.

Chronic Suppurative Otitis Media

- Chronic suppurative otitis media (CSOM) is further clinically subclassified (**Flowchart 2**) as tubotympanic (safe) (**Fig. 15**) and atticoantral (unsafe) types. It can also be classified as cholesteatomatous or noncholesteatomatous CSOM (NCSOM).
- Organisms: Unlike acute OM, the infection in CSOM could be due to aerobic bacteria (like *P. aeruginosa, Escherichia coli, Proteus mirabilis,* or *Klebsiella*) or anaerobic bacteria (like *Bacteroides* species, *Propionibacterium*).
- Besides discharging ears, patient can also present with conductive/total hearing loss (also see Chapter 25).

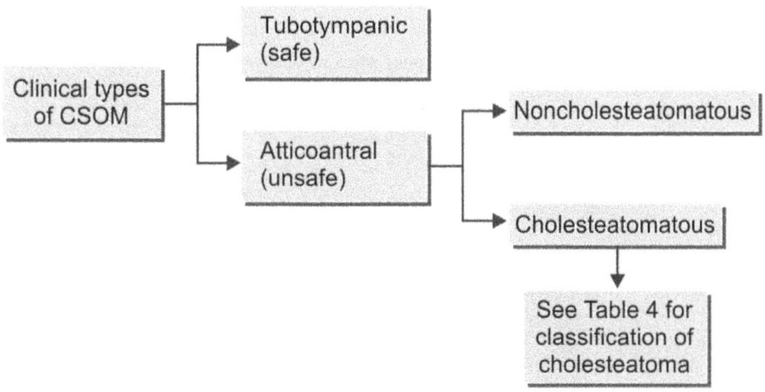

FLOWCHART 2: Classification of chronic suppurative otitis media (CSOM).

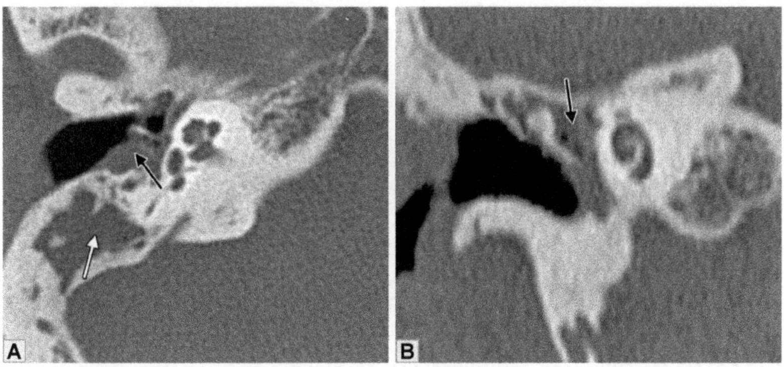

FIGS. 15A AND B: Right safe chronic suppurative otitis media (CSOM): (A) Axial and (B) Coronal HRCT: Soft tissue density in the right middle ear cavity (black arrow) and mastoid (white arrow). No ossicular erosion is noted.

Imaging Findings

- Acute complications and imaging findings in CSOM are similar to that described in acute OM (**Table 3**).
- Acute and chronic complications are listed in **Box 1**.

BOX 1 Complications of chronic suppurative otitis media.

Temporal bone complications	Intracranial complications
• Ossicular destruction	• Meningitis
• Mastoiditis	• Lateral sinus thrombosis
• Postinflammatory ossicular fixation	• Cerebellar abscess
• Lateral semicircular canal fistula (**Fig. 16**)	• Cerebral abscess
• Labyrinthitis ossificans (**Fig. 17**)	• Extradural abscess
• Facial nerve canal erosion (**Fig. 16**)	• Otic hydrocephalus
• Postauricular and zygomatic abscess	
• Petrous apicitis	
• Eroded tegmen, sigmoid sinus plate (**Fig. 17**)	

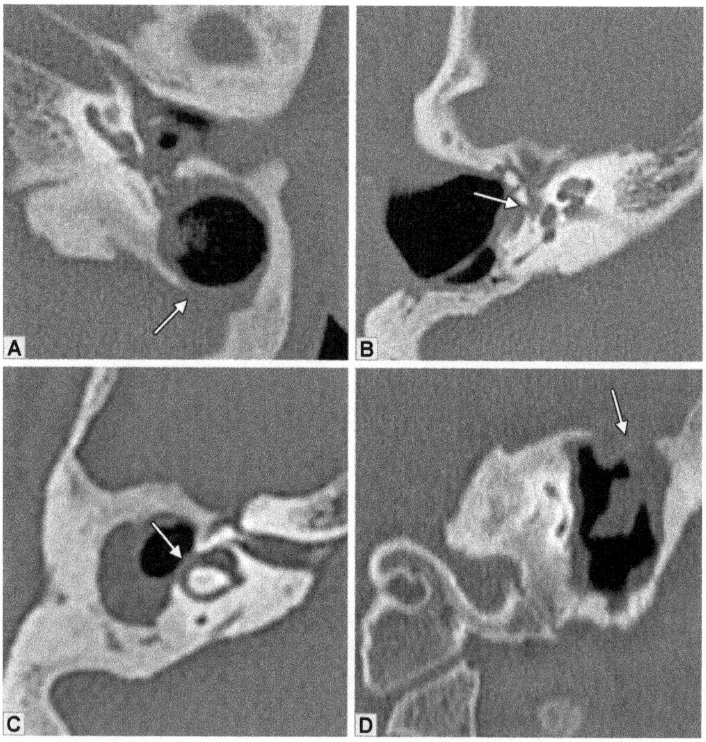

FIGS. 16A TO D: Different complications of chronic suppurative otitis media in different patients: Erosion of: Left sigmoid plate (arrow in A); Tympanic portion of right facial nerve canal (arrow in B); Lateral semicircular canal (labyrinthine fistula) (arrow in C); Tegmen plate (arrow in D).

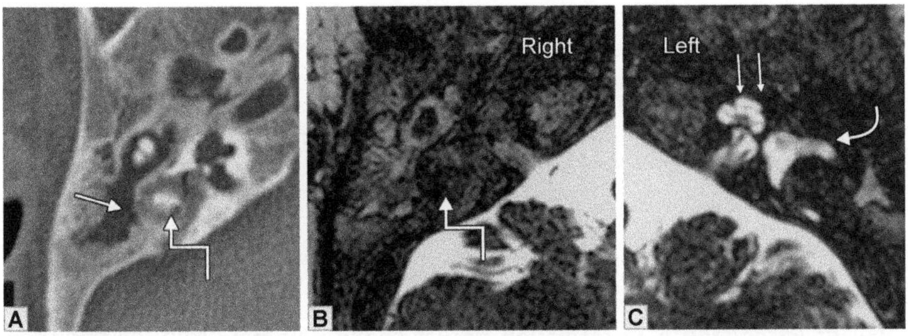

FIGS. 17A TO C: Labyrinthitis ossificans as a complication of long-standing *CSOM*: (A) Axial HRCT: Opacification of the right middle ear (arrow) and ossification of lateral semicircular canal (elbow arrow) and visualized part of posterior semicircular canal. (B) *Heavily T2W MRI*: Loss of normal high signal intensity (SI) in the labyrinthine structures on the right side (elbow arrow in B depicts the expected location of the labyrinth). (C) MRI of the opposite normal side: High SI in the cochlea (double arrows) and visualized part of lateral semicircular canal (curved arrow) on left side.

- Imaging findings of NCSOM are discussed below:
  - Noncholesteatomatous CSOM is characterized by irreversible alterations in the middle ear epithelium that manifest as chronic otorrhoea and perforation of the TM, which mandates surgical correction.
  - The inflammatory process remains confined to middle ear mucosa, and there is no bony erosion.

Cholesteatomatous CSOM

- Cholesteatoma is defined as a mass within the middle ear cleft formed by presence of keratinizing squamous epithelium and accumulation of keratin debris, with or without inflammation around it (**Fig. 18**).
- It has a propensity to gradually enlarge over time due to exfoliation and encapsulation of the tissues.
- Cholesteatoma can be subclassified as congenital or acquired (**Table 4**). It may also be subclassified based on location.
- Based on the location of the cholesteatoma in the middle ear with respect to the TM, it can be classified as pars tensa or pars flaccida cholesteatoma.
  - Pars flaccida (or attic) cholesteatoma (**Fig. 19**):
    - It is related to the upper third of the TM (i.e., pars flaccida or Shrapnell's membrane).
    - It is initially located in the epitympanum in the Prussak space, lateral to the ossicles. (Prussak space—bounded by pars flaccida, neck of malleus, short process of malleus, and lateral malleolar ligament).
  - Pars tensa cholesteatoma (**Fig. 20**):
    - It is related to the lower two-thirds of the TM (i.e., pars tensa). TM is usually perforated.
    - It is initially located in the sinus tympani or facial recess, medial to the ossicles.
    - Once the cholesteatoma is large, it can extend across these spaces and exact site of origin may be hard to establish.

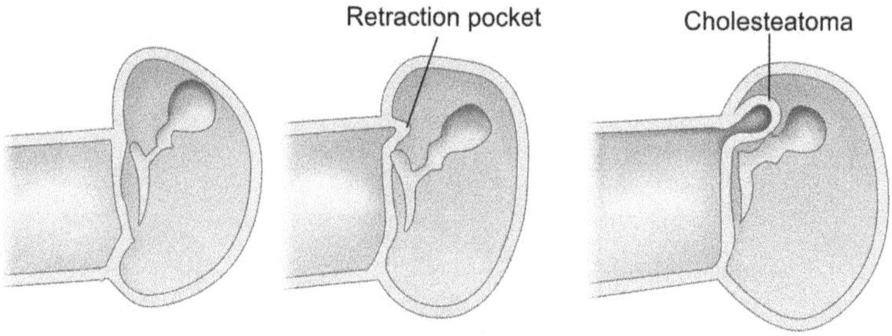

FIG. 18: Pathogenesis of retraction pocket cholesteatoma: When the retraction pocket fails to empty itself and keratin debris starts accumulating, it gets converted to a cholesteatoma.

TABLE 4 **Classification of cholesteatoma.**

Types of cholesteatoma	Subtypes		Description
Congenital			• Present at birth, but can be diagnosed later • Medial to intact tympanic membrane (TM) • More commonly in anterosuperior quadrant, followed by posterosuperior and others
Acquired	Retraction pocket cholesteatoma	Pars tensa	• Retraction pockets can form due to Eustachian tube dysfunction and abnormalities in middle ear (ME) pressure regulation • When the retraction pocket fails to empty itself keratin debris starts accumulating, converted to cholesteatoma (**Fig. 18**)
		Pars flaccida	
		Combined pars tensa and pars flaccida	
	Nonretraction pocket cholesteatoma	Related to TM perforation	It is proposed that squamous epithelium can migrate into the ME through the defect in the TM
		Related to previous trauma or surgery	
Unclassified	Unable to determine the origin		

Staging of Cholesteatoma

- To help in assessing the extent of cholesteatoma, STAM system is used to divide the middle ear into four sites. These are:
  i. **S:** Sites difficult to assess; S1—pro or anterior epitympanum (also called supratubal recess) and S2—sinus tympani
  ii. **T:** Tympanic cavity

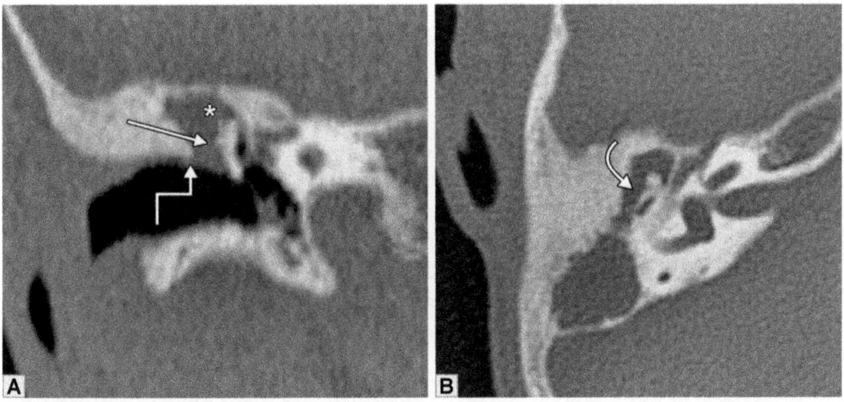

FIGS. 19A AND B: Pars flaccida cholesteatoma: (A) Coronal HRCT: Soft tissue in epitympanum in the Prussak space (asterisk), with eroded head of malleus (long arrow) and blunting of scutum (elbow arrow). (B) Axial HRCT: Soft tissue in epitympanum and antrum with erosion of short process of incus (curved arrow).

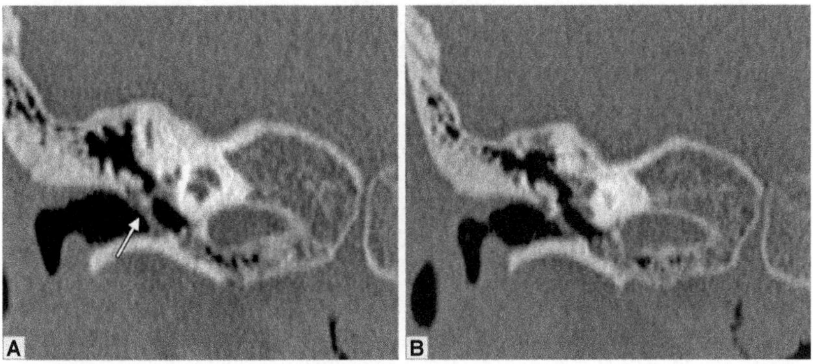

FIGS. 20A AND B: Pars tensa cholesteatoma: Coronal HRCT images reveal soft tissue density in the mesotympanum (arrow) with eroded handle of malleus, suggesting pars tensa cholesteatoma.

  iii. **A:** Attic (posterior border is posterior end of short process of incus)
  iv. **M:** Mastoid (antrum and air cells)
- *The stages are as follows:*
  - Stage I—confined to primary site (i.e., attic for pars flaccid cholesteatoma and tympanic cavity for pars tensa cholesteatoma)
  - Stage II—extends to involve two or more sites
  - Stage III—with extracranial complications like facial palsy, tegmen erosion, postauricular or neck abscess, labyrinthitis or labyrinthine fistula, and adhesive otitis
  - Stage IV—with intracranial complications like meningitis, epidural or subdural or parenchymal abscess, and sigmoid sinus thrombosis

Imaging in Cholesteatomas

Imaging is used in patients with clinically suspected cholesteatoma or in setting of complications.

Plain Radiography

- Plain radiography is of limited value and, less often used now and has been largely replaced by CT and MRI scans.
- Schuller's, Law's, Stenvers, Towne's, and submentovertical views can be used to assess the middle ear and mastoid.
- On plain radiographs (**Figs. 21** and **22**), degree of pneumatization of mastoid air cells, coalescence of mastoid air cells with loss of intervening septa, development of cavities and bone erosions or development of mastoid sclerosis can be assessed.
- Intactness of dural plate (interface with dura) and sinus plate (interface with sigmoid sinus) and low lying dural plate can also be evaluated.

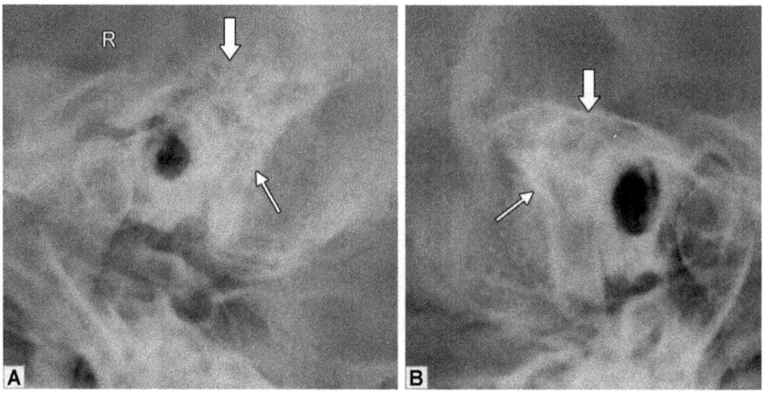

FIGS. 21A AND B: Bilateral sclerosing mastoiditis in a 45-year-old man with chronic ear discharge: *Modified Law's views* of (A) right and (B) left mastoids: Sclerosis of mastoid air cells (Left > Right). No cavity is seen. Sinus (arrow) and dural plates (block arrow) are intact.

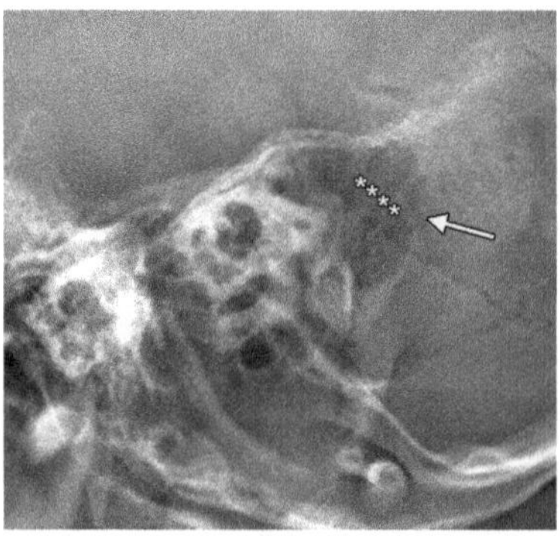

FIG. 22: Cholesteatoma cavity: *Modified Law's view* of the mastoid showing an expansile cavity replacing the mastoid (**) with erosions of the sinus plate (arrow).

High-resolution CT of the Temporal Bone

- High-resolution CT has high sensitivity and high negative predictive value with normal HRCT effectively ruling out a cholesteatoma. However, findings on CT are nonspecific as in addition to cholesteatoma, other conditions like granulation tissue, thick secretions, neoplasms, and cholesterol granuloma may also present with opacification of the middle ear (**Box 2**).
- On CT, cholesteatoma is usually seen as a well-defined, expansile, soft tissue density lesion in the middle ear with retraction of the TM and bone erosions which could involve scutum (lateral wall of the epitympanum), lateral semicircular canal (LSCC), tegmen tympani, long process, lenticular process of the incus, and stapes superstructure.
- Bone erosions favor cholesteatoma over granulation tissue or OM without cholesteatoma. Presence of the bone erosions along with clinical suspicion can help in coming to a diagnosis of cholesteatoma (**Figs. 19** and **23**). However, absence of bone erosion cannot exclude cholesteatoma.
- Congenital cholesteatomas uncommonly cause bone erosion, while pars tensa cholesteatomas cause bone erosion more often than pars flaccida ones.
- Computed tomography helps in detecting the extent of bone erosion and to look for complications like postinflammatory ossicular fixation. But, CT is not accurate in making a definitive diagnosis or assessing the exact extent of disease.
- Large window width (4,000 HU) and a low window level (0–200 HU) settings are best to evaluate the ossicles. Various oblique projections are described along the line of ossicles to delineate them better.
- Erosion of the facial nerve (FN) canal is difficult to distinguish from normal, as the wall of the tympanic portion of FN canal is often so thin that it is not visible at CT. Tympanic portion of the FN canal may be dehiscent in 25–57% of normal population.
- Erosion of the LSCC or cochlear promontory is suspected if patients present with vertigo. In cases of LSCC fistula, patients may present with a pseudoconductive hearing loss owing to the "third window" phenomenon. Detailed discussion of "third window" phenomenon is given in Chapter 21.

BOX 2 **Causes of middle ear soft tissue opacification on high-resolution CT.**

Differentials for soft tissue opacification of middle ear on CT:

- Eustachian tube dysfunction (secretory otitis) (see preceding part of the Chapter)
- Acute inflammation/infection (see preceding part of the Chapter)
- Chronic infection
  - Granulation tissue (**Fig. 24**)
  - Cholesteatoma
- Chronic Inflammation
  - Granulomatous polyangiitis (**Fig. 25**)
  - Langerhans cell histiocytosis
- Cholesterol granuloma
- Traumatic hemotympanum
- Glomus tympanicum
- Middle ear schwannoma

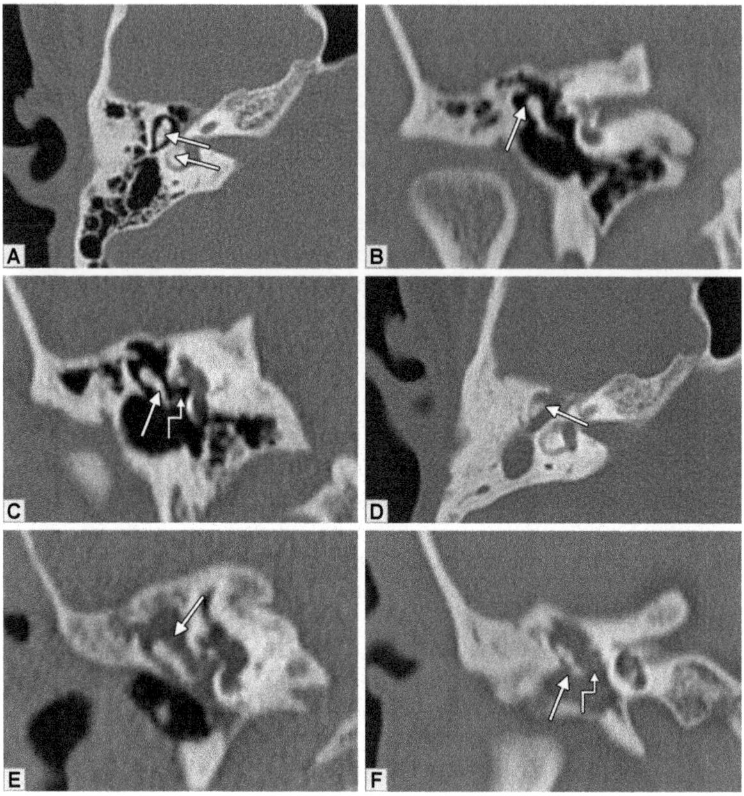

FIGS. 23A TO F: Ossicular erosion in cholesteatoma: (A) Normal axial and (B and C) oblique coronal HRCT images. Normal short process of incus (arrow in A), head of malleus (arrow in D), long process of incus (arrow in C), normal stapes (elbow arrow). Images at comparable sections in a patient with cholesteatoma. An eroded short process of incus (arrow in B); eroded malleus (arrow in E), eroded long process of incus (arrow in F), and absent stapes (elbow arrow in F showing expected location of stapes).

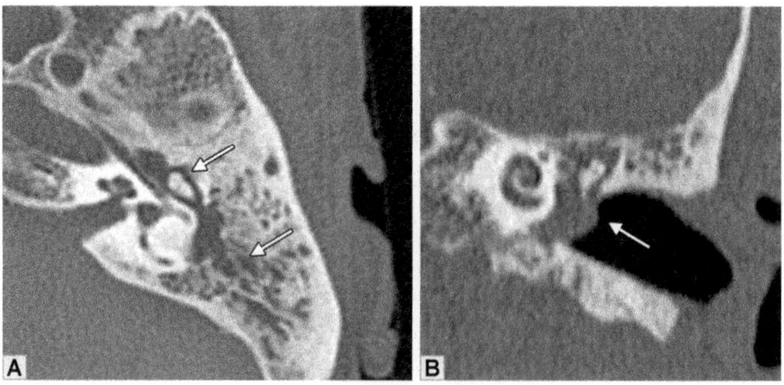

FIGS. 24A AND B: Chronic suppurative otitis media with granulation tissue: (A) Axial HRCT: Opacification of the left mastoid and middle ear (arrows). (B) Coronal HRCT: Left middle ear opacification with bulging tympanic membrane (arrow). Note that there is no scutum or ossicular erosion, and the soft tissue appears dependent.

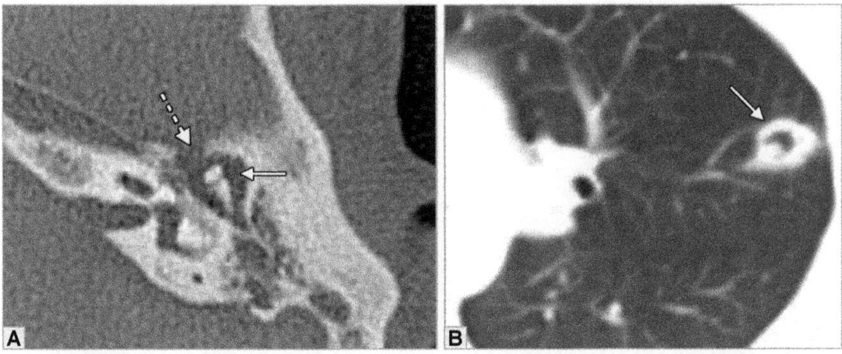

FIGS. 25A AND B: Granulomatous polyangiitis (GPA) as a cause of middle ear soft tissue opacification: (A) Axial HRCT: Left middle ear opacification (arrow) with tegmen erosion (dotted arrow). (B) CT chest: Thick walled cavitating lesion in the left upper lobe.

- If a fragment of stapes is displaced into the vestibule, a fistula at the oval window can be suspected.
- Enhancement pattern is difficult to assess on CT, especially in smaller lesions.

Checklist During Assessment of CT for Suspected CSOM and Cholesteatoma would Include

- Epitympanic lesion in Prussak space and scutum erosion
- Ossicular erosion
- Mesotympanic soft tissue in sinus tympani/facial recess/oval or round window areas
- Intact/eroded tegmen tympani
- Intact/eroded sinodural plate
- Presence or absence of erosion or fistulization with LSCC
- Any dehiscence or erosion of cochlear promontory
- Erosion of bony FN canal
- Any ossification in the labyrinth [labyrinthitis ossificans (LO)]

Magnetic Resonance Imaging

- Magnetic resonance imaging is a problem-solving tool, in temporal bone imaging. It can help to differentiate among different type of effusions and different causes for opacification of middle ear (CT cannot differentiate).
- Cholesteatomas are of mixed iso- to hypointense signal on T1W pulse sequences; and of high intensity on T2W pulse sequences, and do not enhance on postgadolinium images (**Fig. 26**). Only thin peripheral enhancement may be seen.
- While cholesteatoma does not enhance, associated inflammatory/granulation tissue enhances.
- Magnetic resonance imaging is particularly useful for evaluating the extension of a cholesteatoma into the middle and/or posterior fossa, and for demonstrating possible herniation of intracranial contents into the temporal bone, before or after surgery.

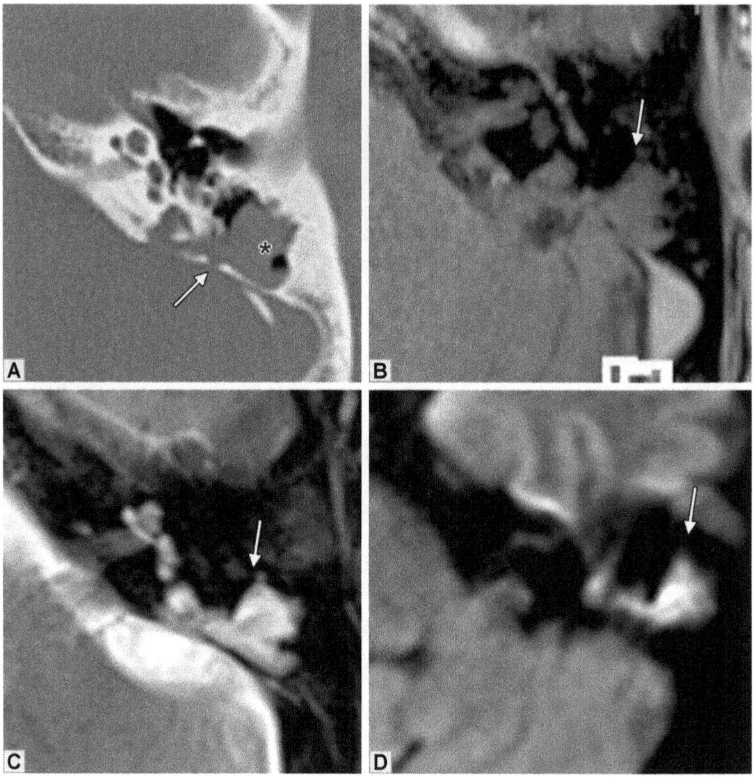

FIGS. 26A TO D: MRI in cholesteatoma: (A) Axial HRCT: Soft tissue in the left mastoid (asterisk) with erosion of the posterior and medial walls (arrow). (B) The lesion is hypointense on T1W, (C) hyperintense on T2W MRI, and (D) shows diffusion restriction (D).

- Diffusion-weighted MR can differentiate between a cholesteatoma, which has a restricted diffusion (**Fig. 26**), and other abnormalities—especially granulation tissue—which have normal diffusion characteristics.
- The nonecho-planar diffusion-weighted sequences are superior to echo-planar diffusion-weighted images.
  - Conventional echo-planar DWI:
    - Poor resolution and susceptibility artifacts at the air-bone interface.
    - Only cholesteatomas larger than 5 mm can be visualized.
    - Smaller residual cholesteatomas and early recurrences can be missed.
  - Nonecho-planar-based DWI sequences (turbo or fast spin echo based):
    - Higher resolution, generate thinner slices.
    - No susceptibility artifacts.
    - Enable visualization of cholesteatomas as small as 2 mm.
- In case of a labyrinthine fistula, enhancement of the membranous labyrinth on contrast-enhanced MRI.

TABLE 5 Differentiating points between granulation tissue and cholesteatoma.

Granulation tissue	Cholesteatoma
• Absence of significant hearing deficit • Poorly marginated soft tissue	• Sharply marginated, expansile soft tissue in nondependent location
• Tympanic membrane (TM) usually intact	• TM perforation or retraction
• Bone erosion not a feature	• Bone erosion
• Contrast-enhanced CT (CECT)—can enhance	• CECT—enhancement difficult to assess in smaller lesions • Larger lesions can show lack of enhancement or mild peripheral enhancement
• CEMRI—enhancement present	• Delayed CEMRI—nonenhancing (can show peripheral enhancement)
• MRI-DWI: No restricted diffusion	• MRI-DWI: Restricted diffusion

- Signal loss within the perilymphatic and endolymphatic spaces on the thin slice heavily T2W sequences would suggest labyrinthitis which can be detected on MRI even before ossification sets in (CT can detect only after ossification has set in).

Granulation Tissue Versus Cholesteatoma

This distinction is a key imaging question. **Table 5** below summarizes the points that help the differentiation of the two entities.

SPECIFIC COMPLICATIONS

Some other selected entities are described in detail.

Postinflammatory Ossicular Fixation

- *Synonym*: Chronic adhesive OM
- Ossicular fixation of a chronic complication of CSOM
- High-resolution CT plays an important role in the differentiation of postinflammatory ossicular fixation from other pathologic conditions. For example, in case of an intact TM, the differentiation of postinflammatory ossicular fixation from otosclerosis may be difficult clinically, because both typically present with a dry ear and conductive hearing loss.
- *Ossicular fixation can be of three different types*: (1) Fibrous; (2) Tympano-sclerotic; and (3) Ossifying.

Fibrous Tissue Fixation

- *Fixation of the malleus head and neck*: This is to be looked as Prussak space.
- High-resolution CT reveals noncalcified soft tissue debris encasing ossicular chain.
- Findings are nonspecific, but can be assumed in a patient with a history of CSOM with a dry ear and with conductive hearing loss.
- Stapedial fixation appears as peristapedial tenting.

Tympanosclerosis

- Appears as calcific foci within the middle ear with sites of involvement being TM, ossicles, surface of ligaments, stapes footplate, or even muscle tendons.
- High-resolution CT reveals: Unifocal or multifocal, punctate or diffuse calcified densities on the TM or middle ear structures (also see Chapter 21).
- Calcified debris may be seen on the stapedial crura.
- Subtle findings:
  - Stapes is "too well seen" because of increased density.
  - Can easily be missed when not compared with the contralateral side.

Ossifying

It is the least common manifestation with formation of lamellar new bone (mostly seen in the epitympanum).

Labyrinthitis Ossificans

- Represents pathologic ossification of the membranous labyrinth as a response to an insult to the inner ear.
- Most commonly results from an inflammatory process of the inner ear.
- It can be related to otomastoiditis (tympanogenic), secondary to meningitis (meningogenic), or can be associated with temporal bone trauma, surgery, temporal bone tumors, or autoimmune inner ear disease.
- Patients present with profound sensorineural hearing loss.
- Three stages have been proposed for LO—acute inflammatory, followed by fibroblastic and finally ossification.
- Labyrinthitis ossificans may complicate or preclude cochlear implantation.
- Computed tomography and MRI findings in LO are detailed in **Table 6** and **Figure 19**.

TABLE 6 **Imaging findings in labyrinthitis ossificans (LO).**

Phase of LO	HRCT temporal bone	MRI
Acute inflammatory	Can appear normal	• Enhancement within the membranous labyrinth on thin section fat-suppressed postcontrast images, due to breach in the blood labyrinth barrier • There can also be loss of normal high signal intensity (SI) of the fluid in the membranous labyrinth (cochlea/semicircular canals/vestibule). Best seen on heavily T2-weighted (T2W) images
Fibroblastic	Can appear normal or show mild increase in density within the labyrinth	Variable degree and extent of loss of normal T2W high SI of the fluid in the membranous labyrinth
Ossific	Variable degrees and extent of ossification with obliteration of bony labyrinth (cochlea, semicircular canals or vestibule)	Same as above

POSTCHOLESTEATOMA SURGERY IMAGING: HRCT VERSUS MRI

- Computed tomography has a good negative predictive value and a pneumatized middle ear without any soft tissue can exclude any recurrence. But, when middle ear is opacified, CT has a limited role in looking for recurrence as postoperative changes, postoperative packing material, granulation tissue, postoperative collections, and scars can all cause opacification of the middle ear and differentiating between these entities on CT is not possible.
- As on preoperative imaging, nonecho-planar-based DWI and post-gadolinium T1W images (45 min delayed images can be done to look for scar tissue enhancement) have the best sensitivity and specificity to detect residual or recurrent cholesteatoma. Similar to preoperative imaging recurrent cholesteatoma shows restricted diffusion and no enhancement (**Fig. 27**).

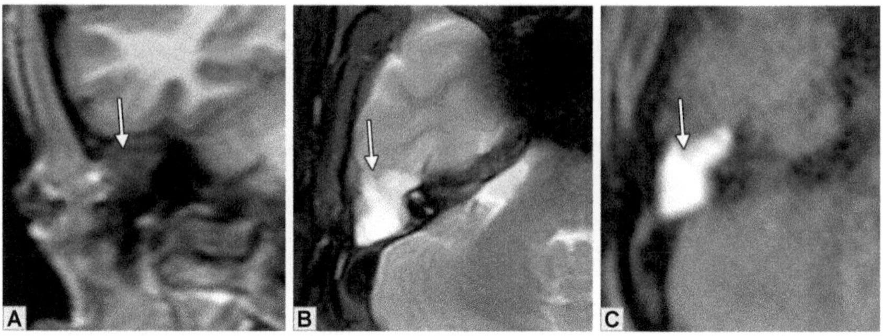

FIGS. 27A TO C: MRI in recurrent cholesteatoma: Follow up imaging a few years after initial surgery for cholesteatoma. A lesion in right mastoid, which is (A) hypointense on T1W, (B) hyperintense on T2W, and (C) restricted diffusion on diffusion-weighted imaging MR images confirming recurrent cholesteatoma.

MIDDLE EAR INFECTIONS IN IMMUNOCOMPROMISED PATIENTS

- Immunocompromised patients are predisposed to recurrent middle ear infection.
- More than 10 episodes of acute OM in a year is taken as a diagnostic criteria for immune-compromised state.
- Middle ear infections are associated with defects of humoral (B-cell) immunity.
- In addition to usual bacterial infections, such patients are predisposed to fungal infections as well.

In conclusion, imaging plays an important role in the diagnosis and extent assessment in external and middle ear infections. Illustrative cases with reporting template are given in Chapter 10.

REFERENCES

1. Baráth K, Huber AM, Stämpfli P, Varga Z, Kollias S. Neuroradiology of cholesteatomas. AJNR Am J Neuroradiol. 2011;32(2):221-9.
2. Bhalla AS, Singh A, Jana M. Chronically Discharging Ears: Evaluation with High Resolution Computed Tomography. Pol J Radiol. 2017;82:478-89.
3. Mehrotra P, Elbadawey MR, Zammit-Maempel I. Spectrum of radiological appearances of necrotising external otitis: a pictorial review. J Laryngol Otol. 2011;125(11):1109-15.
4. Ozgen B, Oguz KK, Cila A. Diffusion MR Imaging Features of Skull Base Osteomyelitis Compared with Skull Base Malignancy. Am J Neuroradiol. 2011;32(1):179-84.
5. Vazquez E, Castellote A, Piqueras J, Mauleon S, Creixell S, Pumarola F, et al. Imaging of Complications of Acute Mastoiditis in Children. Radiographics. 2003;2:359-72.
6. Yung M, Tono T, Olszewska E, Yamamoto Y, Sudhoff H, Sakagami M, et al. EAONO/JOS Joint Consensus Statements on the Definitions, Classification and Staging of Middle Ear Cholesteatoma. J Int Adv Otol. 2017;13(1):1-8.

9

Infectious Diseases: Surgical Perspective

Shuchita Singh, Kapil Sikka

- Otitis media (OM) has been an important cause of middle ear (ME) disease. Despite the indispensable contribution of antibiotics, OM still remains a common disease in our country leading to morbidity.
- Chronic suppurative otitis media (CSOM) refers to a focal or generalized chronic inflammatory process involving the ME cleft. It may be infectious or noninfectious.
- It can be subdivided into two categories: Cholesteatomatous CSOM or noncholesteatomatous CSOM (NCSOM). Both of them are refractory to clinical treatment, and are the most frequent indications of mastoidectomy.
- Noncholesteatomatous CSOM is characterized by irreversible alterations in the ME epithelium that manifests as chronic otorrhea and perforation of the tympanic membrane (TM), which mandates surgical correction.
- Presence of keratinized stratified squamous epithelium in any region of the ME cleft is mandatory for it to be labeled it as cholesteatoma, which can be further subclassified as acquired or congenital.

CLINICAL PRESENTATION

Acute Otitis Media

Acute otitis media (AOM) universally presents with ear pain; other possible symptoms being fever and irritability. There can often be other accompanying symptoms like cough and nasal discharge. Discharge from the ear can be present in AOM with perforation of the ear drum, and/or acute otitis externa.

Chronic Otitis Media

- Chronic suppurative otitis media presents with a chronically discharging ear (>12 weeks), with a possible history of recurrent AOM, or traumatic TM perforation.
- The external auditory canal (EAC) may possibly be edematous but is not usually tender. The discharge can be serous or purulent; and may even be cheese-like.

- On examination, granulation tissue is often seen in the medial canal or ME space. The TM is perforated; and the ME mucosa seen through it appears edematous or erythematous.
- Cholesteatoma has the propensity to grow, migrate, and cause osseous erosion and are thus locally destructive.
- Both NCSOM and CSOM occur in poorly pneumatized mastoids.
- Chronic suppurative otitis media does not present with ear pain or fever typically. Presence of ear pain in CSOM points toward complications.
- Features of impending complications include:
  - Ear pain
  - Fever
  - Scanty blood-stained discharge
  - Vertigo
  - Facial weakness
  - Sensorineural hearing loss
  - Significant headache
  - Seizures
  - Postaural swelling ± fistula
- The complicated CSOM poses a management challenge.

PREOPERATIVE IMAGING

- Various radiological modalities have been used to assess disease extent in CSOM; including radiographs, computed tomography (CT), and magnetic resonance imaging (MRI).
- High resolution CT (HRCT) is the most commonly used modality nowadays due to the explicit anatomic information it provides.
- The role of CT in the preoperative evaluation of CSOM is controversial. Some otologists advocate its use regularly to evaluate the extension of the disease, identify the important landmarks and thus predict any potential risk of complications.
- Another school of thought reserves its utilization for revision cases and also those cases having suspicion of complication, recurrence, or diagnostic doubt.

Indications of Preoperative Imaging in CSOM

The indications of preoperative imaging include:

- Suspected neurological complications of CSOM
- Preoperative facial paralysis
- Vertigo with positive fistula test
- Revision mastoidectomy
- Postaural swelling
- Postaural fistula
- Severe headache with seizures
- Fever with headache and diplopia

Detailed imaging evaluation has been discussed in Chapter 8.

Crucial Information to be Looked for in Preoperative Imaging

Information given by radiology helps us to determine the extent of soft tissue involvement of the antrum, middle ear, and the posterior tympanic space, which is of utmost importance to the operating surgeon in deciding between a canal wall up or canal wall down procedure.

- Presence of *Korner's septum* and its relation with facial nerve—chances of facial nerve injury is more.
- *Dural plate*—whether it is low lying or dehiscent
- *Sinus plate*—whether it is forward lying or dehiscent
- *Lateral semicircular canal (LSCC)*—location of the canal, whether there is any erosion of the canal along with the location of the erosion—LSCC is the single most common location for the cholesteatoma-induced labyrinthine fistulas because of its anatomic position in the antrum.
- *Facial canal*—erosion; the tympanic segment of the facial nerve is the most susceptible to erosion.
- *Scutum*—whether intact or eroded.
- *Ossicles*:
    - The incus is the most frequently eroded ossicle followed by the malleus and stapes.
    - The presence of malleus could be predicted with greatest accuracy.
    - The stapes is not consistently visualized by CT, but when seen usually appears as a soft tissue density in the oval window niche.
    - Displacement of the ossicular chain.
    - Whether the soft tissue mass is lying medial to ossicles.
- *Mastoid antrum*—depth, pneumatization, and erosion of the septa
- *Lateral cortical wall*—whether eroded
- *Carotid canal*—anomalous position
- *Jugular bulb*—high riding jugular bulb, erosion of the jugular bulb
- *Tegmen tympani*—erosion, extent of dehiscence
- *Intracranial involvement*—abscess, meningitis, and otitic hydrocephalus
- *Internal jugular vein (IJV)* thrombophlebitis and lateral sinus thrombophlebitis
- *Mastoid abscess*

Normal Anatomic Variants

Normal anatomic variants which may pose a danger during surgery are:

- High jugular bulb or jugular bulb diverticulum
- Bulging sigmoid sinus
- Large vestibular aqueduct
- External auditory canal atresia
- Cochlear deformities
- Lateral semicircular canal malformation

MANAGEMENT

Management of Acute Suppurative Otitis Media

- In majority of patients, acute suppurative otitis media (ASOM) will resolve spontaneously within 24 hours, nearly all within 3 days.
- All patients should be treated with simple analgesics in the first instance. Antibiotics should be reserved only for complicated features.
- Grommets can also be used to treat recurrent AOM in some instances.

Management of Chronic Otitis Media

Conservative management should be the first-line treatment in chronic OM, which should include:

- Aural toilet and syringing of affected ear (warm saline with 1.5% acetic acid).
- Medical treatment with antibiotics and antihistaminics; both systemic as well as topical use.
- Nasal decongestants (both nasal as well as systemic use) to reduce Eustachian tube edema.
- Treatment of respiratory infections and allergies; and appropriate precautions.

Indications of Surgical Intervention

- Acute suppurative otitis media: Surgery should be reserved for complicated or refractory cases.
- In chronic OM, surgery is the treatment of choice in cholesteatomatous CSOM. In NCSOM, surgery is advocated in complicated cases or cases that are refractory to medical/conservative management.

TYPES OF SURGICAL INTERVENTIONS FOR CSOM

The main surgical technique employed in CSOM is "mastoidectomy." Various surgical techniques used in the management of CSOM are summarized below:

- The term refers to surgical removal of the mastoid air cells.
- It can be done as part of treatment for mastoiditis, CSOM, or cholesteatoma.
- Indications other than infectious causes include: For gaining access to ME in various procedures, as well as in cochlear implant surgery.
- The different types of mastoidectomy procedures are: Simple, cortical, radical, and modified radical mastoidectomy (MRM).

Simple Mastoidectomy (Fig. 1A)

It consists of opening the mastoid cortex and identifying the aditus and antrum. An incision given behind the ear and the mastoid bone is opened to remove the infected cells. A small incision is made within the TM to drain excess fluid.

Cortical Mastoidectomy

- It is also called as "Schwartze procedure."
- Herein, the mastoid air cells are removed without affecting the ME. The mastoid cortex is opened and the aditus and antrum are identified, and the patency of aditus is checked.

Radical Mastoidectomy (Fig. 1B)

- Posterior and superior canal wall (of bony EAC) are removed; meatoplasty and complete exteriorization of ME are performed. The TM and ossicles are not reconstructed, thus exteriorizing the ME and the mastoid.
- The Eustachian tube is often obliterated with soft tissue to reduce the risk of a chronic otorrhea. A skin graft can be placed in the ME to reduce the risk of mucosalization and otorrhea.

Modified Radical Mastoidectomy

- Modified radical mastoidectomy differs from radical mastoidectomy in that the ossicles and the TM remnants are preserved.
- The posterior and superior canal wall are preserved.
- It offers the scope for possible hearing reconstruction at a later stage.

Types of MRM

It can further be divided into following types:

- *Canal wall down mastoidectomy* (**Fig. 1C**):
  - Complete mastoidectomy is performed in addition to removal of the posterior and superior osseous EAC.
  - The TM is reconstructed to separate the mucosal-lined ME space from the mastoid cavity and ear canal and a meatoplasty is done.
- *Canal wall up mastoidectomy* (**Fig. 1D**):
  - Necessitates removal of all of the mastoid air cells along the tegmen, sigmoid sinus, presigmoid dural plate, and posterior wall of the EAC.
  - Herein, the posterior wall of the EAC is preserved, posterior and superior canal wall are kept intact and the ME is accessed through facial recess.
  - Since the normal EAC anatomy is maintained with preservation of posterior wall, the problems associated with a mastoid cavity are less common with this procedure.
  - This is also the common approach for cochlear implantation.
- *Bondy's procedure*:
  - This procedure is employed for treatment of diseases involving the epitympanum.
  - Diseased areas as well as portions of the adjacent superior and posterior canal are simply exteriorized without affecting the uninvolved ME.

In conclusion, surgery is required for cholesteatomatous CSOM; but at the same time it may be a challenging task due to high recurrence rates.

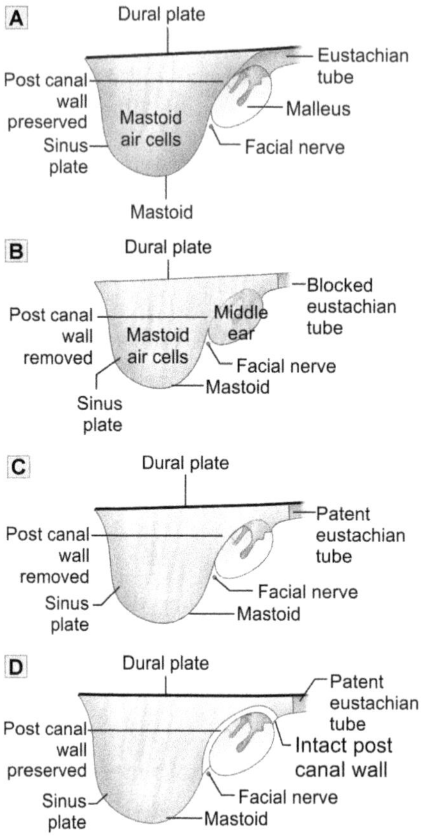

A. Simple mastoidectomy:
- Removal of disease from mastoid antrum and air cells
- Outer cortical bone and septum removed
- Posterior canal wall, middle ear preserved

B. Radical mastoidectomy:
- Mastoid, middle ear disease removed
- Posterior canal wall removed
- Cavity communicating with EAC

C. Modified radical mastoidectomy (MRM) canal wall down procedure:
- Posterior canal wall removed
- Middle ear, mastoid converted to single cavity
- Eustachian tube patent, hearing intact

D. MRM canal wall up procedure:
- Similar to canal wall down procedure; but with better hearing result
- Eustachian tube kept patent
- Middle ear space better preserved

FIGS.1A TO D: Diagram of various types of mastoidectomy (shaded area denotes the surgically removed part).

REFERENCES

1. Mittal R, Lisi CV, Gerring R, Mittal J, Mathee K, Narasimhan G, et al. Current concepts in the pathogenesis and treatment of chronic suppurative otitis media. J Med Microbiol. 2015;64(10):1103-16.
2. Schilder AG, Marom T, Bhutta MF, Casselbrant ML, Coates H, Gisselsson-Solén M, et al. Panel 7: Otitis Media: Treatment and Complications. Otolaryngol Head Neck Surg. 2017;156(4_suppl):S88-105.
3. Islam MA, Haque S, Ahmed K, Bari MS, Hoque MM, Khan MK, et al. Outcome of Surgery in Chronic Inactive Mucosal Otitis Media. MMJ. 2018;27(3):617-25.
4. Heah H, Soon SR, Yuen HW. A case series of complicated infective otitis media requiring surgery in adults. Singapore Med J. 2016;57(12):681-5.
5. Altuna X, Navarro JJ, Goiburu M, Palicio I. Management of chronic otitis media by subtotal petrosectomy. Utilidad de la petrosectomía subtotal en el tratamiento de la otitis media crónica. Acta Otorrinolaringologica Espanola. 2016;67(5):249-53.
6. Orhan KS, Çelik M, Polat B, Aydemir L, Aydoseli A, Sencer A, et al. Endoscope-Assisted Surgery for Petrous Bone Cholesteatoma with Hearing Preservation. J Int Adv Otol. 2019;15(3):391-5.

10

Reporting Template with Illustrative Cases

(Infections of External and Middle Ear)

Smita Manchanda, Ashu Seith Bhalla

REPORTING TEMPLATE

	Right	*Left*

External Ear

- Tympanic membrane (TM) (Intact or Not)
- Soft tissue density (Present/Absent)

Middle Ear

- Soft tissue density (Present/Absent)
- Location of soft tissue density:
  - Prussak space
  - Anterior epitympanic recess
  - Sinus tympani
  - Facial nerve recess
- Ear ossicles (Intact or Eroded):
  - Malleus
  - Incus
  - Stapes
- Bone erosion:
  - Scutum
  - Tegmen tympani
  - Tegmen mastoideum
  - Sigmoid plate
  - Lateral semicircular canal (SCC)
  - Facial nerve canal

Inner Ear

- Internal auditory canal (Normal or Widened)
- Cochlea (Normal or Not)
- Vestibule (Normal or Not)
- Mastoid air cells (Pneumatized/Opacified/Sclerotic)

Any Other Finding

Key: A: Absent; E: Eroded; I: Intact; N: Normal; NI: Not intact; Op: Opacified; P: Present; Pn: Pneumatized; Sc: Sclerotic

Impression

Mention cholesteatomatous/noncholesteatomatous chronic suppurative otitis media (CSOM) and complications, if any.

CASE 1 (FIGS. 1A TO F)

A 15-year-old presenting with right ear ache and scalp swelling.

Erosion of the mastoid wall laterally with presence of enhancing scalp abscess (**Fig. 1E**).

	Right	*Left*
External Ear		
• TM (Intact or Not)	I	I
• Soft tissue density (Present/Absent)	P	A
Middle Ear		
• Soft tissue density (Present/Absent) (**Fig. 1A**)	P	A
• Location of soft tissue density:		
○ Prussak space	A	A
○ Anterior epitympanic recess (**Fig. 1C**)	P	A
○ Sinus tympani (**Fig. 1D**)	A	A
○ Facial nerve recess (**Fig. 1D**)	P	A
• Ear ossicles (Intact or Eroded):		
○ Malleus	I	I
○ Incus	I	I
○ Stapes	I	I
• Bone erosion:		
○ Scutum	I	I
○ Tegmen tympani	I	I
○ Tegmen mastoideum	I	I
○ Sigmoid plate	I	I
○ Lateral SCC	I	I
○ Facial nerve canal	I	I
Inner Ear		
• Internal auditory canal (Normal or Widened)	N	N
• Cochlea (Normal or Not)	N	N
• Vestibule (Normal or Not)	N	N
• Mastoid air cells (Pneumatized/ Opacified/Sclerotic) (**Fig. 1B**)	Sc	Pn

Key: A: Absent; E: Eroded; I: Intact; N: Normal; NI: Not intact; Op: Opacified; P: Present; Pn: Pneumatized; Sc: Sclerotic

Impression

- Right noncholesteatomatous CSOM
- Mastoid wall erosion and scalp abscess

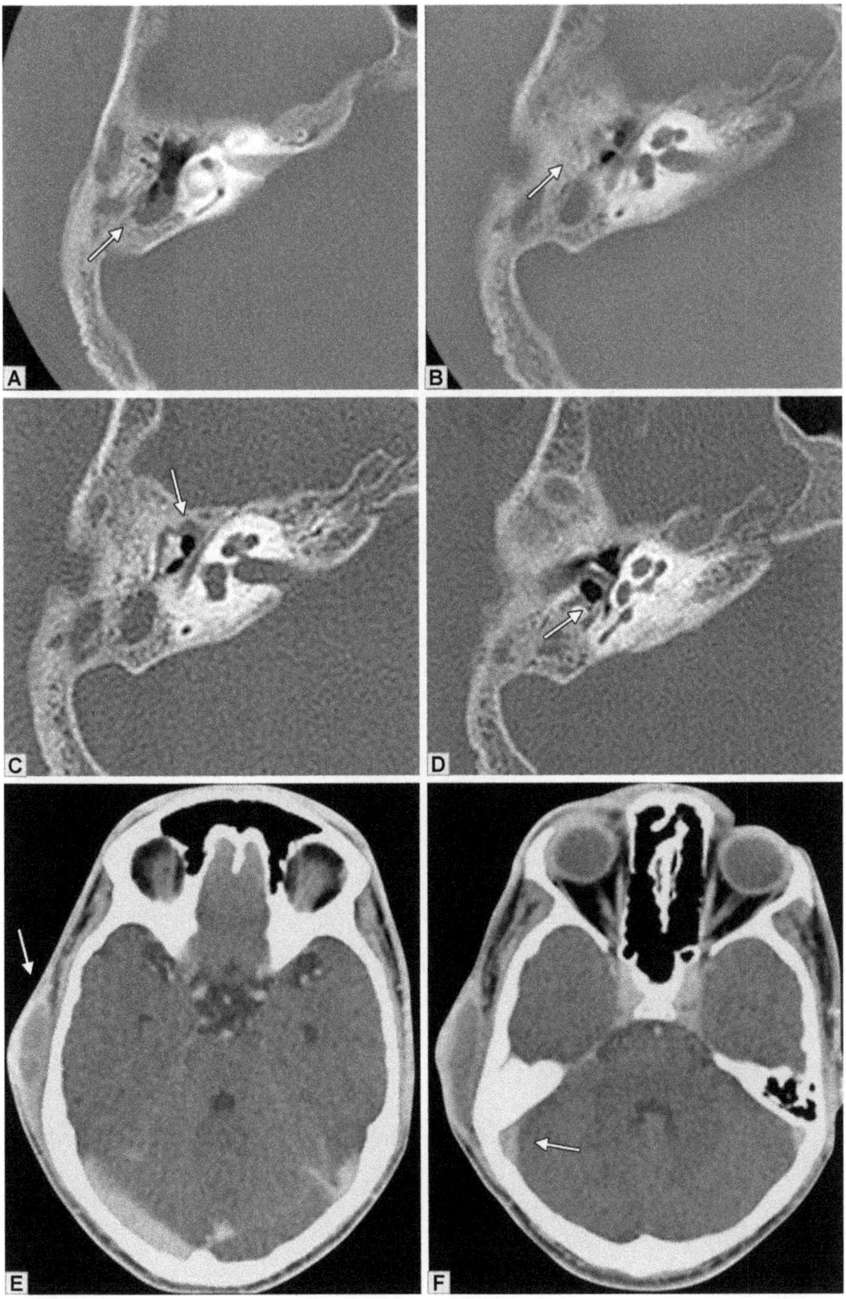

FIGS. 1A TO F: (A to D) Axial HRCT superior to inferior. (E and F) Axial contrast-enhanced computed tomography (CECT) superior to inferior.

CASE 2 (FIGS. 2A TO D)

A 17-year-old male presenting with discharging right ear.

	Right	*Left*
External Ear		
• TM (Intact or Not)	***Thickened***	I
• Soft tissue density (Present/Absent) (**Fig. 2B**)	P	A
Middle Ear		
• Soft tissue density (Present/Absent)	P	P
• Location of soft tissue density (**Fig. 2A**):		
○ Prussak space (**Fig. 2C**)	P	P
○ Anterior epitympanic recess	P	A
○ Sinus tympani	P	A
○ Facial nerve recess	P	A
• Ear ossicles (Intact or Eroded) (**Fig. 2D**):		
○ Malleus	E	I
○ Incus	E	I
○ Stapes	E	I
• Bone erosion:		
○ Scutum (**Fig. 2C**)	E	I
○ Tegmen tympani (**Fig. 2C**)	E	I
○ Tegmen mastoideum	I	I
○ Sigmoid plate	I	I
○ Lateral SCC	I	I
○ Facial nerve canal	I	I
Inner Ear		
• Internal auditory canal (Normal or Widened)	N	N
• Cochlea (Normal or Not)	N	N
• Vestibule (Normal or Not)	N	N
• Mastoid air cells (Pneumatized/ Opacified/Sclerotic)	Op	Op

Key: A: Absent; E: Eroded; I: Intact; N: Normal; NI: Not intact; Op: Opacified; P: Present; Pn: Pneumatized; Sc: Sclerotic

Impression

- Right cholesteatomatous CSOM and left noncholesteatomatous CSOM
- Erosion of right sided ossicles, scutum and tegmen tympani

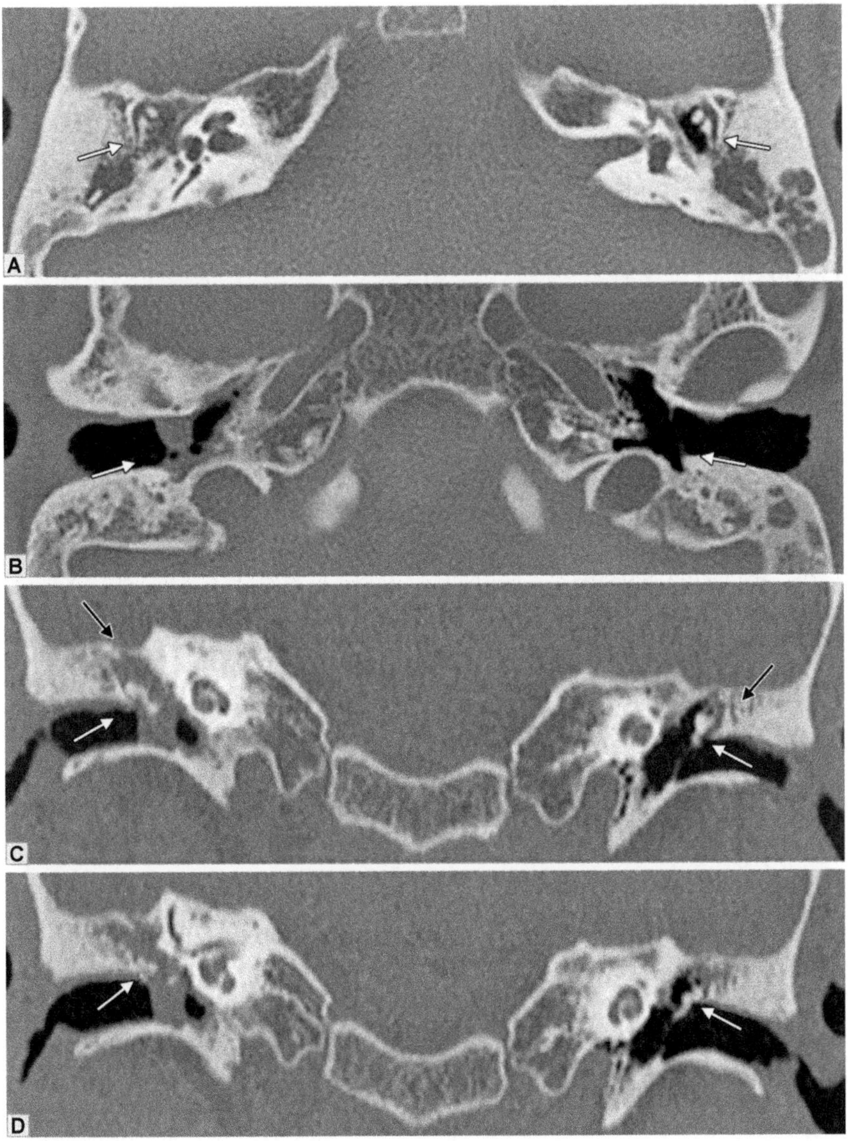

FIGS. 2A TO D: (A and B) Axial HRCT superior to inferior. (C and D) Coronal HRCT anterior to posterior.

CASE 3 (FIGS. 3A TO D)

A 5-year-old case of bilateral (B/L) CSOM presenting with right-sided facial palsy.

Ossification is noted in the cochlea and vestibule with obliteration of middle and apical turns and stenosis of basal turn. Vestibule is also irregular with partial obliteration of all three SCCs (**Figs. 3A** to **D**).

	Right	*Left*
External Ear		
• TM (Intact or Not)	I	I
• Soft tissue density (Present/Absent)	A	A
Middle Ear		
• Soft tissue density (Present/Absent) (**Fig. 3A**)	P	P
• Location of soft tissue density (**Fig. 3C**):		
○ Prussak space	P	P
○ Anterior epitympanic recess	P	P
○ Sinus tympani	P	P
○ Facial nerve recess	P	A
• Ear ossicles (Intact or Eroded) (**Fig. 3D**):		
○ Malleus	E	E
○ Incus	E	E
○ Stapes	E	E
• Bone erosion:		
○ Scutum	E	E
○ Tegmen tympani	I	I
○ Tegmen mastoideum	I	I
○ Sigmoid plate	I	I
○ Lateral SCC (**Fig. 3B**)	E	I
○ Facial nerve canal (**Fig. 3B**)	E	I
Inner Ear		
• Internal auditory canal (Normal or Widened)	N	N
• Cochlea (Normal or Not) (**Fig. 3C**)	Sc	N
• Vestibule (Normal or Not) (**Fig. 3B**)	Sc	N
• Mastoid air cells (Pneumatized/Opacified/Sclerotic)	Sc	Op

Key: A: Absent; E: Eroded; I: Intact; N: Normal; NI: Not intact; Op: Opacified; P: Present; Pn: Pneumatized; Sc: Sclerotic

Impression

Bilateral cholesteatomatous CSOM:

- Erosion of right ossicles, scutum, lateral SCC, and facial nerve canal and labyrinthitis ossificans
- Erosion of left ossicles and scutum

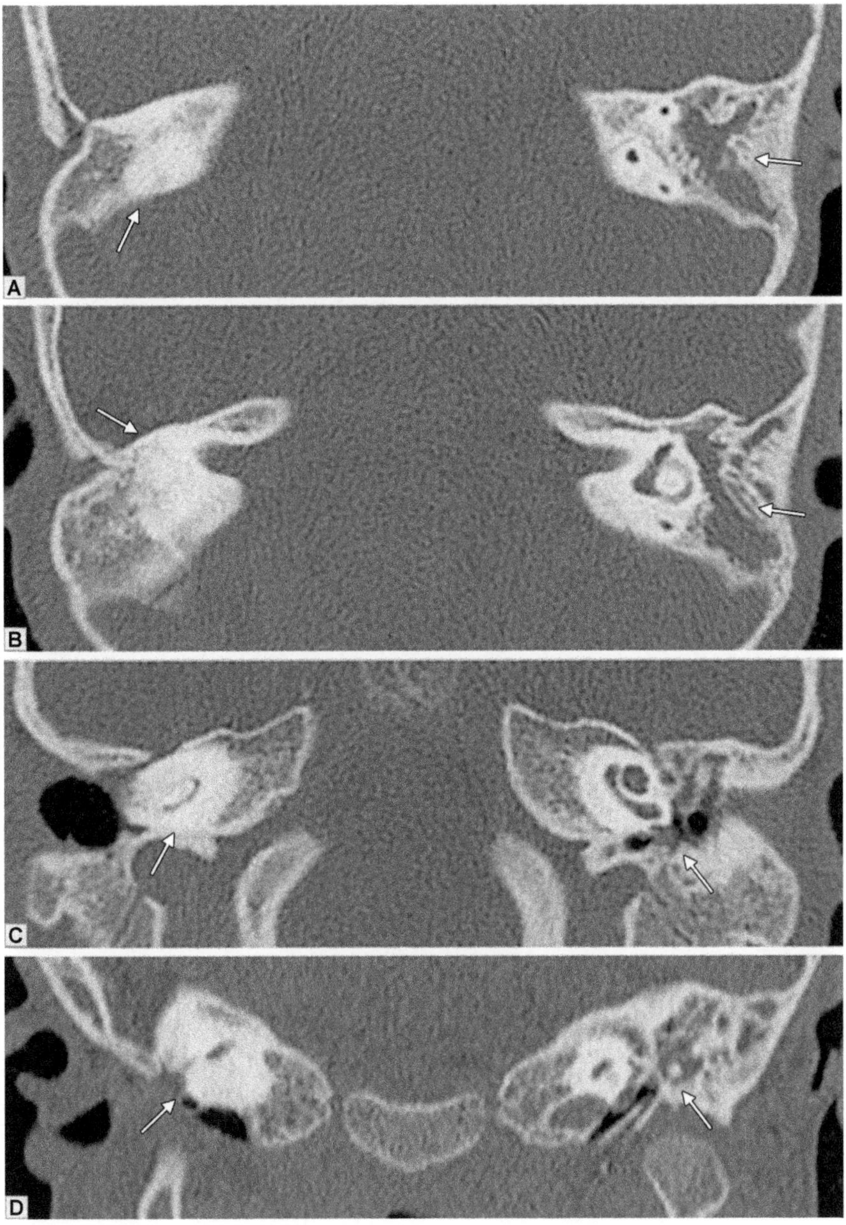

FIGS. 3A TO D: (A to C) Axial HRCT superior to inferior. (D) Coronal HRCT.

CASE 4 (FIGS. 4A TO F)

- Postoperative case of right CSOM with persistent ear discharge
- Inferior displacement of dural plate (**Fig. 4E**)

	Right	*Left*
External Ear		
• TM (Intact or Not)	NI	I
• Soft tissue density (Present/Absent) (**Fig. 4A**)	P	A
Middle Ear		
• Soft tissue density (Present/Absent) (**Fig. 4A**)	P	A
• Location of soft tissue density:	Post op	A
○ Prussak space		
○ Anterior epitympanic recess		
○ Sinus tympani		
○ Facial nerve recess		
• Ear ossicles (Intact or Eroded):	Post op	I
○ Malleus	I	
○ Incus	I	
○ Stapes	I	
• Bone erosion:		
○ Scutum	E	I
○ Tegmen tympani	I	I
○ Tegmen mastoideum	I	I
○ Sigmoid plate	I	I
○ Lateral SCC (**Fig. 4B**)	E	I
○ Facial nerve canal (**Fig. 4C**)	E	I
Inner Ear		
• Internal auditory canal (Normal or Widened)	N	N
• Cochlea (Normal or Not)	N	N
• Vestibule (Normal or Not) (**Fig. 4F**)	N	N
• Mastoid air cells (Pneumatized/Opacified/Sclerotic)	Post op	Pn

Key: A: Absent; E: Eroded; I: Intact; N: Normal; NI: Not intact; Op: Opacified; P: Present; Pn: Pneumatized; Sc: Sclerotic.

Impression

- Postoperative case (for right CSOM) with recurrent right cholesteatomatous CSOM
- Erosion of vestibule, lateral SCC, and facial nerve canal

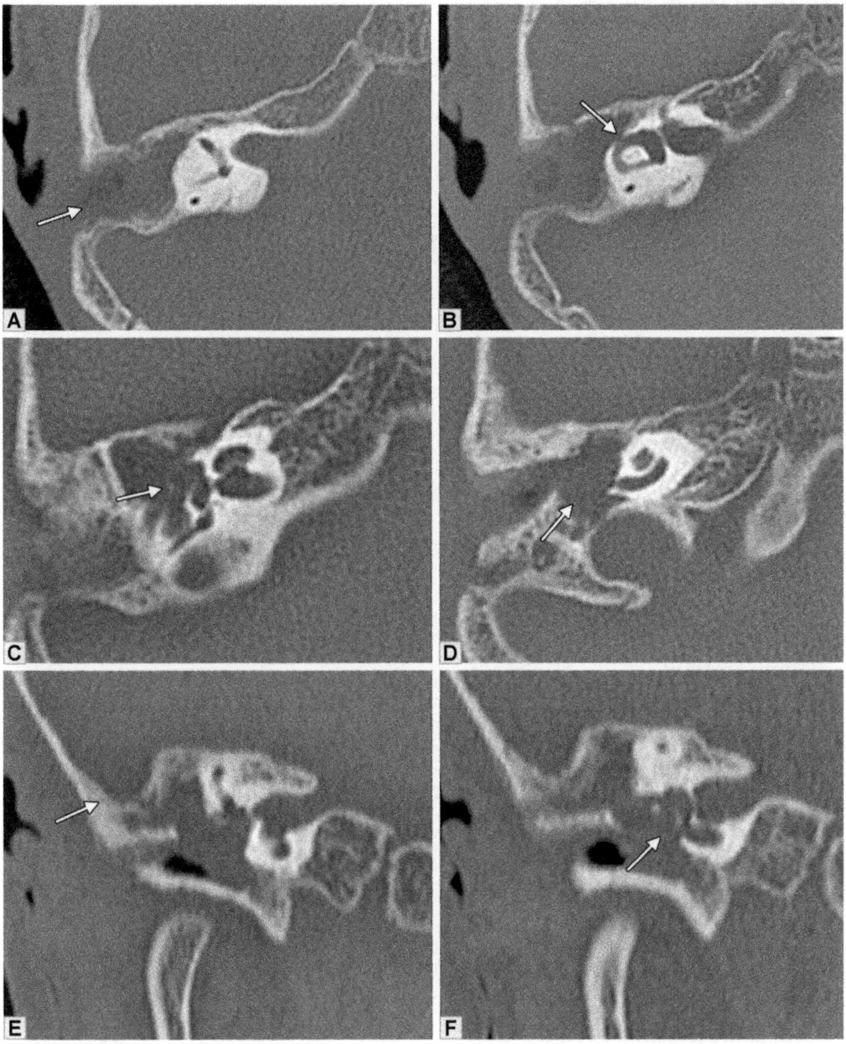

FIGS. 4A TO F: (A to D) Axial HRCT superior to inferior. (E and F) Coronal HRCT anterior to posterior.

CASE 5 (FIGS. 5A TO E)

A 17-year-old postoperative case of left CSOM presenting with ear bleed. Pack seen in the left external ear (**Fig. 5D**).

	Right	*Left*
External Ear		
• TM (Intact or Not)	I	I
• Soft tissue density (Present/Absent)	A	P
Middle Ear		
• Soft tissue density (Present/Absent)	P	P (Post op)
• Location of soft tissue density (**Fig. 5A**):		
○ Prussak space	A	
○ Anterior epitympanic recess	A	
○ Sinus tympani	P	
○ Facial nerve recess	P	
• Ear ossicles (Intact or Eroded):		
○ Malleus	I	E
○ Incus	I	E
○ Stapes	I	E
• Bone erosion:		
○ Scutum (**Fig. 5B**)	I	P (Post op)
○ Tegmen tympani (**Fig. 5C**)	I	E
○ Tegmen mastoideum (**Fig. 5C**)	I	E
○ Sigmoid plate (**Fig. 5A**)	I	E
○ Lateral SCC	I	I
○ Facial nerve canal	I	I
Inner Ear		
• Internal auditory canal (Normal or Widened)	N	N
• Cochlea (Normal or Not)	N	N
• Vestibule (Normal or Not)	N	N
• Mastoid air cells (Pneumatized/Opacified/Sclerotic)	Op	Post op

Thrombosis of left sigmoid sinus (**Fig. 5D**) and proximal internal jugular vein (IJV) (**Fig. 5E**).

Key: A: Absent; E: Eroded; I: Intact; N: Normal; NI: Not intact; Op: Opacified; P: Present; Pn: Pneumatized; Sc: Sclerotic

Impression

- Postoperative case (for left CSOM) with recurrent left cholesteatomatous CSOM and right noncholesteatomatous CSOM
- Erosion of left ossicles, tegmen tympani, tegmen mastoideum, and sigmoid plate and thrombosis of left sigmoid sinus and proximal IJV

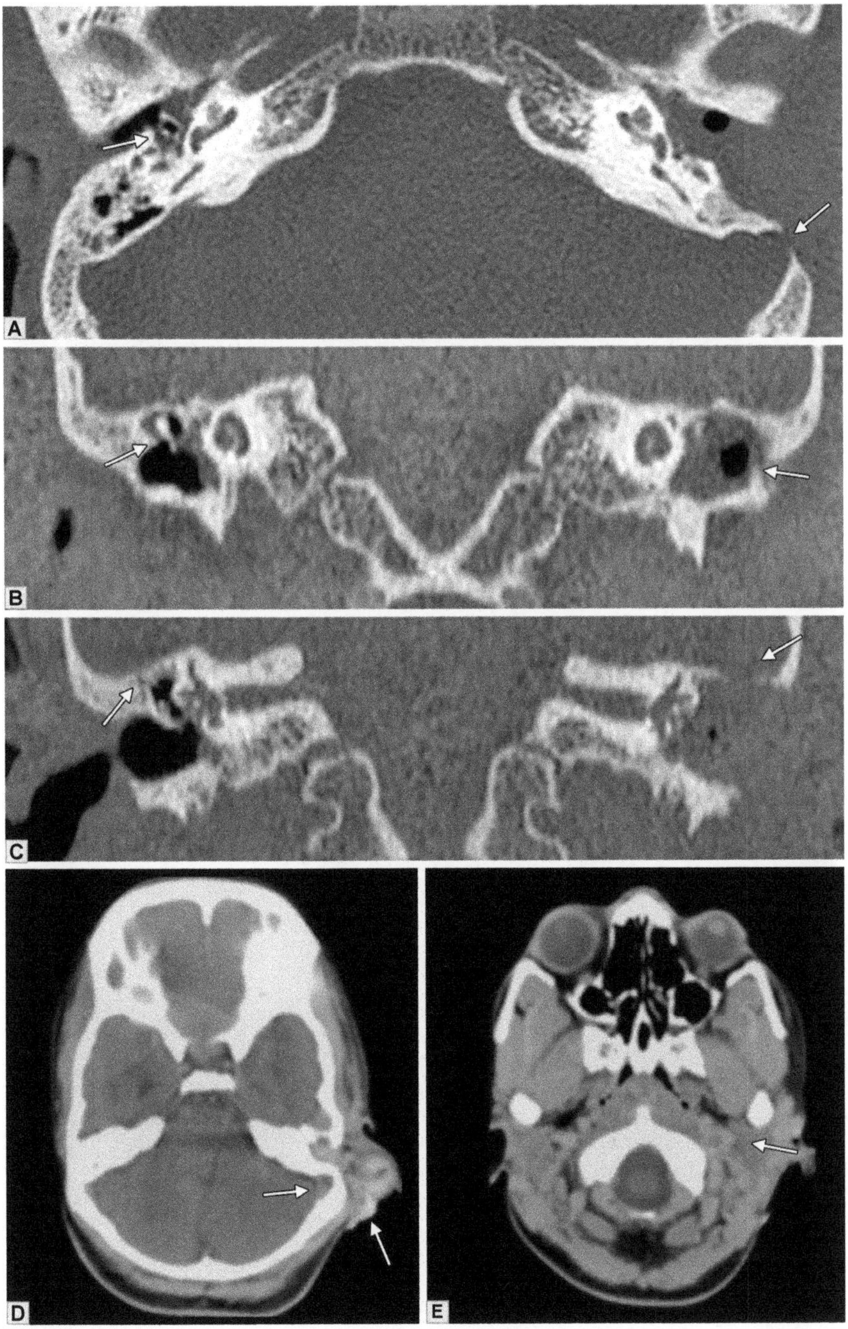

FIGS. 5A TO E: (A) Axial HRCT. (B and C) Coronal HRCT anterior to posterior. (D and E) contrast-enhanced computed tomography (CECT) axial plane, superior to inferior.

4
SECTION

Inner Ear, Internal Auditory Canal and Cochlear Implant

11

Congenital Anomalies of Inner Ear

Manisha Jana, Ashu Seith Bhalla

- Embryology
- Classification
- Specific Anomalies Based on Sennaroglu Classification
- Other Classification Systems
  - INCAV System
  - SMS Classification
- Syndromes and IEM

Congenital inner ear malformations (IEMs) are a very heterogeneous group consisting of many diseases entities. The clinical presentations are also variable; although sensorineural hearing loss (SNHL) remains the most common one. This chapter will discuss the various IEMs and their implications in cochlear implantation (CI).

EMBRYOLOGY

- Inner ear develops from the otic placode (thickening of surface ectoderm) at 4 weeks. The otic placode gets detached from ectoderm and invaginates into mesoderm, to form otic vesicle (**Fig. 1**).
- Otic vesicle then divides into utricular and saccular portions. Utricle, semicircular canals (SCCs), and endolymphatic duct develop from utricular portion. Saccule and cochlea develops from saccular portion.

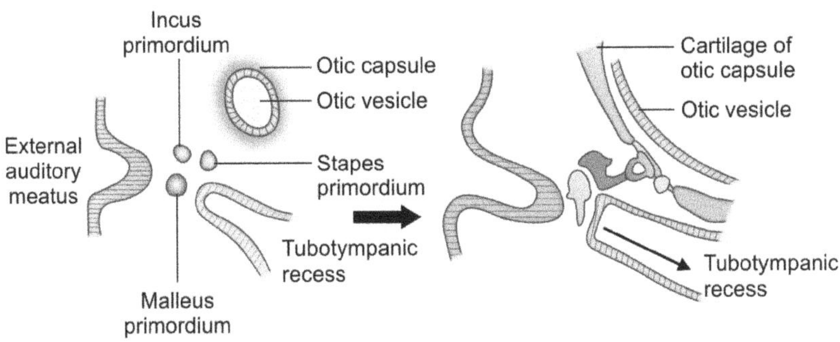

FIG. 1: Embryology of ear development.

CLASSIFICATION

- Congenital anomalies of the inner ear can be either bony or membranous otic capsule anomaly. Bony otic capsule anomaly is rare, seen in 10–20% cases; and can be detected on CT or MRI.
- Membranous otic capsule anomalies are commoner (80–90%). Usually, the bony labyrinth is normal and no abnormalities detected on CT.
- Several classification systems have been used over the years. The most commonly used ones are referred to in this chapter (**Tables 1** and **2**).
- A newer classification based on cochlear morphology was proposed by Sennaroglu et al. in 2002 (**Table 2**).
- Embryologically, the anomalies can be graded from most severe to least severe, depending on the stage of insult. Michel's anomaly is the severest; where the insult happens at third gestational week.
- As the arrest or aberrant development occurs at more advanced gestational ages, less severe anomalies result. Least severe of them are cochlear hypoplasia (CH) and incomplete partition type-II (IP-II) (classic Mondini) deformity.
- In groups 1–4 the cochlea and vestibule are not well defined; while in groups 5–8 cochlear and vestibule are well defined and these groups mainly comprise of hypoplasia/IP.

TABLE 1 **Classification based on polytomography (Jackler et al., 1987).**[1]

Malformations limited to membranous labyrinth	Complete membranous labyrinthine dysplasia (Siebenmann–Bing)
	Limited membranous labyrinthine dysplasia: • Cochleosaccular dysplasia (Scheibe) • Cochlear basal turn dysplasia (Alexander)
Malformations of the osseous and membranous labyrinth	
Complete labyrinthine aplasia (Michel)	
Cochlear anomalies	Cochlear aplasia
	Cochlear hypoplasia
	Incomplete partition (Mondini)
	Common cavity
Labyrinthine anomalies	Semicircular canal dysplasia
	Semicircular canal aplasia
Aqueductal anomalies	Enlarged vestibular aqueduct
	Enlarged cochlear aqueduct
Internal auditory canal (IAC) anomalies	Narrow IAC
	Wide IAC

Source: Modified from Jackler RK, Luxford WM, House WF. Congenital malformations of the inner ear: a classification based on embryogenesis. Laryngoscope. 1987;97(3 Pt 2, Suppl 40):2-14.

TABLE 2 **Classification by Sennaroglu et al. (2002).**[2]

Cochlear malformations	Michel anomaly
	Cochlear aplasia
	Common cavity deformity
	Cochlear hypoplasia
	Incomplete partition type-I (IP-I)
	Incomplete partition type-II (IP-II) (classic Mondini)
Vestibular malformations	Michel anomaly, common cavity, dilated vestibule, absent vestibule, and hypoplastic vestibule
Semicircular canal (SCC) malformations	Absent, hypoplastic, or enlarged SCC
Internal auditory canal malformations	Absent, narrow or enlarged
Vestibular and cochlear aqueduct findings	Normal or enlarged

Source: Modified from Sennaroglu L, Saatci I. A new classification for cochleovestibular malformations. Laryngoscope. 2002;112(12):2230-41.

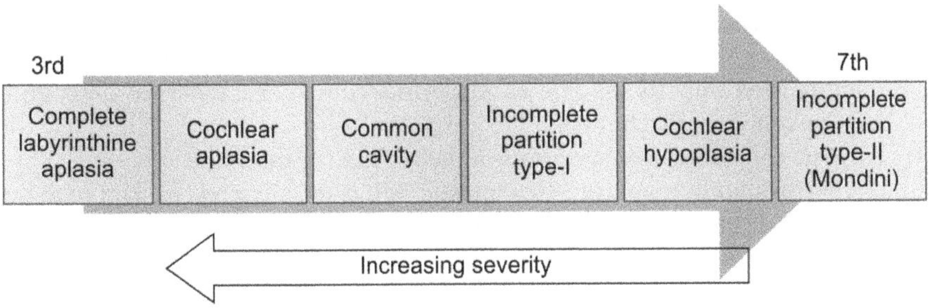

SPECIFIC ANOMALIES

Group 1: Complete Labyrinthine Aplasia

Synonym: Michel anomaly or Michel deformity

- This anomaly was first described by P Michel in 1863. It occurs as a result of failure of development of otic capsule at a very early stage (3rd week of gestation)
- It is a very rare anomaly (1% of all congenital inner ear anomalies); characterized by complete absence of all cochlear and vestibular structures.[3] In addition SCC and the aqueducts (cochlear and vestibular) are also absent.
- Audiometry reveals no response; or profound SNHL on low frequencies.
- May be unilateral (contralateral inner ear dysplasia) or bilateral.
- Narrow internal auditory canal (IAC) may be seen on CT.
- MRI shows absent vestibulocochlear (8th) nerve (VCN).
- *Imaging*: Characteristic features include hypoplastic petrous bone, absent round and oval window, and flat medial wall of middle ear (ME) (**Fig. 2**).

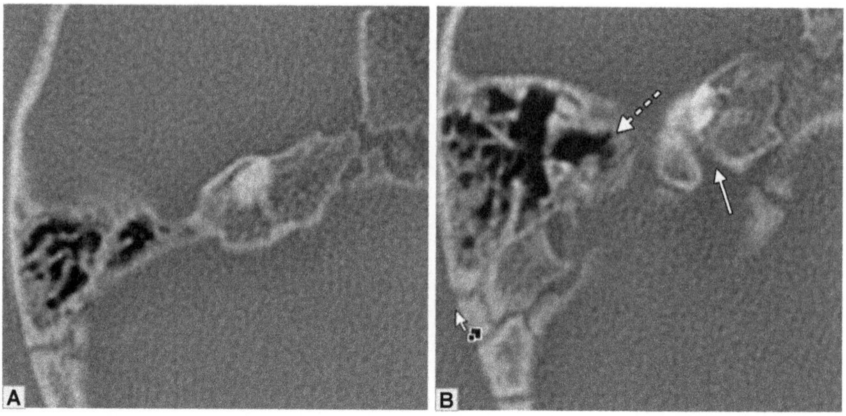

FIGS. 2A AND B: Group 1 IEM, complete labyrinthine aplasia type B: Axial HRCT cranial to caudal sections reveal:
- Petrous bone is present but otic capsule hypoplastic.
- Narrow IAC (arrows).
- Complete absence of labyrinthine structures.
- Note the flat medial wall of middle ear (dotted arrow).

- *Associations*: Hypoplastic ME and mastoid, dysplastic stapes, anomalous course of facial nerve (FN), and platybasia. While the tympanic and mastoid segments of FN canal are identified in all subtypes, the labyrinthine segment may be seen only in subtype C. Abnormal course of transverse sinus and jugular vein may also be seen.
- Subtypes of complete labyrinthine aplasia (CLA) are as follows:
  a. Petrous bone is aplastic/hypoplastic. ME is usually present, and may be located close to the posterior fossa.
  b. Herein, the petrous bone is present. However, there is aplasia or hypoplasia of the otic capsule.
  c. Petrous bone and otic capsule are present.
- Suitability for cochlear implant: CLA is an absolute contraindication for cochlear implant. It is an indication for auditory brainstem implants (ABI).

Differential Diagnosis

Labyrinthitis Ossificans

Differentiating these two depends on the presence of bulge of cochlear promontory in medial wall of ME. Whereas the bulge is present in labyrinthitis ossificans (LO); it is absent in CLA (also see Chapter 20).

Group 2: Rudimentary Otocyst

- In this malformation, there is a small rudimentary (few mm only) otic capsule present (**Fig. 3**).
- Malformed SCC may be present.
- Internal auditory canal is absent, as is the cochlear nerve (CN); and hence there is no communication between the otocyst and brainstem.

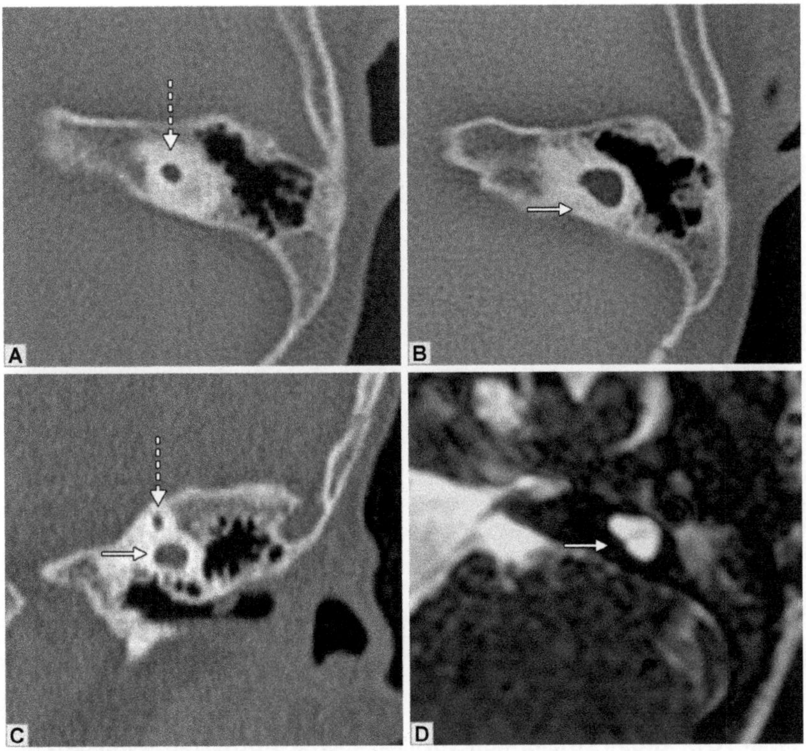

FIGS. 3A TO D: Group 2 IEM: Left rudimentary otocyst: (A and B) Axial, (C) coronal HRCT and (D) axial CISS images reveal:
- Rudimentary cystic structure (arrow) without any communication with the IAC.
- IAC is absent.
- No differentiation into cochlea and vestibule.
- Dysplastic superior SCC (dotted arrow) and absent lateral and posterior SCC.

Group 3: Cochlear Aplasia

- It results from failure of development of otic capsule at a stage later than Michel's anomaly (3rd to 4th week of gestation)
- This is a rare anomaly (3% of all IEM) and is characterized by absence of cochlea. Dense otic bone is present where cochlea would have been present.
- Vestibule and SCCs are present at their usual location, i.e., adjoining the posterior and lateral part of IAC.
- Facial nerve canal is abnormal in location, with the labyrinthine part being anteriorly displaced (and hence appears in extended location of cochlea). There are two subtypes of this anomaly:
  i. Cochlear aplasia (CA) + normal labyrinth; i.e., vestibule and SCC are normal. They are mostly symmetrical on both the sides.
  ii. Cochlear aplasia + dilated vestibule (CADV): Herein, the vestibule as well as the SCCs are dilated (**Fig. 4**). It is commonly asymmetric on the two sides. This anomaly is difficult to differentiate from common cavity (CC) (group 4).
- It is an absolute contraindication to cochlear implant.

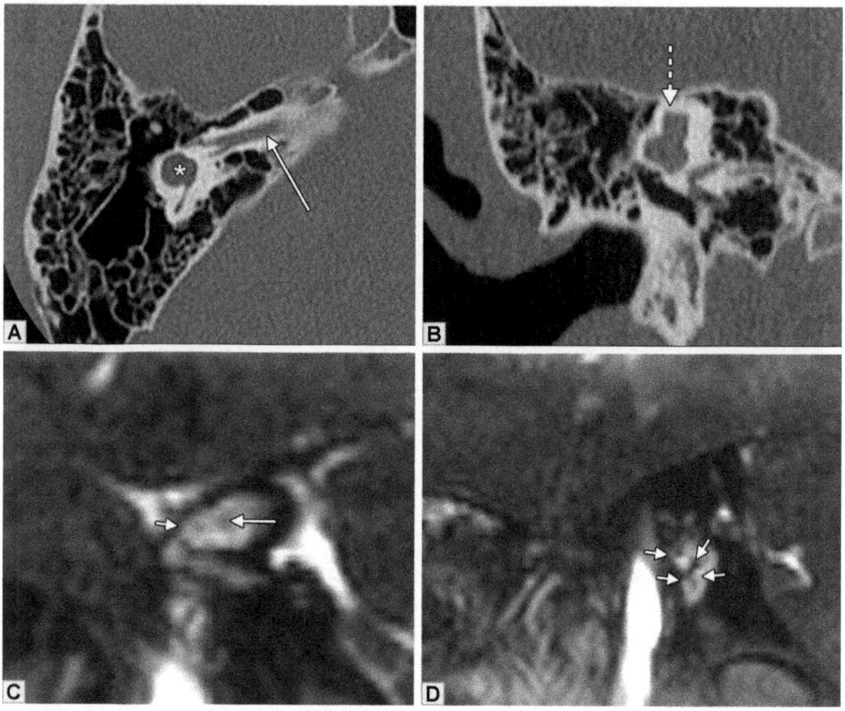

FIGS. 4A TO D: Group 3 B IEM. Right cochlear aplasia with dilated vestibule (CADV) with hypoplasia of cochlear nerve: HRCT axial (A) and coronal (B), and oblique sagittal CISS sequence MR images (C and D) reveal:

- Absent cochlea, dilated vestibule (asterisk) and a narrow IAC (long arrow). The *IAC is located in normal position*.
- The *medial wall of middle ear is flat*.
- Dysplastic SCCs (dotted arrows).
- Right IAC: Presence of facial nerve (small arrow in C) and a fused vestibular nerve (long arrow in C). *Cochlear nerve is absent*.
- Normal left IAC (D) showing normal nerves (small arrows) for comparison.

Differential Diagnosis

Labyrinthitis Ossificans (For Subtype A)

- Differentiating these two depends on the presence of bulge of cochlear promontory in medial wall of ME. Whereas the bulge is present in LO; it is absent in CA.
- Common cavity (for subtype B): Differentiating features are given in **Table 3**.

Group 4: Common Cavity Anomaly

- This anomaly is caused by a disruption in the differentiation of inner ear structure development at a stage later than Michel's anomaly and CA (about 4th week of gestation).

TABLE 3 **Differentiating features of CC from CADV.**

	Common cavity (CC) anomaly	**Cochlear aplasia with dilated vestibule (CADV)**
Cochlea/ vestibule	• One CC, one ovoid structure seen • Semicircular canals (SCCs) if seen are rudimentary	• Cochlea absent • Vestibule dilated • Normal location (posterolateral to fundus of IAC) • SCC height: Normal or enlarged
Internal auditory canal (IAC)	• Posteriorly oriented • Directly enters the CC • Enters the center of CC	• Normal
Cochlear implantation	• Can be done if cochleovestibular nerve is present	• Contraindicated

- It accounts for about one-fourth of all IEM.
- Single cystic CC is seen replacing cochlea and vestibule with no differentiation into cochlea and vestibule. Width of the cystic cavity is usually more than height, round or ovoid in shape with no internal architecture (**Fig. 5**).
- Semicircular canals are commonly malformed; rarely normal.
- The IAC is present but abnormally oriented (posteriorly directed). It enters the center of this CC.
- Cochlear nerve may be present in these cases and is referred to as cochleovestibular nerve (CVN) as it contains both cochlear as well as vestibular fibers.
- Relative contraindication for CI: CI can be performed in CC if CVN is present.

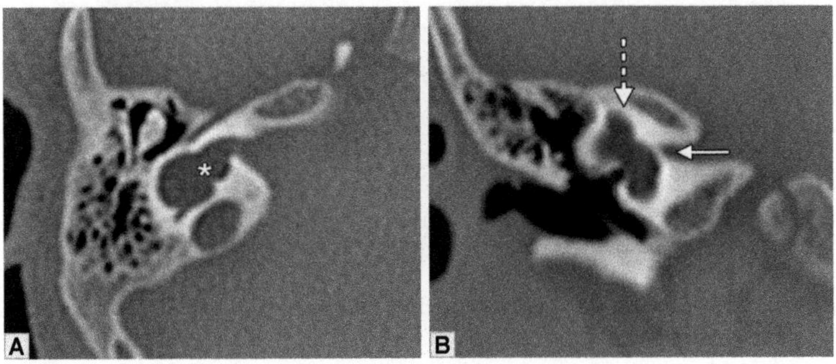

FIGS. 5A AND B: Group 4 IEM: Right-sided common cavity (CC): (A and B) Consecutive axial HRCT reveal:
- Oval cystic structure (asterisk) without any differentiation into cochlea and vestibule.
- IAC enters the cystic structure at the dysplastic SCCs (dotted arrow).

Differential Diagnosis

It is critical to differentiate CC from CADV (**Table 3**), as CI is contraindicated in CADV. If IAC is long and stenotic, CVN is likely to be absent.

Group 5: Cochlear Hypoplasia

- Cochlear hypoplasia results from abnormal development of cochlear duct at 6th week; and comprises of 15% of congenital cochlear anomalies.
- Cochlea and vestibule are differentiated and separated from each other but small in size.
- Cochlea is not only small in size but abnormalities of internal architecture are seen such as deficient bony modiolus (**Figs. 6** to **10**).

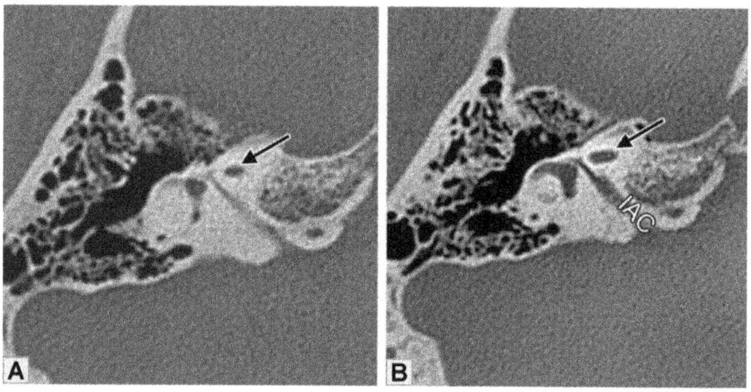

FIGS. 6 A AND B: Group 5 IEM: Right-sided cochlear hypoplasia subtype I (CH-I): HRCT axial images reveal:
- A small cochlear bud (long arrow) is seen to arise from the IAC. IAC is stenotic.
- The vestibule is hypoplastic and semicircular canals are normal.

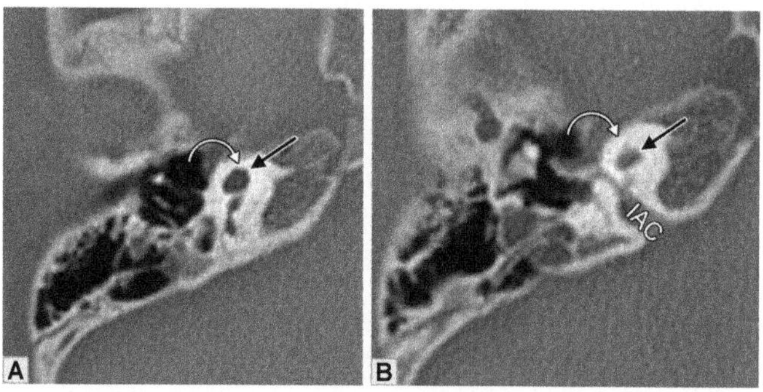

FIGS. 7A AND B: Group 5 IEM: Right-sided cochlear hypoplasia subtype I (CH-I): HRCT axial images reveal:
- A small cochlear bud (black arrow) is seen to arise from the IAC. IAC is stenotic.
- The vestibule is hypoplastic and semicircular canals are absent.
- There is a dense bone (curved arrow) in the place of normal cochlea.

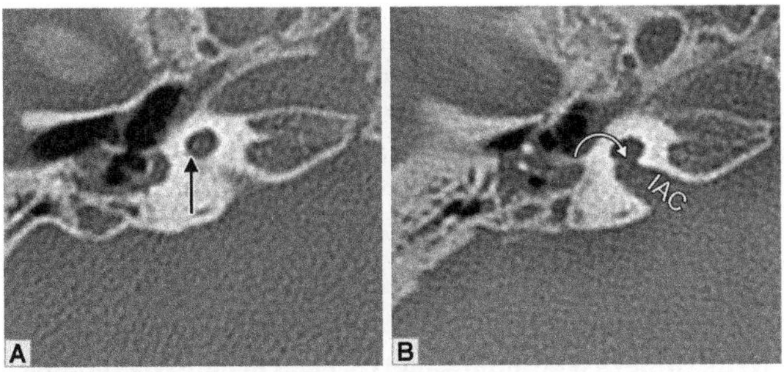

FIGS. 8A AND B: Group 5 IEM: Right-sided cochlear hypoplasia subtype II (CH-II), associated with hypoplasia with absent vestibule and SCC: Axial Images reveal:
- Small cochlea (arrow) with absent modiolus (curved arrow).
- Interscalar septum is also absent.
- Note the short wide IAC and the wide communication of cochlea with IAC.
- Vestibules and SCCs are absent.

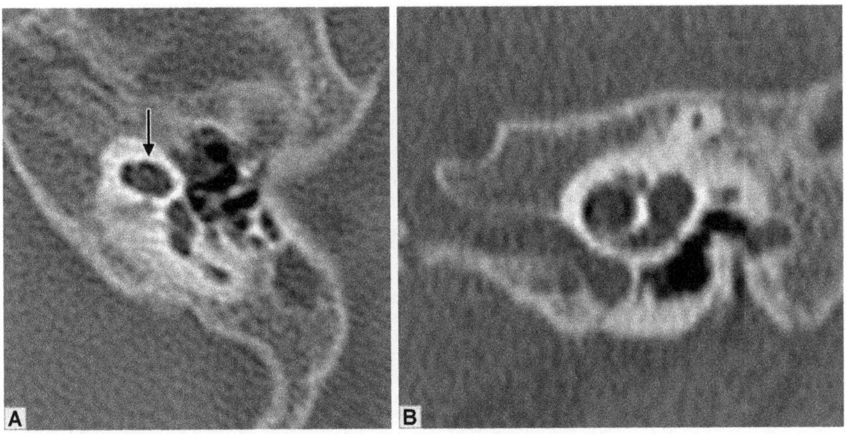

FIGS. 9A AND B: Group 5 IEM: Right-sided cochlear hypoplasia subtype III (CH-III): (A) Axial and (B) standardized cochlear reformatted images reveal:
- Small cochlea (arrow) with "one and a half turns".
- Interscalar septum is normal at the basal part; but not seen at the superior part.
- Vestibule and SCC are normal.

- Vestibule and SCCs may be normal or malformed.
- Cochlear nerve may be absent or hypoplastic. IAC is small.
- Cochlear hypoplasia is a heterogeneous group with wide spectrum. There are four subtypes (**Table 4**).
- The CH-II form is particularly prone to cerebrospinal fluid (CSF) leak or being a "gusher" during CI due to the wide connection with IAC. In fact, the electrode may extend into the IAC (**Fig. 8**).
- The CH-II patients are also prone to recurrent meningitis due to deficiency of stapes footplate.

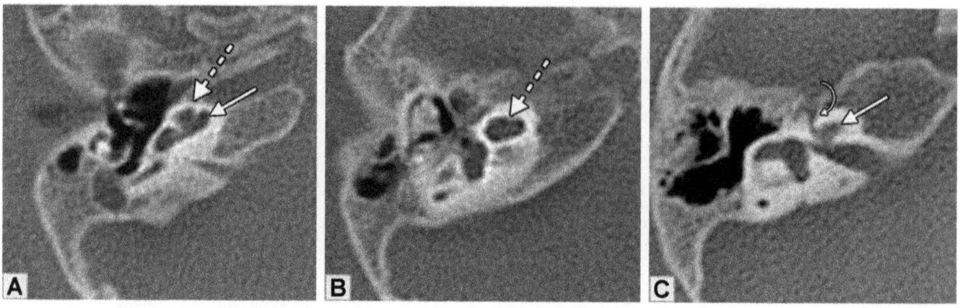

FIGS. 10A TO C: Group 5 IEM: Right-sided cochlear hypoplasia subtype IV (CH-IV): Axial HRCT images reveal:
- Basal turn of cochlea is normal (arrow); however, the middle and apical turns are hypoplastic (dotted arrow).
- Note the anterior location of labyrinthine segment of facial nerve (curved arrow) in relation to cochlea (arrow in C).

TABLE 4 **Morphological features of various subtypes of cochlear hypoplasia (CH).**

Features	CH-I	CH-II	CH-III	CH-IV
Size	Small	Small	Normal	Normal
Shape	Round or ovoid	Normal	Normal	Normal basal turn
Modiolus	Absent	Absent/defective	Short	• Middle and apical turns hypoplastic • Thin, position more anteromedial than normal
Interscalar septum	Absent	Absent/defective	Reduced in length (**Fig. 9**)	
Internal auditory canal	Appears to arise directly from cochlea (**Figs. 6** and **7**)	Wide communication (**Fig. 8**)		
Other anomalies		• Vestibular dilation • Vestibular aqueduct dilation • Stapes footplate defective	Stapes fixation	• Facial nerve labyrinthine segment is located anterior to cochlea (**Fig. 10**) • Stapes fixation

- While CH-II can have a defective stapes, CH-III and CH-IV can be associated with stapes fixation; and hence show mixed hearing loss (HL) on audiometry (**Figs. 9** and **10**).

- Cochlear nerve aplasia/hypoplasia is frequent. Herein, the better side should be chosen for CI. If present, the ABI is required.
- Also, electrodes need to be modified with smaller electrodes required (thin, short).
- Not a contraindication to CI. However, result of CI depends on the number of electrodes that can be accommodated and degree of CN hypoplasia.

Differential Diagnosis

Cochlear hypoplasia III can appear very similar to IP-II, though the term "cochlea with 1.5 turns" ideally refers to CH-III, and not IP-II.

Group 6 (Incomplete Partition Anomalies)

- These are the most common group of anomalies constituting >40% of IEMs.
- These anomalies are characterized by IP of cochlea, i.e., deficiencies in the interscalar (IS) septum, and/or modiolus in varying degrees of severity.
- However, there is clear differentiation between cochlea and vestibule; and the external dimensions, i.e., size of the cochlea, are normal (vs. CH).
- There are three subtypes as detailed in **Table 5**.

TABLE 5 **Clinicoradiological differentiating features of subtypes of incomplete partition type-II (IP-II).**

	IP-I	IP-II	IP-III
Synonym/ association	Cystic cochlea-vestibular malformation (**Figs. 11** to **13**)	Mondini deformity (**Figs. 14** and **15**)	Pseudo-Mondini X-linked deafness (**Fig. 16**)
Modiolus	Completely absent	Apical part defective	Completely absent
Interscalar septum	Completely absent	Apical part defective	Completely absent
Vestibule	Enlarged	Minimal dilation	
Vestibular aqueduct	Enlargement rare	Enlarged	Medially located, dilation may be or may not be present
IAC/cochlea communication	Defect (CSF fills cochlea)	Absent	Defect present and bulbous IAC
Stapes	Footplate absent	Normal	Normal
Complications	Recurrent meningitis, gusher	Progressive hearing loss	• Gusher • Facial nerve stimulation (half band electrodes with smooth lateral end preferred)
Cochlear nerve	Present or aplastic	Present	Present

(CSF: cerebrospinal fluid; IAC: internal auditory canal)

Incomplete Partition Type I

- It is caused by abnormal differentiation of inner ear structure development at a stage later than Michel's anomaly, CA, and CC anomaly (about 5th week of gestation).
- Rare, consists of 6% of all congenital inner ear anomalies.
- Two cystic structures in place of cochlea and vestibule. The vestibule is often dilated, modiolus is absent (**Figs. 11** to **13**). IAC is always dilated. Cribriform plate between base of cochlea and IAC may be deficient.

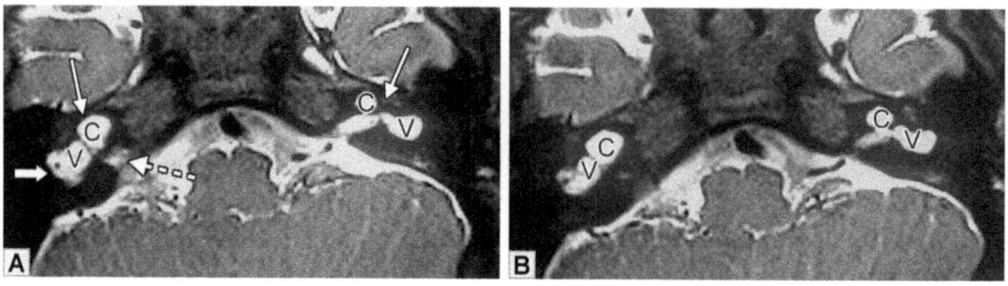

FIGS. 11A AND B: Group 6 IEM: Incomplete partition type-I (IP-I) on MRI: T2-weighted MRI axial images reveal:
- Cystic structure in both ears with "figure of eight" appearance (arrow).
- Malformed cochlea (C) without bony modiolus, and a deformed dilated vestibule (V).
- SCCs are absent on left side, dysplastic on right side (block arrow).
- Right IAC is dilated (dotted arrow).

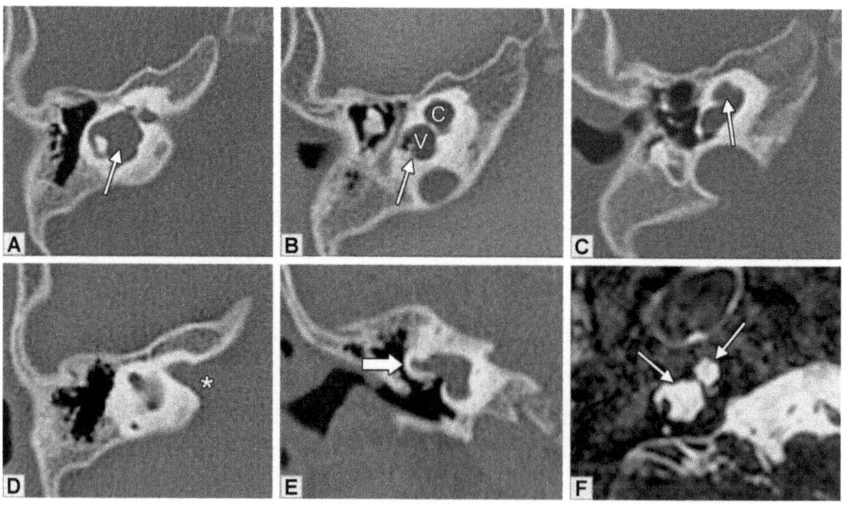

FIGS. 12A TO F: Group 6 IEM: Right-sided incomplete partition type-I (IP-I): (A to D) HRCT axial, (E) coronal, and (F) CISS axial MR images reveal:
- A cystic cochlea without any internal architecture (C), and a dilated vestibule (V); producing a "figure of eight" appearance.
- The IAC is dilated (asterisk). The semicircular canals are dysplastic (block arrow).
- The cochlea and vestibule appear hyperintense, without any internal architecture on MRI (arrows in F).

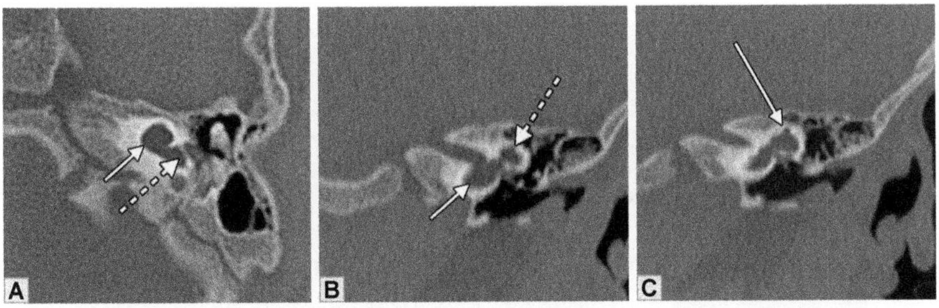

FIGS. 13A TO C: Group 6 IEM: Left-sided incomplete partition type-I (IP-I) with semicircular canal (SCC) dysplasia (cystic cochleovestibular dysplasia): (A) HRCT axial, (B and C) coronal images reveal:

- Two cystic rudimentary structures in the location of cochlea (arrow) and vestibule (dotted arrow). The superior SCC is stunted (long arrow). Other SCC is not visualized.

- Not a contraindication to CI, but predisposes to meningitis and CSF leak after CI due to defective cribriform plate.
- Incomplete partition type-I malformation is associated with a high-risk of recurrent meningitis (even without CI surgery). This is due to wide communication between IAC and cochlea, as a consequence of which CSF fills the cochlea. Further the stapes footplate is absent, hence any infection of ME spreads to the CSF readily though the oval window. In fact, a large cyst has been at surgery in the region of the stapes footplate.

Differential Diagnosis: Common Cavity

- In CC, there is no differentiation into cochlea and vestibule.
- In IP-I, cochlea is separately identifiable from vestibule, giving rise to "figure of eight" appearance.

Incomplete Partition Type II

Synonym: Mondini deformity

- Incomplete partition type-II malformation is characterized by deficiency in apical part of modiolus and IS septum, resulting in fusion of apical and middle turns; basal turn is normal (**Figs. 14** and **15**).
- This is the most common IEM.
- Cochlea consists of one and a half turns; middle and apical turns fuse.
- It is hypothesized that an enlarged vestibular aqueduct (EVA) leads to transmission of CSF pulsations to cochlea, resulting in defective development of the modiolus. This also results in "third window effect" (also see Chapter 26).
- Hence during CI surgery CSF pulsation may be observed at round window.
- Hearing loss in IP-II is progressive and hearing can be normal at birth. Head trauma accelerates progression, and hence affected children are cautioned accordingly.

Differential Diagnosis: CH-III

Since the size of cochlea is normal in IP-II, the term "cochlea with 1.5 turns" should not be used (reserved for CH-III).

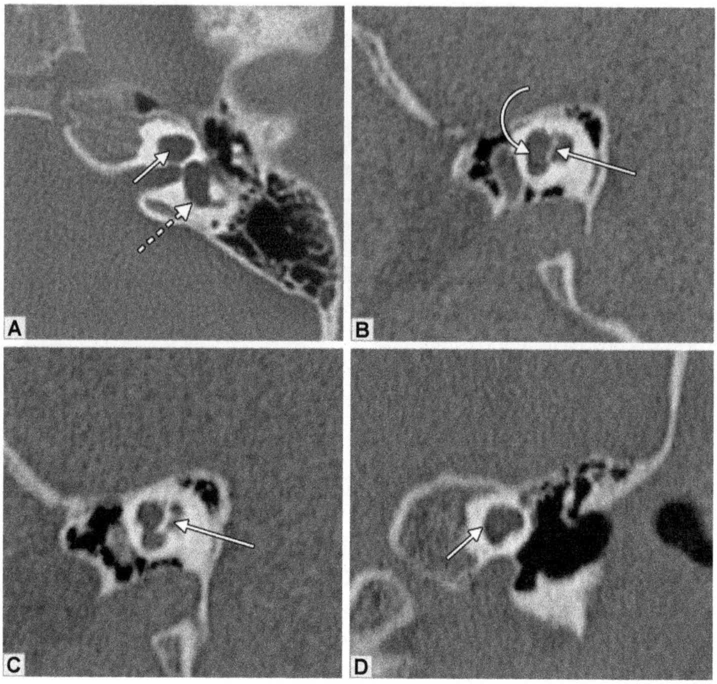

FIGS. 14A TO D: Group 6 IEM: Left-sided incomplete partition type-II (Mondini dysplasia): (A) HRCT axial, (B and C) sagittal, and (D) coronal images reveal:

- A dilated cochlea (arrow) and vestibule (dotted arrow).
- The modiolus is present; osseous spiral lamina (long arrow) seen near basal turn but not seen at cochlear apex (curved arrow).

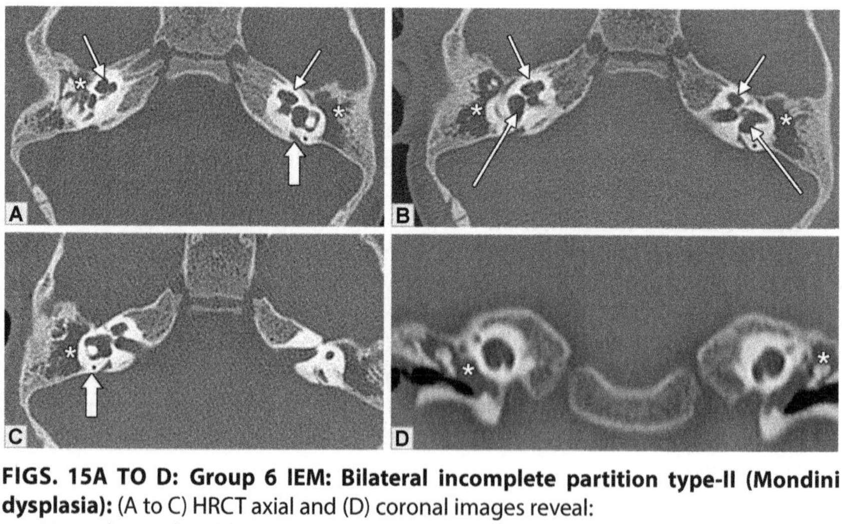

FIGS. 15A TO D: Group 6 IEM: Bilateral incomplete partition type-II (Mondini dysplasia): (A to C) HRCT axial and (D) coronal images reveal:

- Normal size of cochlea on both the sides (arrow).
- The vestibule (long arrow) and vestibular aqueduct (block arrow) are dilated.
- Note soft tissue opacification of bilateral middle ear (asterisk) due to congenital cholesteatoma.

Incomplete Partition Type III

- Incomplete partition type-III is a rare IEM seen in X-linked deafness.
- Herein, primarily the bony labyrinth (otic capsule) is thin, while the membranous labyrinth is normal. The IS septum is normal but modiolus is absent (**Fig. 16**).
- Wide communication between a bulbous IAC and cochlea leads to a high-risk of CSF leak (gusher) during CI.
- The FN (labyrinthine segment) has an abnormal course, i.e., just above cochlea; while normally it courses around the basal turn (as seen in axial CT).
- Due to a deficient membranous labyrinth patients may have associated conductive HL. However, this is not due to stapedial fixation and stapedectomy should not be attempted during CT, as there is a risk of gusher. More CSF will leak and worsen the HL.

Group 7: Enlarged Vestibular Aqueduct (EVLA/EVA)

Synonyms: Large vestibular aqueduct syndrome (LVAS),[4] large endolymphatic sac anomaly (LESA)

- An anomaly is placed into this group if vestibular aqueduct (VA) is dilated but cochlea and vestibule are normal (vs. IP-II) (**Figs. 17** and **18**).
- A dilated VA results in CSF pressure being transmitted to cochlea, and HL due to "third window phenomenon."

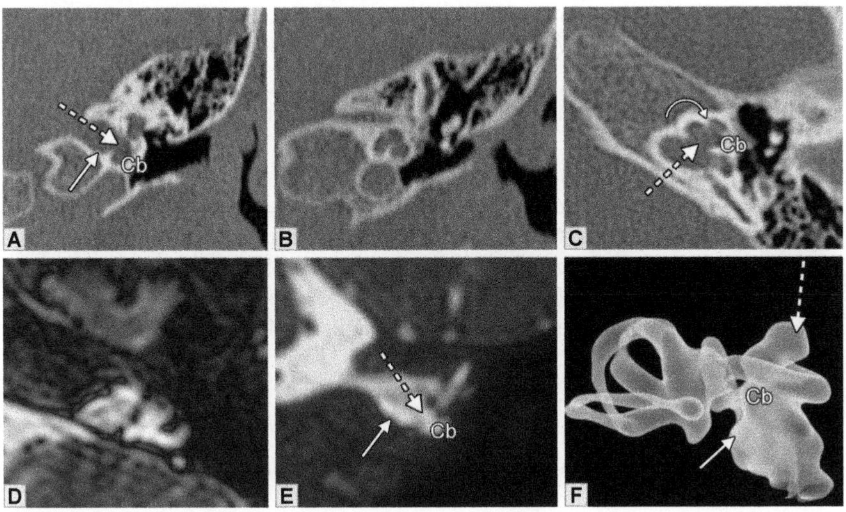

FIGS. 16A TO F: Group 6 IEM: Left-sided incomplete partition type-III (IP-III): (A and B) Coronal HRCT, (C) axial HRCT, (D and E) axial and coronal CISS MRI, and (F) VRT images reveal:

- Bulbous dilation of the IAC at the end (arrows).
- Deficient modiolus, leading to a wide communication (dotted arrow) of basal turn of cochlea (Cb) and IAC.
- Vestibule is normal (D).
- Poorly formed interscalar septum (curved arrow), leading to a rounded configuration of middle and apical turns of cochlea on VRT images (dotted arrow in F).

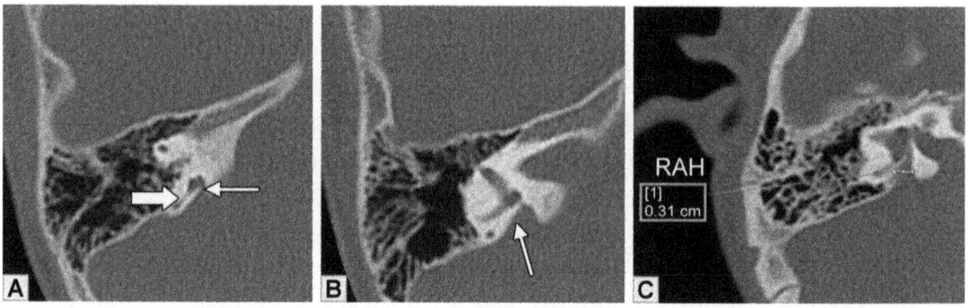

FIGS. 17A TO C: Group 7 IEM, Right sided enlarged vestibular aqueduct (EVA).
- Axial HRCT images show dilated vestibular aqueducts. The dimension of aqueduct is to be measured midway (arrows) between the crus and the external opening. The posterior SCC (block arrow) serves as the internal reference. A diameter more than the posterior SCC is abnormal.
- Measurement of dilated vestibular aqueduct (C) (3.1 mm at the mid part).

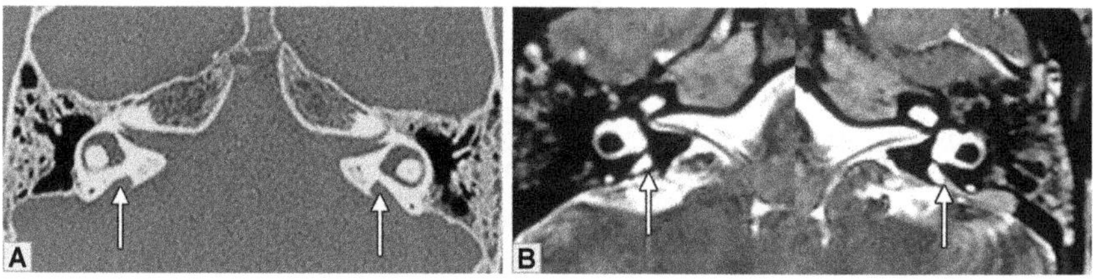

FIGS. 18A AND B: Group 7 IEM: Bilateral enlarged vestibular aqueduct (EVA). (A) Axial HRCT and (B) CISS MR images show dilated vestibular aqueducts (arrows in A) and endolymphatic sac (arrows in B). The vestibule and cochlea are normal.

- The SNHL is mostly progressive but can also be sudden. Pattern of HL is also variable.
- Criteria for a dilated VA:
  - *Visual approximation*: VA larger than the adjacent posterior SCC.
  - *Valvassori criteria*: Measure size of VA at midpoint of posterior labyrinth and operculum. Normal is <1.5 mm; dilated ≥1.5 mm (**Fig. 17**).
  - *Cincinnati criteria*: Midpoint of VA ≥1 mm or operculum ≥2 mm.
  - Midpoint diameter measured in Pöschl plane (45° oblique) >0.9 mm.

Vestibule and Semicircular Canal Anomalies

- Isolated vestibular anomalies are rare.
- Isolated SCC anomalies are commoner than vestibular anomalies, but these are also uncommon.
- Semicircular canal development starts from 6th to 8th week gestational age and completed by 19th to 22nd week. The order of development is superior, posterior, and lateral at the last.
- Hence, whenever the superior SCC and posterior SCC are dysplastic, lateral SCC (LSCC) is very rarely normal (**Figs. 19** and **20**).
- *Exception to this rule*: Isolated posterior SCC aplasia in Alagille syndrome and Waardenburg syndrome.
- Most often associated with other inner ear anomalies (**Fig. 21**).

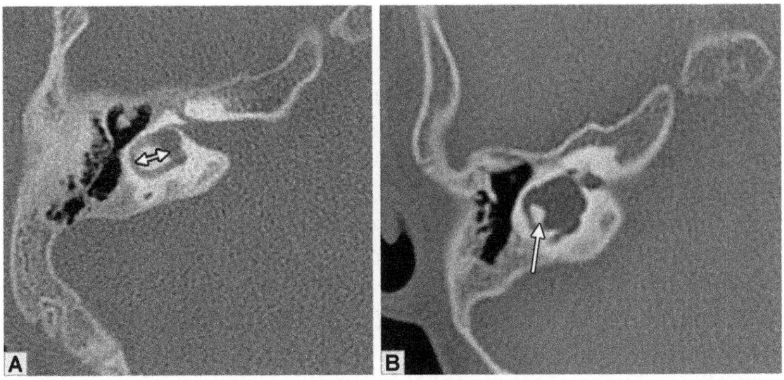

FIGS. 19A AND B: Measurement for semicircular canal (SCC) dysplasia: (A) The bony island which needs to be measured is shown with double-sided arrow in a normal temporal bone. (B) Decreased width of the island in SCC dysplasia.

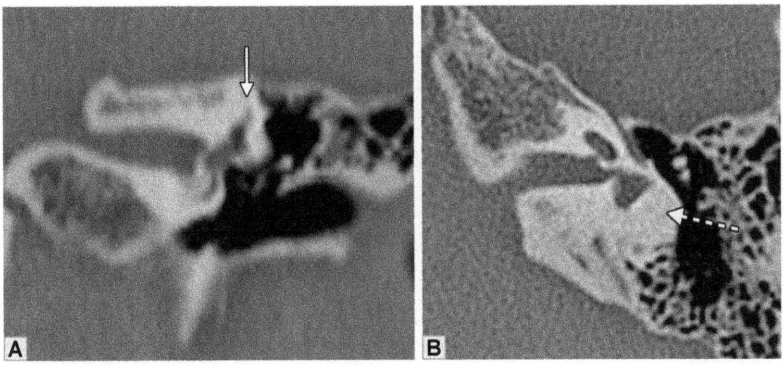

FIGS. 20A AND B: Left-sided semicircular canal (SCC) dysplasia: (A) Coronal and (B) axial HRCT images reveal:

- Left superior SCC (arrow in A) is small.
- Nonvisualized lateral SCC (dotted arrow in B).

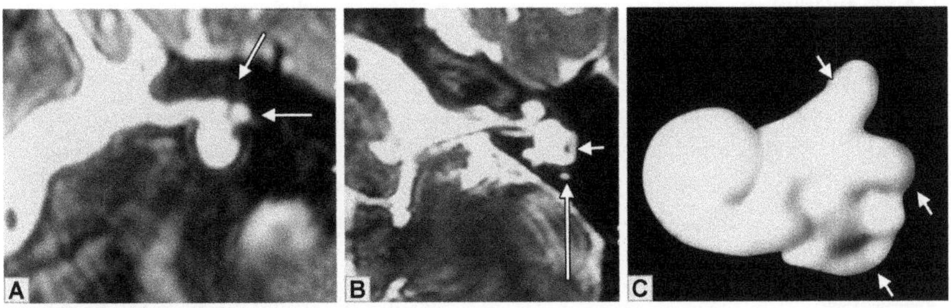

FIGS. 21A TO C: Left sided semicircular canal dysplasia associated with type I incomplete partition:

- Coronal (A) and axial (B) CISS images reveal: Two cystic structures in place of cochlea and vestibule, without any internal architecture. Vestibule is dilated.
- Lateral SCC is small (long arrows). Note the small hypointense bony island of LSCC (small arrow). Superior SCC is also not visualized (long arrow in B).
- VRT image showing dysplastic SCCs on left ear (arrows in C).

- Dysplasia of SCC is more common than aplasia. Dysplastic SCCs are short and wide.
- *Measurement of dysplasia*: Measurement of the width of bony island of LSCC on axial HRCT (normal 2.6–4.8 cm) is a sensitive measurement of dysplasia (**Fig. 19**).
- In "LSCC-vestibular canal dysplasia", a severe form of SCC dysplasia, the vestibule is dilated and forms a common lumen with the LSCC.
- Cochlea may be normal or malformed, depending on the gestational age of insult.
- *Semicircular canal aplasia*: Associated with CHARGE syndrome (coloboma, heart anomaly, choanal atresia, growth retardation and genitourinary anomalies), abnormal course of FN, and oval window atresia.

Differential Diagnosis of Canal Aplasia

Labyrinthitis Ossificans: The Differentiating Features are:
- Calcification within the canal can be seen in LO.
- In fibrous obliteration of canal, HRCT shows the SCC.
- Semicircular canal is not visualized in aplasia.

Internal Auditory Canal Anomalies

(Discussed in Chapter 12)

Table 6 and **Figure 22** summarize the different types of IEM in Sennaroglu classification with their close differentials.[5]

TABLE 6 Closely mimicking entities in Sennaroglu classification.

Type	Differential diagnosis	Key differentiating features
1 (CLA)	Labyrinthitis ossificans (LO)	Bulge of promontory present in LO, absent in CLA
3a (CA with normal labyrinth)	LO	Bulge of promontory present in LO, absent in CA with normal
3b (CADV)	Common cavity (CC)	See Table 2
4 (CC)	• CADV • IP-I	• See Table 2 • Figure of eight configuration in IP-I, differentiation into rudimentary cochlea and vestibule; single cystic structure in CC
5 (cochlear hypoplasia III)	IP-II	Size of cochlea is normal in IP-II; reduced in CH-III
SCC aplasia	LO	• Calcification within the canal can be seen in labyrinthitis ossificans • In fibrous obliteration of canal, HRCT shows the SCC • Whereas in aplasia, SCC is not visualized

(CA: cochlear aplasia; CADV: cochlear aplasia with dilated vestibule; CH: cochlear hypoplasia; CLA: complete labyrinthine aplasia; IP-II: incomplete partition type-II; SCC: semicircular canal)

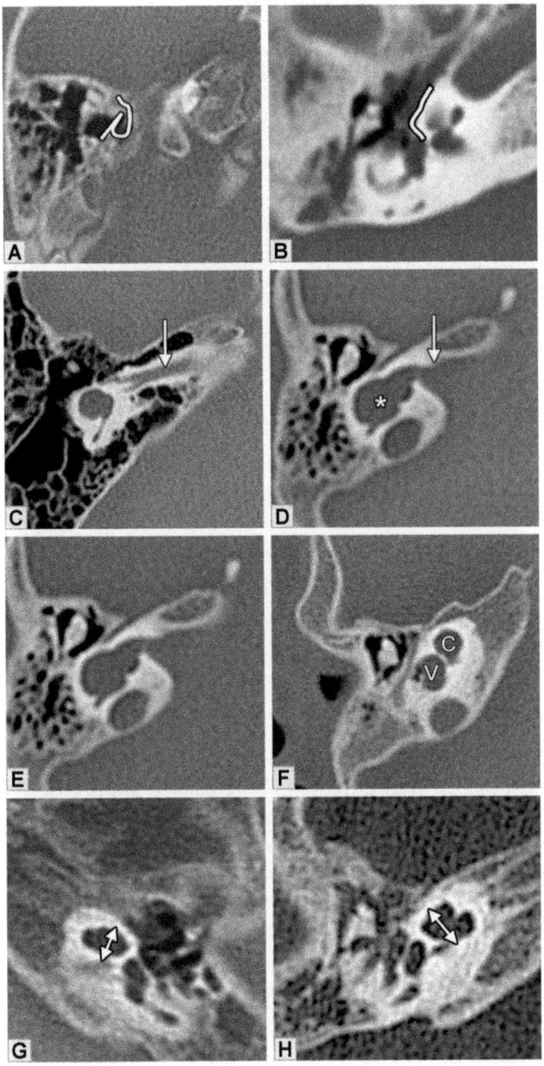

FIGS. 22A TO H: Closely mimicking entities according to Sennaroglu classification: (A) CLA versus (B) LO. The medial wall of ME lacks the bulge of promontory in CLA (marked in A). In LO, the bulge is present (marked in B). Although cochlear basal turn is still appreciable in B; in advanced cases, entire cochlea may be obliterated; thereby making this point of differentiation helpful. **(C) CADV versus (D) CC.** The location of IAC (arrow) is normal in CADV. In CC, the IAC is posterolaterally located (arrow), and enters the center of the cystic structure (asterisk). **(E) CC versus (F) IP-I:** There is no differentiation of the cystic structure into cochlea (C) and vestibule (V) in CC; unlike in IP-I. The cochlea and vestibule in IP-I are malformed, though. **(G) CH-III versus (H) IP-II.** The cochlear size is small in CH-III; compared to the normal size in IP-II. The double-sided arrows give a rough subjective estimate of the cochlear height. Ideally cochlear height should be measured on an oblique coronal image; horizontal cochlear height on axial image at modiolar level (refer to Chapter 14).

OTHER CLASSIFICATION SYSTEMS

While Sennaroglu system remains the most frequently followed classification system; other newer classifications have been proposed by some investigators. Two such systems are discussed below.

INCAV

- This system was introduced in 2016 by Adilbelli et al.,[6] in order to device an easier classification system for both radiologists and ENT surgeons.
- This comprises of five components:
    i. Internal acoustic canal
    ii. Cochlear nerve
    iii. Cochlea
    iv. Vestibular aqueduct
    v. Vestibule

Internal Acoustic Canal (I)

Internal acoustic canal is divided into four types: (1) I0 (normal); (2) I1 (enlarged); (3) I2 (narrow); and (4) I3 (atretic). For ascertaining the size of IAC, the anteroposterior (AP diameter) was considered, with <2 mm or >8 mm being considered as abnormal.

Cochlear Nerve (N)

Cochlear nerve is divided into four types: (1) N0 (normal); (2) N1 (thick); (3) N2 (hypoplastic); and (4) N3 (not detected on MRI). The diameter of the normal CN on MRI typically varies from 1.1 to 1.4 mm if <0.2 mm, it is not detected on MRI. Nerve was labeled as hypoplastic if measuring between 0.2 and 0.6 mm; or based on comparison with FN (if less than FN).

On CT, only two options are given. N0 for normal; and Nx for abnormal.

Cochlea (C)

Cochlea is divided into seven types: C0–C6.

1. C0: Normal
2. C1: Corresponds to IP-II
3. C2: Corresponds to IP-III
4. C3: Hypoplasia, dimensions are reduced. This is again subdivided into A, B, and C subtypes. Type A corresponds to CH-I, type B corresponds to CH-II, and type C corresponds to CH-III.
5. C4: Corresponds to IP-I
6. C5: Corresponds to common cavity
7. C6: Cochlear aplasia

Vestibular Aqueduct (A)

Vestibular aqueduct is categorized into two types: A0 (normal) or A1 (enlarged). On CT, if VA is >1.5 mm it is termed as enlarged. On MRI, if the endolymphatic duct and sac are termed enlarged if they are larger than the adjoining posterior SCC.

Vestibule (V)

Vestibule is divided in seven types:
1. V0: Normal
2. V1: Isolated malformations of SCC
3. V2: Dilated
4. V3: Hypoplasia ± SCC hypoplasia
5. V4: Cochleovestibular anomaly, "figure of eight" appearance
6. V5: Common cavity
7. V6: Absent vestibule

SMS Classification

Another newer simplified classification (the SMS classification) has been proposed by Grover et al. in 2019;[7] keeping in mind the surgical implications of cochleovestibular anomalies. This classification system takes three major parameters into account: (1) The cochlear morphology; (2) The modiolus; and (3) The lamina cribrosa. This has been discussed in **Flowchart 1**.

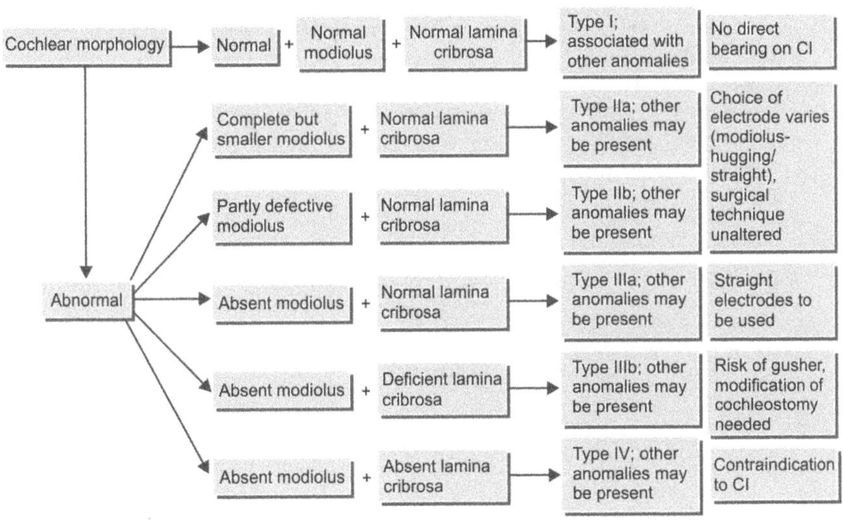

FLOWCHART 1: Algorithmic representation of **SMS classification system.**

SYNDROMES AND IEMS

Various congenital anomalies and syndromes are associated with EVLA. Cochleovestibular malformations are associated in more than one-third of patients.

- *Pendred syndrome*: Euthyroid goiter with SNHL due to IEM, commonly IP-II or EVA
- Choanal atresia
- Coloboma
- CHARGE syndrome
- Branchio-oto-renal syndrome
- Congenital heart defects

In conclusion, the institute should adopt any one classification system, and should be followed by all involved departments.

REFERENCES

1. Jackler RK, Luxford WM, House WF. Congenital malformations of the inner ear: a classification based on embryogenesis. Laryngoscope. 1987;97(3 Pt 2, Suppl 40):2-14.
2. Sennaroglu L, Saatci I. A new classification for cochleovestibular malformations. Laryngoscope. 2002;112(12):2230-41.
3. Joshi VM, Navelkar SK, Kishore GR, Reddy KJ, Vinay Kumar EC. CT and MR Imaging of the Inner Ear and Brain in Children with Congenital Sensorineural Hearing Loss. Radiographics. 2012;32:683-98
4. Berrettini S, Forli F, Bogazzi F, Neri E, Salvatori L, Casani AP, et al. Large vestibular aqueduct syndrome: audiological, radiological, clinical, and genetic features. Am J Otolaryngol. 2005;26:363-71.
5. Sennaroglu L, Bajin MD. Classification and Current Management of Inner Ear Malformations. Balkan Med J. 2017;34(5):397-411.
6. Adibelli ZH, Isayeva L, Koc AM, Catli T, Adibelli H, Olgun L. The new classification system for inner ear malformations: the INCAV system. Acta Otolaryngol. 2017;137(3):246-52.
7. Grover M, Sharma S, Preetam C, Gupta G, Samdani S, Agarwal S, et al. New SMS classification of cochleovestibular malformation and its impact on decision-making. J Laryngol Otol. 2019;133(5): 368-75.

12

Imaging of the Internal Acoustic Canal

Smita Manchanda, Ajay Garg

- Normal Anatomy
- Congenital IAC Malformations
  - Atresia/Stenosis
  - Dilatation
  - Abnormal Orientation
  - Duplication Anomalies
- Vascular Loops
- Tumors of the IAC
- Abnormal Enhancement in IAC (Apart from Tumors)
- Cochlear Nerve Abnormalities

- The internal acoustic canal (IAC) is an important bony canal in the temporal bone through which the seventh and eighth cranial nerve complexes pass. It transmits nerves and vessels from the posterior cranial fossa to the cochleovestibular apparatus.
- The chapter will first discuss the normal anatomy, followed by common pathologies: Both congenital and acquired.

NORMAL ANATOMY

Internal acoustic canal is a bony canal in the posterior portion of the temporal bone. The embryology, structure, and normal dimensions are detailed below.[1,2]

- *Embryology*:
  - Fibers of the vestibulocochlear nerve (VCN) grow to contact the cochlea and vestibule; and by the 8 week of gestation, they are surrounded by the chondrification process of the mesoderm.
  - This mesoderm transforms into cartilage and bone which form the IAC.
- *Structure*:
  - *Porus acusticus internus [internal auditory meatus (IAM)]* is the medial open aperture located near the center of the posterior surface of the petrous part of the temporal bone.
  - The *fundus* is the lateral end, limited by a thin bony plate the *lamina cribrosa* which separates fundus from cochlea and vestibule.
  - The *falciform crest or transverse crest* separates superior from inferior part, whereas the *Bill's bar* separates anterosuperior from posterosuperior section.
  - *Contents*: The contents of the IAC include—neural structures: Coated by arachnoid membrane; and its lining (dural sheet); VCN (cochlear, superior, and inferior vestibular nerve, singular nerve); facial nerve (FN) (and intermedius portion); labyrinthine artery and the vestibular ganglion.

- *The specific contents with location of nerves are as follows (**Fig. 1**)*:
  - Anterosuperior part—FN
  - Anteroinferior—cochlear nerve (CN)
  - Posterosuperior section—superior vestibular nerve
  - Posteroinferior—inferior vestibular nerve, singular nerve
- *Normal dimensions*:
  - *Shape*: The IAC can have variable shapes with cylindrical being the most common (50%). It can also be ovoid with greatest height in middle part (25%) or have a wedge-shaped appearance (25%).[1]
  - *Length*: The distance from the midpoint of the opening of the IAC to the extremity of the canal in its most concave portion is the length. Normal dimension is 4–15 mm, average 8 mm.
  - *Diameter (**Fig. 2**)*: A perpendicular straight line drawn at the midpoint of the IAC length from the anterior to the posterior wall is used to measure the diameter. Normal range is 2–8 mm, average 5 mm with intraindividual difference between both sides not more than 1 mm.

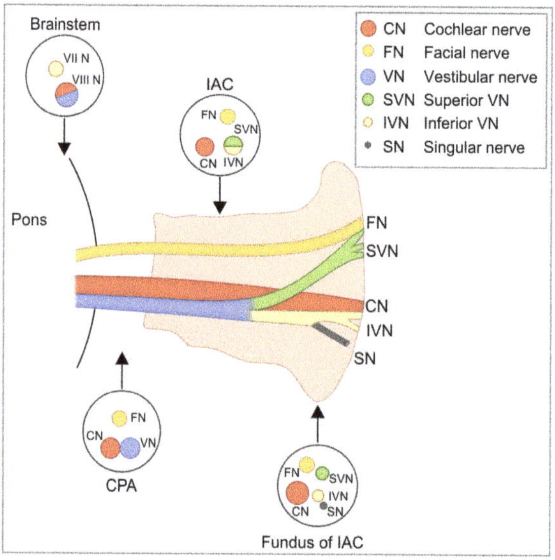

FIG. 1: Anatomy of nerves coursing through IAC.

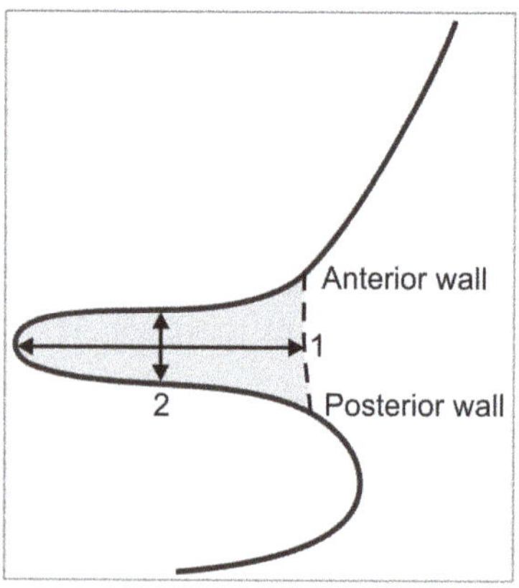

FIG. 2: Measurement of dimensions of the IAC: (1) Longitudinal length of the canal; (2) Anteroposterior diameter of the canal.

CONGENITAL IAC MALFORMATIONS

The reported malformations of the IAC include atresia or stenosis, dilatation, abnormal orientation, and duplication anomalies.

Atresia/Stenosis of the IAC

- Internal auditory meatus stenosis accounts for 12% of all congenital temporal bone malformations.[1]
- Embryology: Stenosis of IAC results from altered VCN development. This can be secondary to failure of chemotactic mechanisms or a lack of end-organ targets, the cochlea or vestibule.
- Minimal diameter required for the neurovascular bundle running through the IAC is about 2 mm and a diameter of 2 mm or less is regarded as significant. Hence a canal <2.0 mm in diameter is suggestive of a stenosis.
- It is usually associated with hypoplasia/aplasia of the nerves:
    - Cochlear nerve hypoplasia—CN with its diameter smaller than that of the FN.
    - Cochlear nerve aplasia—CN not detected with MRI (**Figs. 3** and **4**).
- Internal acoustic canal anomalies are frequently associated with other inner ear anomalies (**Figs. 5** and **6**).

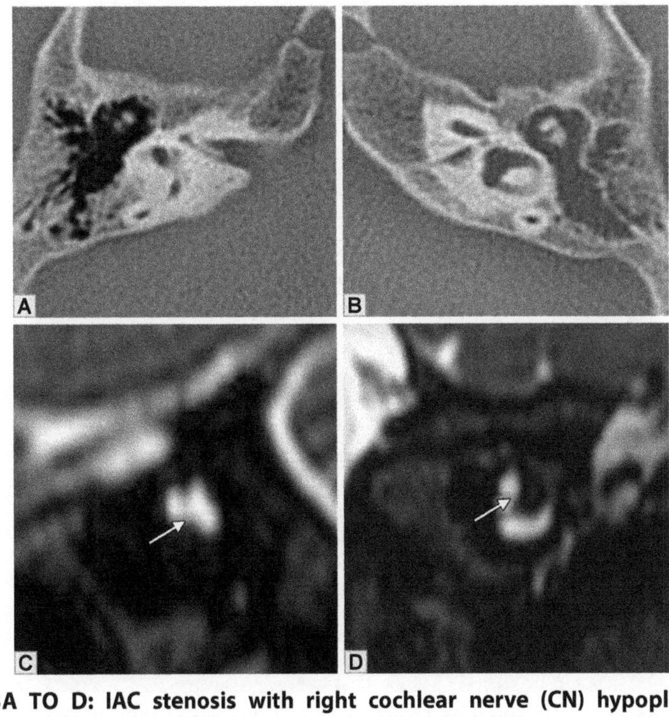

FIGS. 3A TO D: IAC stenosis with right cochlear nerve (CN) hypoplasia and left CN aplasia: (A) Mild narrowing of right IAC; (B) Marked narrowing of left IAC; (C) Right CN hypoplasia [small hypointense structure (arrow) inferior to the facial nerve]; (D) Left CN aplasia (arrow).

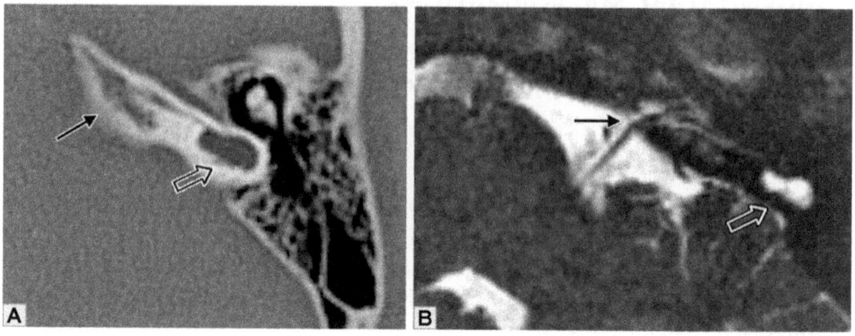

FIGS. 4A AND B: IAC stenosis with common cavity and cochlear nerve aplasia: (A) Deformed and markedly narrow left IAC (arrow) with undifferentiated cochlea and vestibule (open arrow) suggestive of common cavity; (B) Axial constructive interference in steady state: Absence of CN within the atretic IAC (arrow). The common cavity (open arrow) is also well seen.

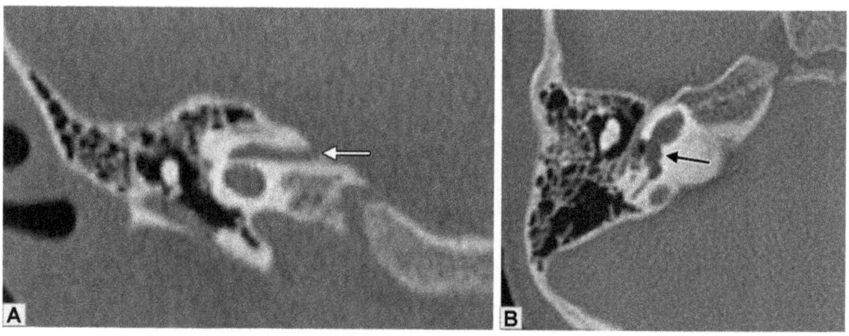

FIGS. 5A AND B: IAC stenosis with common cavity: (A) Coronal HRCT shows narrow right IAC (arrow); (B) Axial plane reveals a single cavity representing the undifferentiated cochlea and vestibule suggestive of common cavity (arrow).

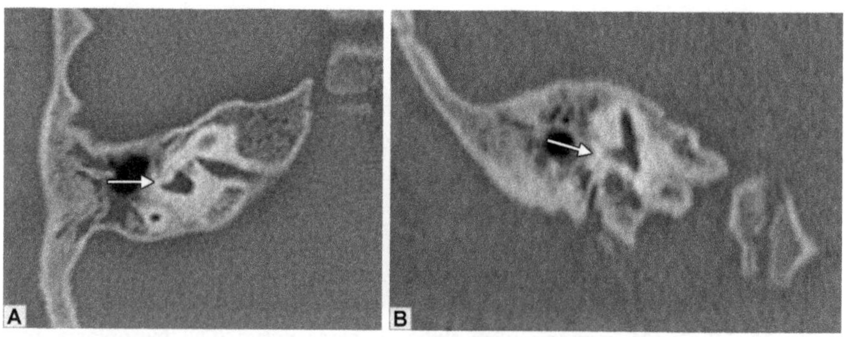

FIGS. 6A AND B: IAC stenosis lateral semicircular canal (LSCC) hypoplasia: (A) Narrow IAC with a short LSCC confluent with the vestibule (arrow); (B) Coronal plane also shows the right LSCC hypoplasia (arrow).

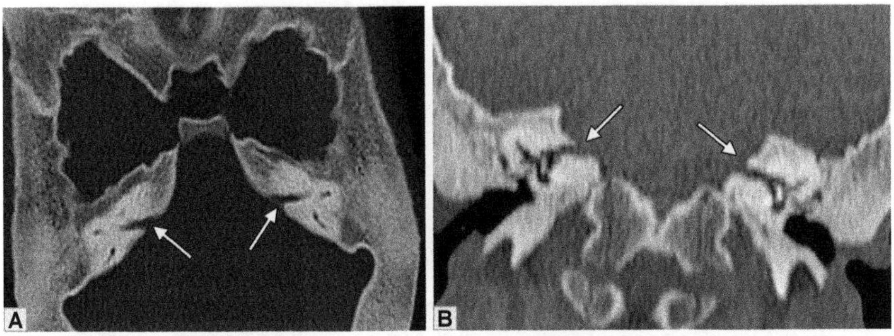

FIGS. 7A AND B: IAC stenosis in case of sclerosing dysplasia: (A) Axial and (B) coronal HRCT. There is significant narrowing of the bilateral IAC in this known case of sclerosing dysplasia. Note the generalized increase in bone density and diffuse calvarial thickening.

- In cases of maldeveloped labyrinth, IAC is narrow and tapering laterally.
- Unilateral/bilateral internal auditory canal anomalies may occasionally be associated with middle or external ear anomalies and rarely associated with systemic disease (**Figs. 7A** and **B**).

Dilatation of the IAC

- The IAC is dilated if the diameter is >8 mm. It is usually asymptomatic and is unlikely to be recognized as abnormal.
- There is no adequate embryological explanation for the abnormally dilated IAC.
- Dilatation may be associated with thinning or bony defect between the IAC and perilymph space of the inner ear. There may be bony fundus defects with the wall of the vestibular labyrinth or the margin of the basal turn of the cochlea.
- Clinical significance of dilated IAC is the risk of perilymph hydrops and "*stapes gusher*" during stapes surgery (**Figs. 8A** to **D**)
- If the IAC is abnormally dilated, careful assessment of the bony partition between the IAC and the cochlea/vestibule should be done (**Figs. 9A** and **B**)
- The causes of widening at the lateral end include tumors like acoustic neuroma, chronic hydrocephalus, and dural ectasia (neurofibromatosis secondary to localized increased pressure).

Abnormal Orientation of the Canal

The upward pointing with compression of the nerve structures may be associated with craniosynostosis syndromes.

Duplication of the IAC

- This is a rare anomaly with a thick bony septum dividing the canal into two compartments and can be incomplete or complete (**Fig. 10A** and **B**).

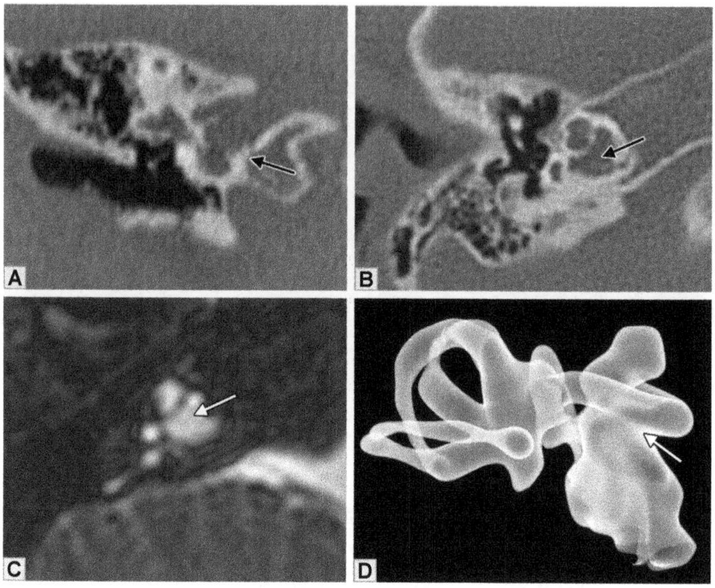

(CSF: cerebrospinal fluid; VRT: volume-rendering technique)

FIGS. 8A TO D: Dilated IAC with abnormal communication with cochlea: (A) Coronal HRCT shows dilated IAC and a bony defect between the fundus and the basal turn of cochlea (arrow); (B) Axial section reveals the abnormal communication between the dilated fundus and basal turn of cochlea (arrow); (C) Axial CISS shows the abnormal communication (arrow) between the dilated IAC and cochlea; (D) VRT image of the inner ear showing the communicating CSF (in IAC) and perilymph space (in cochlea).

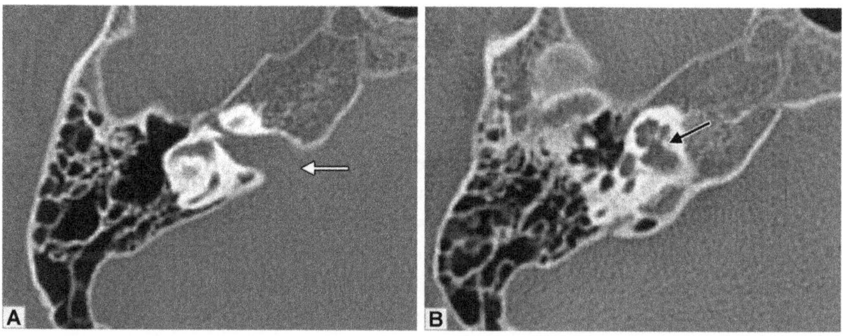

FIGS. 9A AND B: Dilated IAC with intact bony partition: (A) Dilated IAC (arrow); (B) Intact bony partition between the IAC and cochlea (arrow).

- These may be unilateral or bilateral.
- Duplication anomalies have separate bony canals for the seventh and eighth nerves.
- The separate canal is usually stenotic and is often associated with complete sensorineural hearing loss (SNHL).

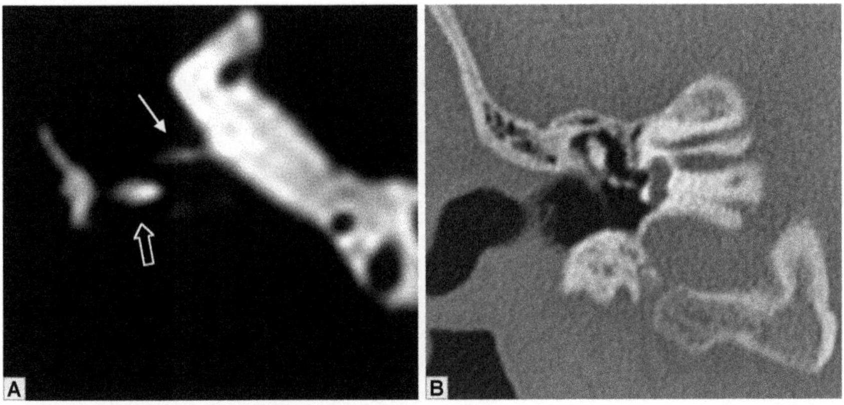

FIGS. 10A AND B: Duplication of IAC: (A) Coronal CISS: Two CSF-containing canals in the region of the IAC. The superior and anterior canal (arrow) appears narrower than the inferior canal (open arrow); (B) HRCT image in the coronal oblique plane: Two separate bony canals in the entire extent.

VASCULAR LOOPS

- Vascular loops of anterior inferior cerebellar artery (AICA) in contact with VCN/FN are a normal variant.
- Vascular cross-compression is characterized by compression of a cranial nerve by a vessel. Excitation of the nerve fibers can occur at the root entry zone (REZ) of the cranial nerve. The REZ of VCN can be located as distally as within the IAC (implies that VCN is predisposed to AICA compression along its entire intracranial length, from the brainstem into the IAC).[3]
- Symptoms occur due to abnormal contact between the nerve and compressing artery, leading to decrease in the inner ear circulation. These include hearing loss, recurrent vertigo, continuous disequilibrium, motion intolerance, pulsatile tinnitus, and hemifacial spasm.
- Reporting of vascular loops on MRI should include anatomical type (**Table 1**) and type of structural relationship between the vessel and nerve (**Table 2**).

TABLE 1 **Anatomical classification of the AICA loop according to Chavda in McDermott, et al.[3]**

Type	Location
I	Within the CPA but does not enter the IAC (**Figs. 11A** and **B**)
II	Enters the IAC and extends <50% of its total length (**Fig. 12**)
III	Extends >50%, into the total length of the IAC (**Figs. 13A** and **B**)

(AICA: anterior inferior cerebellar artery; CPA: cerebellopontine angle; IAC: internal acoustic canal)

Source: McDermott AL, Dutt SN, Irving RM, Pahor AL, Chavda SV. Anterior inferior cerebellar artery syndrome: fact or fiction. Clin Otolaryngol. 2003;28:75-80.

TABLE 2 **Relationship between AICA and VCN on MRI as described by Sirikci A.**[4]

Type	Name	Finding
1	Point compression	The AICA compresses only a limited portion of the VCN (**Fig. 13**)
2	Longitudinal	The AICA approaches the VCN as both traverse parallel to each other (**Fig. 12**)
3	Loop compression	Vascular loop of the AICA encircles the VCN (**Figs. 11** and **12**)
4	Indentation	The AICA compresses the VCN so as to make an indentation in the nerve

(AICA: anterior inferior cerebellar artery; VCN: vestibulocochlear nerve)

Source: Sirikci A, Bayazit Y, Ozer E, Ozkur A, Adaletli I, Cüce MA, et al. Magnetic resonance imaging based classification of anatomic relationship between the cochleovestibular nerve and anterior inferior cerebellar artery in patients with non-specific neuro-otologic symptoms. Surg Radiol Anat. 2005;27(6):531-5.

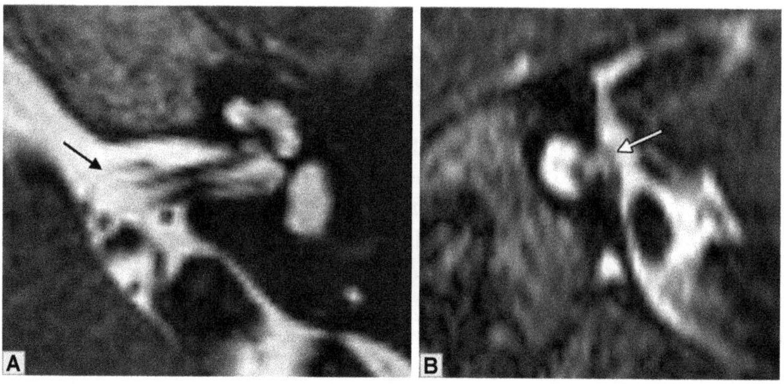

FIGS. 11A AND B: Vascular loop type I: (A) Axial CISS: anterior inferior cerebellar artery (AICA) loop (arrow) within the cerebellopontine cistern (type I); (B) Sagittal oblique section just proximal to the porus acusticus: Vessel (arrow) is encircling the nerve (loop compression type).

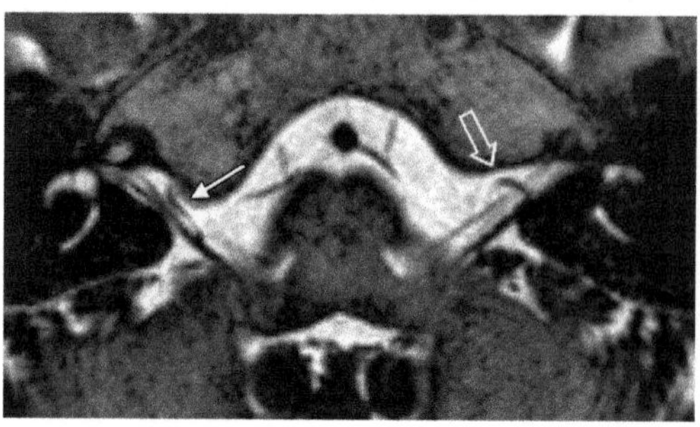

FIG. 12: Vascular loop type II: Axial T2 CISS: AICA loop within the IAC <50% of its depth bilaterally (Type II). Right longitudinal type vascular loop: Nerve and vessel (arrow) traverse parallel to each other. Left loop compression type vascular loop: Vessel (open arrow) encircles the nerve.

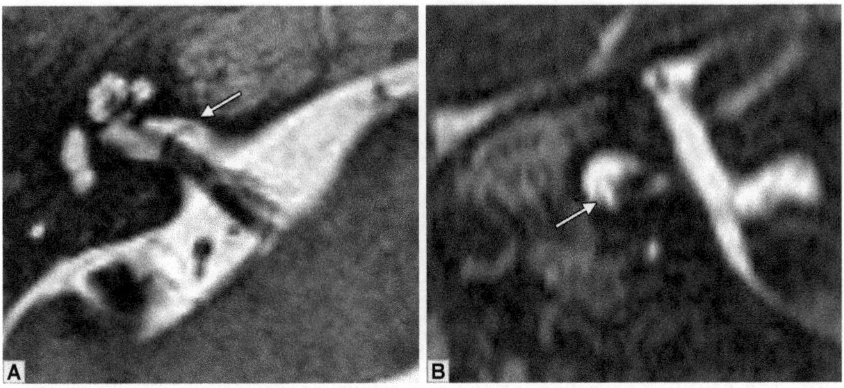

FIGS. 13A AND B: Vascular loop type III: (A) Axial CISS: AICA loop (arrow) extending to >50% of the depth of IAC (type III); (B) Sagittal oblique CISS: Vessel (arrow) compresses the nerve at a single point (point compression type).

TUMORS OF THE INTERNAL ACOUSTIC CANAL

Tumors in the IAC may include primarily intrameatal tumors or extension of lesions in the cerebellopontine (CP) angle. A complete discussion of CP angle tumors is beyond the scope of the chapter and common entities predominantly involving the IAC are discussed here. The most common tumor of this region is the schwannoma.

- *Schwannoma*:
  - It is a benign tumor arising from the nerve sheath and can arise from the FN (facial schwannomas) or the VCNs (vestibular schwannomas)—please refer to Chapter 16 for a detailed description of facial schwannomas. Vestibular schwannomas usually arise from the inferior or superior division of the vestibular nerve; cochlear schwannomas being rare. Hence, commonly schwannomas in this region are referred to as vestibular schwannomas. Acoustic schwannoma, though a misnomer, is often used synonymously with vestibular schwannomas.
  - It is the most common tumor of the internal auditory canal and CP angle region.
- *Types of IAC schwannomas*:
  - *Cerebellopontine angle schwannomas (**Figs. 14A** and **B**)*:
    - Usually of vestibular division and originate near the vestibular ganglion. These are usually aligned parallel to the petrous surface.
    - The comet tail or ice cream cone appearance is typical; with cone or tail representing the intracanalicular extension and the ice cream or comet being the cisternal component.
  - *Typical intracanalicular IAC schwannoma (**Figs. 15A** and **B**)*:
    - Seen classically as a focal, lobulated, intracanalicular mass and are usually vestibular in origin.
    - Treatment is surgical resection with preservation of hearing and FN function.

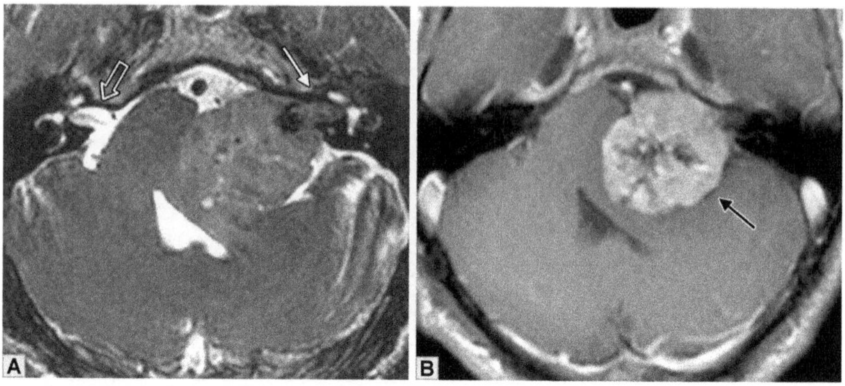

FIGS. 14A AND B: Cerebellopontine angle schwannoma: (A) Axial T2 CISS reveals a large heterogeneous extra-axial mass in the left cerebellopontine cistern causing mass effect on the pons and the fourth ventricle with extension of the mass into the left IAC (white arrow). Note the normal CSF signal intensity in the right IAC (open arrow); (B) Axial postgadolinium T1-weighted image shows intense heterogeneous contrast enhancement of the mass (black arrow).

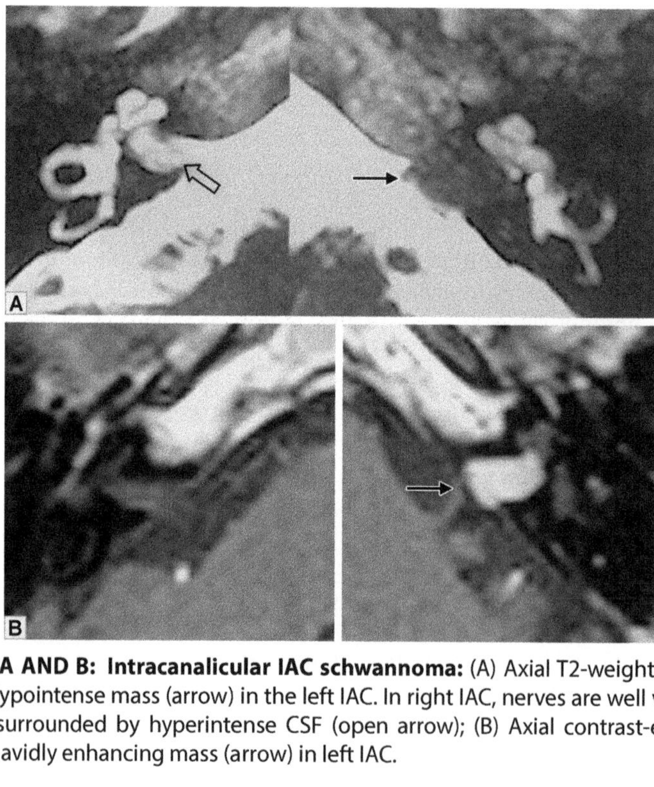

FIGS. 15A AND B: Intracanalicular IAC schwannoma: (A) Axial T2-weighted image (T1WI): Hypointense mass (arrow) in the left IAC. In right IAC, nerves are well visualized and are surrounded by hyperintense CSF (open arrow); (B) Axial contrast-enhanced T1WI: An avidly enhancing mass (arrow) in left IAC.

- *Dumbbell schwannoma of the IAC:*
  - These are distinct from the dumbbell tumor of the CP angle which has a component in the CP angle and another in the IAC. Herein, the two components are in the IAC and the ear.
  - It is like a dumbbell-shaped mass with two globular segments, one in the fundus of IAC and the other in the membranous labyrinth or the geniculate ganglion of the FN.
  - Types: It can be of the following types:
    - Transmodiolar—extends into the cochlea (**Fig. 16**)
    - Transmacular—extends into the vestibule (**Fig. 16**)
    - Facial—extends along the FN (labyrinthine segment) (**Figs. 17** and **18**)
  - Clinical relevance of identifying these dumbbell lesions:
    - Extension into the labyrinth: Hearing preservation surgery is not feasible.
    - Extension to the geniculate ganglion: Need for FN repair.

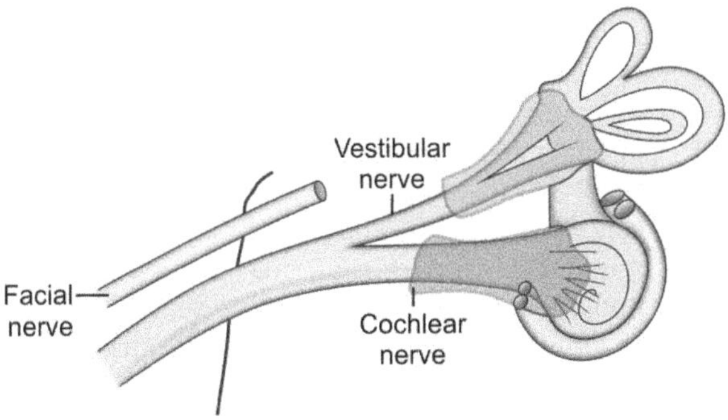

FIG. 16. Dumbbell schwannoma of the IAC (of vestibulocochlear nerve).
- Transmacular—mass extends through the macula into the vestibule.
- Transmodilolar—mass extends through the cochlear aperture and modiolus into the cochlea.

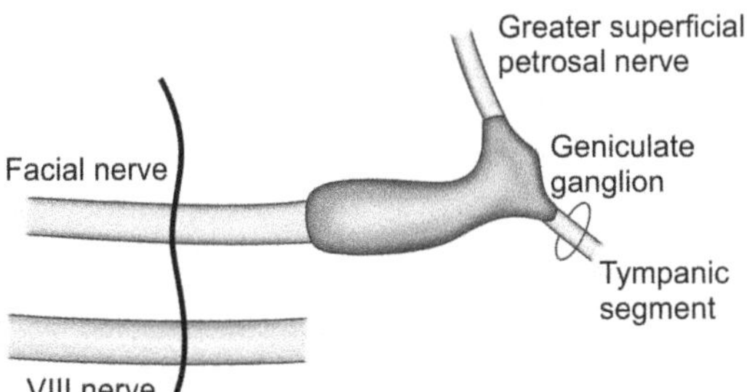

FIG. 17: Dumbbell Schwannoma of IAC (of facial nerve): Mass extends through the enlarged labyrinthine facial canal to involve the geniculate ganglion. Tympanic segment is usually not involved.

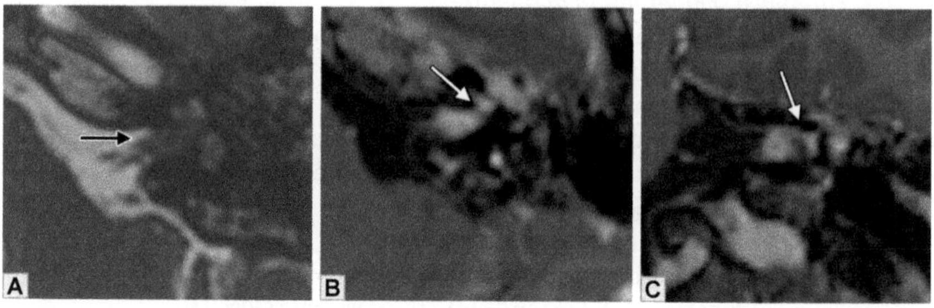

FIGS. 18A TO C: Dumbbell schwannoma of IAC (of facial nerve): (A) Axial CISS: Hypointense mass (arrow) in the left IAC displacing the CSF; Contrast-enhanced T1-weighted images show enhancement into the first genu (arrow in B) and extension along the labyrinthine segment of the facial nerve (arrow in C).

  - *Imaging appearance of vestibular schwannomas*:
    - CT: Isoattenuating lesions on NCCT with homogeneous postcontrast enhancement. Calcifications/hemorrhages are rare.
    - Eighth nerve schwannomas cause bony expansion of IAC whereas facial schwannomas cause a bony expansion of facial canal.
    - MRI: Homogeneous masses which are isointense or slightly hypointense to grey matter on T1-weighted image, hypointense to CSF on T2-weighted image with homogeneous postcontrast enhancement. On MR perfusion, there is low relative cerebral blood volume and myoinositol peak may be present on MRS.
    - Larger schwannomas can appear heterogeneous with necrosis/cystic degeneration.
    - 3D T2-weighted sequences (CISS, FIESTA) are used to demonstrate hypointense lesions along the nerves in the CP cistern and IAC.
    - Diffusion tensor imaging (DTI): Facial nerve DTI-based tracking (**Fig. 19**) can be used for the prediction of position of the FN in patients with large vestibular schwannomas. This allows accurate preoperative planning and can increase the safety of the surgery.
- *Meningiomas*:
  - These tumors arise from arachnoid meningothelial cells and are typically located at the posterior aspect of the temporal bone or at the premeatal area. The extension into the IAC is usually without enlargement of the porus.
  - CT: The mass is hyperdense in 70% of the cases, calcified in about 20% with occasionally adjacent hyperostosis and enostotic spur.
  - MRI reveals a broad-based dural lesion which is isointense with the cortex on all sequences and shows marked homogeneous contrast enhancement. There is a high relative cerebral volume on MR perfusion and alanine peak may be present on MRS.
- *Other intrameatal tumors*:
  - Nonschwannomatous lesions are rare and imitate the symptoms of vestibular schwannomas.

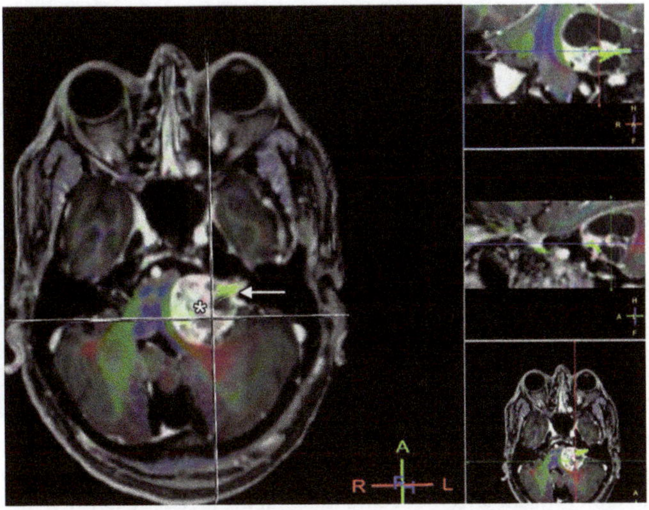

FIG. 19: DTI in vestibular schwannoma: Contrast-enhanced MRI and diffusion tensor imaging brain reveal a large left vestibular schwannoma (*). Large, heterogenous mass with extension into IAC and compression and rotation of the brainstem. Left facial nerve (arrow) is anterior to lesion in the middle third.

- These include meningiomas, arachnoid cysts, metastasis, carcinomatous meningitis, hamartomas, lipomas, neurofibroma, lymphoma, neuritis/arachnoiditis, cavernomas, hemangiomas, hemangioblastomas, labyrinthine artery aneurysms, jugular bulb diverticulum, and traumatic neuromas.
- Preoperative differentiation of rare lesions is challenging.

- *Cystic lesions in the cerebellopontine angle*: This includes epidermoid cyst, arachnoid cyst, neurenteric cyst, dermoid cyst, and cystic component of schwannoma.

ABNORMAL ENHANCEMENT IN IAC (APART FROM TUMORS): NEURITIS

- This may be seen as enhancement of or around the seventh or eighth nerve and/or within the labyrinth (**Figs. 20A** and **B**). Occasionally, mass-like lesion can be seen along the course of the nerve.
- The causes can be infective or malignant and include:[2]
  - Viral infections (herpes simplex, herpes zoster, and cytomegalovirus).
  - Bacterial infection (source can be middle ear/mastoid/skull base osteomyelitis).
  - Leptomeningeal disease (e.g., Lyme disease, sarcoidosis, syphilis, and tuberculosis). Associated meningeal enhancement may be seen in tuberculous meningitis and brainstem involvement at the FN REZ can be seen in Lyme disease.
  - Perineural spread of cancer (very rare).

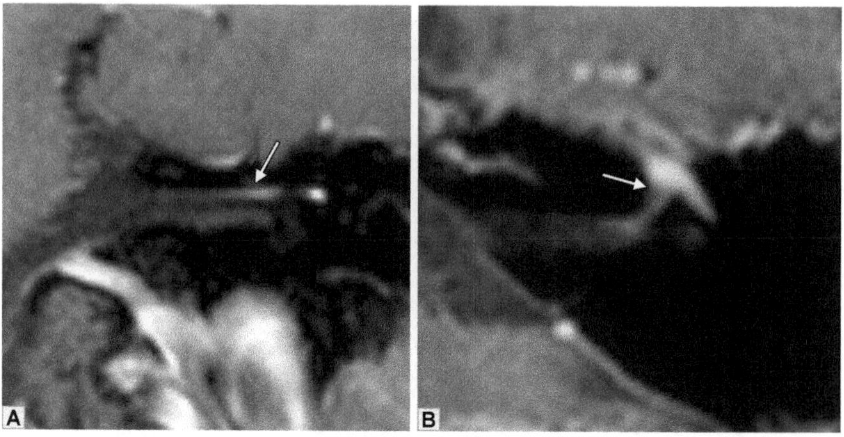

FIGS. 20A AND B: Facial neuritis: (A) Coronal postgadolinium T1WI: Contrast enhancement along the lateral half of the intracanalicular part of the facial nerve (arrow); (B) Axial postgadolinium T1WI: Enhancement extending till the first genu (arrow).

COCHLEAR NERVE ABNORMALITIES

These are discussed as CN or cochleovestibular nerve (CVN) abnormalities, with the latter term being used in cases of common cavity (CC). Also see Chapter 11 for more details.

- *Cochlear nerve*: Cochlear nerve may be normal, hypoplastic, or absent.
  - *Normal*:
    - On axial sections—CN is seen entering cochlea in the inferior sections of the IAC.
    - On parasagittal sections—it is anteroinferior in location within IAC (**Fig. 21A**).
    - Size of nerve:
      - Compared to opposite side if it is normal.
      - Compared to FN (CN appears similar or more in size).
    - Cochlear nerve diameter: Identify the level immediately medial to the fundus of the IAC on the axial slice showing the maximal diameter[5] and measured on the parasagittal plane.
    - Normal size of the CN on MRI: 1.2 ± 0.2 mm in the mid to distal IAC[4]
  - *Absent CN*:
    - No nerve identified in expected location (**Fig. 21B**).
    - There may be an associated inner ear malformation. In cases of cochlear aplasia and cochlear aperture (CA) aplasia, CN is always absent.
    - In cases of CA hypoplasia, there may be aplasia or hypoplasia of CN.
  - *Hypoplasia of CN*: Size is smaller, compared to the opposite side or to the FN (**Figs. 22A** and **B**).
- *Vestibulocochlear nerve (VCN, eighth nerve)*: The normal VCN originates from the brainstem, enters the IAC, and then subdivided into three segments, i.e., CN, superior vestibular nerve, and inferior vestibular nerve.

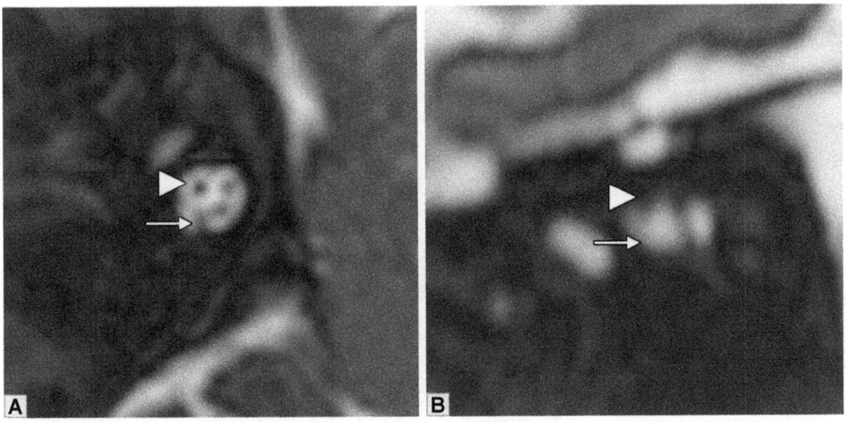

FIGS. 21A AND B: Cochlear nerve (CN) aplasia: (A) *Normal* caliber of CN (arrow); (B) *Aplasia* of CN (arrow) in a case of cochlear aplasia. Facial nerve is normal in both the figures (arrowhead).

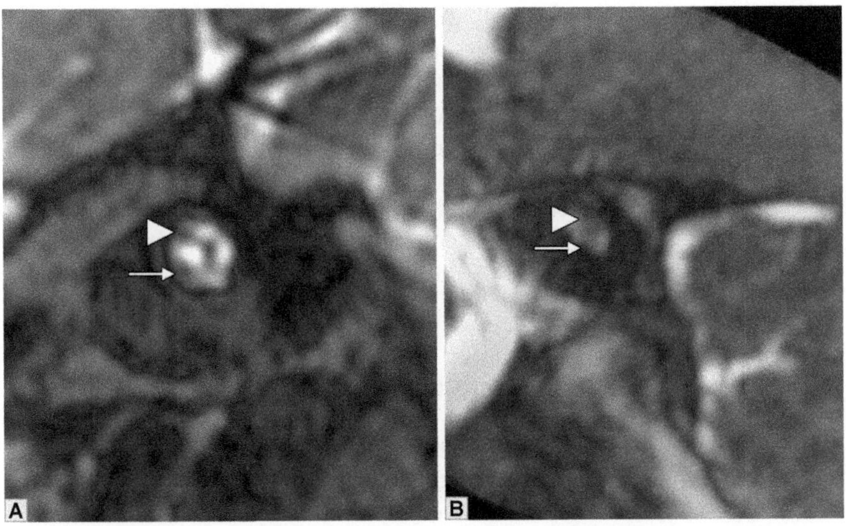

FIGS. 22A AND B: Cochlear nerve (CN) hypoplasia: (A) *Normal* caliber of CN (arrow); (B) Marked *hypoplasia* of CN (arrow) with IAC stenosis and cochlea hypoplasia. Facial nerve is normal in both the figures (arrowhead).

- *Normal VCN*:
  - In cases of CC, the VCN does not divide into its three divisions, and the entire course continues into the CC; and the cochlear and cochleovestibular components cannot be discerned separately.
  - To ascertain if size of VCN is normal compare with opposite side. On comparison, both sides VCN should be similar; and VCN should be 1 ½ to 2 times the size compared with ipsilateral FN (**Fig. 23A**)

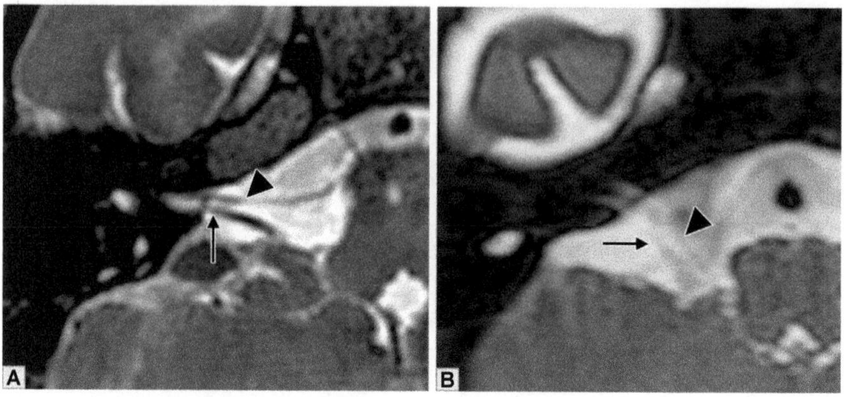

FIGS. 23A AND B: Vestibulocochlear nerve (VCN) hypoplasia: (A) Normal caliber of VCN (arrow); (B) *Hypoplasia* of VCN (arrow) with IAC stenosis. Facial nerve is normal in both the figures (arrowhead).

- VCN diameter: VCN is identified at a level medial to the porus acusticus internus on the slice showing the maximal nerve diameter[5] and the diameter is measured on the parasagittal plane.
- Normal size of the VCN on MRI: 1.8 ± 0.2 mm at the porus acousticus.[5]

- *Hypoplasia of VCN*: If VCN is smaller in size, comparison detailed above (**Fig. 23B**).
- *Absent VCN*: In these instances, only FN is visualized and VCN is absent in its entire course; IAC is often absent. This situation is encountered in Michel deformity.

Cochlear Aperture

- Synonym of Cochlear Aperture (CA): Cochlear fossette/CN canal/bony cochlear nerve canal (BCNC)
- It is the bony canal through which the CN passes from the cochlea into internal auditory canal and it lies at base of modiolus.
- Cochlear aperture is best measured on CT in the mid-modiolar view, while CN is obviously measured on MRI at a similar level (**Figs. 24A** and **B**).
- *Normal measurements*:
  - Done on axial images
  - Section at mid portion of the modiolus
  - Width of canal/diameter: Measured at its midportion
  - Normal range: 1.4–3.0 mm[5]
- *Cochlear aperture abnormalities*:
  - Cochlear aperture abnormalities include hypoplasia (<1.4 mm) (**Fig. 24C**), or aplasia (absence), or enlarged (>3.0 mm) (**Fig. 24D**).
  - *Isolated cochlea*: This is the term used when CA is absent and filled with bone[6] (**Figs. 25A** and **B**).
  - If CA is hypoplastic, CN may be hypoplastic/aplastic.

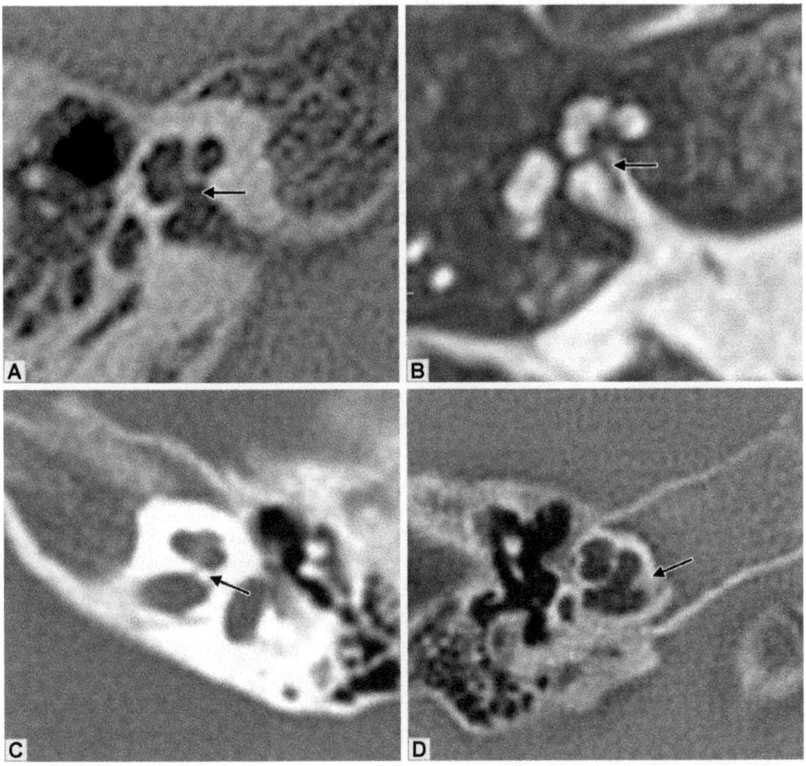

FIGS. 24A TO D: Cochlear aperture: (A) *Normal* cochlear aperture (arrow) in CT in the mid-modiolar axial view; (B) *Normal* cochlear aperture in MRI in the mid-modiolar axial view. CN (arrow) is seen to pass from the cochlea into IAC through the aperture; (C) *Hypoplasia* of cochlea aperture (arrow); (D) *Enlarged* cochlear aperture (arrow).

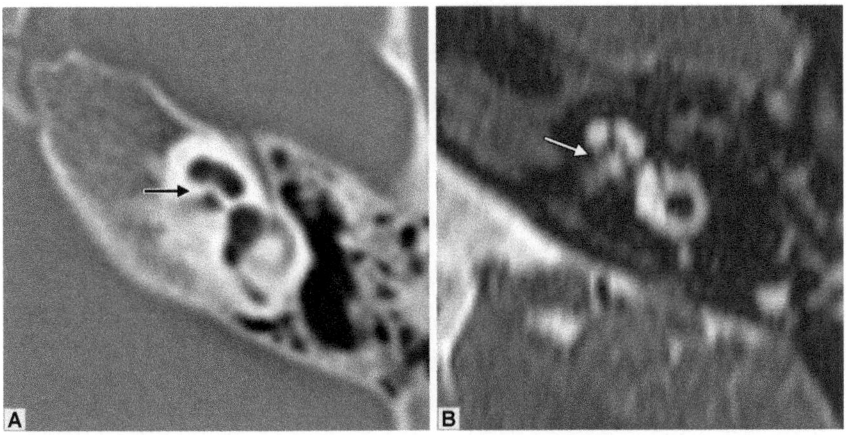

FIGS. 25A AND B: Isolated cochlea: (A) Axial HRCT: Cochlear aperture is absent and filled with bone (arrow); (B) Axial MRI: No communication between cochlea and IAC (arrow).

- If there is CA aplasia, CN is also absent.
- Associations: IAC may be narrow/normal and similarly, cochlea may be abnormal or normal.
- Large CA (>3.0 mm): Associated with risk of Stapes gusher

In conclusion, evaluation of the IAC is an integral part of evaluation of HRCT temporal bone and MRI in cases of inner ear malformations. Further, contrast-enhanced MRI is required in case of tumors and neuritis which can be identified as abnormal enhancement within the IAC.

REFERENCES

1. Sennaro lu L, Bajin MD. Classification and Current Management of Inner Ear Malformations. Balkan Med J. 2017;34:397-411.
2. Verbist BM. Imaging of sensorineural hearing loss: a pattern-based approach to diseases of the inner ear and cerebellopontine angle. Insights Imaging. 2012;3:139-53.
3. McDermott AL, Dutt SN, Irving RM, Pahor AL, Chavda SV. Anterior inferior cerebellar artery syndrome: fact or fiction. Clin Otolaryngol. 2003;28:75-80.
4. Sirikci A, Bayazit Y, Ozer E, Ozkur A, Adaletli I, Cüce MA, et al. Magnetic resonance imaging based classification of anatomic relationship between the cochleovestibular nerve and anterior inferior cerebellar artery in patients with non-specific neuro-otologic symptoms. Surg Radiol Anat. 2005;27(6):531-5.
5. Jaryszak EM, Patel NA, Camp M, Mancuso AA, Antonelli PJ. Cochlear nerve diameter in normal hearing ears using high resolution magnetic resonance imaging. Laryngoscope 2009;119(10): 2042-5.
6. Gupta SS, Maheshwari SR, Kirtane MV, Shrivastav N. Pictorial review of MRI/CT Scan in congenital temporal bone anomalies, in patients for cochlear implant. Indian J Radiol Imaging. 2009;19(2): 99-106.

13

Cochlear Implant: Surgical Perspectives

Kapil Sikka, Hitesh Verma

- Indications for Cochlear Implant
  - Standard Indications
  - Expanded Indications
- Preoperative Evaluation
- Contraindications
- Conditions that Modify Surgical Technique/Type of Implant
- Conditions that Increase Surgical Complications
- Types of Surgical Implants
- Surgical Approach
- Intraoperative Evaluation
- Postoperative Evaluation

- Cochlear implants (CIs) are electronic devices implanted surgically for sound transmission in severe to profound sensorineural hearing loss (SNHL) patients. These act by direct stimulation of the cochlear nerve.
- Cochlear implants have an external and internal component (**Figs. 1** and **2**). The external device changes environmental sound into electric sound and then transmits sound to the internal device. Internal device further sends these electric signals to functional cochlear nerve directly.[1,2]

INDICATIONS FOR COCHLEAR IMPLANT

Standard Indications

The standard indications include:

- Prelingual (before language development) bilateral severe to profound sensorineural deafness (≥70 dB), preferably under 5 year of age.
- Postlingual (after language development) bilateral severe to profound sensorineural deafness in a child.

Expanded Indications

The expanded indications include:

- Single-sided deafness where other ear is normal or near normal.
- Less than profound hearing loss where higher frequencies are more severely affected than lower frequencies. In such situations, smaller electrode CIs can stimulate basal frequencies and hearing aids can stimulate apical (electroacoustic stimulation).
- Tinnitus.

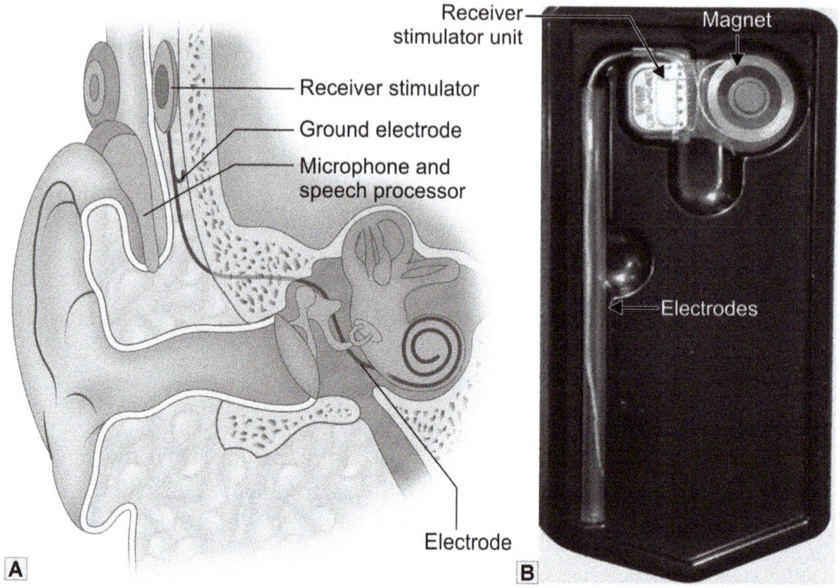

FIGS. 1A AND B: (A) Schematic diagram, and (B) photograph of the **parts of a cochlear implant**. The internal parts comprise of the internal magnet, receiver stimulator, and the electrode array.

Source: Dr Arvind K Kairo.

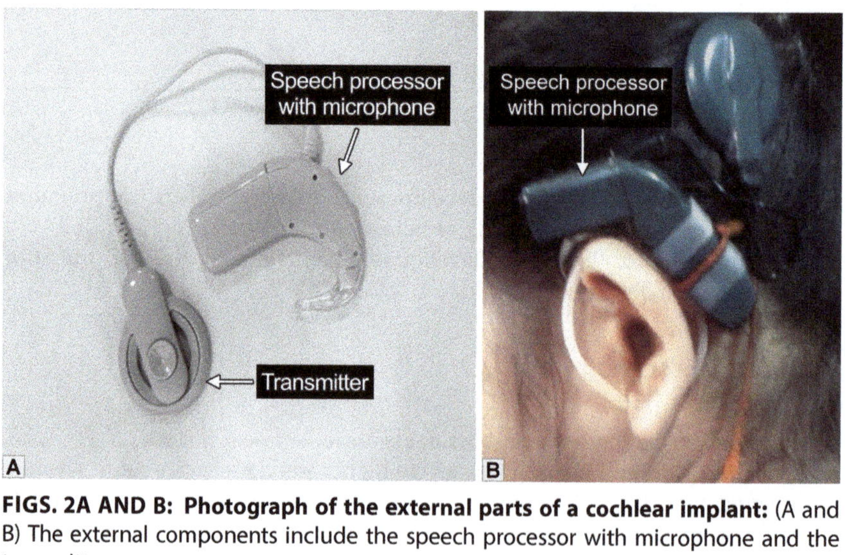

FIGS. 2A AND B: Photograph of the external parts of a cochlear implant: (A and B) The external components include the speech processor with microphone and the transmitter.

PREOPERATIVE EVALUATION FOR COCHLEAR IMPLANT

- *History and evaluation*: Detailed history and complete medical evaluation are required to check suitability for CI surgery.
- *Audiological and hearing aid evaluation*: The audiological work-up includes pure tone audiogram (PTA), aided audiogram, and brainstem-evoked response audiometry (BERA). PTA, being a subjective test, may not be feasible in very young children and decision making in such cases lies on careful assessment by interdisciplinary team and reliance on behavioral and objective tests. Speech tests with hearing aids are also advised as preoperative evaluation. The response with hearing aids is evaluated for 3–6 months with regular speech therapy and speech evaluation.[2-4]
- Counseling for CI surgery and postoperative management.
- *Radiology*: HRCT and MRI of temporal bone with 3D reconstructions of inner ear is proposed to see anatomical detail, any variation in anatomy, selection of surgical approach, exclude any contraindications to surgery, and predict prognosis of surgery.

CONTRAINDICATIONS FOR COCHLEAR IMPLANT

Based on the preoperative evaluation (history, audiometry, and imaging findings), the need and suitability of CI surgery should be assessed. Contraindications to surgery should be carefully excluded.

- *Absolute contraindications*:
    - Absent cochlea and cochlear nerve
    - Active middle ear infection
- *Relative contraindications/difficult situations*:
    - Labyrinthine ossificans (obliterated basal turn of cochlea)
    - Advanced otosclerosis
    - Severe cochlear malformations with absent modiolus
    - Severe mental retardation and other learning disabilities
    - Organic brain dysfunction
    - Psychosis
    - Unrealistic expectations

CONDITIONS THAT MODIFY SURGICAL TECHNIQUE/TYPE OF COCHLEAR IMPLANT

Further, there are findings on imaging that are not a contraindication, but require modifications of technique or type of implant. These include:

- Partial and total cochlear ossification, basal turn ossification
- Hyperostosis of round window niche
- Endolymphatic sac dilatation
- Abnormal cochlear segmentation
- Deficient modiolus
- Dilated vestibule and semicircular canal

CONDITIONS THAT INCREASE SURGICAL COMPLICATIONS

Similarly certain findings on imaging alert the surgeons to increased risk of complications, such as:

- Hypocellular mastoid
- Middle ear infection
- Aberrant and dehiscent facial nerve course
- Abnormal position of sigmoid plate and dural plate
- Dehiscent jugular bulb
- Aberrant carotid and persistent stapedial artery

TYPES OF SURGICAL IMPLANTS

Surgical implants can be of different types, namely CI, middle ear implant, and brainstem implant.

Cochlear Implant

- These are the most commonly used type.
- Indicated in severe to profound bilateral SNHL where implant is placed in inner ear via cochleostomy or through round window.
- The implants prepared by various companies have different number of electrodes varying from 16 to 24.
- The compressed array and split array form of CIs are indicated in ossification of labyrinth where complete insertion is not possible.

Cochlear Implant Electrodes and Processors

- The most widely available implants are by three vendors: Cochlear Ltd. (Australia), MedEl (Austria), and Advanced Bionics (USA).
- Different companies manufacture different electrode and processor portfolios.[4] The common electrode portfolios are:
  - *Cochlear:*
    - Cochlear™ Nucleus® CI24RE (ST) straight electrode, which is the most widely used.
    - Nucleus® CI24RE (CA) perimodiolar electrode. This variant has a stylet for insertion and is modiolus hugging.
    - Nucleus Hybrid L24 is indicated in patients with significant residual hearing.
    - Nucleus Profile with Slim Modiolar electrode (CI 532) is a recent slim implant.
  - *MedEl:*
    - MedEl provides Flex series based on length. The sizes being Flex soft (31.5 mm), Flex 28, Flex 24, and Flex 20 to be used based on length (mm) required.

- MedEl also provides the FORM series of electrodes designed for malformed cochleae; and for instances where leakage of cerebrospinal fluid (CSF) is expected. This electrode has an integrated SEAL designed to close off the cochlear opening and hence plugs the leak.

○ *Advanced Bionics:*
- HiFocus 1J electrode is the Lateral wall electrode.
- Hifocus Midscala is the "atraumatic" midscale electrode.

Middle Ear Implant

- Usage of middle ear implant is much rarer compared to CIs.
- The implant is placed in middle ear by transmastoid facial recess approach.
- It attaches with one of the ossicle of middle ear or placed over round window niche.
- This is indicated in moderate-to-severe mixed and sensorineural deaf adult patient where conventional hearing aids are not effective.

Brainstem Implant

- The electrodes are placed directly over cochlear nucleus on brainstem. These are more complex and expensive compared to CIs, and is indicated in patients with damaged or absent cochlear nerves on both sides; either developmentally or accidentally.
- This is also indicated where there is no lumen for CI insertion, e.g., complete cochlear ossification after meningitis.

SURGICAL APPROACHES

The various surgical approaches toward placement of a CI are as described here.[3,5]

Transmastoid-facial Recess Approach (Figs. 3A to C)

- Also see Chapter 14.
- The middle ear is approached posterior to pinna. The surgical steps include cortical mastoidectomy and middle ear entry through facial recess.
- The implant inserted in inner ear via round window or cochleostomy (anterior-inferior to the round window niche).
- This approach is followed by most of CI surgeons.

Transcanal Approach

The middle ear is approached superior to pinna. The tympanomeatal flap is elevated and incudostapedial joint and round window niche are exposed. The middle ear is approached from above and outside canal wall.

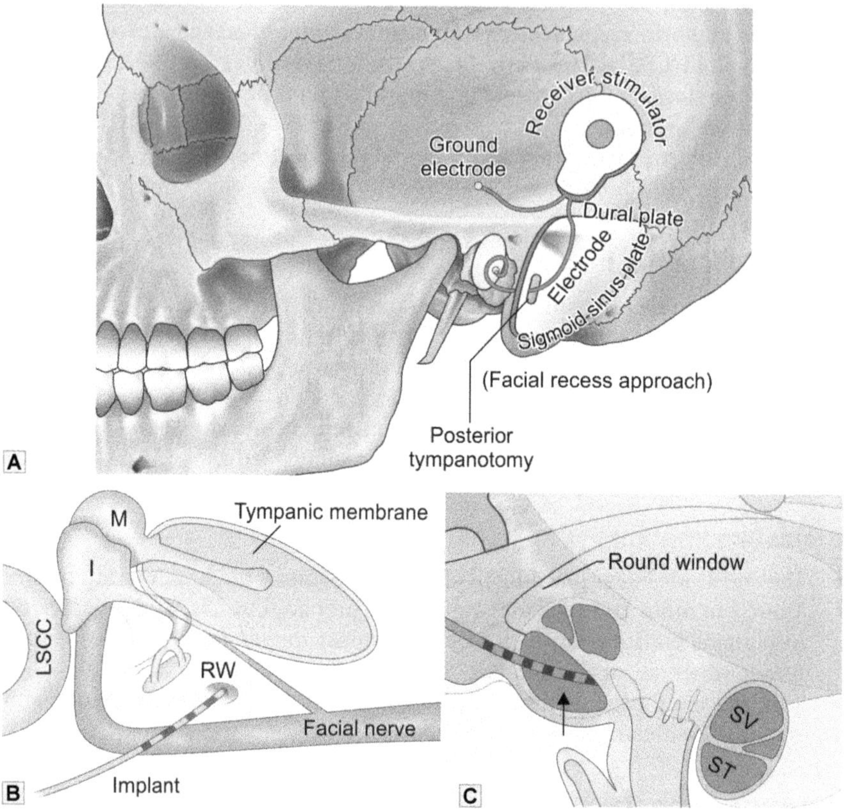

(LSCC: lateral semicircular canal; ST: scala tympani; SV: scala vestibuli)

FIGS. 3A TO C: Facial recess approach to cochlear implant surgery: (A) The external approach to surgery. (B) The site of round window (RW) cochleostomy (arrow). (C) The ideal placement of the electrode in the scala tympani chamber (arrow).

Source: Dr Arvind K Kairo.

Middle Cranial Fossa Approach

- In this technique, the middle ear is approached from floor of middle cranial fossa. Drilling of internal auditory meatus is continued till the identification of most superficial portion of basal turn of cochlea and cochleostomy is performed.
- This approach is less preferred due to complex anatomy and more chances of complications.
- It is indicated in cases where inner ear access is not possible by above-mentioned approaches, or in some cases where posterior canal wall is violated by previous cholesteatoma surgery.

INTRAOPERATIVE EVALUATION

- Plain radiological assessment is required for confirmation of correct insertion of implants. In cases of malformations advanced radiological investigations are suggested for confirmation of proper insertion of electrodes.
- Neural response telemetry (NRT) is an electric method to assess correct insertion of electrodes, functioning of device, and average voltage of stimulation.[6]

POSTOPERATIVE EVALUATION

- Besides regular clinical follow-up, audiometry analysis, and speech counseling, NRT is also indicated for functional evaluation of implants.
- Postoperative radiography is performed for the assessment of position of implant (**Figs. 4A** and **B**).
- Other indications for postoperative radiological assessment include implant malfunction (accidentally or because of trauma) or when patient is complaining of implant-related complication. In such situations, CT is the preferred imaging modality.
- Implant-related complications include:
  - Flap-related complications (necrosis and infection)
  - Facial nerve stimulation
  - Tinnitus and vertigo (transient)
  - Electrode migration
  - Magnet dislocation

In conclusion, a successful CI program requires well-coordinated functioning of multiple departments.

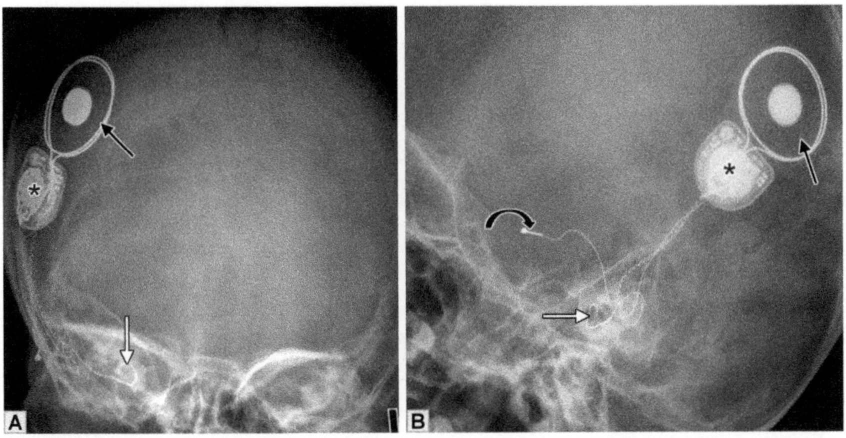

FIGS. 4A AND B: Postoperative radiographs: (A) Anteroposterior, and (B) lateral views revealing the parts of a cochlear implant; the internal receiver-stimulator (asterisk), the transmitter and the internal magnet (arrow), the electrode array (block arrow), and the ground electrode (white arrow).

REFERENCES

1. Roche JP, Hansen MR. On the Horizon: Cochlear Implant Technology. Otolaryngol Clin North Am. 2015;48(6):1097-16.
2. Marshall A, Broomfield S. Cochlear Implants. In: Watkinson JC, Clarke RW (Eds). Scott-Brown's Otorhinolaryngology Head & Neck Surgery. 8th edition. Boca Raton, FL: CRC Press; 2018. pp. 1157-66.
3. Wackym PA, Tran A. Cochlear Implantation: Patient Evaluation and Device Selection. In: Flint PW, Haughey BH, Lund V, Niparko JK, Robbins KT, Thomas JR, Lesperance M, et al. (Eds). Cummings Otolaryngology Head and Neck Surgery, 6th edition. Philadelphia: Elsevier Saunders; 2015. pp. 2428-43.
4. Naples JG, Ruckenstein MJ. Cochlear Implant. Otolaryngol Clin North Am. 2020;53(1):87-102.
5. Balkany TJ, Brown KD. Medical and Surgical Considerations in Cochlear Implantation. In: Flint PW, Haughey BH, Lund V, Niparko JK, Robbins KT, Thomas JR, et al. (Eds). Cummings Otolaryngology Head and Neck Surgery, 6th edition. Philadelphia: Elsevier Saunders; 2015. pp. 2444-54.
6. Miyazaki H, Caye-Thomasen P. Intraoperative Auditory System Monitoring. Adv Otorhinolaryngol. 2018;81:123-32.

14

Imaging in Cochlear Implant

Manisha Jana, Ashu Seith Bhalla, Surabhi Vyas

Imaging of cochlear implant (CI) patients is crucial in the preoperative setting. It is also employed in intraoperative as well as postoperative scenarios.

PREOPERATIVE IMAGING

Role of Imaging

The role of preoperative imaging is:

- *Choosing the optimal treatment method*: Hearing aid vs. CI vs. auditory brainstem implant (ABI) is based on clinical situation as well as imaging findings (e.g., inner ear, cochlear nerve status, etc.) (also see Chapter 13)
- In case of planned CI, detecting inner ear malformations, status of cochlear nerve, and anatomic variations for the purpose of:
  - Selecting the ear to undergo surgery
  - Deciding the surgical approach
  - Helping to choose correct electrodes
  - Predicting the outcome
  - Predicting complications (e.g., anomalous facial nerve course, inner ear malformations at risk of cerebrospinal fluid (CSF) leak/"gusher").

Imaging Modalities

- *High-resolution CT* (HRCT) and *MRI* of the temporal bone and inner ear are two cornerstones of preoperative imaging in CI. The two are complementary; having their own benefits and drawbacks. *HRCT* is usually the first imaging modality. A dedicated HRCT scan with 0.6 mm slice collimation and high kernel reconstruction algorithm are the basic requirements of CT acquisition. Reconstruction in various planes other than coronal and sagittal planes are often needed, and is detailed later (also refer to Chapter 1). While CT is ideal for assessing bony inner ear, middle ear anatomy, and aeration and mastoid pneumatization; it cannot visualize the cochlear nerve or other nerves in the internal auditory canal (IAC).

- *Magnetic resonance imaging* of inner ear essentially requires a heavily T2-weighted (T2W) sequence such as CISS (constructive interference in steady state). The prime utility of MRI lies in the identification of the intracanalicular and cisternal part of the eighth nerve. It also provides netter details of the internal architecture of cochlea and scala chambers. As in CT, multiplanar and 3D reconstructions are immensely useful.
- The choice of imaging modality varies from center to center. At our institution, both are routinely used in all patients. The rationale behind this approach lies in the fact that in a certain number of patients with eighth nerve deficiency have a normal IAC and cochlear aperture; CT alone may not be adequate in predicting the outcome of surgery. Although some authors advocate the use of MRI alone.

Basic Surgical Steps

- Cochlear implantation is a demanding surgical procedure; so the preoperative imaging needs to be accurate, as emphasized in previous chapter. However, in order to learn CI preoperative imaging essentials; one must have a preliminary knowledge about the surgical steps in CI. **Flowchart 1** details the basic surgical step and the linked critical preoperative imaging evaluation.
- In the subsequent section, we shall discuss the structure-wise assessment relevant to CI. Most often, a subjective assessment of individual structures suffices. However, if an abnormality is suspected, it should be reported in terms of predefined measurements; which are well described in literature[1] and will be discussed below. The readers are also advised to refer to Chapters 3 and 4 for more anatomic details.

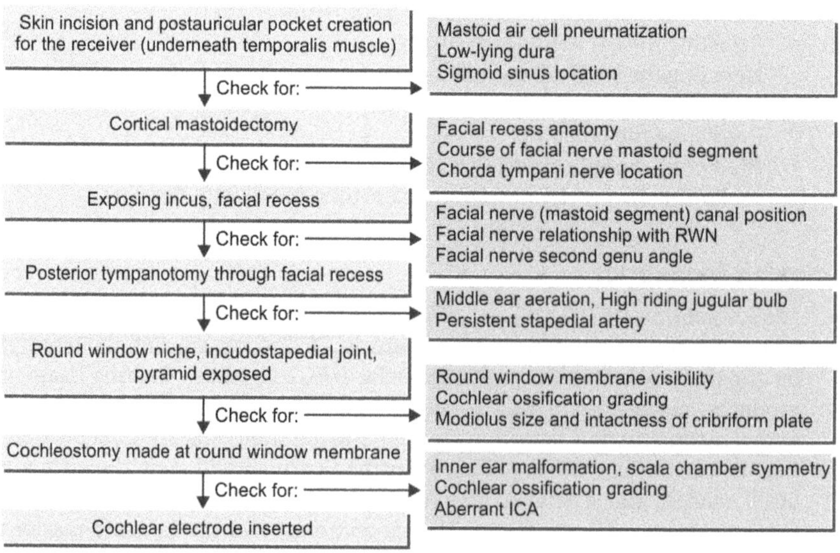

FLOWCHART 1: Key surgical steps in cochlear implant (CI).

Structure-wise Assessment

In structure-wise assessment, a subjective assessment should be done as a first step. Quantitative measurement may not be required in normal cases. Detailed measurement of individual structures can be reserved for the situations when the subjective assessment reveals a gross abnormality.

Mastoid

Bilateral mastoids should be evaluated for following:

- *Pneumatization* (**Figs. 1A** to **C**): The extent of pneumatization is labeled as: Pneumatic (or cellular), sclerotic, diploeic, hypocellular, or mixed pattern. Sclerotic contracted mastoid makes cortical mastoidectomy challenging.[1,2]
- Effusion/*mastoiditis*
- Presence of *Korner's septum* (a division between superficial and deep portion of mastoid). If present, it can misdirect toward mastoid antrum during surgery.
- Presence of persistent/enlarged *emissary veins.*

Sigmoid Sinus Location

- As sigmoid sinus (SS) is an immediate posterior relation of the mastoid, its position also needs to be ascertained. If anteriorly displaced (as will happen if the mastoid is sclerosed and thus contracted), there is a risk of injury to SS during cortical mastoidectomy.
- In fact SS may be so anterior so as to reach up to the posterior wall of external auditory canal (EAC).
- The position of the SS has also been graded by Sun DII et al.[3] The *classification* is based on location of the most protruding part of the SS in relation to following 3 lines (**Fig. 2**).
    - 1: Passes through the common crus of posterior semicircular canal (PSCC) and superior semicircular canal (SSCC).
    - 2: Through tympanic segment of facial nerve.
    - 3: Along the malleal-incudal axis.

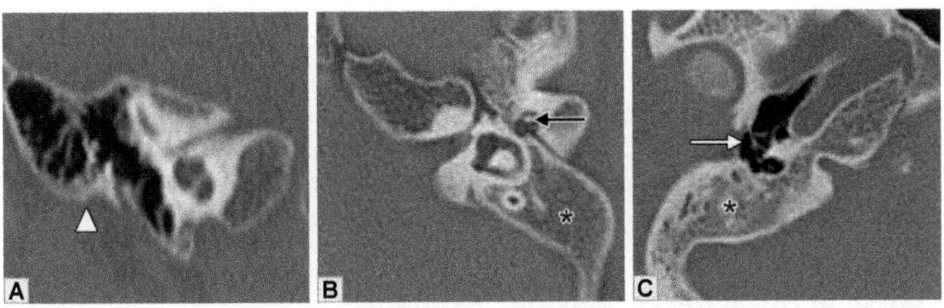

FIGS. 1A TO C: Variable mastoid pneumatization: (A) Coronal HRCT: Right external auditory canal (EAC) atresia with pneumatized mastoid (arrowhead); (B) Axial HRCT: Left EAC atresia with small middle ear (arrow); and sclerotic mastoid (asterisk); (C) Axial HRCT: Right EAC atresia with good volume middle ear (arrow), and sclerotic mastoid (asterisk).

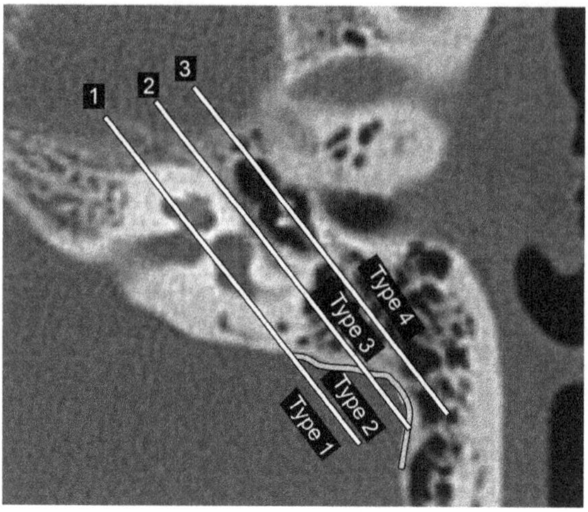

FIG. 2: Sigmoid sinus (SS) location: Based on the most protruding part of the SS in relation to the lines 1, 2, and 3; four different types have been defined. In the given example, type 3 location of sigmoid sinus has been shown.

Types based on position of most protruding part of SS:
- Type 1: Posterior/medial to line 1
- Type 2: Between lines 1 and 2
- Type 3: Between lines 2 and 3
- Type 4: Anterior/lateral to line 3

Types 3 and 4 indicate a contracted mastoid, and are associated with a difficult mastoidectomy.

- Another measurement reported is the distance from anterior wall of SS to posterior wall of EAC; with increased surgical difficulty if it is <9 mm.[4]

Low-lying Dura

- A sclerosed mastoid is also associated with lower position of the dura, which increases surgical difficulty during mastoidectomy.
- *Quantitative measurement*: On coronal image, a line is drawn tangential to the upper border of petrous bone. Distance from this line to the tegmen (also will be the level of temporal meninges) is measured. If this distance is ≥7 mm, it implies a low-lying dura (**Fig. 3**).[4]

Middle Ear Aeration

- Active middle ear infection is a contraindication to implantation.
- Clinical feature of otitis media combined with middle ear opacification on imaging requires preoperative medical management to reduce chances of implantation-induced complication such as meningitis and labyrinthitis.

Course of Facial Nerve (Mastoid Segment)

- In cortical mastoidectomy and posterior tympanotomy approach, the posterior wall of middle ear is opened at the space between mastoid segment

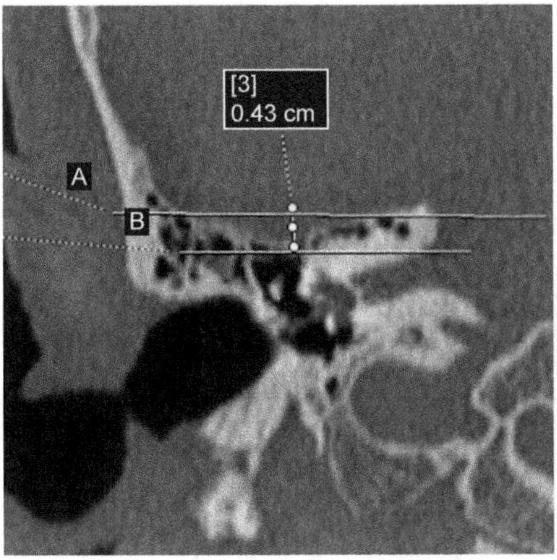

FIG. 3: Measurement for low-lying dura on a coronal HRCT image. Distance between the line A (tangential to the upper border of petrous temporal bone) and line B (tegmen tympani). If ≥7 mm indicates a low-lying dura. In this patient it is <7 mm (normal).

of facial nerve and chorda tympani nerve. This approach (through facial recess) gives a direct access to the round window niche (RWN) and cochlea; thereby avoiding cochleostomy.

- Success of this approach depends on the relationship between the RWN and facial nerve mastoid segment. This can be measured by a method described by Mandour et al.[5]
- *Quantitative assessment*: Two lines are drawn on axial image: First one tangential to the junction of the bony and cartilaginous part of posterior wall of EAC; and the tympanic annulus. This is called the *EAC line*. Another line (*RW line*) is drawn from the posterior edge of RWN along the anterolateral part of the mastoid segment of facial nerve (**Fig. 4**).
- Normal RW line is situated posterior and parallel to EAC line. Anteriorly placed RW line indicates a difficult posterior tympanotomy.
- On oblique sagittal image, *second genu angle* can be measured. This refers to the angle between the tympanic and mastoid segment of facial nerve. Normal value is approximately 110–117°.[6] An increased angle indicates wide space between chorda tympani and the mastoid part of facial nerve; which in turn results in superior visualization of RWN at surgery.[7] An angle <92° is associated with poor visualization of RWN.
- An abnormal location or size of facial nerve canal (**Figs. 5A** and **B**) should also be noted in preoperative imaging report.

Round Window Niche Status

- Round window is a 1.5-mm wide, 2-mm long area which connects the cochlea and middle ear. It has round window membrane (*RWM*, a three-layered central component); and *RWN* which is the surrounding bone overhanging from the cochlear promontory.

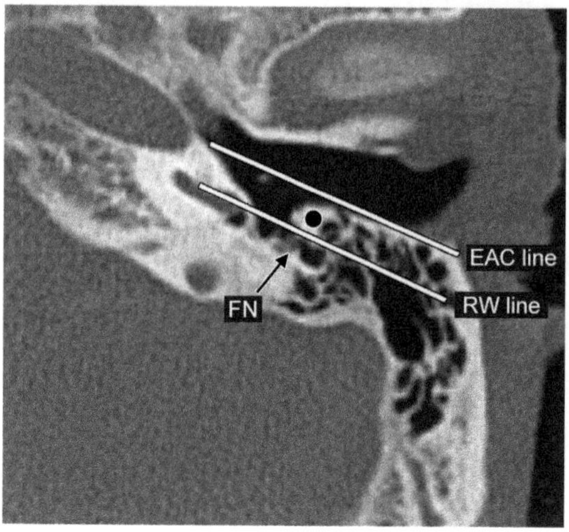

FIG. 4: Facial nerve mastoid segment (axial scan): Normally, the EAC line lies anterolateral to the RW line. Normal position of mastoid part of facial nerve is shown with an arrow. Abnormally anterior location of facial nerve is shown with black dot.

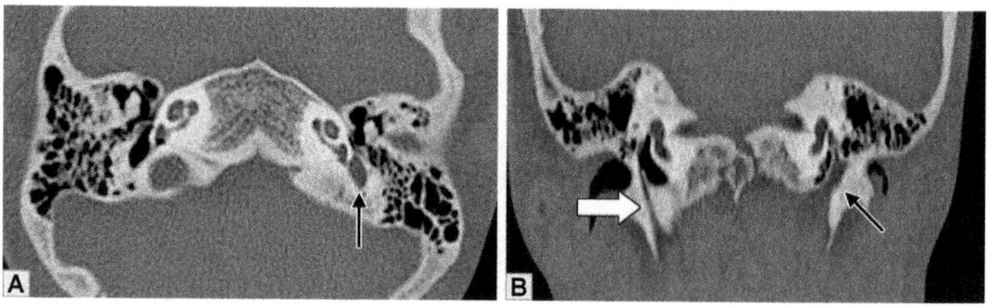

FIGS. 5A AND B: Abnormal facial nerve canal (mastoid segment): HRCT (A) axial and (B) coronal images reveal abnormal dilatation of the left-sided facial nerve canal (arrow). Note the normal right-sided vertical part of facial nerve canal (block arrow).

- *Round window membrane* is the preferred site for entering the cochlea, as opening a membranous area is technically easier compared to drilling the promontory in cochleostomy.
- Variable morphology of *RWN* affects the visibility of RWM (**Figs. 6A** and **B**) and therefore, difficulty encountered during surgery.
- Congenital atresia or stenosis of round window is a rare abnormality. Acquired stenosis of RWN may occur in otosclerosis, Paget disease, postmeningitis labyrinthitis. (also see Chapter 21)
- Round window ossification requires excessive drilling.
- Stenosis of RWN requires variation in standard surgical technique or in implants selection. On axial sections, *Modified Park's ratio* can be measured to express the RWM visibility. It is the ratio expressed as: number of sections where RWM is completely covered by RWN/total number of sections where RWM is seen. A higher ratio indicates poor visibility of RWM.[2,7]

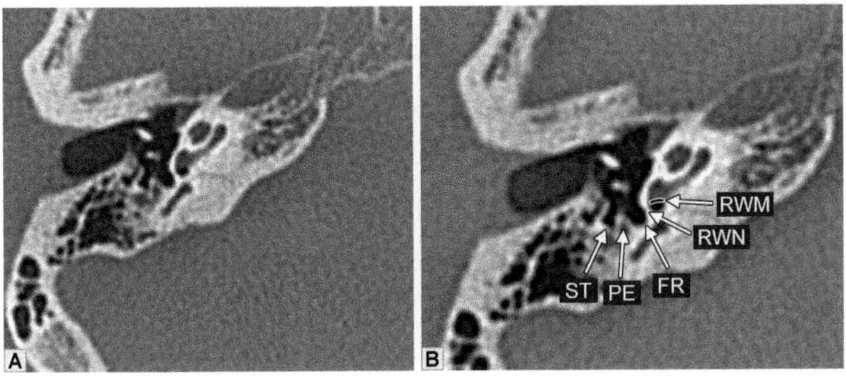

FIGS. 6A AND B: Anatomy of round window: Axial HRCT images at the level of round window niche (A) and (B) annotated image.

Relevant Vascular Anatomy

Jugular Bulb

- Normally the jugular bulb lies at a level inferior to the floor of IAC. It is best addressed in coronal plane. It is separated from the middle ear by a thin cortical bone called sigmoid plate.
- If the highest point of jugular bulb lies at the same level/higher than the floor of ipsilateral IAC, or above the PSCC; it is termed "high jugular bulb."
- If the highest point of jugular bulb is at the level of basal turn of cochlea, it is termed *"high-riding jugular bulb."* High-riding jugular bulb can have either an intact or absent sigmoid plate. In the latter scenario, it is termed as dehiscent jugular bulb.[8]
- A high-riding jugular bulb (**Figs. 7A** and **B**) may cause mechanical obstruction to the RWN; and thereby poses both surgical challenge and risk (posterior tympanotomy/round window approach).

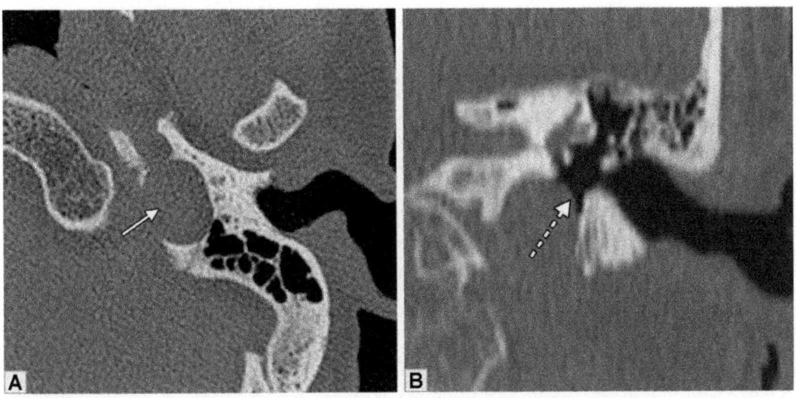

FIGS. 7A AND B: Dehiscent high riding jugular bulb: HRCT axial bone window (A) High location of jugular bulb (arrow). HRCT coronal image (B) Jugular bulb dehiscence (dotted arrow).

Aberrant Carotid Artery

- Within the petrous temporal bone, the carotid canal lies anteromedial to the cochlea.
- *Quantitative assessment*: An objective measurement of the distance from cochlea, termed as cochlea-carotid interval, can be measured on coronal HRCT images (**Figs. 8A** and **B**). Normal values may range from 1.2 to 1.4 mm.[9] When the two structures come in very close contact, the cortical bone between them may be absent.
- An aberrant course of internal carotid artery (ICA) (**Figs. 9A** and **B**) includes posterolateral to the cochlea, or very close to the inferior surface of basal turn of cochlea.
- In such cases, inadvertent injury to the carotid may happen during electrode insertion.

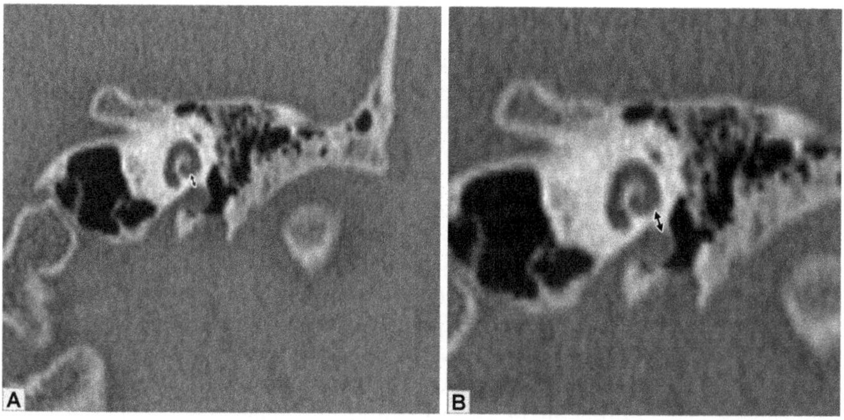

FIGS. 8A AND B: Cochlea-carotid distance on coronal HRCT image (shown with an arrow in A). Further magnified version of the same section (B).

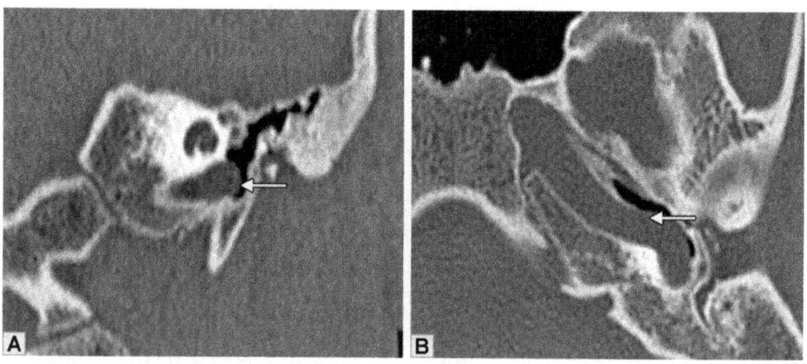

FIGS. 9A TO B: Aberrant course of ICA: HRCT coronal (A) and axial (B) images: Aberrant location of the left internal carotid artery canal (arrow).

Persistent Stapedial Artery

Persistence of stapedial artery is usually an asymptomatic congenital anomaly, detected only on imaging. In the embryonic stage, stapedial artery continues as the middle meningeal artery which later pierces the dura and becomes intracranial. In case of its persistence, middle meningeal artery arises from it. The imaging findings include:

- A canal running parallel to the horizontal part of facial nerve canal, or
- Enlarged facial nerve canal (horizontal part)
- Thin linear structure within the middle ear, close to the promontory
- Absence of the foramen spinosum

Internal Auditory Canal and Cochlear Nerve

- Please refer to Chapter no 12 for details.
- *IAC*:
    - Normally, IACs of both sides show reasonable symmetry in size. An IAC is labeled as stenotic if the diameter is <4 mm.
    - Usual site of measurement of IAC diameter is at the midpoint of the internal aperture and the ampulla.
    - A narrow IAC is often associated with cochlear nerve hypoplasia and therefor, a poor outcome. However, a normal IAC does not imply normal cochlear nerve.
- *Cochlear nerve*:
    - Normal cochlear nerve is larger in size than superior and inferior vestibular nerves; and mostly same size/larger than facial nerve (**Figs. 10A** and **B**).
    - A thin cochlear nerve indirectly indicates reduced number of ganglion cells; and hence poor outcome.

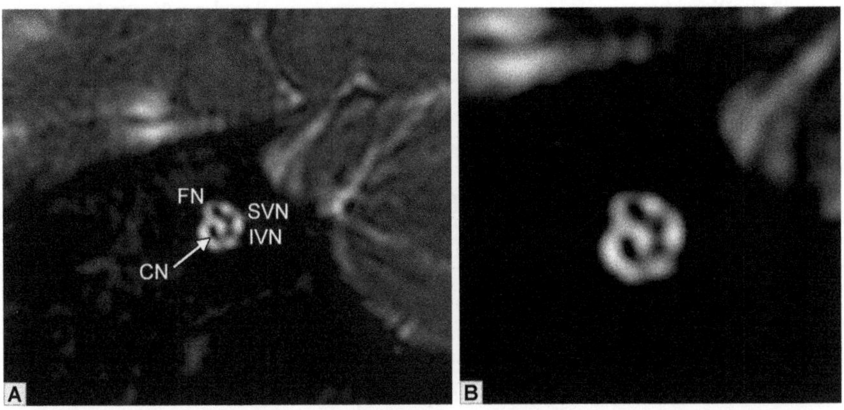

(CN: cochlear nerve; FN: facial nerve; IVN: inferior vestibular nerve; SVN: superior vestibular nerve)

FIGS. 10A AND B: Normal cochlear nerve on an oblique sagittal heavily T2-weighted (T2W) MR image (A). Note that the cochlear nerve is the biggest amongst all four nerves in the IAC. Further magnified version (B) of the same section.

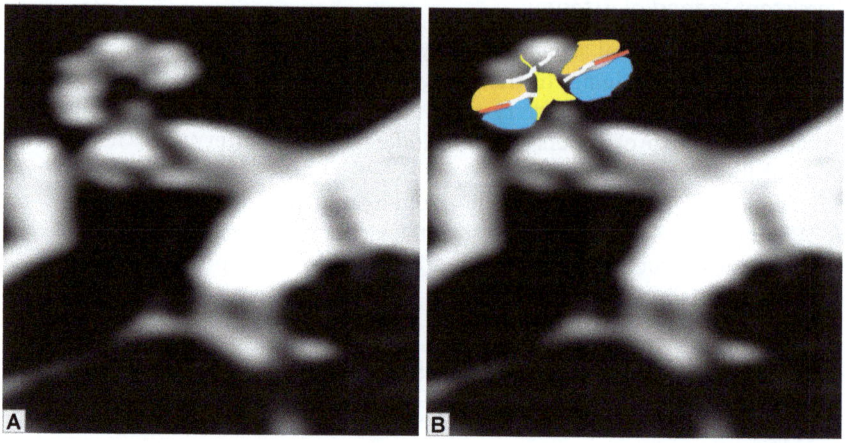

FIGS. 11A AND B: Cochlear anatomy on heavily T2W axial MR image. *Modiolus* is marked in yellow. White line: Osseous spiral lamina. Red line: Basilar membrane. *Scala tympani* is marked in blue, *scala vestibuli* in orange.

   - It is important to differentiate cochlear nerve aplasia from hypoplasia as the former is an absolute contraindication to CI; while in latter it can be done with guarded prognosis.
   - Cochlear nerve hypoplasia is almost invariably associated with a narrow IAC.
- *Cochlear aperture*:
   - It refers to a small aperture (**see Figs. 11A** and **B**) at the fundus of the IAC, through which cochlear nerve enters the cochlea. A small cochlear aperture on CT indirectly indicates hypoplasia or absence of cochlear nerve. When it is absent, the condition is termed "isolated cochlea."
   - Although the criteria for a normal aperture size are not well defined in the literature, an aperture with a diameter smaller than 2 mm is usually considered abnormal.
   - A narrow/stenotic aperture is associated with poor outcome; whereas wide aperture and an absent modiolus is associated with intraoperative CSF gushers.

Inner Ear Anatomy and Abnormalities

- See Chapter 11 for details. Herein the aspects pertinent to CI are discussed.
- *Cochlea:* Normal cochlea is a spiral structure with 2.5–2.75 turns. It contains a central trapezoid-shaped bony structure called the modiolus which harbors the spiral ganglion. Osseous spiral lamina is attached to the modiolus in a spiral fashion and divides the cochlea into scala tympani (inferiorly located), scala media, and scala vestibule (superiorly located).
- Preferred site for cochlear electrode insertion is scala tympani. Cochlear aperture refers to a small aperture at the fundus of the IAC, through which cochlear nerve enters the cochlea.[10] Detailed evaluation of inner ear structures helps to establish preoperative etiology of SNHL, risk of intraoperative gusher, selection of side of ear, and prognostication of outcome of surgery.[2,11]

Points needed to check on radiology are as follows:

- *Number of cochlear turns*: Dictates the number of electrodes which can be accommodated.
- *Status of modiolus and posterior membranous labyrinth (**Figs. 11A** and **B**)*: Modiolus thickness less than 3 mm is suggestive of absent cochlear nerve which is a contraindication for surgery.
- *Scala chamber symmetry (**Figs. 11A** and **B**)*:
  - The anatomy is best demonstrated on axial heavily T2W MR sequence (CISS). Identifying the basilar membrane is crucial in separately denoting these two chambers; which, in turn, is important in deciding the electrode trajectory.
  - A CI bypasses the hair cells and directly stimulates the spiral ganglion in the modiolus. The preferred site of electrode insertion is scala tympani through an anteroinferior round window cochleostomy. In cases of ossification at the RWM; round window cochleostomy may not be feasible. In such cases, a scala vestibuli insertion may be performed. Cochleostomy of the superior part of RWM will damage the osseous spiral lamina; whereas cortical bone at the interval between oval and round window leads to access to scala vestibuli.
  - However, it should be kept in mind that in case of scala vestibuli insertion of electrode in the basal turn will not stimulate the spiral ganglia of basal turn; rather the spiral ganglion of middle turn of cochlea will be stimulated.
- *Ossification of cochlea*: Cochlear ossification does not preclude cochlear implantation; but the degree/severity of ossification dictates the method of cochleostomy. MRI superior to CT in early cases of labyrinthitis ossificans (**Figs. 12A** and **B**); when the T2WI hyperintense signal of cochlea is lost.
- *Cochlear measurements*:
  - Prior to CI surgery; it is crucial to have a detailed imaging evaluation which should include several specified measurements. The key imaging

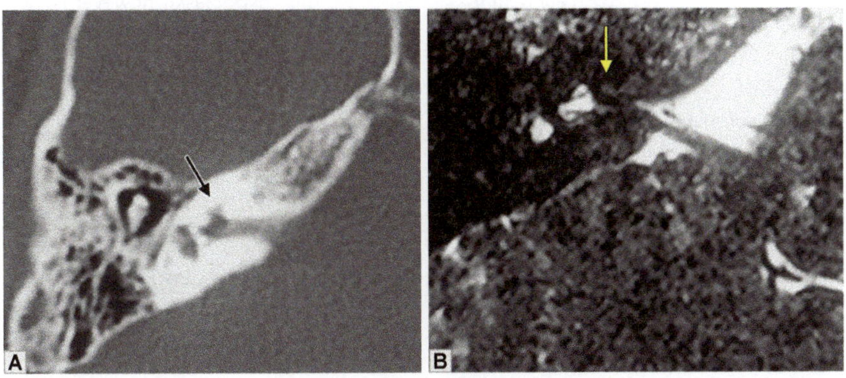

FIGS. 12A AND B: Advanced labyrinthitis ossificans precluding cochlear implantation. (A) Axial HRCT: Ossification in right cochlea and vestibule (black arrow); (B) Axial constructive interference in steady state (CISS) image: Loss of normal hyperintense signal of cochlea (yellow arrow). Implant surgery is not possible and risky in such cases.

planes are axial, coronal, and standardized cochlear view.[12] The steps of viewing in a standardized cochlear reformat is given in **Figures 13A** to **C**.
  - This is important in order to select the most appropriate electrode type, and also to assess the risk of several complications. Various measurements are described on different planes; and detailed in **Table 1** and **Figures 14A** to **E**.
- *Anomalies*: Inner ear anomalies and their relevance in CI are listed in **Table 2**.

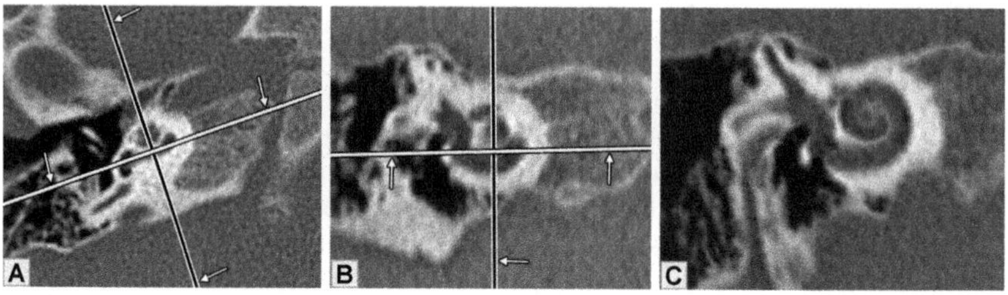

FIGS. 13A TO C: Steps of standardized cochlear reformat: (A) Identification of basal turn of cochlea on axial image; (B) Coronal image perpendicular to the basal turn of cochlea is identified; (C) Image manipulated till the lateral and superior semicircular canal, and cochlea are visible in the same plane. Viewed in the minimum intensity projection mode (minIP) of thickness 1.3–1.5 mm.

TABLE 1 **High-resolution CT measurements in preoperative evaluation of cochlear implant (CI).**

Imaging plane	Parameter	Normal value	Implications
Axial (at the level of basal turn of cochlea)	Horizontal cochlear length (HCL)	8.17 ± 0.35 mm	Reduced in malformations
Axial (modiolar level)	Horizontal cochlear height (HCH)	2.83 ± 0.21 mm	Reduced in malformations (hypoplasia), however, is prone to measurement errors
Oblique coronal	Cochlear height (CH)	3.2–3.9 mm	Reduced in malformations; of specific use in CH and IP-II
	Cochlear nerve foramen diameter (CND)	1.8–1.9 mm	
Standardized cochlear reformat	Cochlear length (CL)	8.10–9.59 mm	Smaller CL (<8.1 mm) and smaller CH (3.2 mm) indicates hypoplasia IP-II: CH values are normal or increased, CL maintained; middle and apical turns fused

Continued

Continued

Imaging plane	Parameter	Normal value	Implications
	Cochlear width (CW)	5.33–7.27 mm	Usually changes proportionately with CH
Curved MPR (Nowadays, calculated using specific formulae)	Cochlear duct length (CDL)		Reduced in hypoplasia and has direct impact on electrode selection. The insertion depth depends on the CDL

Other inner ear structures that need to be evaluated include cochlear aperture, round window niche (discussed above), vestibular aqueduct, and endolymphatic sac (discussed in Chapter 11).

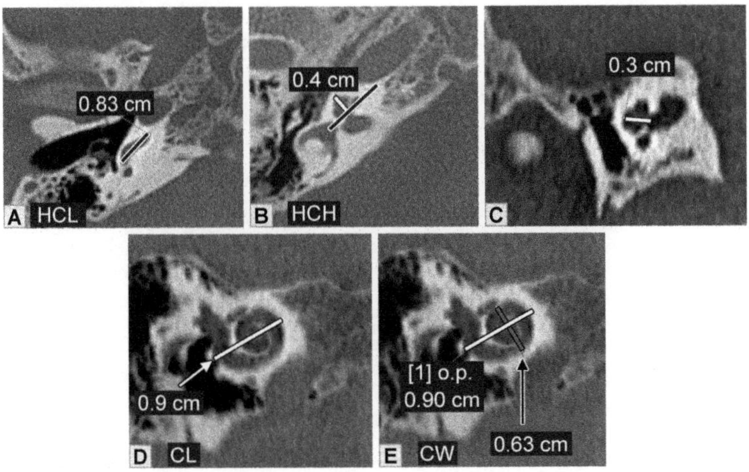

FIGS. 14A TO E: Cochlear measurements shown on a normal cochlea. (A) HCL: Measured on axial image at the level of basal turn of cochlea; (B) HCH: Measured on axial image at modiolar level; (C) CH: Measured on oblique coronal image, perpendicular to modiolus and till the apex of cochlea; (D) CL and (E) CW: Measured on standardized cochlear reformat.

TABLE 2 **Inner ear malformations and their implications for CI (Figs. 16 to 19).**

	Name	Audiology	Implication for CI
Group 1	CLA	• No response • Profound SNHL on low frequencies	• CI not possible • Indication for ABI
Group 2	Rudimentary otocyst	Similar to group 1	Similar to group 1
Group 3	Cochlear aplasia	Similar to group 1 and 2	Similar to group 1 and 2

Continued

Continued

	Name	Audiology	Implication for CI
Group 4	Common cavity (**Figs. 15A** to **D**)	Profound SNHL	• In CVN present and response to trial hearing aid present: consider for CI • If not—contralateral ABI
Group 5	Cochlear hypoplasia CH I to IV (**Figs. 16A** to **D**)	• Variable hearing loss • Normal to profound SNHL • Conductive also if stapes are abnormal	• CI if cochlear nerve present, using smaller electrodes • ABI if absent • Stapedectomy in case with fixation • CH II prone to "gusher"
Group 6	Incomplete partition (IP): • IP-I (**Figs. 17A** to **D**) • IP-II (**Figs. 18A** to **D**) • IP-III	• Severe/ profound SNHL • Variable • Normal to profound • Air bone gap + • Profound SNHL/mixed HL	• CI if cochlear nerve present (gusher risk) • ABI in CI aplasia • CI can be done, gusher risk • CI can be done, gusher risk
Cochlear nerve (CN/CVN) abnormalities		Severe to profound SNHL	Trial of CI—if hypoplastic ABI (absent nerve, late presentation)

(ABI: auditory brainstem implant; CI: cochlear implant; CLA: complete labyrinthine aplasia; CVN: cochleovestibular nerve; SNHL: sensorineural hearing loss)

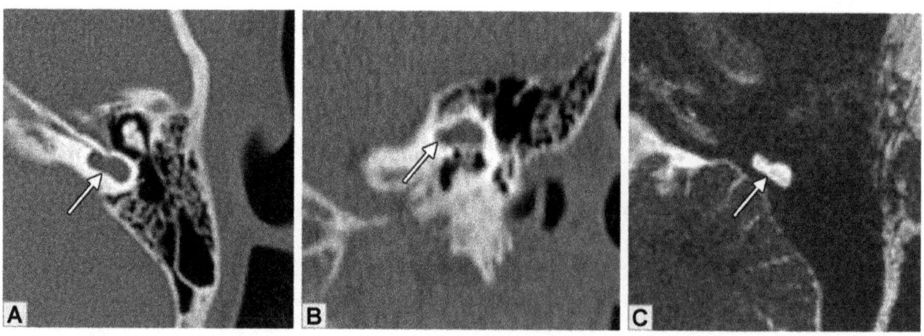

FIGS. 15A TO C: Group 4 inner ear malformation: Common cavity anomaly in a 4-year-old girl *precluding cochlear implantation*. HRCT temporal bone (A) axial and (B) coronal images and (C) axial CISS MR image of left ear reveal presence of one cystic structure without differentiation into cochlea and vestibule (arrow), and a narrow internal auditory meatus (IAM). The cochlear nerve was also absent.

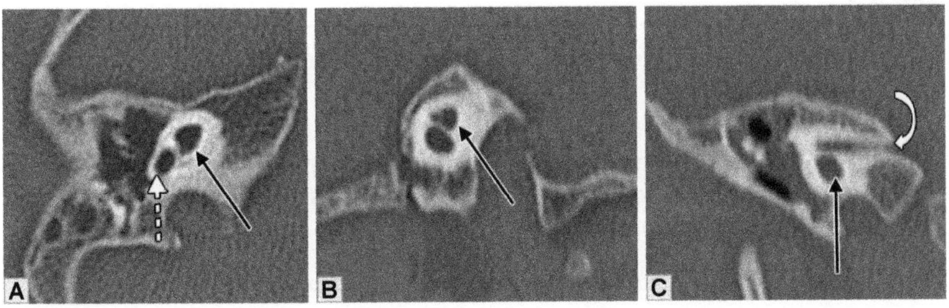

FIGS. 16A TO C: Group 5 inner ear malformation. Right cochlear hypoplasia: HRCT axial (A), sagittal (B) and coronal (C) image.
- Small cochlear bud (long arrow) arising from the vestibule (dotted arrow). Vestibule is hypoplastic; SCC absent.
- IAC is small (curved arrow). This is not a *contraindication to implantation*, but the hearing results will be limited.

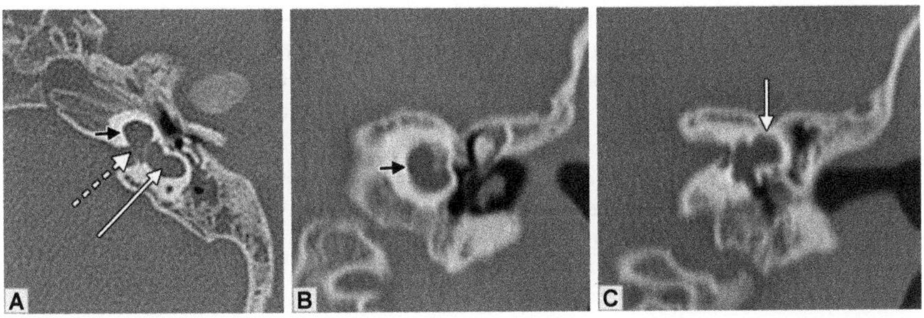

FIGS. 17A TO C: Left incomplete partition type I (cystic cochleovestibular dysplasia) *precluding cochlear implantation.* HRCT axial (A) and coronal (B and C) images.
- Cystic cochlea without any internal architecture (small arrow in A and B), and a dilated vestibule (long arrow in A).
- Cribriform plate is partly dehiscent (dotted arrow in A).
- Semicircular canal dysplasia (arrow in C).

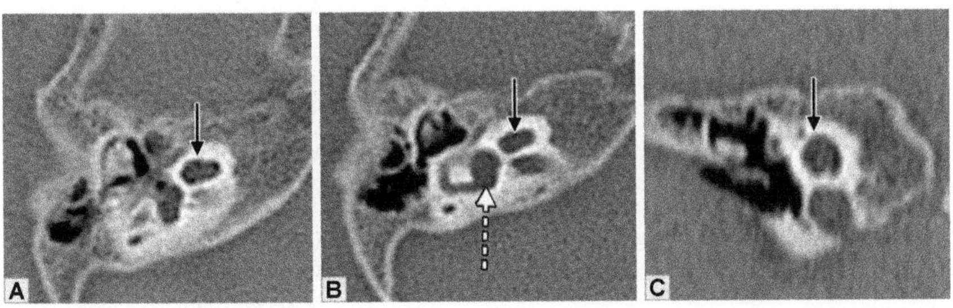

FIGS. 18A TO C: Right incomplete partition type II (Mondini dysplasia): *Not a contraindication to implantation.* HRCT (A and B) axial and (C) coronal images. Confluence of middle and apical turns of cochlea (arrow in A to C). Dilated vestibule (dotted arrow).

RECAP

As discussed earlier in **Flowchart 1**, a step-wise review of important anatomic details is given in **Table 3**.

TABLE 3 **Step-wise summary of cochlear implantation surgery and required anatomic details on HRCT/MRI (besides description of inner ear malformations).**

Steps	Anatomic details required	Implications
Postauricular pocket creation for the receiver (underneath temporalis muscle)	Local soft tissue status	Risk of infection
Cortical mastoidectomy	• Mastoid air cell pneumatization • Low-lying dura • Sigmoid sinus location	• Difficult mastoidectomy, injury to sigmoid sinus • Inadvertent injury • Inadvertent injury
Exposing incus, facial recess	• Facial recess anatomy • Course of facial nerve mastoid segment • Chorda tympani nerve location	• Difficult exposure • Difficult window for tympanotomy and risk of injury to facial nerve
Posterior tympanotomy through facial recess*	• Facial nerve (mastoid segment) canal position and relationship with RWN • Facial nerve second genu angle	• Difficulty in round window visibility • Difficulty in round window visibility
Round window niche (RWN), incudostapedial joint, pyramid exposed	• Middle ear aeration • High riding jugular bulb • Variant anatomy (persistent stapedial artery)	• Difficulty in round window visibility/chance of infection • Inadvertent injury, mechanical obstruction to round window niche • Inadvertent injury/difficulty in round window access
Cochleostomy made	• Round window membrane visibility • Cochlear ossification grading • Modiolus size and intactness of cribriform plate	• Difficulty in cochleostomy • Choosing site of cochleostomy, and modification of electrode type • Risk of gusher
Cochlear electrode inserted	• Inner ear malformation • Cochlear ossification grading • Scala chamber symmetry • Aberrant internal carotid artery	• Modification of electrode type/risk of gusher or meningitis • Modification of electrode type • Type of electrode insertion (scala tympani vs. scala vestibuli) • Risk of inadvertent injury

* Earlier, a separate cochleostomy anteroinferior to the round window membrane was used for cochlear electrode insertion. However, round window insertion (through its anteroinferior quadrant) is the preferred route nowadays; as it assures a superior access to scala tympani through a small incision. Several other sites of cochleostomy are known. However, details are beyond the scope of this chapter.

STRUCTURED REPORTING FORMAT

Please refer to Chapter 15.

INTRAOPERATIVE IMAGING

Plain radiological assessment is required for confirmation of correct insertion of implants. In cases of malformations advanced radiological investigations are required for confirmation of proper insertion of electrodes. (also see Chapter 13)

POSTOPERATIVE IMAGING

- Required in implant malfunction (trauma, malposition, infection, or other implant-related complications) HRCT is ideal modality (**Figs. 19A** to **D**).
- MRI suitability: Vendor instruction should be followed. Implants with detachable magnets are available. Internal implant dislocation is serious complication which needs revision of surgery.

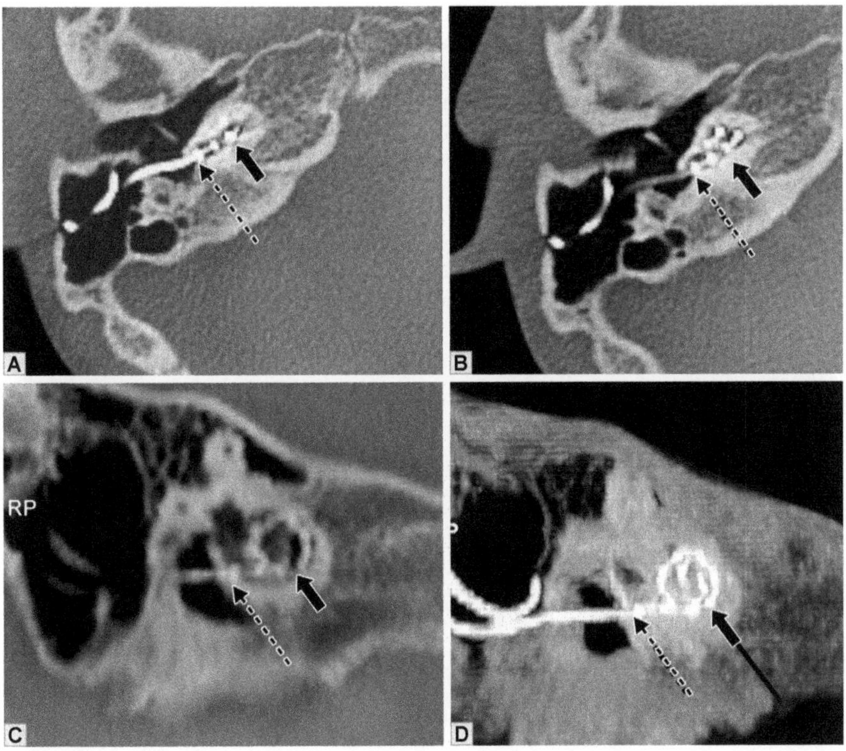

FIGS. 19A TO D: Normal position of cochlear implant on CT: (A and B) Axial HRCT images and (C and D) MIP images. Electrodes are arranged along the turns of cochlea (block arrow). Reference electrode is present at cochleostomy site (dotted arrow).

REFERENCES

1. Young JY, Ryan ME, Young NM. Preoperative imaging of sensorineural hearing loss in pediatric candidates for cochlear implantation. Radiographics. 2014;34(5):E133-49.
2. Alam-Eldeen MH, Rashad UM, Awad Ali AH. Radiological requirements for surgical planning in cochlear implant candidates. Indian J Radiol Imaging. 2017;27:274-81.
3. Sun D-Il, Lee DH, Jang KH, Park YS, Yeo SW, Choi J, et al. A suggested new classification system for the anatomic variations of the sigmoid sinus: a preliminary study. Int Adv Otol. 2009;5:1-5.
4. Pereira AR Júnior, Pinheiro SD, Vieira de Castro JD, Ximenes Filho JA, Rabelo de Freitas M. Mastoidectomy: anatomical parameters x surgical difficulty. Int Arch Otorhinolaryngol. 2012;16(01): 57-61.
5. Mandour MF, Khalifa MA, Khalifa HA, Tomoum MO. A novel radiologic check test of round window accessibility for cochlear implantation: Our experience in 198 cases. Clin Otolaryngol. 2017;42(05):1108-11.
6. Sayit AT, Gunbey HP, Sa lam D, Gunbey E, Karda S, Çelenk C. Association between facial nerve second genu angle and facial canal dehiscence in patients with cholesteatoma: evaluation with temporal multidetector computed tomography and surgical findings. Braz J Otorhinolaryngol. 2019;85(3): 365-70.
7. Hasaballah MS, Hamdy TA. Evaluation of facial nerve course, posterior tympanotomy width and visibility of round window in patients with cochlear implantation by performing oblique sagittal cut computed tomographic scan temporal bone. Egyptian J Otolaryngol. 2014;30:317-21.
8. Sasindran V, Joseph A, Abraham SS, Hiremath SB. High-riding jugular bulb: A rare entity. Indian J Otol. 2014;20(3):129-31.
9. Young RJ, Shatzkes DR, Babb JS, Lalwani AK. The Cochlear-Carotid Interval: Anatomic Variation and Potential Clinical Implications. AJNR Am J Neuroradiol. 2006;27(7):1486-90.
10. Glastonbury CM, Davidson HC, Harnsberger HR, Butler J, Kertesz TR, Shelton C. Head and neck: Imaging findings of cochlear nerve deficiency. AJNR Am J Neuroradiol. 2002;23:635-43.
11. Fatterpekar GM, Mukherji SK, Alley J, Lin Y, Castillo M. Hypoplasia of the bony canal for the cochlear nerve in patients with congenital sensorineural hearing loss: Initial observations. Radiology. 2000;215:243-6.
12. Escude B, James C, Deguine O, Cochard N, Eter E, Fraysse B. The size of cochlea and predictions of insertion depth angles for cochlear implant electrodes. Audiol Neurotol 2006;11(suppl):27-33.

15

Reporting Template and Illustrative Cases

Smita Manchanda, Manisha Jana

- The following describes the reporting template for evaluation of cases of inner ear malformations and cochlear implant reporting.
- The CT measurements (**Figs. 1A** and **B**) for inner ear reporting template should be done as described below.
  - Make the CT true axial before making measurements.
  - To make true axial, make the bilateral head of condyle at same level on coronal section and on sagittal section make the plane along the base of skull.
  - After making true axial image, place one axis along the basal turn of cochlea. Now we get oblique coronal and oblique sagittal planes.
  - *Oblique coronal image*:
    - Oblique coronal image is made by placing the one axis along the basal turn of cochlea and other axis perpendicular to the previous such that it passes through the apex to cochlea.
    - The *cochlear height* is measured at this level by drawing a line perpendicular to cochlear basal turn, from the level of cochlear nerve foramen up to the cochlear apex.
    - Normal range is 3.28–3.90 mm.

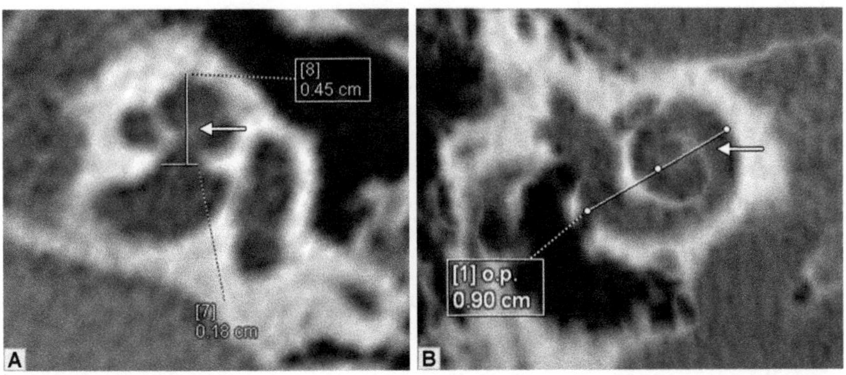

FIGS. 1A AND B: Measurement of cochlear height and cochlear length on CT image: (A) The ***cochlear height*** is measured on the oblique coronal plane by drawing a line perpendicular to cochlear basal turn, from the level of cochlear nerve foramen up to the cochlear apex (4.5 mm in this case); (B) The ***cochlear length*** is measured on the standardized cochlear image as the length of line passing from the midpoint of round window through cochlear modiolus and intersecting with cochlear anterior edge (9.0 mm in this case).

- *Standardized cochlear image*:
  - On the oblique sagittal image place the axis such that it passes through superior and inferior segments of basal turn of cochlea. This gives the double oblique coronal reformatted image of cochlea. This is viewed in the minimum intensity projection (minIP) with slice thickness increased to 1.3–1.5. All turns of cochlea, round window and oval window are seen in a single image to call it as standard minIP cochlear image.
  - The *cochlear length* is measured at this level as the length of line passing from the midpoint of round window through cochlear modiolus and intersecting with cochlear anterior edge.
  - Normal range is 8.10–9.59 mm.

REPORTING TEMPLATE CT

	Right	Left
1. External ear		
2. Middle ear:		
a. Soft tissue		
b. Ossicles		
3. Facial nerve canal		
4. Any mastoiditis		
5. Semicircular canal (SCC):		
a. Lateral SCC		
b. Superior SCC		
c. Posterior SCC		
6. Endolymphatic sac/duct		
7. Vestibule		
8. Cochlea:		
a. Turns		
b. Sclerosis		
c. Modiolus		
d. Cochlear height (mm)		
e. Cochlear length (mm)		
9. Cochlear aqueduct patency		
10. Round window patency		
11. Oval window patency		
12. Internal auditory canal (IAC) width (mm)		
13. Carotid canal location		
14. Jugular bulb location		
15. Any other finding		

Key: N: Normal; Ab: Abnormal; P: Present; A: Absent; I: Intact; E: Eroded; S: Stenosis; D: Dilatation; Dy: Dysplasia

IMPRESSION: Mention according to classification system as given by Sennaroglu L, et al. (Refer to Chapter 11)

REPORTING TEMPLATE MRI

	Right	Left
1. External ear		
2. Middle ear:		
a. Soft tissue		
b. Ossicles		
3. Facial nerve canal		
4. Any mastoiditis		
5. SCC:		
a. Lateral SCC		
b. Superior SCC		
c. Posterior SCC		
6. Endolymphatic sac/duct		
7. Vestibule		
8. Cochlea:		
a. Turns		
b. Sclerosis		
c. Modiolus		
9. Cochlear aqueduct patency		
10. Round window patency		
11. Oval window patency		
12. IAC width (mm)		
13. Carotid canal location		
14. Jugular bulb location		
15. Facial nerve		
16. Cochlear nerve		
17. Vestibular nerve		
18. Any other finding		

Key: N: Normal; Ab: Abnormal; P: Present; A: Absent; I: Intact; E: Eroded; S: Stenosis; D: Dilatation; Dy: Dysplasia

IMPRESSION: Mention according to classification system as given by Sennaroglu L, et al. (Refer to Chapter 11) and the size of cochlear nerves.

CASE 1 (FIGS. 2A TO F)

A 5-year-old female presenting with right sensorineural hearing loss (SNHL).

	Right	Left
1. External ear	***TM retraction***	N
2. Middle ear:		
a. Soft tissue	N	N
b. Ossicles (**Fig. 2C**)	N	N
3. Facial nerve canal (**Fig. 2E**)	N	N
4. Any mastoiditis	A	A
5. SCC:		
a. Lateral SCC (**Fig. 2D**)	***Dy***	N
b. Superior SCC	N	N
c. Posterior SCC	N	N
6. Endolymphatic sac/duct	N	N
7. Vestibule (**Figs. 2A** and **F**)	***Common cavity***	N
8. Cochlea (**Figs. 2A** and **F**):	***Common cavity***	N
a. Turns	A	N
b. Sclerosis	A	A
c. Modiolus	A	N
d. Cochlear height (mm)	-	3.7
e. Cochlear length (mm)	-	8.9
9. Cochlear aqueduct patency	A	N
10. Round window patency (**Fig. 2D**)	N	N
11. Oval window patency (**Fig. 2B**)	N	N
12. IAC width (mm)	4	4.2
13. Carotid canal location	N	N
14. Jugular bulb location	N	N
15. Any other finding	-	

Key: N: Normal; Ab: Abnormal; P: Present; A: Absent; I: Intact; E: Eroded; S: Stenosis; D: Dilatation; Dy: Dysplasia

IMPRESSION: Right common cavity

- **Lateral SCC dysplasia**

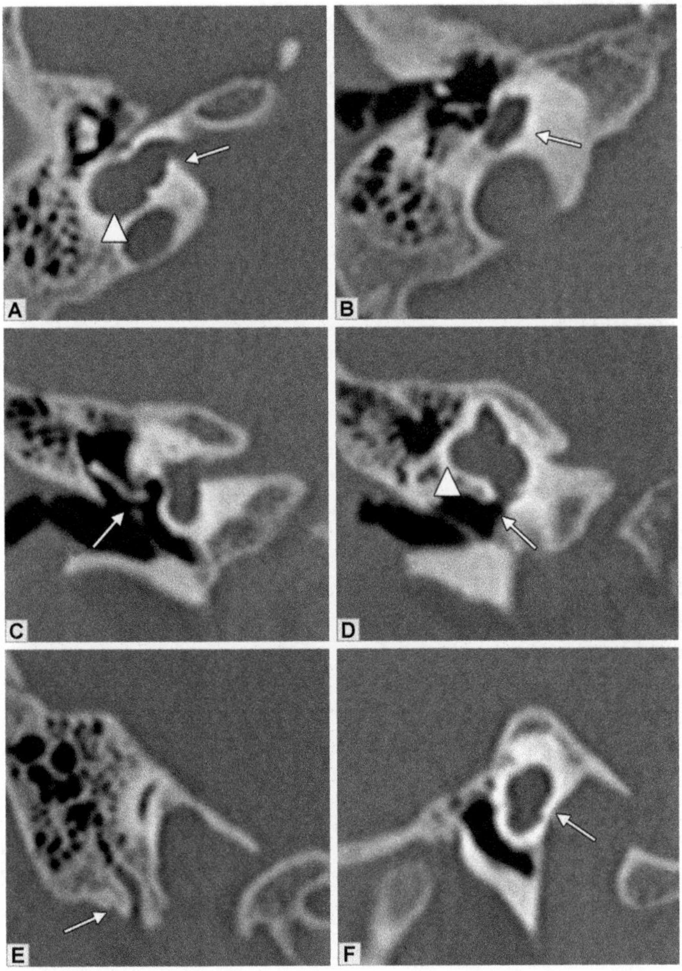

(IAC: internal auditory canal; SCC: semicircular canal)

FIGS. 2A TO F: Right common cavity: (A and B) Axial: Oval cystic structure (arrowhead in A and arrow in B) without any differentiation into cochlea and vestibule. IAC enters at the center of the cystic structure (arrow in B); (C) Coronal: Normal ossicles (arrow); (D) Coronal: Normal round window (arrow). Lateral SCC dysplasia (arrowhead); (E) Coronal: Facial canal (arrow); (F) Right sagittal oblique: Common cavity (arrow).

CASE 2 (FIGS. 3A TO D)

A 3-year-old female presenting with left hearing loss.

	Right	Left
1. External ear	***Soft tissue***	N
2. Middle ear:		
a. Soft tissue	***P***	A
b. Ossicles	I	I
3. Facial nerve canal (**Fig. 3C**)	N	N
4. Any mastoiditis	P	A
5. SCC (**Fig. 3D**):		
a. Lateral SCC	N	N
b. Superior SCC	N	N
c. Posterior SCC	N	N
6. Endolymphatic sac/duct	N	N
7. Vestibule (**Fig. 3A**)	N	N
8. Cochlea (**Fig. 3B**):	N	**Small**
a. Turns	N	2
b. Sclerosis	A	A
c. Modiolus	N	P
d. Cochlear height (mm)	3.9	2.1
e. Cochlear length (mm)	8.9	6.7
9. Cochlear aqueduct patency	A	A
10. Round window patency	A	A
11. Oval window patency	A	A
12. IAC width (mm)	4.2	4.5
13. Carotid canal location	N	N
14. Jugular bulb location	N	N
15. Any other finding	-	

Key: N: Normal; Ab: Abnormal; P: Present; A: Absent; I: Intact; E: Eroded; S: Stenosis; D: Dilatation; Dy: Dysplasia

IMPRESSION: Left type IV cochlear hypoplasia

- **Right noncholesteatomatous CSOM**

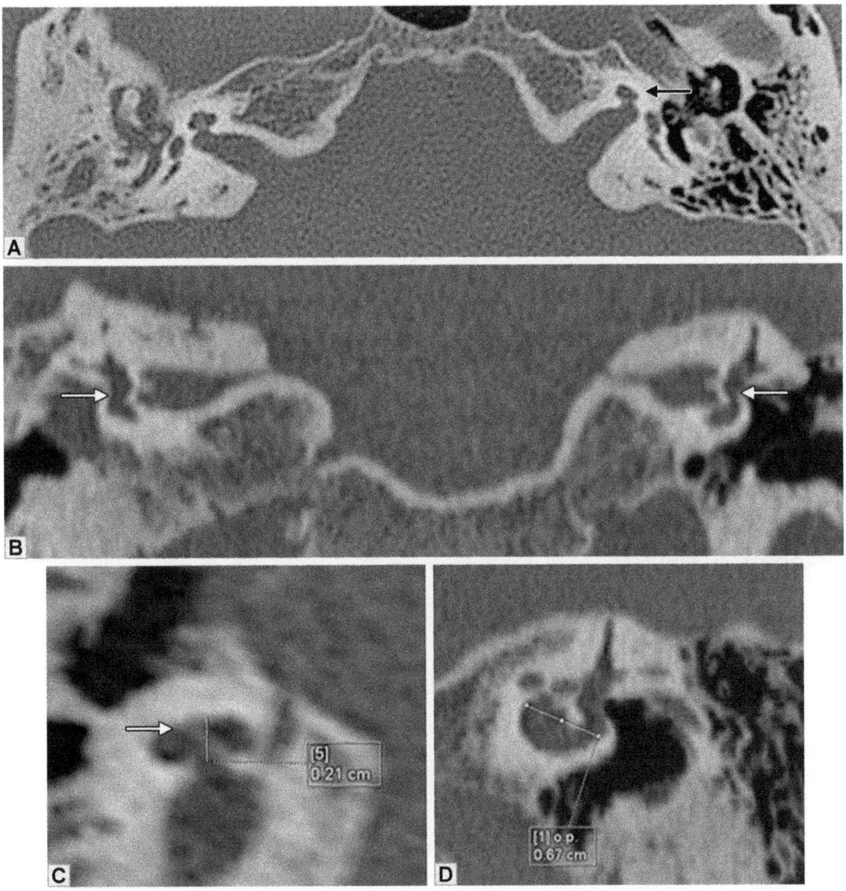

FIGS. 3A TO D: Left type IV cochlear hypoplasia: (A) Axial: Left cochlear hypoplasia (arrow); (B) Coronal: Bilateral vestibule normal (arrows); (C) Oblique coronal image (left): Cochlear height is 2.1 mm. Hypoplastic apical and middle turns (arrow); (D) Standardized cochlear image (left): Cochlear length is 6.7 mm. Basal turn of cochlea normal.

CASE 3 (FIGS. 4A TO D)

A 4-year-old female presenting with right congenital hearing loss.

	Right	Left
1. External ear	N	N
2. Middle ear (**Fig. 4B**):		
a. Soft tissue	***P***	***P***
b. Ossicles	I	I
3. Facial nerve canal	N	N
4. Any mastoiditis	***P***	***P***
5. Semicircular canal:		
a. Lateral SCC (**Fig. 4C**)	N	N
b. Superior SCC	N	N
c. Posterior SCC	N	N
6. Endolymphatic sac/duct (**Fig. 4A**)	***D***	***D***
7. Vestibule (**Figs. 4B**)	***D***	***D***
8. Cochlea (**Fig. 4D**):		
a. Turns	***Fusion of middle and apical turns***	***Fusion***
b. Sclerosis	***A***	A
c. Modiolus	***P but deficient***	***P but deficient***
d. Cochlear height (mm)	4.1	3.9
e. Cochlear length (mm)	7.5	7.7
9. Cochlear aqueduct patency	N	N
10. Round window patency	N	N
11. Oval window patency	N	N
12. IAC width (mm)	5.5	4.1
13. Carotid canal location	N	N
14. Jugular bulb location	N	N
15. Any other finding	-	

Key: N: Normal; Ab: Abnormal; P: Present; A: Absent; I: Intact; E: Eroded; S: Stenosis; D: Dilatation; Dy: Dysplasia

IMPRESSION: Bilateral incomplete partition type II deformity

- **Bilateral noncholesteatomatous CSOM**

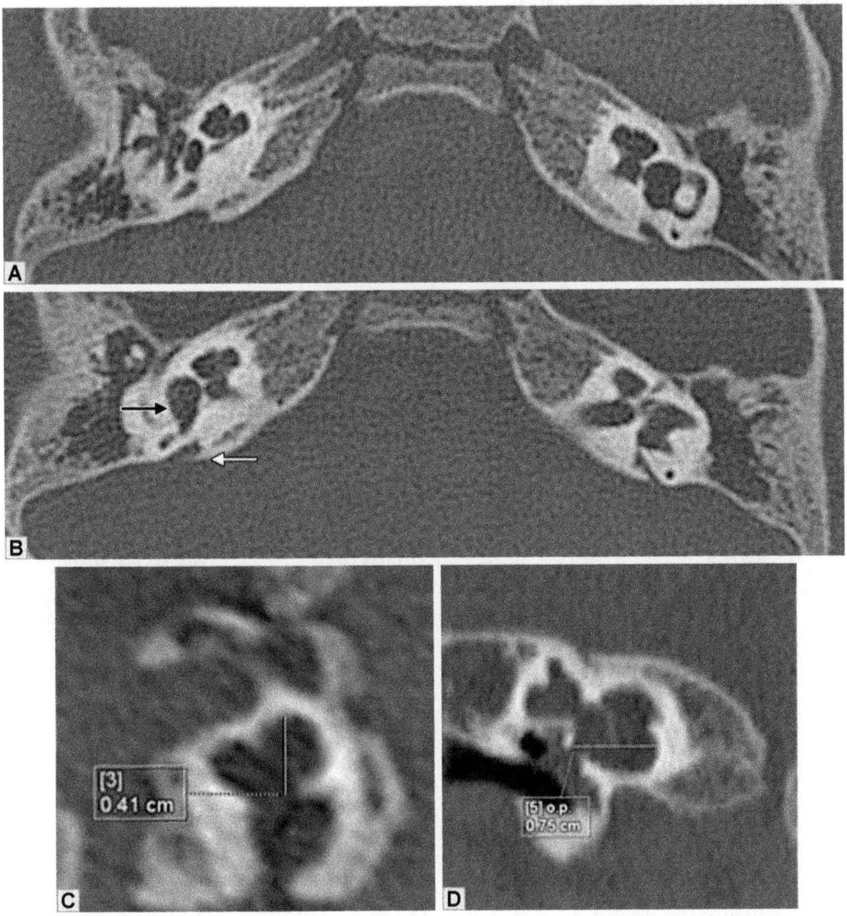

FIGS. 4A TO D: Bilateral incomplete partition type II anomaly: (A) Axial: Normal size of bilateral cochlea; (B) Axial: Bilateral vestibule dilated (black arrow). Vestibular aqueduct dilatation (white arrow); (C) Oblique coronal image (right): Cochlear height is 4.1 mm; (D) Standardized cochlear image (right): Cochlear length is 7.5 mm.

CASE 4 CT (FIGS. 5A TO D)

A 4-year-old male presenting with bilateral mixed hearing loss.

	Right	Left
1. External ear	N	N
2. Middle ear (**Fig. 5A**):		
a. Soft tissue	A	A
b. Ossicles	I	I
3. Facial nerve canal	N	N
4. Any mastoiditis	A	A
5. Semicircular canal:		
a. Lateral SCC	N	N
b. Superior SCC	N	N
c. Posterior SCC	N	N
6. Endolymphatic sac/duct	N	N
7. Vestibule	N	N
8. Cochlea:		
a. Turns	***Basal turn communicating with IAC*** (**Fig. 5C**)	***Basal turn communicating*** **with IAC** (**Fig. 5D**)
b. Sclerosis	A	A
c. Modiolus (**Fig. 5B**)	**A**	**A**
d. Cochlear height (mm)	3.9	3.9
e. Cochlear length (mm)	9.2	9.1
9. Cochlear aqueduct patency	N	N
10. Round window patency	N	N
11. Oval window patency	N	N
12. IAC width (mm) (**Fig. 5B**)	8.8	8.7
13. Carotid canal location	N	N
14. Jugular bulb location	N	N
15. Any other finding	-	

Key: N: Normal; Ab: Abnormal; P: Present; A: Absent; I: Intact; E: Eroded; S: Stenosis; D: Dilatation; Dy: Dysplasia

IMPRESSION: Bilateral incomplete partition type III (pseudo-Mondini) anomaly

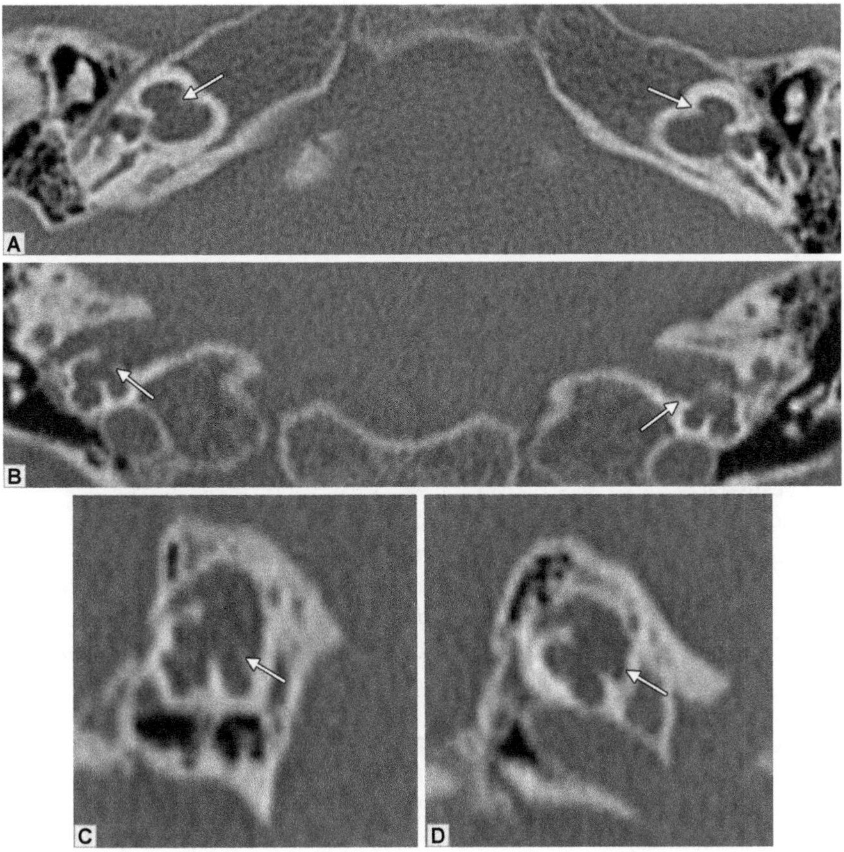

FIGS. 5A TO D: Bilateral incomplete partition type III anomaly (CT): (A) Axial: Wide cochlear aperture (arrows); (B) Coronal: Absent modiolus (arrows); (C) Right sagittal oblique: Basal turn communicating with IAC (arrow); (D) Left sagittal oblique: Basal turn communicating with IAC (arrow).

CASE 4 MRI (FIGS. 6A TO F)

A 4-year-old male presenting with bilateral mixed hearing loss.

	Right	Left
1. External ear	N	N
2. Middle ear:		
a. Soft tissue	A	A
b. Ossicles	I	I
3. Any mastoiditis	A	A
4. Semicircular canal:		
a. Lateral SCC	N	N
b. Superior SCC	N	N
c. Posterior SCC	N	N
5. Endolymphatic sac/duct	N	N
6. Vestibule	N	N
7. Cochlea:		
a. Turns	***Basal turn communicating with IAC*** (**Figs. 6B, C** and **E**)	***Basal turn communicating with IAC*** (**Figs. 6B, D** and **F**)
b. Sclerosis	A	A
c. Modiolus	A	A
8. Cochlear aqueduct patency	N	N
9. Round window patency	N	N
10. Oval window patency	N	N
11. IAC width (mm)	8.8	8.7
12. Carotid canal location	N	N
13. Jugular bulb location	N	N
14. Facial nerve canal	N	N
15. Facial nerve (**Fig. 6A**)	N	N
16. Cochlear nerve (**Fig. 6A**)	1.3 mm	1.2 mm
17. Vestibular nerve (**Fig. 6A**)	N	N
18. Any other finding	-	

Key: N: Normal; Ab: Abnormal; P: Present; A: Absent; I: Intact; E: Eroded; S: Stenosis; D: Dilatation; Dy: Dysplasia

IMPRESSION: Bilateral incomplete partition type III (pseudo-Mondini) deformity

- **Normal visualization of facial and vestibulocochlear nerves**

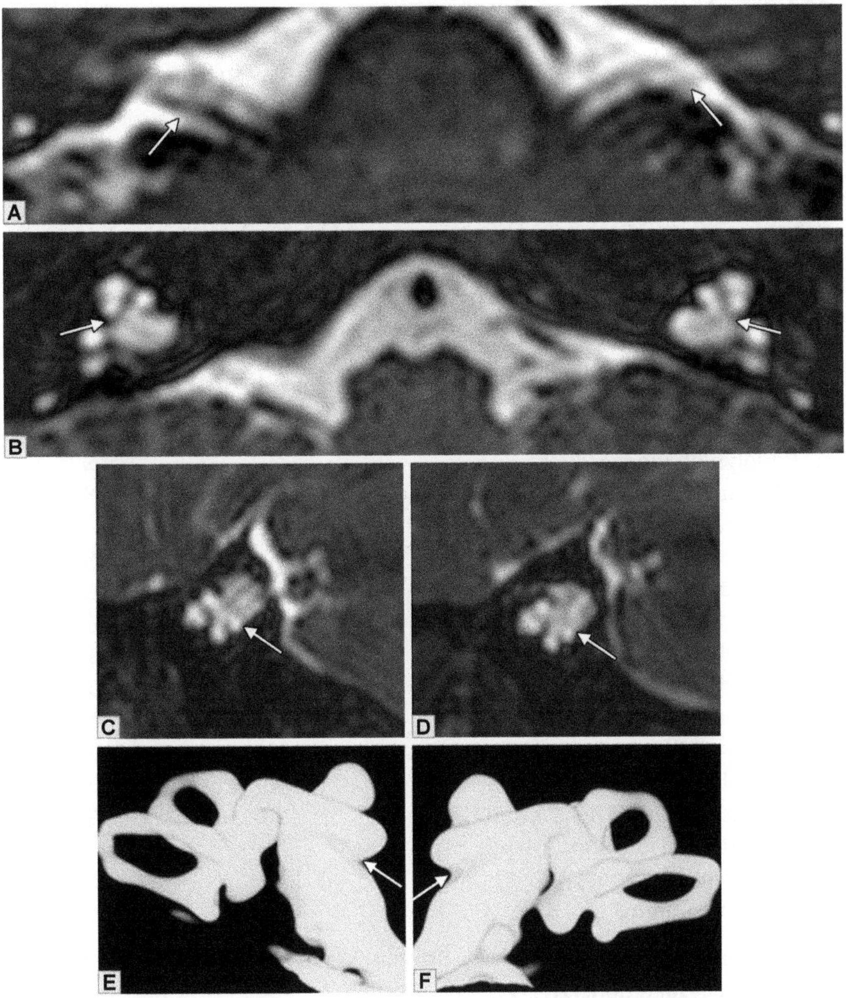

(CISS: constructive interference in steady state; IAC: internal auditory canal; VRT: volume-rendering technique)

FIGS. 6A TO F: Bilateral incomplete partition type III anomaly (MRI): (A) Axial CISS: Bilateral vestibulocochlear nerves in cisternal segments (arrows); (B) Axial CISS: Absent modiolus (arrows); (C) Right sagittal oblique: Basal turn communicating with IAC (arrow); (D) Left sagittal oblique: Basal turn communicating with IAC (arrow); (E and F) Right and left VRT. Basal turn communicating with IAC (arrows).

CASE 5 CT (FIGS. 7A TO C)

A 5-year-old female presenting with bilateral congenital SNHL.

	Right	Left
1. External ear	N	N
2. Middle ear:		
a. Soft tissue (**Figs. 7B** and **C**)	A	***P***
b. Ossicles	I	I
3. Facial nerve canal	N	N
4. Any mastoiditis (**Figs. 7B** and **C**)	A	***P***
5. Semicircular canal:		
a. Lateral SCC	N	N
b. Superior SCC	N	N
c. Posterior SCC	N	N
6. Endolymphatic sac/duct	N	N
7. Vestibule	N	N
8. Cochlea:		
a. Turns	N	N
b. Sclerosis	A	A
c. Modiolus	P	P
d. Cochlear height (mm)	3.8	3.7
e. Cochlear length (mm)	9.0	8.9
9. Cochlear aqueduct patency	N	N
10. Round window patency	N	N
11. Oval window patency	N	N
12. IAC width (mm) (**Figs. 7A** and **C**)	***1.8***	***0.6***
13. Carotid canal location	N	N
14. Jugular bulb location	N	N
15. Any other finding	-	

Key: N: Normal; Ab: Abnormal; P: Present; A: Absent; I: Intact; E: Eroded; S: Stenosis; D: Dilatation; Dy: Dysplasia

IMPRESSION: Bilateral IAC stenosis

- **Left noncholesteatomatous CSOM**

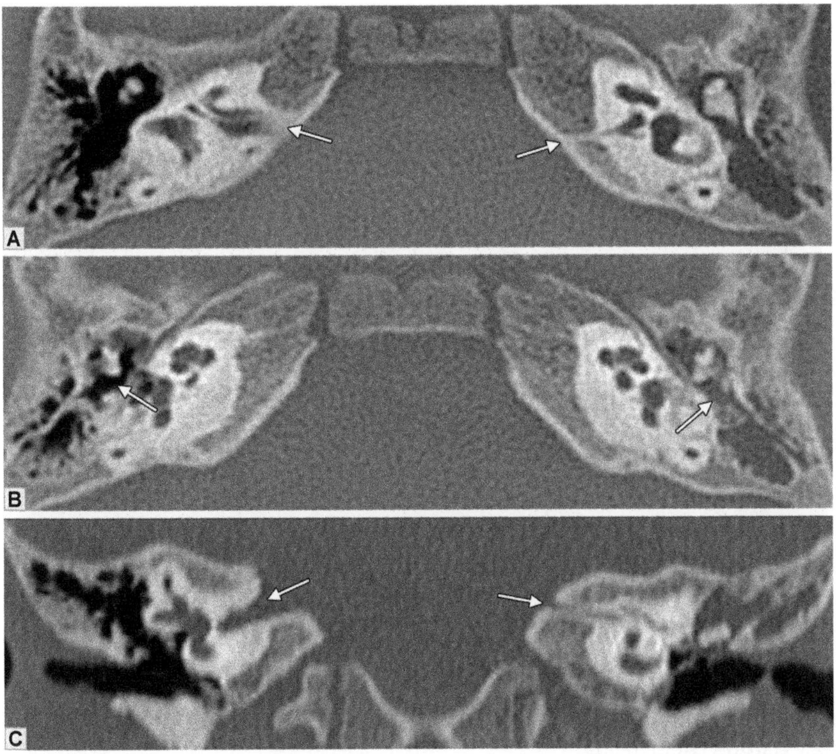

FIGS. 7 A TO C: Bilateral IAC stenosis (CT): (A) Axial: Narrow caliber of bilateral IAC (arrows); (B) Axial: Left otomastoiditis (arrows). Right middle ear cavity normal; (C) Coronal: Bilateral IAC stenosis (arrows).

CASE 5 MRI (FIGS. 8A TO D)

A 5-year-old female presenting with bilateral congenital SNHL.

	Right	Left
1. External ear	N	N
2. Middle ear:		
a. Soft tissue	A	P
b. Ossicles	I	I
3. Any mastoiditis (**Fig. 8B**)	A	P
4. Semicircular canal:		
a. Lateral SCC	N	N
b. Superior SCC	N	N
c. Posterior SCC	N	N
5. Endolymphatic sac/duct	N	N
6. Vestibule	N	N
7. Cochlea:		
a. Turns	N	N
b. Sclerosis	A	A
c. Modiolus	P	P
8. Cochlear aqueduct patency	N	N
9. Round window patency	N	N
10. Oval window patency	N	N
11. IAC width (mm)	***1.8***	***0.6***
12. Carotid canal location	N	N
13. Jugular bulb location	N	N
14. Facial nerve canal	N	N
15. Facial nerve	N (**Figs. 8A** and **C**)	N (**Figs. 8A** and **D**)
16. Cochlear nerve	***Hypoplasia 4 mm*** (**Figs. 8A** and **C**)	***Aplasia*** (**Figs. 8A** and **D**)
17. Vestibular nerve	Hypoplasia	Aplasia
18. Any other finding	-	

Key: N: Normal; Ab: Abnormal; P: Present; A: Absent; I: Intact; E: Eroded; S: Stenosis; D: Dilatation; Dy: Dysplasia

IMPRESSION: Bilateral IAC stenosis

- **Hypoplasia of right cochlear nerve**
- **Aplasia of left cochlear nerve**
- **Left noncholesteatomatous CSOM**

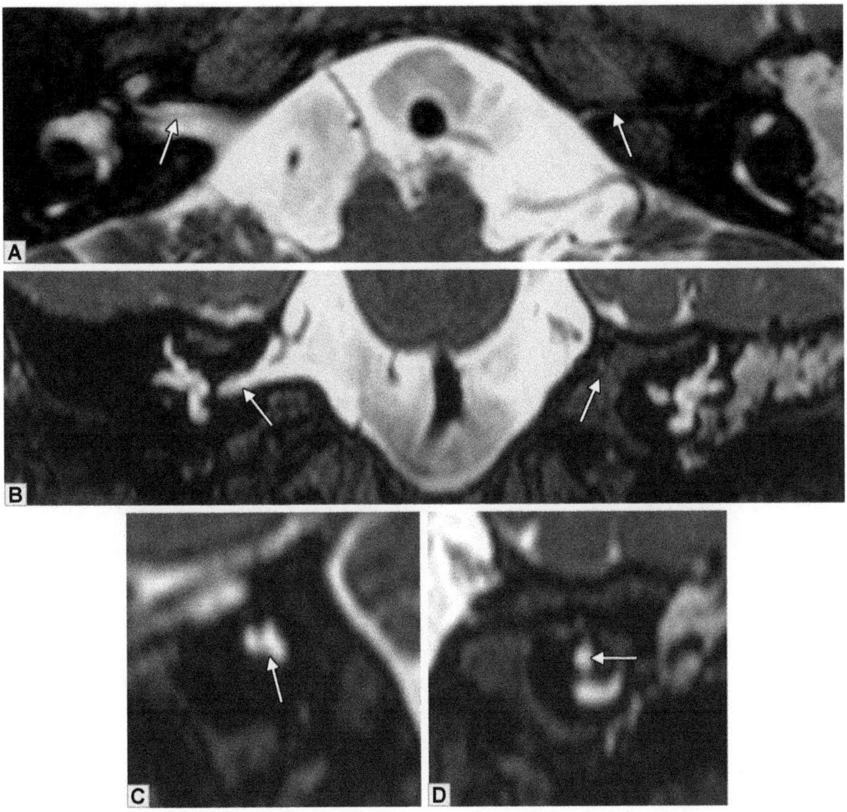

FIGS. 8A TO D: Bilateral IAC stenosis (MRI): (A) Axial: Hypoplasia of vestibulocochlear nerves (arrows); (B) Coronal: Marked stenosis of IAC (Left > Right); (C) Right sagittal oblique: Right cochlear nerve hypoplasia (arrow); (D) Left sagittal oblique: Left cochlear nerve aplasia (arrow).

5
SECTION

Tumors

16

Tumors and Tumor-like Conditions

Chandrashekhara SH, Aanchal Kakkar, Manisha Jana

- Temporal bone tumors are classified based on location, origin, histologic findings, and benign or malignant criteria.
- We should be aware of various pseudo lesions and benign lesions mimicking temporal bone tumors.
- Temporal bone tumors are generally difficult for clinical access, hence imaging is invaluable component of their evaluation.

CLASSIFICATION OF TEMPORAL BONE TUMORS

The recent WHO classification of ear tumors is summarized in **Tables 1** and **2**.[1]

- It is noteworthy that compared to the previous version; there has been a number of changes in the classification of EAC tumors in the recent WHO classification (also see **Table 3**).
- Entities such as exostosis and osteoma have been excluded from the list.

TABLE 1 **WHO 2017 classification of tumors of the EAC, and their histological and immunohistochemical (IHC) features (Figs. 1A to I).**

	Origin	Histopathological features	IHC and genetic profile
Squamous cell carcinoma	Squamous epithelium of the EAC	Atypical keratinocytes in nests, sheets, and single cells with abundant eosinophilic cytoplasm, large nucleus with vesicular chromatin and prominent nucleolus;	Positive for cytokeratin, CK5/6, p40, p63

Continued

Continued

	Origin	Histopathological features	IHC and genetic profile
		dyskeratotic cells, intercellular bridges, keratin pearls, and squamous eddies may be present; spindle cell and acantholytic features may also occur. May be well, moderately, or poorly differentiated	
Adenocarcinomas			
Ceruminous adeno-carcinoma	Ceruminous glands of the EAC	Infiltrative tumor with solid, cystic, glandular, cribriform, and single-cell architecture; comedo-necrosis and PNI indicative of carcinoma; cells show apocrine features: decapitation secretion; ceroid pigment is absent	Biphasic pattern: CK7, CD117 in luminal cells; p63, p40, CK5/6, SMA in abluminal cells; GATA3 positivity indicates apocrine differentiation
Adenoid cystic carcinoma	Ceruminous glands of the external auditory canal	Tubular, cribriform, and solid architecture; basaloid cells with scant cytoplasm, and angulated hyperchromatic nuclei	Biphasic pattern: CK7, CD117 in luminal cells; p63, p40, CK5/6, SMA in abluminal cells; MYB positive; translocations in *MYB/MYBL1* genes
Mucoepider-moid carcinoma	Ceruminous glands of the external auditory canal	Solid-cystic tumor with variable proportion of squamoid, intermediate and mucin-producing cells; may be low-, intermediate-, or high grade	CK7 in mucous cells; p40 and p63 in intermediate cells; p40, p63, and CK5/6 in squamoid cells; *CRTC1-MAML2* gene fusions
Ceruminous adenoma	Ceruminous glands of the external auditory canal	Unencapsulated proliferation of bilayered glandular structures lined by inner cuboidal cells with granular eosinophilic cytoplasm and outer flattened basal/myoepithelial cells; luminal cells contain ceroid pigment, may show decapitation secretion; limited pleomorphism, infrequent mitoses, no necrosis	Biphasic pattern: CK7, CD117 in luminal cells; p63, p40, CK5/6, SMA in abluminal cells; GATA3 positivity indicates apocrine differentiation

(EAC: external auditory canal; PNI: perineural invasion; SMA: smooth muscle actin)

TABLE 2 **WHO 2017 classification of tumors of the middle and inner ear, and their histological and immunohistochemical (IHC) features (Figs. 1A to I).**

Type	Origin	Histopathological features	IHC and genetic profile
Squamous cell carcinoma (SCC)	Squamous epithelium within the middle ear	Similar to SCC of external auditory canal	
Aggressive papillary tumor	Origin from the endolymphatic sac has been suggested	Infiltrative tumor with papillary and glandular structures lined by low cuboidal to columnar cells with eosinophilic cytoplasm and monomorphic nuclei	Stain with cytokeratin, EMA, and S100
Endolymphatic sac tumor	Papillary epithelium of the endolymphatic sac	Broad papillary and cystic structures lined by flat, low cuboidal, or columnar cells with clear to pale eosinophilic cytoplasm and bland, eccentric nuclei; follicular structures containing colloid-like secretions resemble thyroid tissue	• CK, EMA, CK5/6, CK7, GFAP positive; TTF-1, CD10, CA-IX, and PAX8 negative • Germline and somatic mutations of *VHL* gene
Otosclerosis	Otic capsule	Masses of immature trabecular bone with evidence of remodeling	-
Cholesteatoma	Congenital: epidermoid formation; acquired: ingrowth of squamous epithelium into the middle ear	Keratinizing squamous epithelium, abundant anucleate keratin flakes	-
Vestibular schwannoma	Vestibulocochlear nerve	Alternating Antoni A and B areas; Antoni A: cellular areas with spindle cells showing nuclear palisading and Verocay bodies; Antoni B: microcystic or reticular appearance	S100, SOX10 positive
Meningioma	Meningothelial cells	Infiltrative tumor with cells in nests and lobules, with syncytial appearance; nuclei frequently show intranuclear inclusions	EMA, progesterone receptor

Continued

Continued

Type	Origin	Histopathological features	IHC and genetic profile
Middle ear adenoma	Dual mucin-secreting and neuroendocrine differentiation	Infiltrative tumor with varying architecture: trabecular, glandular, solid, acinar, cribriform, nested, sheeted, single-cell in a fibrotic stroma; inner flattened cells, outer cuboidal to columnar cells	CK, chromogranin, synaptophysin positive; CK7 in luminal cells; CK5/6, p63, p40 in abluminal cells
Middle ear paraganglioma*	Paraganglia in the adventitia of the jugular bulb or on the medial promontory wall of the middle ear	Nested architecture, i.e., Zellballen pattern; chief cells have pale eosinophilic to amphophilic, mildly granular cytoplasm, nuclei with stippled chromatin and abrupt nuclear pleomorphism; slender sustentacular cells at the periphery of nests	Synaptophysin, chromogranin, CD56 in chief cells; S100 in sustentacular cells; Germline mutations in *SDHx* genes

* Not classified under ear tumors, but under paraganglion tumors.

- Otosclerosis and cholesteatoma have been included in this classification, due to their aggressive behavior.[1-3]

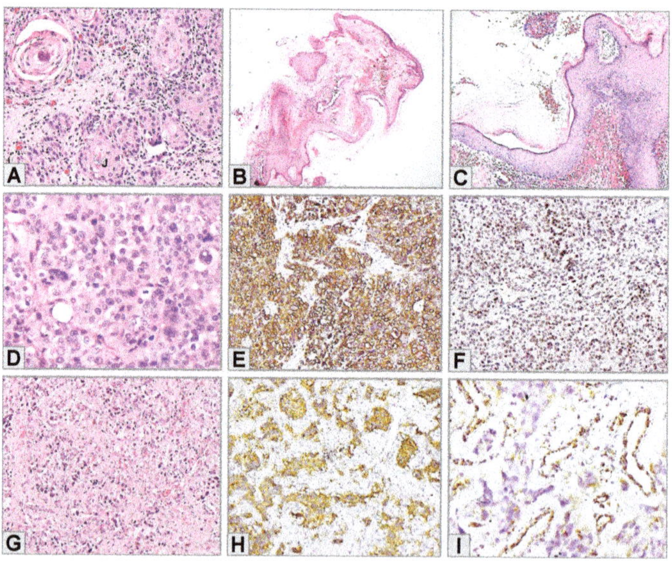

FIGS. 1A TO I: Squamous cell carcinoma of the external auditory canal with keratin pearls (A). Cholesteatoma showing proliferating squamous epithelium (B) with abundant keratin flakes (C). Ceruminous adenocarcinoma showing cells with abundant eosinophilic cytoplasm and frequent mitoses (D), immunopositive for cytokeratin (E), and GATA3 (F). Paraganglioma showing irregular nests of cells (G) that stain positively with synaptophysin (H) and show loss of SDHB staining indicative of *SDHx* gene mutation (I).

TABLE 3 Changes in classification of ear tumors from WHO 2005 to WHO 2017.

WHO 2005	WHO 2017	Change
Tumors of the external ear	Tumors of the EAC	Change in terminology
Benign tumors of ceruminous glands: • Adenoma • Chondroid syringoma • Syringocystadenoma papilliferum	Ceruminous adenoma	Ceruminous pleomorphic adenoma and ceruminous syringocystadenoma papilliferum are considered subtypes of ceruminous adenoma, as they show histological features of the named tumor as well as features of ceruminous differentiation
Cylindroma	-	Excluded as it is a skin adnexal tumor not unique to the EAC
Embryonal rhabdomyosarcoma	Excluded	Not unique to the EAC*
Osteoma and exostosis	Excluded	Not unique to the temporal bone*
Fibrous dysplasia	Excluded	Not unique to the temporal bone*
Angiolymphoid hyperplasia with eosinophilia	Excluded	Not unique to the external auditory canal[#]
Idiopathic pseudocystic chondromalacia	Excluded	Nonneoplastic
Chondrodermatitis nodularis chronica helicis	Excluded	Nonneoplastic
Tumors of the middle ear, and Tumors of the inner ear	Tumors of the middle and inner ear	Clubbed together, as the site of origin cannot always be determined
Adenoma of the middle ear	Middle ear adenoma	Minor change in terminology
Papillary tumors: Aggressive papillary tumor • Schneiderian papilloma • Inverted papilloma	Aggressive papillary tumor	Schneiderian papilloma and inverted papilloma excluded: insufficient evidence to support their occurrence in the middle ear
Lipoma of the internal auditory canal	Excluded	Not unique to the inner ear*
Hemangioma	Excluded	Not unique to the inner ear*
Hematolymphoid tumors: • B-cell chronic lymphocytic leukemia/small lymphocytic lymphoma • Langerhans cell histiocytosis	Excluded	Not unique to the ear*

Continued

Continued

WHO 2005	WHO 2017	Change
Secondary tumors	Excluded	Not unique to the ear
-	Otosclerosis	Included as uncontrolled growth and invasion of normal structures in the cochlear and vestibular otic capsules suggests behavior like that of a neoplasm
-	Cholesteatoma	Nonneoplastic; included due to its propensity to cause erosion of local structures and recur following surgery are indicative of aggressive and destructive behavior

(EAC: external auditory canal)

* Described elsewhere in the WHO Head and Neck fascicle.

Described in WHO skin tumors and WHO soft tissue tumors fascicles.

IMAGING

For evaluation of suspected tumor of temporal bone—CT and MRI are complimentary.

Computed Tomography

- Computed tomography (CT) provides information regarding the bony invasion by tumor, pattern of destruction, and also characterizes the tumors based on tumor morphology (matrix).
- High-resolution CT (HRCT) is essential for the evaluation of bony structures.
- Contrast CT is advocated for evaluation of temporal bone tumors.
- It is mandatory to view all the data set in both soft tissue and high-resolution bone algorithm.
- Multiplanar reconstructions, in particular coronal sections, provide extra information regarding extension of tumor and invasion of adjacent structures, facial nerve, and membranous labyrinth.
- Dual energy CT may be useful for artifact reduction and bone removal for better assessment of tumors.

Magnetic Resonance Imaging

- Magnetic resonance imaging (MRI) is the modality of choice for the evaluation of mass lesions involving internal auditory canal (IAC) and cerebellopontine angle (CPA).

- Various pulse sequences can be used. 3T MRI is better.
- Intravenously (IV) administered gadolinium—to visualize enhancement of tumor, soft tissues, meninges, and surrounding vascular structures.
- Usually, MRI is performed using dedicated multichannel head coil and high field strength.
- While scanning, both temporal bones should be imaged to compare both sides. Entire skull base should be included so that intracranial extension can be evaluated.

MRI Protocol

- It is better to begin the study with brain examination using either T2-weighted fast spin-echo (T2W FSE) or FLAIR (fluid-attenuated inversion recovery) sequence.
- Heavily thin T2W sequence 3D turbo spin echo (TSE)/FSE T2W sequence is acquired for the evaluation of fluid content and signal intensity (SI) characteristics in membranous labyrinth.
- Thin sections T1-weighted (T1W) sequences before and after intravenous administration of gadolinium: 1 mm (or even submillimetric) axial 3D T1W gradient echo sequence or a thin-slice (2 mm or less) axial and coronal SE T1W sequence can be used. Fat saturation techniques should be applied in one direction after contrast administration.
- Magnetic resonance angiogram should be done in suspected cased of glomus tumor or in patients of pulsatile tinnitus.
- Diffusion weighted imaging (DWI), preferably non-echo planar imaging (EPI) is added to evaluate the suspected tumoral or pseudotumoral lesion of temporal bone.
- Using DWI, we can differentiate between congenital or acquired cholesteatoma and epidermoid cysts.
- Coronal non-EPI method is better than axial technique due to reduced artifact from adjacent air.
- Recent advances in tractography may help in the delineation of facial nerve prior to tumor surgery.

EXTERNAL AUDITORY CANAL TUMORS

The external ear comprises of the pinna (auricle) and the external auditory canal (EAC). A discussion of tumors of pinna is beyond the scope of this chapter; as mostly they do not require imaging. The major entities are listed in **Box 1**.

BOX 1 Tumors of the external auditory canal.

- Benign: Ceruminous adenoma
- Malignant:
  - Squamous cell carcinoma
  - Adenocarcinoma (ceruminous, adenoid cystic, and mucoepidermoid)

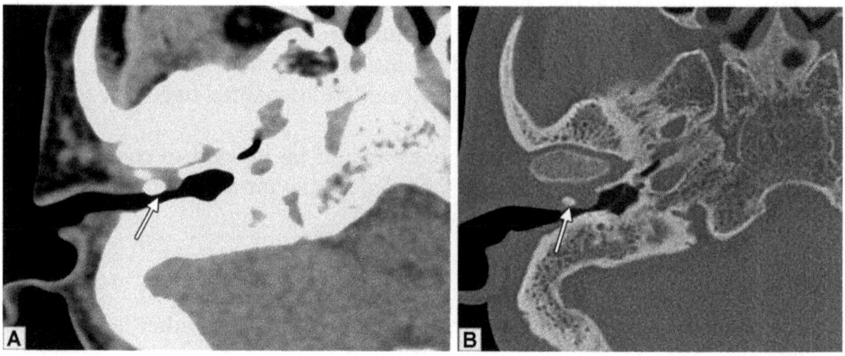

FIGS. 2A AND B: Right external auditory canal (EAC) ceruminous adenoma: HRCT (A) temporal bone axial soft tissue window and (B) bone window images showing soft tissue lesion with small calcification (arrow) in the anterior wall of right EAC.

Benign Tumor: EAC Adenoma (Ceruminous Adenoma)

- This is a rare EAC tumor and clinically can mimic a boil.
- Computer tomography may show a well-defined low attenuation lesion in the EAC (**Figs. 2A** and **B**).

Malignant Tumors of External Auditory Canal

- Malignant tumors of EAC are rare, and occur in older individuals (50–70 years).
- Most frequent primary malignant neoplasms of EAC are squamous cell carcinoma, basal cell carcinoma, adenoid cystic carcinoma, and ceruminous gland carcinoma.
- The risk factors include chronic ear infection and prior radiotherapy (for conditions such as nasopharyngeal carcinoma).

Imaging

- *Computed tomography is useful f*or early disease confined to the EAC or ME; detects erosion of the bony EAC (**Figs. 3** to **6**).
- *MRI*: It may demonstrate earliest sign of intracranial extension, which is seen as mild dural thickening and enhancement in vicinity of tegmen tympani. Spread into the labyrinth and perineural involvement of 7th and 8th cranial nerves are better appreciated.
- *The pathways of tumor spread are described in* ***Figure 7****, and the staging is discussed in Chapter 17.*
- Stylomastoid foramen should always be included in scanning volume to evaluate its fatty content with central hypointense facial nerve.
- Adenoid cystic carcinomas have propensity for skip metastases; thus, careful evaluation of entire course of facial nerve is mandatory.
- Prognosis of primary malignant tumors of the EAC depends on local invasion and extent.

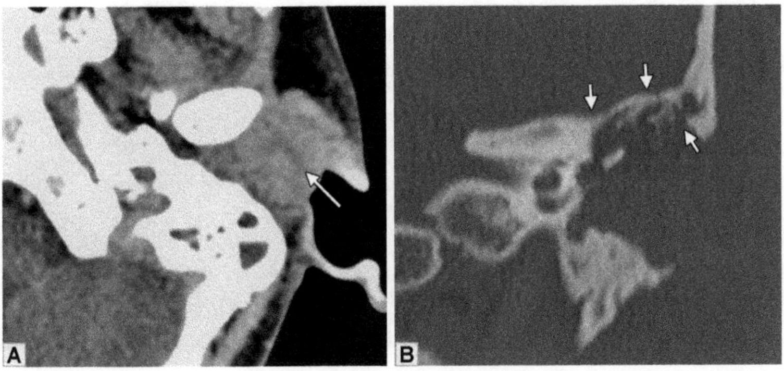

FIGS. 3A AND B: Left external auditory canal (EAC) carcinoma: CT (A) temporal bone axial image: Heterogeneously enhancing mass in the left EAC (arrow); (B) Coronal bone window image: Adjacent bony erosion (small arrows) by the mass.

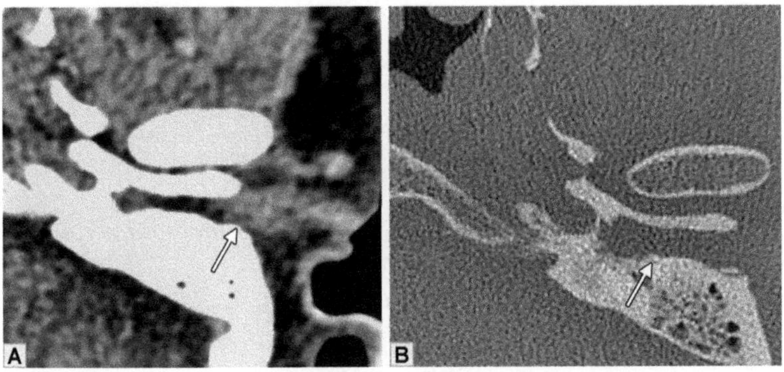

FIGS. 4A AND B: Left external auditory canal (EAC) carcinoma: HRCT (A) temporal bone axial soft tissue and (B) bone window images demonstrating heterogeneously enhancing mass in the left EAC (arrow), extending into middle ear, causing mild bony erosion (T3 stage).

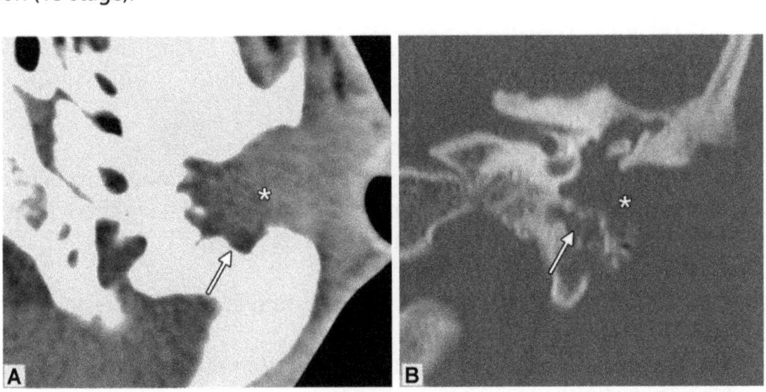

FIGS. 5A AND B: Recurrent left external auditory canal (EAC) carcinoma: HRCT (A) axial soft tissue window and (B) coronal bone window images demonstrate heterogeneously enhancing mass (asterisk) in the left EAC extending into middle ear cavity, causing bony destruction (arrow) of EAC.

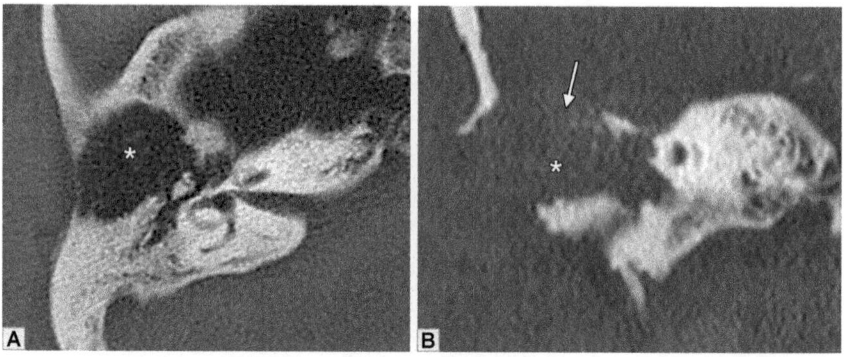

FIGS. 6A AND B: Squamous cell carcinoma of right external auditory canal (EAC): HRCT (A) axial and (B) coronal bone window images show large destructive soft tissue mass (asterisk) in right EAC with extension into middle ear cavity, causing bony destruction, including tegmen tympani (arrow) (T4 stage).

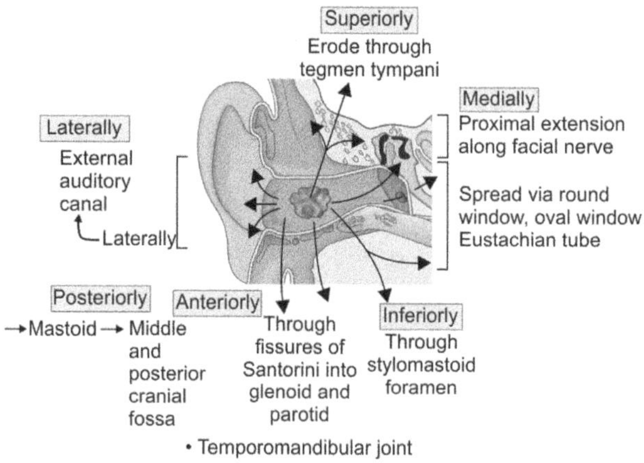

FIG. 7: Pathways of spread for external auditory canal (EAC) carcinoma.

Differential Diagnosis

- *Necrotizing external otitis*:
  - It is commonly seen in diabetics.
  - It may demonstrate extensive cellulitis and inflammatory changes, sometimes abscess formation involving the adjacent deep cervical spaces, most commonly the parotid space (see Chapter 8).
- *Osteoradionecrosis (ORN)*:
  - *Osteoradionecrosis* results from complication after radiotherapy for head and neck tumors.
  - The temporal bone is particularly susceptible due to its relatively poor blood supply.
  - It may be seen as diffuse permeative demineralization of the skull base. It may involve the mastoid air cells with disruption of the air cell septation, and associated radiation-induced otomastoiditis.

EAC Conditions Excluded from WHO 2017 Classification

Several disease entities have been omitted from the recent classification (**Table 2**); however some of them worth mentioning are discussed briefly.

Exostoses and Osteoma

These are benign bony tumors of the EAC, and exostoses are far more common than osteomas.

Exostoses

- Exostoses are broad-based lesions in medial half of EAC, near the tympanic annulus.
- There is a clear relation between exostoses and history of repetitive exposure to cold water, such as in surfing, swimming, and diving (*Surfer's* or *swimmer's* ear).
- It is often bilateral and asymptomatic.
- On CT, a broad-based bony well-demarcated lesion is seen. CT shows the extent and eventual retro-obstructive pathologic findings in middle ear.
- Magnetic resonance imaging is not required.

Osteomas

- Osteomas are more rare and are situated in lateral part of EAC
- These are mostly unilateral.
- Osteomas are layered as normal bone, including central bone marrow (**Figs. 8** and **9**).
- Osteomas may also arise in middle ear and mastoid and even in petrous bone pyramid near porus of internal acoustic canal.
- Large EAC osteomas may cause obstruction of epithelial migration and debris impaction, predisposing to cholesteatoma formation.

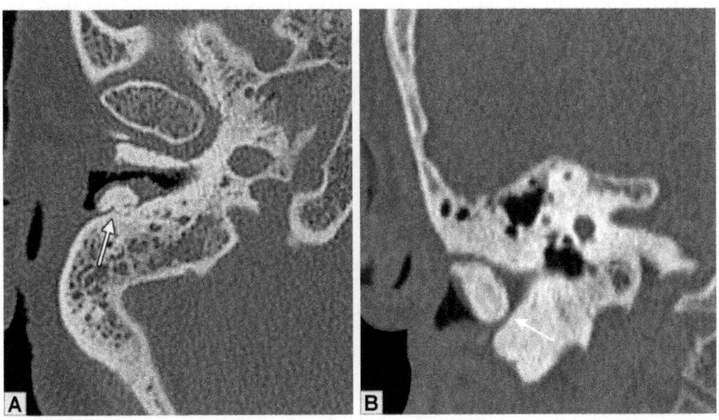

FIGS. 8A AND B: Right external auditory canal (EAC) osteoma: HRCT temporal bone (A) axial and (B) coronal reformatted images demonstrate ossified lesion (arrow) in the right EAC suggesting osteoma.

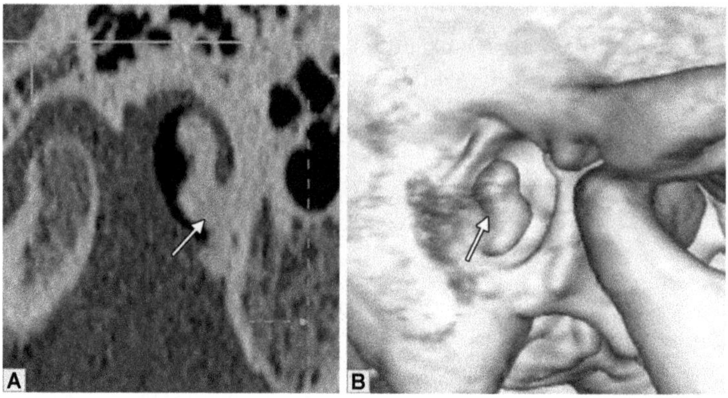

FIGS. 9A AND B: Right external auditory canal (EAC) osteoma: HRCT temporal bone sagittal reformat (A) and VRT (B) image demonstrating ossified lesion arising from the posterior wall of right EAC suggesting osteoma.

Secondary Tumors of External Auditory Canal

- External auditory canal can be involved secondarily due to contiguous/metastatic spread of primary tumors arising elsewhere.
- *Direct invasion*: From parotid malignancy. Primary tumors arising in squamous and mastoid parts of the temporal bone can also involve the EAC.
- *Metastatic tumor*: Breast carcinoma, malignant melanoma
- When tumors become large, exact origin may be difficult to determine
- *Differential diagnosis*: When extending into temporomandibular joint (TMJ) and deep spaces of neck, differentiation from necrotizing external otitis on imaging can be difficult.

MIDDLE AND INNER EAR TUMORS

A list of middle and inner ear tumors is given in **Box 2**. In this section, we shall discuss the common tumors of middle and inner ear.

BOX 2 Middle and inner ear tumors.

- Benign:
  - Otosclerosis
  - Cholesteatoma
  - Middle ear adenoma
  - Vestibular schwannoma
  - Meningioma
  - Middle ear Paraganglioma/glomus tympanicum (listed as paraganglion tumors)
- Intermediate/borderline:
  - Endolymphatic sac tumor
  - Aggressive papillary tumor
- Malignant
- Squamous cell carcinoma

Otosclerosis

This has been included in the list of tumor owing to its uncontrolled growth and invasion of normal structures in the cochlear and vestibular otic capsules; like that of a neoplasm (Discussed in Chapter 20).

Cholesteatomas

- This is a nonneoplastic lesion; yet included in the list owing to its aggressiveness and tendency to recur after surgery.
- It is most frequently found in middle ear and mastoid cavity.
- In rare cases, they originate in EAC.
- Congenital and acquired cholesteatomas have been reported in cases of congenital stenosis or atresia.
- Imaging findings are nonspecific-soft tissue mass in EAC with associated bony erosion on CT (**Figs. 10A** and **B**).
- Usually, margins of bony erosion are sharp and regular. In case of associated periostitis, the margins become irregular and differentiating from malignant tumor is difficult.
- It is known that accumulated keratin in cholesteatoma sac causes clear hyperintensity on B1000 DWI imaging; thus, non-EPI DWI sequences aid in making diagnosis.

Vestibular Schwannoma

This has been discussed in Chapter 12.

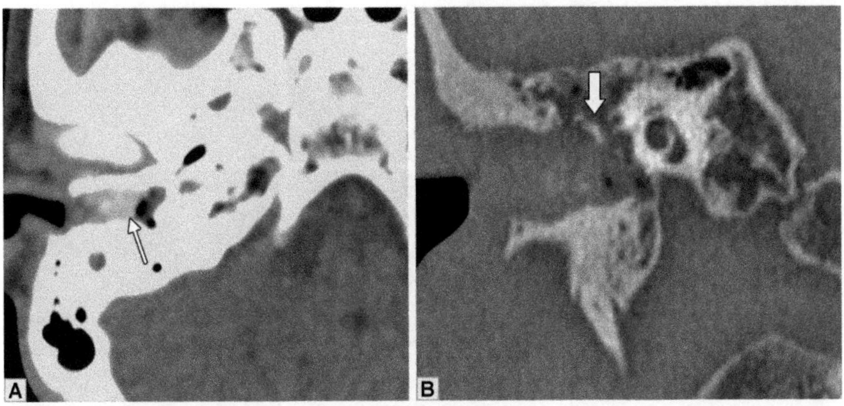

FIGS. 10A AND B: External auditory canal (EAC) cholesteatoma with otitis media: CT (A) axial soft tissue window, (B) coronal bone window images showing hyperdense soft tissue (arrow) in right middle ear and EAC with ossicular erosion (block arrow).

Meningioma

- *Meningioma of temporal bone can be of three subtypes*: Tegmen tympani, jugular fossa, and IAC meningioma.[4,5]
- Origin of tegmen tympani meningioma is middle cranial fossa dura, with inferomedial spread through tegmen tympani.
- Bony changes are characterized by lack of frank bone destruction and sclerosis. Irregular bone deposition occurring along inner and outer table with spiculated margins is considered highly typical of meningioma.
- Tegmen tympani and jugular foramen (JF) meningiomas are characterized by an enhancing mass in the middle ear cavity without erosive or destructive changes of involved bone or ossicles.
- Petroclival meningiomas can arise from the petrous apex or clivus and may extend to cavernous sinus (**Figs. 11** and **12**).
- On MRI, they are seen as strongly enhancing dural-based lesion; slight hyperintense on T2W, isointense on T1W.
- Flow voids are usually absent.

Differentials for Meningioma

- *For tegmen tympani meningioma*: Granulation tissue, facial nerve hemangioma, and facial schwannoma
- *For jugular fossa meningioma*: Glomus jugulare and paraganglioma (PG)
- *For IAC meningioma*: Schwannoma (*see Chapter 12, and question no. 20 in Chapter 29*).

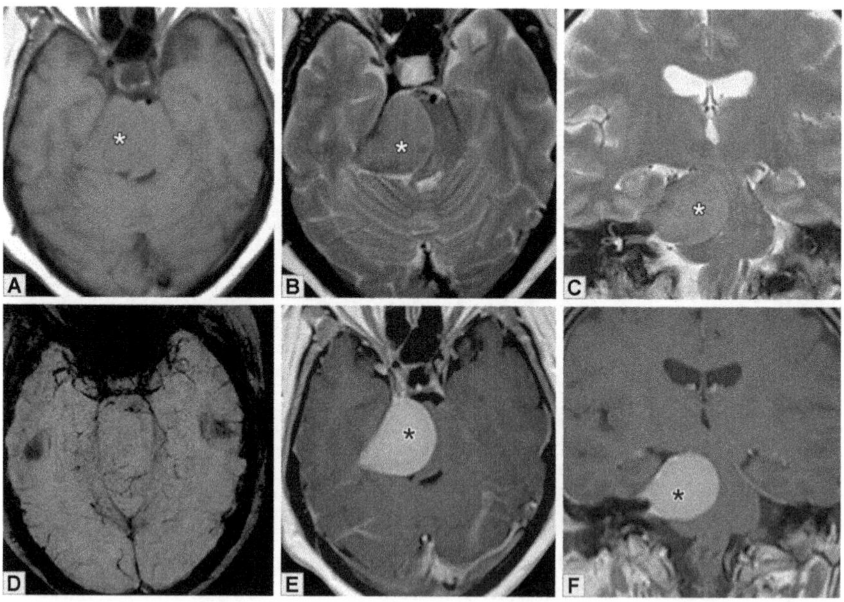

FIGS. 11A TO F: Petrous apex meningioma: The mass (asterisk) is (A) isointense on T1-weighted (T1W), (B and C) hypointense on T2-weighted (T2W), and (E and F) show strong postcontrast enhancement.
Courtesy: Professor Ajay Garg.

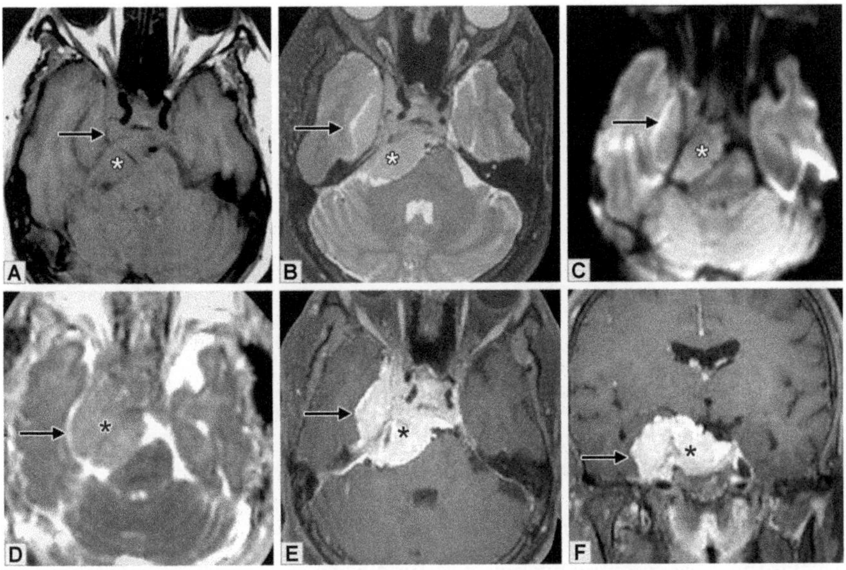

FIGS. 12A TO F: Petroclival meningioma: A large mass (asterisk) is seen along petrous apex and clivus. It is (A) isointense on T1-weighted (T1W), (B) hypointense on T2W, (C and D) not showing diffusion restriction; and (E and F) shows intense contrast enhancement. Note the invasion of right cavernous sinus by the mass (arrow).
Courtesy: Professor Ajay Garg.

Paragangliomas

- *Synonym*: Glomus tumors; they arise from the chromaffin cells of the parasympathetic ganglia in head and neck.
- It is the most common primary tumor of the middle ear and the second most common tumor of the temporal bone
- It is a benign tumor, usually associated with the jugular bulb adventitia and glomus formations of inferior tympanic branch of 9th nerve (Jacobson's nerve) or mastoid branch of 10th nerve (Arnold's nerve).
- Slow growing, locally destructive nonmetastasizing, spreading along paths of less resistance.
- Only 1–3% are endocrinologically functional.
- Multiple endocrine neoplasia type 2, von Hippel-Lindau disease (VHL), and neurofibromatosis type I are associated with increased risk of PGs.
- Based on location, these are of three types (**Fig. 13**):
  1. *Tumors arising from the glomus bodies affiliated with the jugular bulb:* Glomus jugulare
  2. *Tumors arising from the middle ear*: Glomus tympanicum
  3. *Tumors involving both middle ear and JF:* Glomus jugulotympanicum

Classification

- The Glasscock-Jackson classification has separate systems for glomus tympanicum and glomus jugulare.

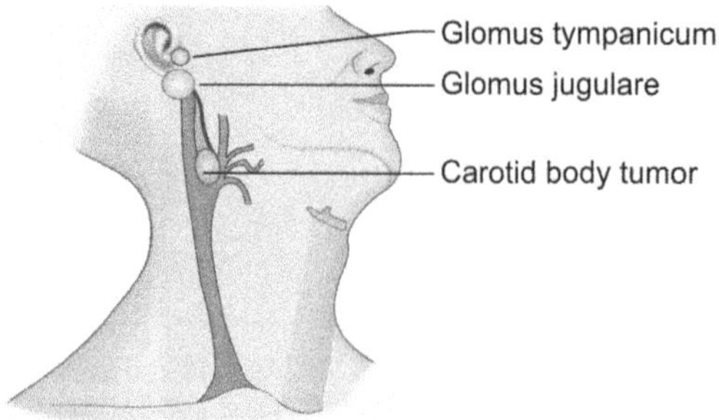

FIG. 13: Types of head and neck paraganglioma.

- Fisch's system utilizes a single system that is applicable to both types of glomus tumors.
- These are detailed in Chapter 17.

Glomus Tympanicum Tumor

- It is the most common neoplasm of middle ear.
- Because surgical intervention or biopsy can potentially be harmful, it is essential that radiologist knows cross-sectional imaging signs of these tumors and can differentiate from anatomic variants.
- The most frequent age is 50–60 years of age, with a female preponderance.
- *Clinical features*: Conductive hearing loss, pulsatile tinnitus, reddish-blue mass behind the tympanic membrane. Clinically, it is difficult to differentiate between glomus tympanicum tumor, glomus jugulotympanicum tumor, and vascular variants [e.g., high riding dehiscent jugular bulb, aberrant internal carotid artery (ICA)]

Imaging

Computed Tomography

- *Glomus tympanicum tumor (GT)* is usually a small-sized intensely enhancing soft tissue mass abutting the promontory of the middle ear[6] (**Figs. 14A** and **B**).
- The enhancement can be difficult to demonstrate due to small size, and surrounding bony structures. Use of dual energy CT is immensely helpful in this regard.
- In larger tumors, ossicles may show erosion and displacement.
- Inferior wall of middle ear cavity is usually intact.
- The air or bone between the tumor and the jugular bulb confirms the diagnosis of a tympanicum (vs. jugulare).
- If mass is sufficiently large to fill epitympanum, attic and antrum, retention of fluid in mastoid can be found.
- Bone erosion is usually not present.

Magnetic Resonance Imaging

- Better evaluates the relationship of the tumor to adjacent jugular vein, carotid artery, and membranous labyrinth in large tumors.

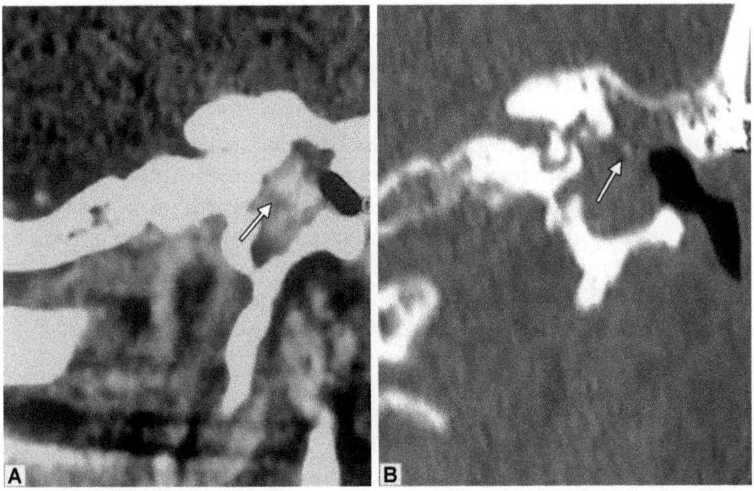

FIGS. 14A AND B: Glomus tympanicum: HRCT temporal bone (A) coronal reformatted soft tissue window, and (B) coronal reformatted bone window images demonstrating enhancing mass in the left middle ear cavity (arrow) with adjacent mild bony erosion (*Glasscock–Jackson classification Type 3*).

- Contrast-enhanced T1W images strongly enhance mass located anteriorly in signal void of temporal bone pyramid.
- Signal intensity on T2W images may vary but are predominantly intermediate.
- Diffusion-weighted image variable; can show either facilitated or restricted diffusion or heterogeneous.

Angiogram

Owing to its small size, angiographic visualization of the mass is difficult.

Differentials of Glomus Tympanicum

- Otitis media
- Langerhan's cell histiocytosis (LCH)
- Cholesteatoma
- Aneurysm

Glomus Jugulare/Glomus Jugulotympanicum

- *Origin*: Glomus bodies in relation to the jugular bulb
- *Clinical features*: Tinnitus and hearing loss
- *Associations*: Pheochromocytoma, parathyroid adenoma, thyroid carcinoma, neurofibromatosis-1
- *Complication*: It may undergo malignant change and metastasize to regional lymph nodes.

Imaging

Computed Tomography

- On CT, they appear as a heterogeneous, intensely enhancing mass in jugular bulb region.[6]
- Erosion of corticojugular spine of JF is characteristic.
- Ossicular destruction may be seen (incus most commonly involved).
- Erosion of posteromedial surface of petrous temporal bone may also be seen.
- *Glomus jugulotympanicum*: Moth-eaten erosion of JF, with extension of soft tissue mass to middle ear (**Fig. 15A**).
- *Dual-energy CT*: Superior detection of adjacent bone and structures invasion. Iodine map images increase the conspicuity of the lesion.

Magnetic Resonance Imaging

- Unenhanced T1-weighted images reveal a mass in jugular fossa with *salt and pepper* appearance (**Figs. 15B** and **16**).
- *Pepper*: Signal voids of large feeding arteries.
- *Salt*: Subacute hemorrhage in tumor.
- *Magnetic resonance angiography (MRA) (**Fig. 15C**)*: Preintervention imaging.
- *Magnetic resonance venography (MRV)*: For sigmoid sinus and IJV involvement.
- *DWI*: PGs show restricted diffusion; ADC values are lower compared to other benign tumors.
- *Dynamic CE-MRI*: They show early contrast enhancement and washout pattern, similar to malignancy.

Angiography

- Hypervascular mass with persistent homogenous reticular stain and arteriovenous shunting.

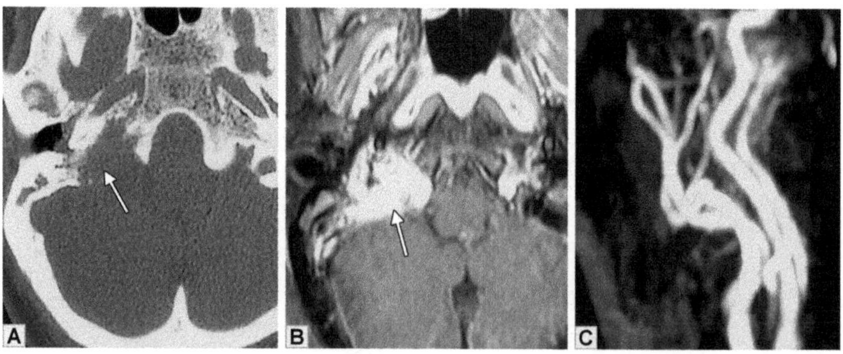

FIGS. 15A TO C: Glomus jugulotympanicum: HRCT temporal bone axial bone window CT image (A) postcontrast TSE T1W MRI image, (B) and MRI angiogram, (C) showing intensely enhancing mass (arrow in B) in the tympanic region, causing adjacent bony erosion (arrow in A) with prominent blood supply (*Glasscock-Jackson classification Type 3*).

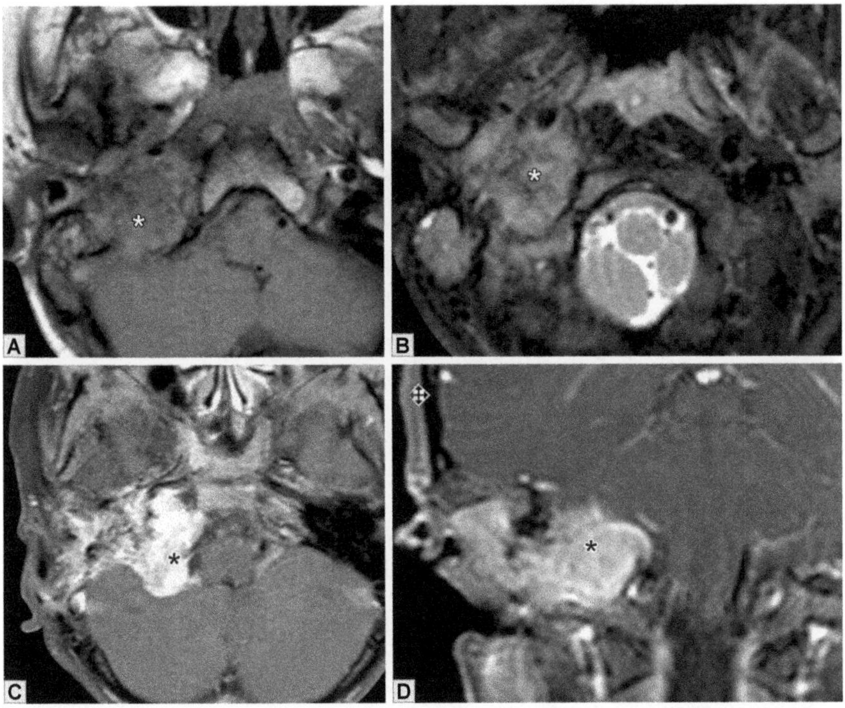

FIGS. 16A TO D: Glomus jugulotympanicum: Axial (A) TSE T1W, (B) TSE T2W, and (C) postcontrast TSE T1W fat-suppressed images; and (D) coronal postcontrast TSE T1W fat-suppressed MRI images showing irregular intensely enhancing T2W hyperintense mass (asterisk) in the right jugulotympanic region with intracranial extension (*Glasscock–Jackson classification Type 4*).

- Invasion/occlusion of jugular bulb by thrombus/tumor.
- Supplied by tympanic branch of ascending pharyngeal artery, meningeal branch of occipital artery, posterior auricular artery via stylomastoid branch, ICA, and internal maxillary artery (**Fig. 17**).
- Performed for preoperative embolization. Another utility is to demonstrate intracranial collateral vessels in case of ICA involvement.

Mimics/Differentials

- The differentials include chordoma, meningioma, schwannoma, neurofibroma, primary or metastatic carcinoma, and lymphoma.
- Care should be taken not to misinterpret normal flow-related signal in large jugular bulb as glomus jugulare or jugulotympanicum tumor.
- Mega jugular bulb can, in case of bony plate deficiency, protrude into middle ear resulting in blue discoloration of tympanic membrane.
- In case of contact with incudostapedial joint, this large protruding dehiscent jugular bulb can even lead to conductive hearing loss.

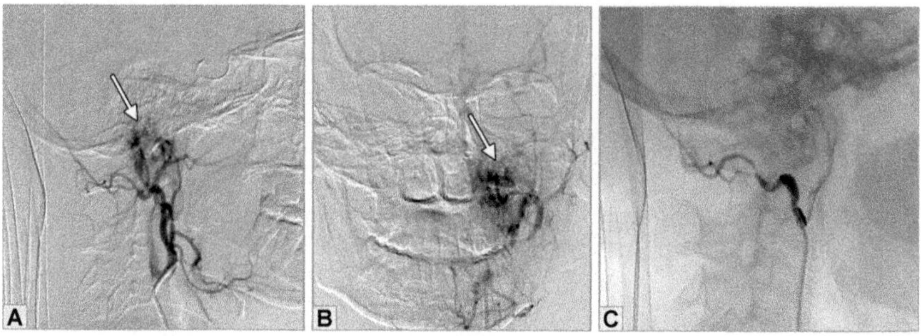

FIGS. 17A TO C: Angiographic appearance of glomus jugulotympanicum. Lateral (A) and AP (B) DSA images of a 30 years old lady showed a hypervascular lesion; evident by significant arterial blush (arrow). The arterial supply was from posterior auricular and occipital arteries. Post-embolization image (C) shows non-visualization of the arterial blush.

Endolymphatic Sac Tumor

- Temporal bone tumors originate from epithelial lining of the endolymphatic sac.
- They are rare, slow growing, highly locally aggressive but do not metastasize.
- *Location:* Posterior petrosal bone region and may involve the dura (**Fig. 18**)
- *Association:* von Hippel–Lindau disease (11–16% of VHL patients); 30% of tumor in VHL are bilateral (**Figs. 19A** to **E**).
- *Clinical features*: Hearing loss, tinnitus, facial nerve palsy (when tumor becomes large, involving the facial nerve canal), and vertigo.

Imaging

Computed Tomography

- These are seen as enhancing solid cystic mass, causing adjacent bony destruction with areas of new bone formation.
- *Patterns of bone destruction*: These tumors are surrounded by thin shell of reactive bone; geographic "moth-eaten" pattern; and spiculated pattern (**Figs. 20** and **21**).
- Hyperenhancing tumor
- These may show calcifications and reactive bone formation.

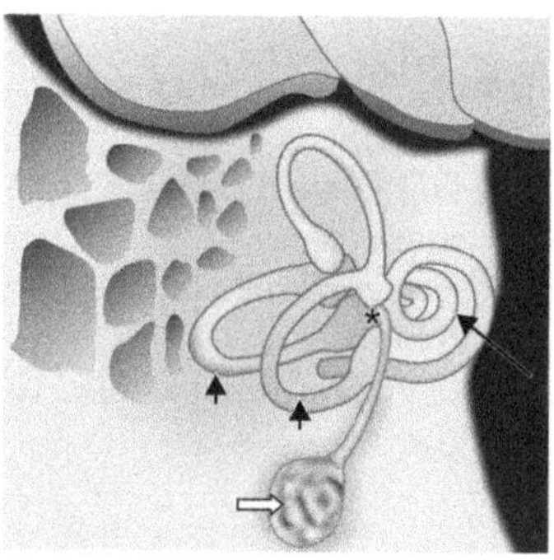

FIG. 18: Diagram showing the location of **endolymphatic sac tumor** in relation to cochlea (arrow), vestibule (asterisk), and semicircular canals (arrows).

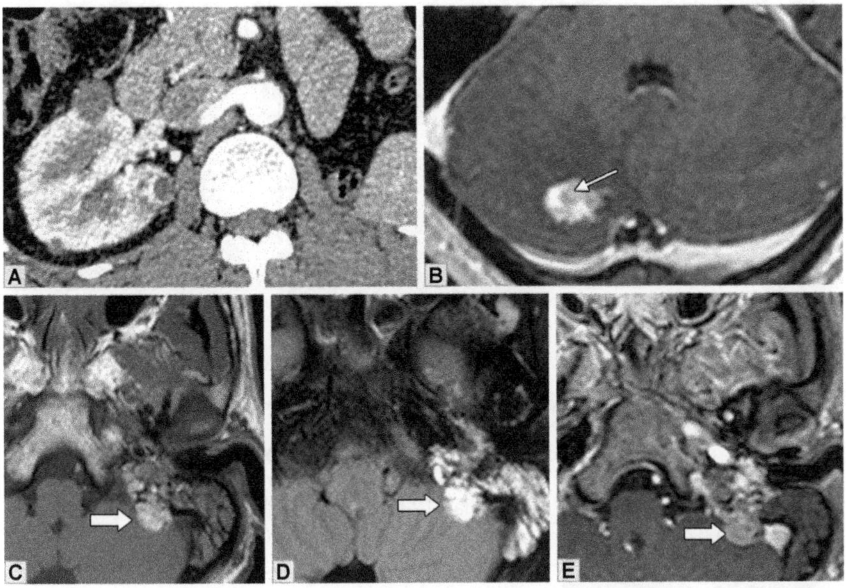

FIGS. 19A TO E: Endolymphatic sac tumor in von Hippel–Lindau syndrome: (A) Axial contrast-enhanced CT abdomen showing multiple right renal simple cysts with retroperitoneal lymph nodes. (B) Axial postcontrast TSE T1W image showing enhancing mass (hemangioblastoma) in right cerebellum. Axial (C) TSE T1W, (D) TSE T2W, (E) and postcontrast TSE T1W MRI images revealing the intensely enhancing retrolabyrinthine mass (block arrow) with underlying bone involvement. The mass is heterogeneously hyperintense on T2WI, and also shows patchy areas of hyperintensity on T1WI.

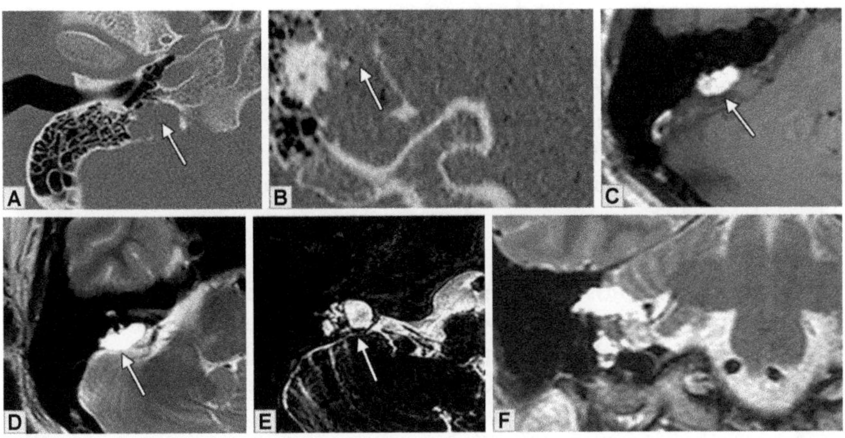

FIGS. 20A TO F: Endolymphatic sac tumor: Axial CT bone window (A), coronal CT bone window (B), axial TSET1W (C), axial TSET2W (D), axial heavily T2W (CISS) (E), coronal T2W MRI (F) images showing retrolabyrinthine mass (arrows) with underlying bone erosion

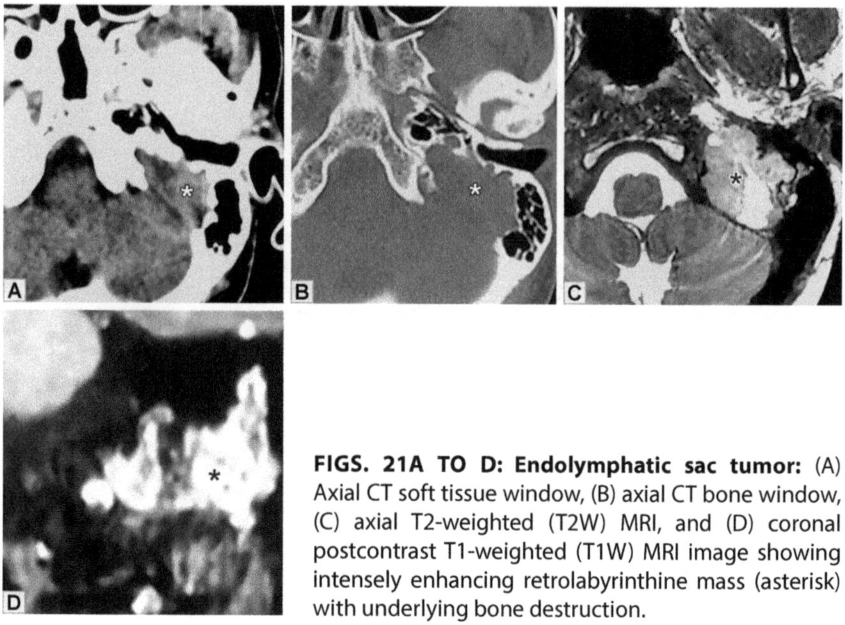

FIGS. 21A TO D: Endolymphatic sac tumor: (A) Axial CT soft tissue window, (B) axial CT bone window, (C) axial T2-weighted (T2W) MRI, and (D) coronal postcontrast T1-weighted (T1W) MRI image showing intensely enhancing retrolabyrinthine mass (asterisk) with underlying bone destruction.

Magnetic Resonance Imaging

- Heterogeneous, intensely enhancing tumor (**Figs. 19** and **20**).
- *T1-weighted images*: Hypo- to isointense with few areas of hyperintensity representing hemorrhage, cholesterol clefts, and proteinaceous cysts
- *T2-weighted images*: Heterogeneously hyperintense
- *Gradient-weighted images*: May show foci of hemorrhage
- *Postcontrast T1WI*: Intense postcontrast enhancement

Angiography

- These tumors are highly vascular, getting arterial supply from the branches of the external carotid artery (ascending pharyngeal and stylomastoid); however ICA and anterior inferior cerebellar arteries may also contribute. Early venous drainage is unusual.
- Preoperative embolization is helpful and helps in surgical excision.

Differential Diagnosis

- *Jugulotympanic PGs*-mostly infralabyrinthine in location, in contrast to endolymphatic sac tumors which are retrolabyrinthine. The absence of serpentine flow voids with sparing of JF is characteristic of endolymphatic sac tumor (ELST) in contrast to PG. The differentiating features are summarized in **Table 4**.
- *Intratemporal benign tumors like hemangiomas:* Location is a differentiating feature with ELST being common in retrolabyrinthine region, where as other benign tumors may be seen elsewhere in temporal bone.

TABLE 4 **Differentiating features of jugulotympanic paragangliomas and ELST.**

	Paragangliomas	ELST
Location	Labyrinthine	Retrolabyrinthine
Epicenter	Anteriorly around jugular bulb	Around vestibular aqueduct
Intratumoral bleed (T1W hyperintensity)	Less common	Commoner
Calcification	Absent	Present
Characteristic "*salt and pepper*" appearance	Present	Absent

(ELST: endolymphatic sac tumor; T1W: T1-weighted)

- Choroid plexus papillomas involving the foramina of Luschka or CPA and typically do not show bony erosion.
- Chondrosarcoma may arise in the petro-occipital fissure and show chondroid matrix.

Other Important Tumor/Tumor-like Conditions not in the WHO 2017 Classification

Many of the commonly encountered tumors do not feature in the recent WHO classification. However, for completion of the imaging discussion, they will be discussed here.

Facial Nerve Schwannoma

- They are the second most common primary middle ear tumor; and can arise anywhere along the facial nerve. Common age of presentation is 3rd–6th decades, and has no sex predilection.
- Predilection for geniculate ganglion (**Figs. 22A** to **D**) but can also originate in tympanic (**Fig. 23**) or mastoid segment (**Fig. 24**).
- *Clinical features*: Depend the segment of facial nerve involved. Common being facial palsy, hearing loss, tinnitus, hemifacial spasm, and otalgia.

Imaging

Computed Tomography

- Primary finding on CT is of enlargement of bony delineation of involved segment of facial nerve. Demonstrate benign appearing bony scalloping, expansion and remodeling of surrounding bony boundaries (**Fig. 22A**). Aggressive bony destruction is unusual.
- Enhancement can be difficult to demonstrate on CT, and is variable.

Magnetic Resonance Imaging

- Superior for the evaluation of tumor extension and relationship with other adjacent structures. CT and MRI are often complimentary.

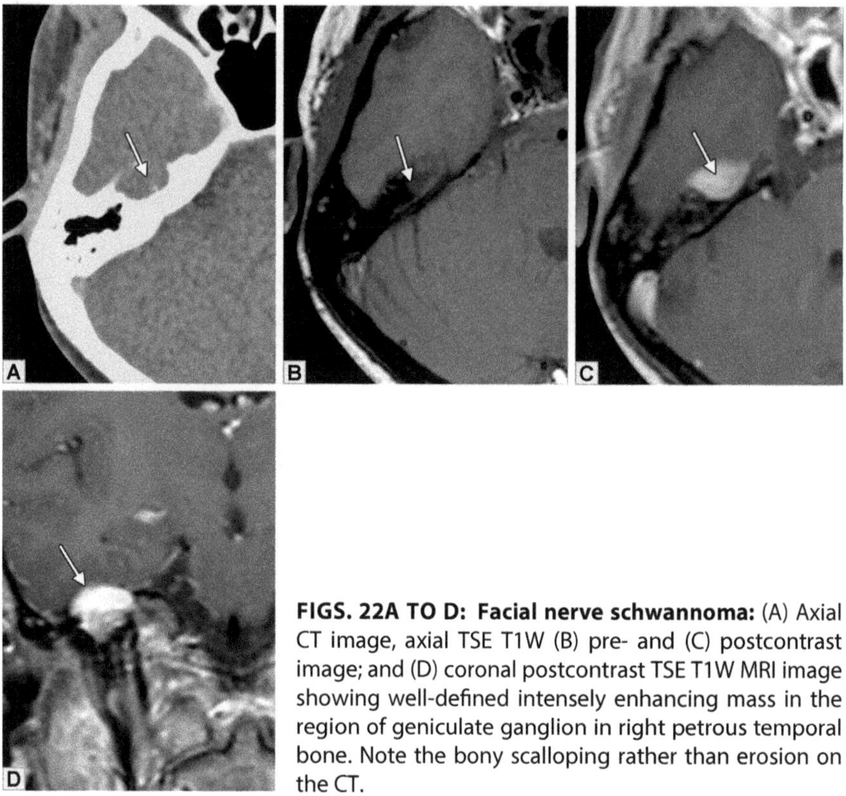

FIGS. 22A TO D: Facial nerve schwannoma: (A) Axial CT image, axial TSE T1W (B) pre- and (C) postcontrast image; and (D) coronal postcontrast TSE T1W MRI image showing well-defined intensely enhancing mass in the region of geniculate ganglion in right petrous temporal bone. Note the bony scalloping rather than erosion on the CT.

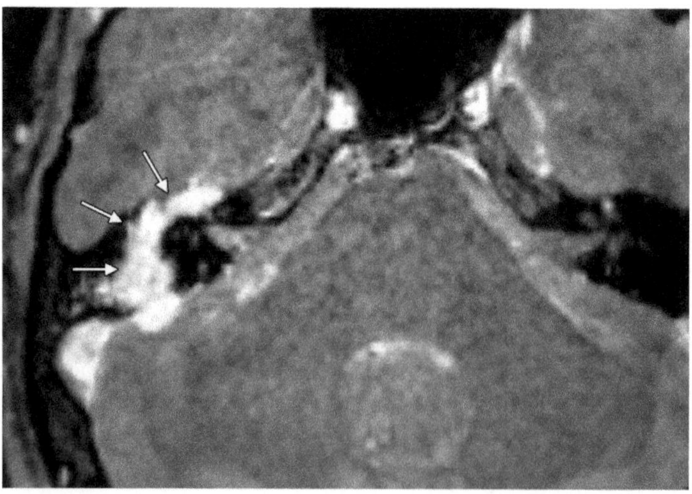

FIG. 23: Facial nerve schwannoma: Axial postcontrast T1-weighted (T1W) MRI image showing irregular intensely enhancing mass along the *horizontal (tympanic)* segment of the facial nerve on right side.

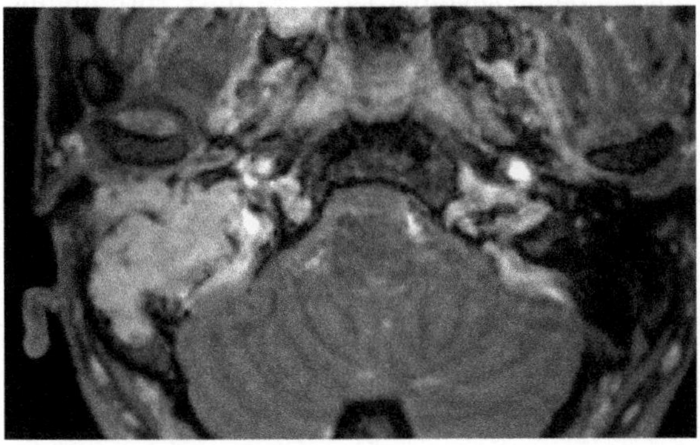

FIG. 24: Facial nerve schwannoma: Axial post-contrast T1-weighted (T1W) MRI image showing large irregular intensely enhancing mass in right *mastoid temporal* bone.

- Facial nerve schwannoma (FNS) is seen as a well-defined lesion which is iso- to hypointense relative to gray matter on T1-weighted images, hyperintense on T2W images and show homogenous contrast enhancement (**Figs. 22** to **24**).
- Larger FNS can undergo a cystic degeneration and heterogeneous SI.
- To differentiate it from congenital cholesteatoma, DWI, preferably non-EPI sequence, can be performed. In case of FNS or hemangioma, no clear hyperintensity on B1000 image contrary to congenital cholesteatoma.
- MRI can also detect and differentiate other inflammatory conditions and Bell's palsy.
  - Focal nodular swelling of facial nerve can be found in fundus of IAC, giving rise to pseudotumoral swelling in cases of idiopathic facial nerve palsy or Bell's paralysis.
  - This is caused by retrograde swelling of nerve before narrowest part of its entire course: Bony canal of labyrinthine segment of facial nerve.

Facial Nerve Schwannoma Involving Various Segments

- *Cerebellopontine angle—IAC segment*: Difficult to distinguish from acoustic schwannomas. When large, they may be seen as a "dumbbell" shaped mass extending from the IAC fundus through the labyrinthine segment and into the geniculate fossa.

  Tumoral nodular lesion in fundus of the IAC is more likely to be vestibulocochlear schwannoma than FNS.

  Parasagittal reformations of high-resolution, 3D, T2W sequence are of help in localizing lesion.
  - Anterior upper quadrant of IAC-FNS
  - Posterior inferior-inferior vestibular nerve schwannoma (*see Chapter 12*)
- It is very difficult to differentiate FNS from vestibular schwannoma (VS) at IAC. However anterosuperior location may be suggestive of FNS.
- *Geniculate ganglion*: Imaging reveals a middle cranial fossa mass with enlargement of the geniculate fossa (containing the first genu of facial nerve).
- Facial nerve schwannomas arising from the greater superficial petrosal nerve usually cause scalloping of the anterior margin of geniculate fossa and the adjacent bony petrous apex (**Figs. 22A** to **D**).

- *Tympanic segment*: As the tympanic segment lacks the thick surrounding bony architecture of the labyrinthine segment of the facial nerve canal, these tumors usually are multilobular instead of fusiform shape (**Fig. 23**). They sometimes erode lateral semicircular canal forming the fistula.
- *Mastoid segment*: As mastoid segment of the facial nerve is surrounded by fragile, thin-walled bony septations, they are seen as irregular, "invasive" tumors (**Fig. 24**).

Differentials of Intratemporal Facial Nerve Schwannoma

- *Cholesteatoma*: Restriction of diffusion in cholesteatoma can differentiate it from FNS.
- *Facial nerve hemangioma*: Absence of calcifications differentiates FNS from facial nerve hemangioma.
- Perineural spread from parotid malignancy; direct invasion of naso- or oropharyngeal carcinomas.
- Hematogenous spread from breast, bronchus, or prostate carcinoma.

Langerhan's Cell Histiocytosis

- Langerhan's cell histiocytosis occurs in children. Its aggressive-looking appearance makes differentiation from rhabdomyosarcoma (RMS) difficult.
- Temporal bone involvement can be solitary (in 5–25%), or as a part of systemic disease. Cranial nerve deficit is uncommon.
- Although extensive osseous destruction with associated soft tissue mass lesion is seen on CT, involvement of auditory ossicles and inner ear is not frequent (**Figs. 25** and **26**).
- Magnetic resonance imaging—nonspecific: variable SI on T1W and high SI on T2W with strong contrast enhancement.
- Another major imaging feature, unlike RMS, is fact that LCH lesions are often bilateral.

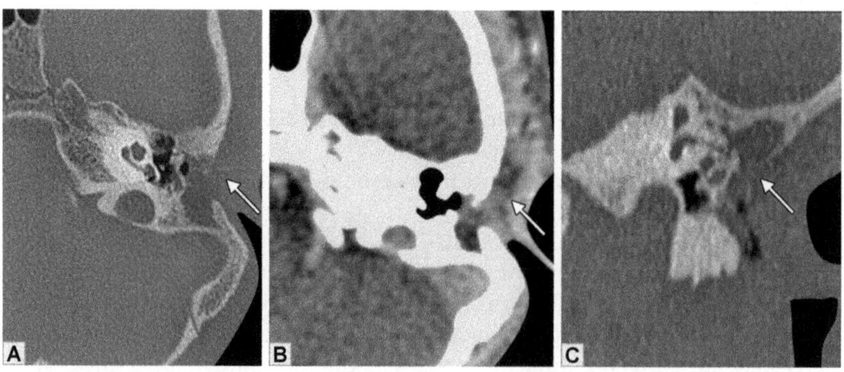

FIGS. 25A TO C: Langerhan's cell histiocytosis: HRCT axial (A) bone window, (B) soft tissue window, and (C) coronal bone window images demonstrating lytic lesion (arrows) involving the temporal bone with small soft tissue component, extending into left external auditory canal (EAC).

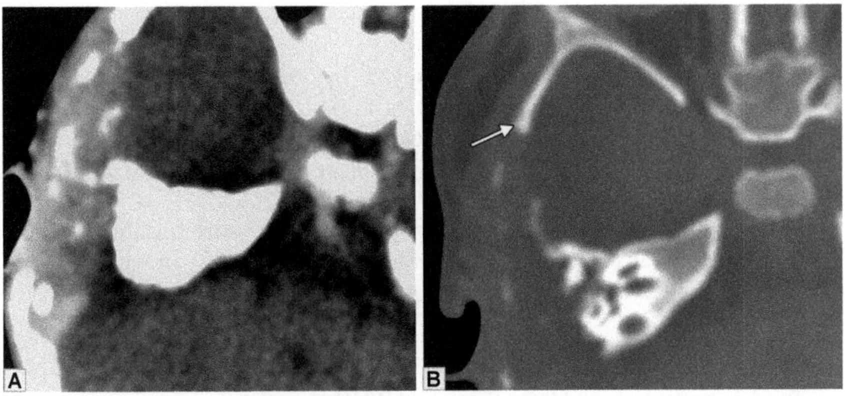

FIGS. 26A AND B: Langerhan's cell histiocytosis in a 4-year-old male child. HRCT axial (A) soft window and (B) bone window images show lytic lesion involving right squamous and mastoid temporal bone with small soft tissue component. Note the sharp margin of the bone erosion (arrow in B).

Rhabdomyosarcoma

- Rhabdomyosarcoma has been excluded from the list of tumors of ear; as it is not unique to the ear. However, for completion's sake, this will be discussed here.
- This is a common malignant head and neck tumor in children. Other locations are orbit, paranasal sinuses, or nasopharynx.
- Rhabdomyosarcoma originates from intrinsic middle ear or Eustachian tube musculature. More commonly involves the mastoid bone than middle ear and petrous apex.
- *Imaging*: Aggressive-looking mass in middle ear with extensive bone destruction. Ossicular destruction is uncommon.
- Magnetic resonance imaging—nonspecific, hyperintensity on T2W and moderate intensity on T1W with strong contrast enhancement.
- Metastasis occurs more commonly to lungs and bones, less commonly to lymph nodes.
- Imaging-based differential is mainly LCH. Occurrence of neurologic "alarm" symptoms of cranial nerve palsy is far less frequent in LCH, and also LCH is often bilateral.

Other Tumors

- *Non-Hodgkin's lymphoma*: Imaging highly nonspecific, relatively homogeneous soft tissue mass destroying all bony structures
- Malignant osseous and soft tissue tumors: Ewing's sarcoma, fibrosarcoma, osteosarcoma, and chondrosarcoma
- Tumors showing calcification—chondrosarcoma and osteosarcoma
- Benign osseous lesions—osteoblastoma, giant cell tumor, and hemangiomas
- Amongst the other osseous lesions, such as Paget's disease, can also affect skull base and temporal bone.

Secondary Tumors

- Temporal bone can also be involved by contiguous involvement in malignancies, or in hematogenous metastases.
- Breast, lung, kidney, prostate carcinoma, and melanoma may involve temporal bone. Lesions can be lytic, blastic, or mixed depending on primary type of tumor.
- Temporal bone can be directly invaded by surrounding tumors. Nasopharyngeal carcinoma may invade temporal bone, growing through foramina and fissures, and following course of vessels and nerves.

Fibrous Dysplasia

- This has been excluded from the recent WHO classification as it is not unique to the ear and can occur at other areas of head and neck as well.
- Fibro-osseous lesions include fibrous dysplasia and ossifying fibroma.
- Lesions show ground glass attenuation on CT; hyperintense on T2W MRI.
- Intense enhancement after gadolinium administration (**Figs. 27** and **28**).
- Can cause narrowing of the EAC or skull base foramen (due to bony expansion)
- Multiple cranial nerve encroachment may be a complication.
  Tumor mimics such as keratosis obturans are described in Chapter 19 and 20.

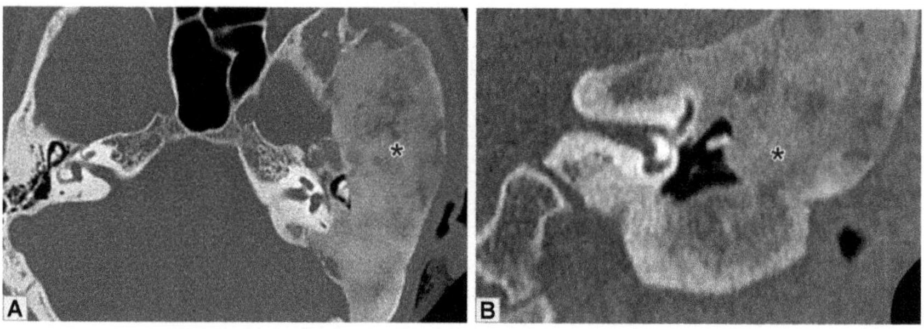

FIGS. 27A AND B: Temporal bone fibrous dysplasia: HRCT (A) axial and (B) coronal images reveal bony expansion with ground glass attenuation (asterisk) involving squamous, petrous, and mastoid part of left temporal bone, narrowing the external auditory canal (EAC) and also encroaching on the middle ear cavity.

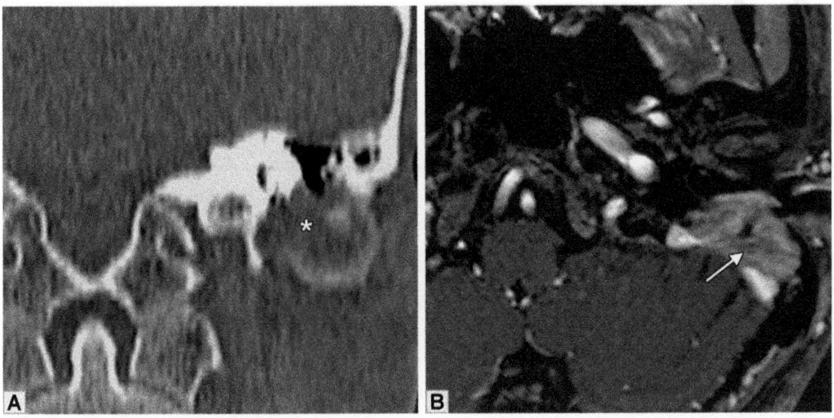

FIGS. 28A AND B: Mastoid fibrous dysplasia: HRCT (A) coronal bone window, and axial postcontrast TSE T1W MRI images reveal expansile bony lesion in the left temporal bone which show ground glass attenuation on CT (asterisk) and heterogeneous contrast enhancement (arrow) on MRI.

In conclusion, temporal bone tumors are a very diverse group of disease entities; and reaching at a definitive diagnosis often requires multimodality imaging.

REFERENCES

1. El-Naggar AK, Chan JKC, Grandis JR, Takata T, Slootweg PJ (Eds). WHO Classification of Head and Neck Tumours, 4th edition. IARC: Lyon; 2017.
2. Barnes L, Eveson JW, Reichart P, Sidransky D (Eds). World Health Organization Classification of Tumors. Pathology and Genetics of Head and Neck Tumours, 3rd edition. IARC: Lyon; 2005.
3. Thompson LD. Update From the 4th Edition of the World Health Organization Classification of Head and Neck Tumours: Tumours of the Ear. Head Neck Pathol. 2017;11(1):78-87.
4. Juliano AF, Ginat DT, Moonis G. Imaging review of the temporal bone: part I. Anatomy and inflammatory and neoplastic processes. Radiology. 2013;269(1):17-33.
5. De Foer B, Kenis C, Vercruysse JP, Somers T, Pouillon M, Offeciers E, et al. Imaging of temporal bone tumors. Neuroimaging Clin N Am. 2009;19(3):339-66.
6. Lee KY, Oh YW, Noh HJ, Lee YJ, Yong HS, Kang EY, et al. Extraadrenal paragangliomas of the body: Imaging Features. AJR Am J Roentgenol. 2006;187(2):492-504.

17

Temporal Bone Tumors: Surgical Perspective

Arvind Kumar Kairo, Suresh C Sharma

The pathological classification and imaging of temporal bone tumors including ear have been covered in Chapter 16. This chapter will discuss the management of two entities: (1) External auditory canal (EAC) carcinoma and (2) Paragangliomas.

EXTERNAL AUDITORY CANAL CARCINOMA

- External auditory canal carcinoma is a rare and aggressive tumor,[1,2] presenting in the fifth to seventh decades.[2]
- Early detection can have a considerable impact on outcome. It should be suspected in a patient with long-standing otorrhea, otalgia, or a mass in the EAC (**Fig. 1**). Another important clinical differential diagnosis is malignant diagnosis externa.
- Most common histopathological subtype is squamous cell carcinoma (60–80%).
- Common temporal bone tumor histologic types, including both primary temporal bone tumors and those which affect it secondarily, are squamous cell carcinoma (39%), basal cell carcinoma (14%), and adenoid cystic carcinoma (7%).
- Carcinoma of pinna is considered cutaneous carcinoma and has different staging and prognosis.

Risk Factors

Risk factors[2] for EAC squamous cell carcinoma include:

- Chronic suppurative otitis media (CSOM)
- Chronic dermatitis (higher risk in those with seborrheic form)

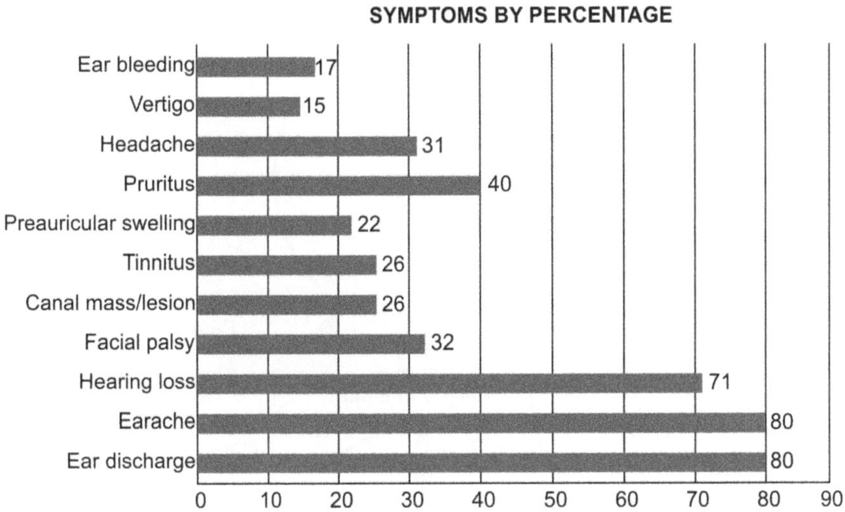

FIG. 1: Symptoms of temporal bone carcinoma.
Source: Modified from Lovin BD, Gidley PW. Squamous cell carcinoma of the temporal bone: A current review. Laryngoscope Investig Otolaryngol. 2019;4(6):684-92.

- Cholesteatoma
- Human papillomavirus
- Previous radiation exposure

Biomarkers

The biomarkers associated with EAC carcinoma include:
- Mammary serine protease inhibitor (MASPIN) a tumor suppressor gene.
- Endoglin (CD105), a proliferation-associated protein expressed in angiogenic endothelial cells.
- Epidermal growth factor receptor (EGFR)

Spread of EAC Carcinoma

- Lymphatic drainage of EAC goes to intraparotid lymph nodes, preauricular lymph nodes, upper deep cervical, and deep internal jugular node (**Fig. 2**).
- Lymphatic drainage of middle ear and mastoid goes to Eustachian tube area and next to deep upper jugular node and retropharyngeal node.

Staging Systems

University of Pittsburgh TNM staging system is based on radiological findings and has good clinic-pathological correlation (**Table 1**).[3,4] This staging system was given for squamous cell carcinoma, but currently it is used to stage other tumor histologic types also.[1]

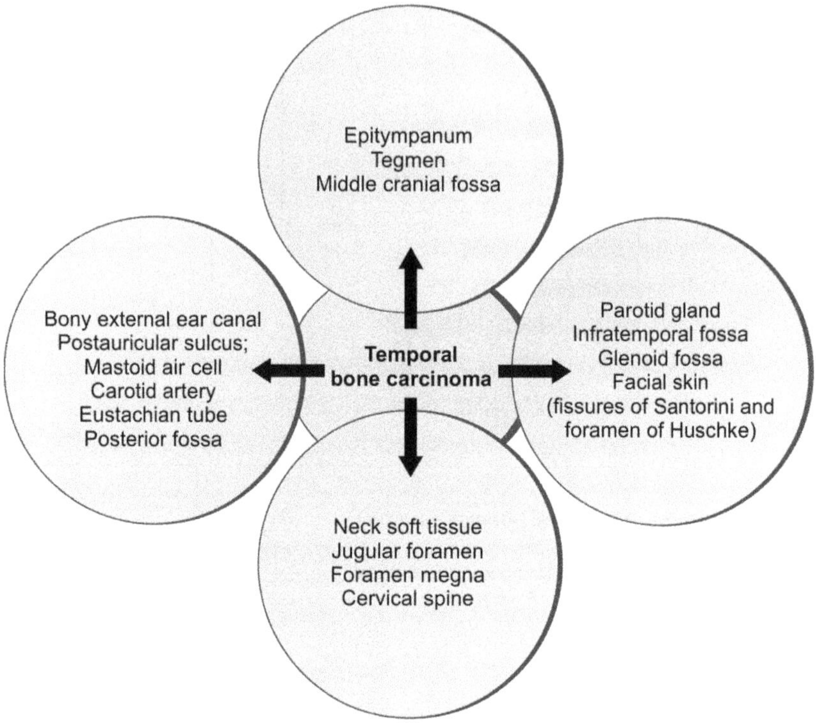

FIG. 2: Spread of external auditory canal carcinoma.

TABLE 1 **Pittsburgh staging system (Modified, Moody et al.).**

T classification[4]	N classification	Overall stage
T1: Tumor limited to the EAC without bony erosion or evidence of soft tissue involvement	**N0:** No regional nodes involved	**Stage I: T1N0**
T2: Tumor limited to the EAC with bone erosion (not full thickness) or limited soft tissue involvement (<0.5 cm)		**Stage II: T2N0**
T3: Tumor eroding through the osseous EAC (full thickness) with limited soft tissue involvement (<0.5 cm), or tumor involvement in the middle ear and/or mastoid		**Stage III: T3N0**

Continued

Continued

T classification[4]	N classification	Overall stage
T4: Tumor eroding the cochlea, petrous apex, medial wall of the middle ear, carotid canal, jugular foramen, or dura; or with extensive soft tissue involvement (>0.5 cm), such as involvement of the TMJ or styloid process; or evidence of facial paresis	**N1:** Single metastatic regional node <3 cm in size	**Stage IV:** T4N0 and any T N+
	N2a: Single ipsilateral metastatic node 3–6 cm in size	
	N2b: Multiple ipsilateral metastatic lymph nodes	
	N2c: Contralateral metastatic lymph node	
	N3: Metastatic lymph node >6 cm in size	

Management

Surgery

For resectable tumors, the various surgical options are (**Fig. 3**):[2]

- Sleeve resection
- Lateral (partial) temporal bone resection (en bloc LTBR)
- Modified lateral (partial) temporal bone resection
- Subtotal temporal bone resection (STBR)
- Total temporal bone resection (TTBR)

Sleeve Resection

- Cartilaginous portion and some or all of the bony canal wall skin are circumferentially removed without bone removal.[2]

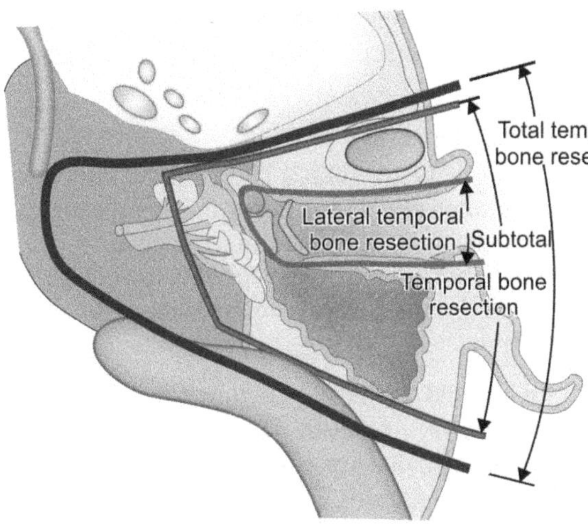

FIG. 3: Types of surgeries for external auditory canal carcinoma.
Source: Modified from Gulya AJ. The glomus tumor and its biology. Laryngoscope. 1993;103(Suppl 60):7-15.

- It is done only in tumors which are confined to the skin and soft tissue of the cartilaginous portion of the EAC; and the bony-cartilaginous junction is not involved.
- It is not an oncological sound procedure for squamous carcinoma.[5]

Lateral Temporal Bone Resection (LTBR)

- This is used when bony and cartilaginous canal are involved but have not violated the annulus.
- Herein, entire EAC is removed en bloc along with the tympanic membrane, malleus, and incus.

Modified Lateral Temporal Bone Resection

- This procedure is used if the tumor has invaded the tympanic cavity or the mastoid air cells.
- If the facial nerve looks involved, it should be sent for biopsy to ascertain perineural tracking.

Subtotal Temporal Bone Resection (STBR)

Herein, entire temporal bone lateral to the petrous carotid artery is removed in an en bloc fashion.

Total Temporal Bone Resection (TTBR)

- The internal and external carotid arteries are divided, as well as cranial nerves 9th (glossopharyngeal), 10th (vagus), and 11th (spinal accessory), and the internal jugular vein.
- The pterygoid muscles are divided.
- A craniotomy is performed, and the middle and posterior fossa dura are exposed.
- Involvement of surrounding structure may require additional surgeries with previously mentioned surgeries like parotidectomy mandibular condylectomy, neck dissection.[5,6]
- Most important factors which determine the poorer outcome are involved margins.

Adjunctive Surgical Procedures

Adjunctive procedures over LTBR/STBR/TTBR (if these structures are directly involved) include craniotomy, dural resection, carotid resection, parotidectomy, neck dissection, mandibulectomies, and zygoma resection.

The choice of surgical technique largely depends on the staging (**Table 2**). The final outcome of EAC carcinoma depends on the stage of the disease, as well as type of treatment received.

Contraindications for Curative Surgery

These include: Involvement of cavernous sinus, internal carotid artery, infratemporal fossa or paraspinous musculature, irresectable neck disease, poor patient health, and distant metastases.[1]

Radiotherapy

- Radiotherapy is used either in postoperative setting, or as a stand-alone radiotherapy for advanced, inoperable tumor.

TABLE 2 **Stagewise choice of surgical procedure, and disease outcome.**[4]

		About 2-year survival for squamous cell carcinoma	
Stage	**Surgical intervention**	**Without RT**	**With RT**
T1	Modified LTBR	100%	100%
T2	LTBR	–	80%
T3	LTBR and STBR	0%	75%
T4	LTBR, STBR, and TTBR	0%	9%
Involvement of: • CS • ICA • ITF • PSM	Inoperable		

(CS: cavernous sinus; ICA: internal carotid artery; ITF: infratemporal fossa; LTBR: lateral temporal bone resection; PSM: paraspinous musculature; RT: radiotherapy; STBR: subtotal temporal bone resection; TTBR: total temporal bone resection)

- Indications for postoperative radiotherapy (PORT) are: Lymph node metastasis; perineural invasion; positive margins; recurrent tumors; bone invasion.[1]
- About 5-year cure rate with radiation alone of 28.7% compared with a rate of 59.6% for patients receiving radiation and surgery.[7]

Chemotherapy

- Chemotherapy is used as adjuvant in advanced tumors (T3 and T4), especially as an induction agent.
- Most commonly used drugs are 5-fluorouracil, docetaxel, and cisplatin.
- Good response with bevacizumab and pemetrexed was seen in few case reports.
- Role of immunotherapy is also emerging especially in advanced cutaneous origin temporal bone cancers.

Prognostic Indicators

The prognostic indicators in EAC carcinoma include:

- *Dural involvement*: Survival rates of dural involvement is poorer.
- Nodal metastasis has poorer prognosis.

JUGULOTYMPANIC PARAGANGLIOMAS

- The cranial-cervical (branchiomeric) paraganglions are distributed along the arteries and cranial nerves.[8]
- Paraganglions are ovoid, lobulated structures measuring 0.1–1.5 mm in diameter, vascularized by the inferior tympanic branch of the ascending pharyngeal artery, the number on average three per side, and are found in association with Jacobson's and Arnold's nerves.

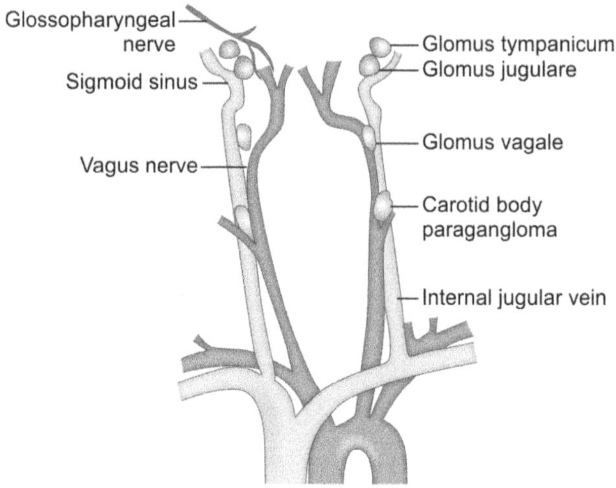

FIG. 4: Types of head and neck paraganglioma.

- Paragangliomas are tumors arising from chief cells of paraganglions and are part of diffuse neuroendocrine system (DNES) formed from neural crest (**Fig. 4**).
- Paragangliomas are slow growing, locally destructive nonmetastasizing, and spreading along paths of less resistance.
- These tumors are classified into three types:
  i. Tumors arising from the glomus bodies affiliated with the jugular bulb: Glomus jugulare (GJ).
  ii. Tumors arising from the middle ear: Glomus tympanicum (GT).
  iii. Tumors involving both middle ear and jugular foramen: Glomus jugulo-tympanicum.

Clinical Presentation

- Paragangliomas typically affect people in their fifth and sixth decades, with a female preponderance.[2]
- Only 1–3% of paragangliomas are functional tumors (secretors), and can present with paraneoplastic syndromes in the form of anemia, gastrointestinal symptoms.[2]
- More aggressive tumors are less likely to be functional (symptoms described in detail in **Fig. 5**).
- Cranial nerve paralysis may be seen in up to a third of jugulotympanic and more than half of intravagal tumors.
- They can be multiple in up to 10% nonfamilial cases. Syndromic associations include multiple endocrine neoplasia (MEN) syndromes.
- Malignancy is rare (1–12%), and malignant tumors may metastasize to lymph nodes, skeleton, lung, liver, and occasionally spleen.

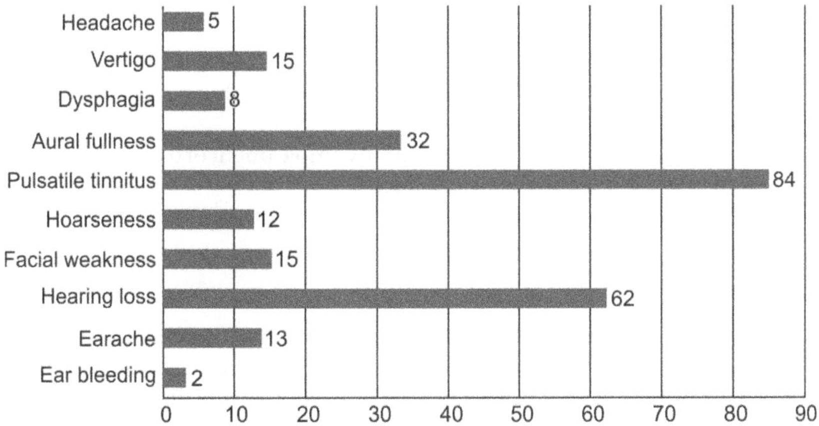

FIG. 5: Symptoms of glomus jugulare by percentage.

Source: Modified from Moody SA, Hirsch BE, Myers EN. Squamous Cell Carcinoma of the External Auditory Canal: An Evaluation of a Staging System. Am J Otol. 2000;21:582-8.

Staging

- These tumors spread across vascular lumina, neurovascular foraminas, Eustachian tube, and direct extension allows it to spread beyond temporal bone (along least resistance pathways).[7] Intracranial extension occurs in 36%.[2]
- Two staging systems are described: Glasscock-Jackson system (**Table 3**) and Fisch staging. Glasscock-Jackson system has separate descriptors for GT and GJ, whereas Fisch system has common classification for both.

TABLE 3 **Glasscock–Jackson glomus tumor classification.**

Glomus tympanicum	Type I	Small mass limited to promontory
	Type II	Tumor completely filling middle ear space
	Type III	Tumor filling middle ear and extending into mastoid process
	Type IV	Tumor filling middle ear and extending into mastoid process or through tympanic membrane to fill EAC; may extend anteriorly to involve ICA
Glomus Jugulare	Type I	Small tumor involving jugulare bulb, middle ear, and mastoid process
	Type II	Tumor extending under IAC; may have intracranial extension
	Type III	Tumor extending petrous apex; may have intracranial extension
	Type IV	Tumor extending beyond petrous apex into clivus or infratemporal fossa; may have intracranial extension

(EAC: external auditory canal; IAC: internal auditory canal; ICA: internal carotid artery)

- Fisch system utilizes a single system that is applicable to both types of glomus tumors:
  - Tumor limited to the middle-ear cleft (GT)
  - Tumor limited to the tympanomastoid area with no infralabyrinthine compartment involvement
  - Tumor involving the infralabyrinthine compartment of the temporal bone and extending into the petrous apex
  - Tumor with intracranial extension

Diagnosis

- These tumors show characteristic imaging findings (Chapter 1). They have high density of somatostatin type 2 receptors.[2] Hence, nuclear medicine-based techniques are widely employed especially to look for multifocal lesions and dissemination. These include:
  - ^{99m}Tc-methoxy isobutyl isonitrile (^{99m}Tc-MIBI)
  - Indium-111 octreotide
  - Iodine 131/132 metaiodobenzylguanidine (MIBG)
- Octreotide has been shown to be both sensitive and specific for the diagnosis and localization of paraganglioma down to a resolution of 1 cm.[8] Ga68 DOTANOC-PET is a very useful imaging modality for detection of these tumors.

Management

Surgery is the definitive (curative) treatment, whereas radiotherapy is primarily used for palliative purposes.

Definitive (Curative) Surgical Management

- In case of multiple/bilateral tumors, the most life-threatening lesion is operated on first.
- In bilateral GJ tumors, if patient emerges neurologically intact after surgery, other side is planned at least after 6 months. Extensive neurological damage mitigates surgery on other side (plan radiotherapy).
- Glomus tympanicum tumors whose borders are clearly seen through the tympanic membrane can be removed transtympanically.[9]
- Preoperative embolization may greatly lessen intraoperative blood loss.[9]
- Glomus jugulare tumors are best removed through Fisch approaches and preauricular infratemporal approach for infratemporal accesses (**Fig. 6**).

Fisch Approaches

Type A Approach

- In this approach, EAC is removed with blind sac closure of EAC and radical mastoidectomy is done.
- The facial nerve should be skeletonized and freed of its bony canal. A new bony canal is drilled in the anterior wall of the epitympanum to receive the freed facial nerve.

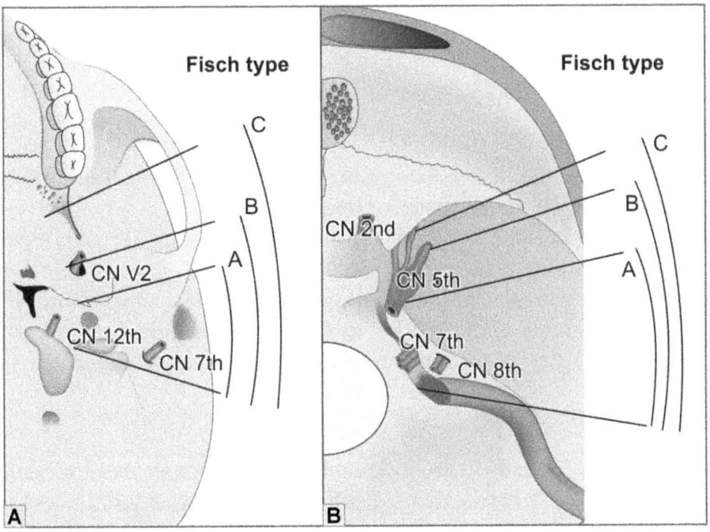

FIGS. 6A AND B: Types of surgeries for glomus tumors: Diagrammatic representation of extent of resection in different types of surgeries as seen from the base of skull (A); and from the cranial aspect (B) (with the brain removed in the image).

- Sigmoid sinus is ligated in lowermost end.
- Dura is elevated superiorly and in posterior area.
- Control on great vessels is made by exposure of jugular bulb and internal carotid artery. Care is to be taken to preserve the blood supply to the brainstem.
- The tumor may be carefully removed. To prevent tumor and air embolism, jugular vein is ligated.
- In intracranial extension, intracranial part is removed separately after removal of extracranial part and achievement of hemostasis. If the size is <2 cm, it is removed in same sitting. Larger lesion may require second stage surgery.

Type B Approach

- Herein, transposition of the facial nerve is usually not required.
- Temporalis muscle is reflected (attachment of coronoid process is kept intact).
- Middle cranial fossa floor, mandibular condyle, is exposed much more (along with superior 4 cm of the infratemporal fossa). Removal of the mandibular condyle may give better exposure to the inferior clivus and upper cervical vertebrae.
- Middle meningeal artery and mandibular nerve are transected (exposure is only posterolateral to the foramen lacerum).
- In cases with extended dissections, superior and inferior petrosal sinuses may be ligated.

Type C Approach

- This is an anterior extension of the type B approach.
- Posterolateral exposure to gain access to the rostral clivus, cavernous sinus, sphenoid sinus, peritubal space, pterygopalatine fossa, and nasopharynx

and to the areas exposed by the type B approach (anterior to the foramen lacerum).
- Pterygoid base and maxillary nerve are also removed.

Preauricular Infratemporal Approach

- Unlike Fisch approaches, this approach is unable to resect lesions extending into the temporal bone or posterior fossa.
- Control on great vessels is made without need for facial nerve transposition; although Eustachian tube may be sacrificed.
- This approach permits access to the petrous apex, clivus, and superior infratemporal fossa and may be extended to include the nasopharynx, parasellar area, pterygopalatine fossa, and anterior infratemporal fossa.

Complications of Surgery

- Complications include cerebrospinal fluid leakage, wound infection, meningitis, massive hemorrhage, aspiration, multiple cranial nerve palsies, and mortality.
- Most common nerve injured is glossopharyngeal (while taking control of ICA).

Palliative (Radiotherapy)

This is reserved for elderly patients, when definitive treatment is contraindicated. External beam radiotherapy and stereotactic radiotherapy can be employed.

To conclude, optimal treatment of temporal bone tumors requires a multidisciplinary team approach. Accurate characterization and staging of the tumors are crucial to successful surgery. Preoperative embolization of jugulotympanic paragangliomas improves operative visualization and reduces perioperative blood loss.

REFERENCES

1. Lovin BD, Gidley PW. Squamous cell carcinoma of the temporal bone: A current review. Laryngoscope Investig Otolaryngol. 2019;4(6):684-92.
2. Gulya AJ. The glomus tumor and its biology. Laryngoscope. 1993;103(Suppl 60):7-15.
3. Gulya AJ, Poe D, Minor LB (Eds). Glasscock-Shambaugh: Surgery of the Ear, 6th Edition. People's Medical Publishing House-USA; 2010.
4. Moody SA, Hirsch BE, Myers EN. Squamous Cell Carcinoma of the External Auditory Canal: An Evaluation of a Staging System. Am J Otol. 2000;21:582-8.
5. Spector GJ, Ciralsky R, Maisel RH, Ogura JH. Multiple glomus tumors in the head and neck. Laryngoscope. 1975;85:1066-75.
6. Borsanyi SJ. Glomus jugulare tumors. Laryngoscope. 1962;72:1336-45.
7. Davis JM, Davis KR, Hesselink JR, Greene R. Malignant glomus jugulare tumor: a case with two unusual radiographic features. J Comput Assist Tomogr. 1980;4:415-7.
8. Irons GB, Weiland LH, Brown WL. Paragangliomas of the neck: clinical and pathologic analysis of 116 cases. Surg Clin North Am. 1977;57:575-83.
9. Flint PW, Haughey BH, Lund VJ, Robbins KT, Niparko JK, Thomas JR (Eds). Cummings Otolaryngology: Head & Neck Surgery, 5th edition. Elsevier Health Sciences; 2010.

18 Reporting Template with Illustrative Cases

(Tumors)

Smita Manchanda, Manisha Jana

REPORTING TEMPLATE

Right *Left*

- External ear:
  - External auditory canal (EAC) wall bony erosion (Absent/Partial/Complete)
  - Soft tissue involvement (Absent/<5 mm/>5 mm)
- Middle ear:
  - Soft tissue density (Present/Absent)
  - Ear ossicles (Intact/Eroded)
  - Bone erosion:
    - Tegmen tympani
    - Sigmoid plate
    - Facial nerve canal
- Inner ear:
  - Internal auditory canal (Normal/Enlarged)
  - Cochlea (Normal/Eroded)
  - Vestibule (Normal/Eroded)
- Mastoid air cells (Normal/Opacified/Sclerotic)
- Petrous apex (Normal/Eroded)
- Clivus (Normal/Eroded)
- Jugular foramen (Normal/Eroded/Enlarged)
- Carotid canal (Normal/Eroded)
- Foramen lacerum (Normal/Eroded)
- Cavernous sinus extension (Present/Absent)
- Intracranial extension (Present/Absent)
- Dural extension
- Extradural (Absent/<2 cm/>2 cm)
- Intradural (A/<2 cm/2–4 cm/>4 cm)
- Infratemporal fossa extension (Present/Absent)
- Lymph nodes [mention separation anxiety disorder (SAD) if involved and unilateral (U/L) or bilateral (B/L)]:
  - Level I
  - Level II
  - Level III
  - Level IV
  - Level V
  - Level VI
- Metastases (mention site)
- Any other finding

Key: A: Absent; C: Complete; E: Eroded; I: Intact; En: Enlarged; N: Normal; Op: Opacified; P: Present; Pa: Partial; Pn: Pneumatized; Sc: Sclerotic

IMPRESSION

Staging (Refer to Chapter 16)

- TNM (for EAC carcinoma)
- Fisch (for glomus jugulotympanicum)

CASE 1 (FIGS. 1A TO F)

A 22-year-old male presenting with right-sided hearing loss.

Mass lesion (measuring 3.5 × 3.3 × 3.0 cm) in the right jugular fossa and middle ear cavity which is of intermediate to hyperintense signal intensity (SI) on T1-weighted image (T1WI) and intermediate to hypointense on T2WI with heterogeneous postcontrast enhancement and extent as described below.

	Right	*Left*
• External ear (**Fig. 1D**):		
○ EAC wall bony erosion (Absent/Partial/Complete)	***Pa***	A
○ Soft tissue involvement (Absent/<5 mm/>5 mm)	***>5 mm***	A
• Middle ear:		
○ Soft tissue density (Present/Absent)	***P***	A
○ Ear ossicles (Intact/Eroded)	I	I
○ Bone erosion:		
– Tegmen tympani	I	I
– Sigmoid plate	I	I
– Facial nerve canal	I	I
• Inner ear:		
○ Internal auditory canal (Normal/Enlarged)	N	N
○ Cochlea (Normal/Eroded)	*E*	N
○ Vestibule (Normal/Eroded)	N	N
• Mastoid air cells (Normal/Opacified/Sclerotic)	***Op***	N
• Petrous apex (Normal/Eroded)	N	N
• Clivus (Normal/Eroded)	N	N
• Jugular foramen (Normal/Eroded/Enlarged)	***En***	N
• Carotid canal (Normal/Eroded)	*E*	N
• Foramen lacerum (Normal/Eroded)	N	N
• Cavernous sinus extension (Present/Absent)	A	A
• Intracranial extension (Present/Absent)	P	P
• Dural extension (**Figs. 1E** and **F**)		
• Extradural (Absent/<2 cm/>2 cm)	<2 cm	A
• Intradural (A/<2 cm/2–4 cm/>4 cm)	A	A
• Infratemporal fossa extension (Present/Absent)	A	A
• Lymph nodes (mention SAD if involved and U/L or B/L):	A	A
○ Level I		
○ Level II		
○ Level III		
○ Level IV		
○ Level V		
○ Level VI		
• Metastases (mention site)	A	A

Key: A: Absent; C: Complete; E: Eroded; En: Enlarged; I: Intact; N: Normal; Op: Opacified; P: Present; Pa: Partial; Pn: Pneumatized; Sc: Sclerotic

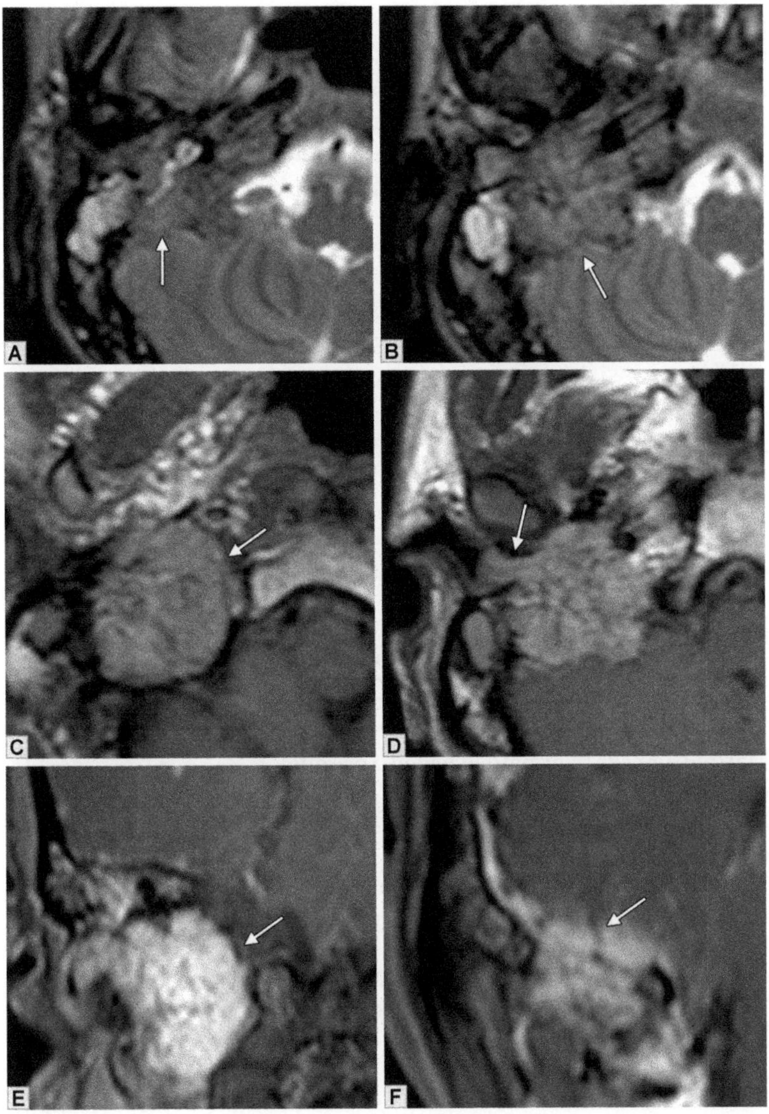

FIGS. 1A TO F: Right glomus jugulotympanicum with extradural extension. Fisch Stage D1. (A and B) Axial T2FS showing T2 hypointense mass with extradural extension (arrows) (C and D) Axial T1 WI. Intermediate SI on T1 WI (arrow in C). Arrow in D shows the EAC extension. (E and F) Coronal Post gad T1 WI showing enhancing mass with extradural extension (arrows).

Impression

Right glomus jugulotympanicum with extradural extension.

Staging

Fisch stage D1.

CASE 2 (FIGS. 2A TO F)

A 50-year-old female presenting with right-sided ear obstruction.

Heterogeneously enhancing mass lesion centered in the right middle ear cavity and jugular fossa (measuring 4.2 × 3.4 × 4.1 cm) with extent as described below.

	Right	*Left*
• External ear (**Figs. 2A** and **B**):		
○ EAC wall bony erosion (Absent/Partial/Complete)	***Pa***	A
○ Soft tissue involvement (Absent/<5 mm/>5 mm)	***>5 mm***	A
• Middle ear:		
○ Soft tissue density (Present/Absent)	***P***	A
○ Ear ossicles (Intact/Eroded)	***E***	I
○ Bone erosion:		
– Tegmen tympani (**Fig. 2F**)	***E***	I
– Sigmoid plate	***I***	I
– Facial nerve canal (**Fig. 2E**)	**E**	I
• Inner ear:		
○ Internal auditory canal (Normal/Enlarged)	N	N
○ Cochlea (Normal/Eroded) (**Fig. 2C**)	***E***	N
○ Vestibule (Normal/Eroded) (**Fig. 2F**)	***E***	N
• Mastoid air cells (Normal/Opacified/Sclerotic) (**Figs. 2C** and **D**)	***Op***	N
• Petrous apex (Normal/Eroded) (**Fig. 2D**)	***E***	N
• Clivus (Normal/Eroded)	***E***	N
• Jugular foramen (Normal/Eroded/Enlarged)	***En***	N
• Carotid canal (Normal/Eroded)	***E***	N
• Foramen lacerum (Normal/Eroded)	N	N
• Cavernous sinus extension (Present/Absent)	A	A
• Intracranial extension (Present/Absent)	***P***	A
• Dural extension (**Fig. 2A**)		
• Extradural (Absent/<2 cm/>2 cm)	***<2 cm***	A
• Intradural (A/<2 cm/2–4 cm/>4 cm)	A	A
• Infratemporal fossa extension (Present/Absent)	***P***	A
• Lymph nodes (mention SAD if involved and U/L or B/L):	A	A
○ Level I		
○ Level II		
○ Level III		
○ Level IV		
○ Level V		
○ Level VI		
• Metastases (mention site)	A	A

Key: A: Absent; C: Complete; E: Eroded; En: Enlarged; I: Intact; N: Normal; Op: Opacified; Pa: Partial; P: Present; Pn: Pneumatized; Sc: Sclerotic

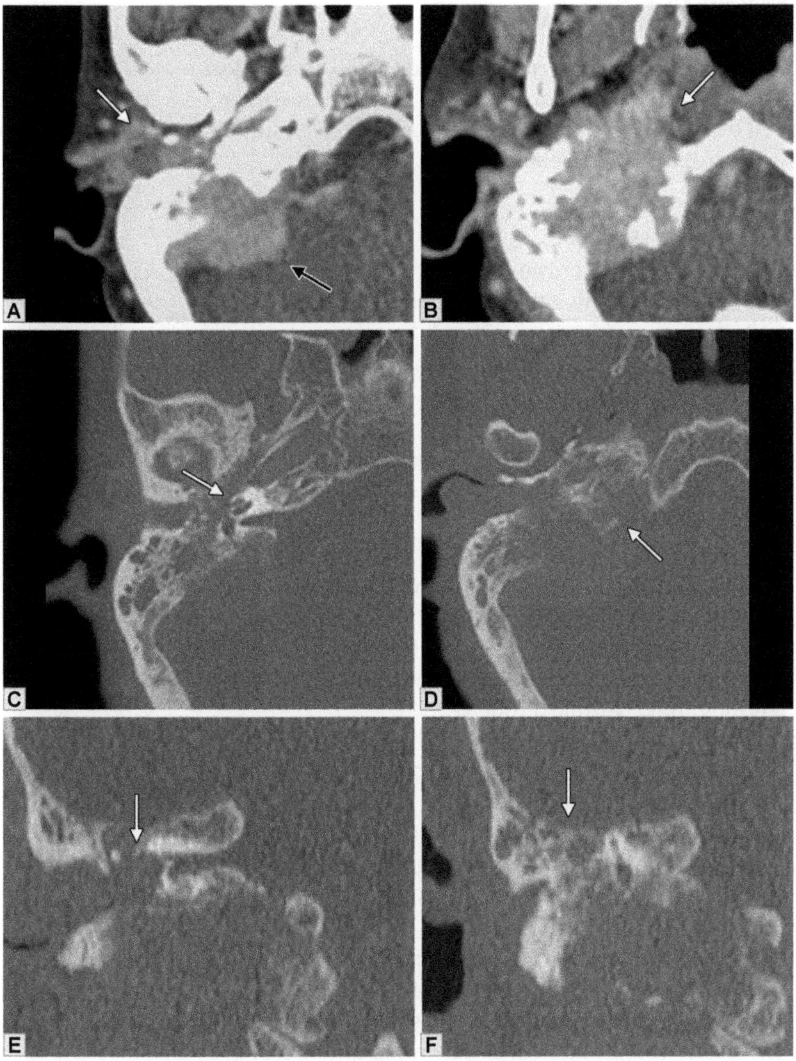

FIGS. 2A TO F: Right glomus jugulotympanicum with extradural extension. Fisch Stage D1. (A) Heterogeneously enhancing mass with extension to external auditory canal (white arrow) with extradural extension (black arrow). (B) Mass extending to nasopharynx (arrow). (C) Erosion of apical turn of cochlea (arrow). (D) Extension to petrous apex (arrow). (E) Erosion of facial canal (arrow). (F) Erosion of tegmen tympani (arrow).

Impression

Right glomus jugulotympanicum with extradural extension.

Staging

Fisch stage D1.

CASE 3 (FIGS. 3A TO F)

A 38-year-old female presenting with left sided hearing loss.

Heterogeneously enhancing mass lesion (measuring 3.5 × 3.2 × 3.4 cm) in the left external ear cavity with extension into the middle ear and infratemporal fossa (**Figs. 3A** to **D**) as detailed below.

	Right	*Left*
• External ear (**Figs. 3A** and **B**):		
○ EAC wall bony erosion (Absent/Partial/Complete)	A	***Pa***
○ Soft tissue involvement (Absent/<5 mm/>5 mm)	A	***>5 mm***
• Middle ear (**Figs. 3C** to **E**):		
○ Soft tissue density (Present/Absent)	A	***P***
○ Ear ossicles (Intact/Eroded)	I	***E***
○ Bone erosion:	I	I
– Tegmen tympani	I	I
– Sigmoid plate	I	I
– Facial nerve canal		
• Inner ear:		
○ Internal auditory canal (Normal/Enlarged)	N	N
○ Cochlea (Normal/Eroded)	N	N
○ Vestibule (Normal/Eroded)	N	N
• Mastoid air cells (Normal/Opacified/Sclerotic) (**Fig. 3F**)	N	***Op***
• Petrous apex (Normal/Eroded)	N	N
• Clivus (Normal/Eroded)	N	N
• Jugular foramen (Normal/Eroded/Enlarged)	N	N
• Carotid canal (Normal/Eroded)	N	N
• Foramen lacerum (Normal/Eroded)	N	N
• Cavernous sinus extension (Present/Absent)	A	A
• Intracranial extension (Present/Absent)	A	A
• Dural extension:		
○ Extradural (Absent/<2 cm/>2 cm)	A	A
○ Intradural (A/<2 cm/2–4 cm/>4 cm)	A	A
• Infratemporal fossa extension (Present/Absent)	A	***P***
• Lymph nodes (mention SAD if involved and U/L or B/L) (**Figs. 3A** and **B**):	A	P
○ Level I		
○ Level II		
○ Level III		
○ Level IV		
○ Level V		
Few Left LN (SAD 1.3 cm)		
○ Level VI	A	A
• Metastases (mention site)		

Key: A: Absent; C: Complete; E: Eroded; En: Enlarged; I: Intact; N: Normal; Op: Opacified; P: Present; Pa: Partial; Pn: Pneumatized; Sc: Sclerotic

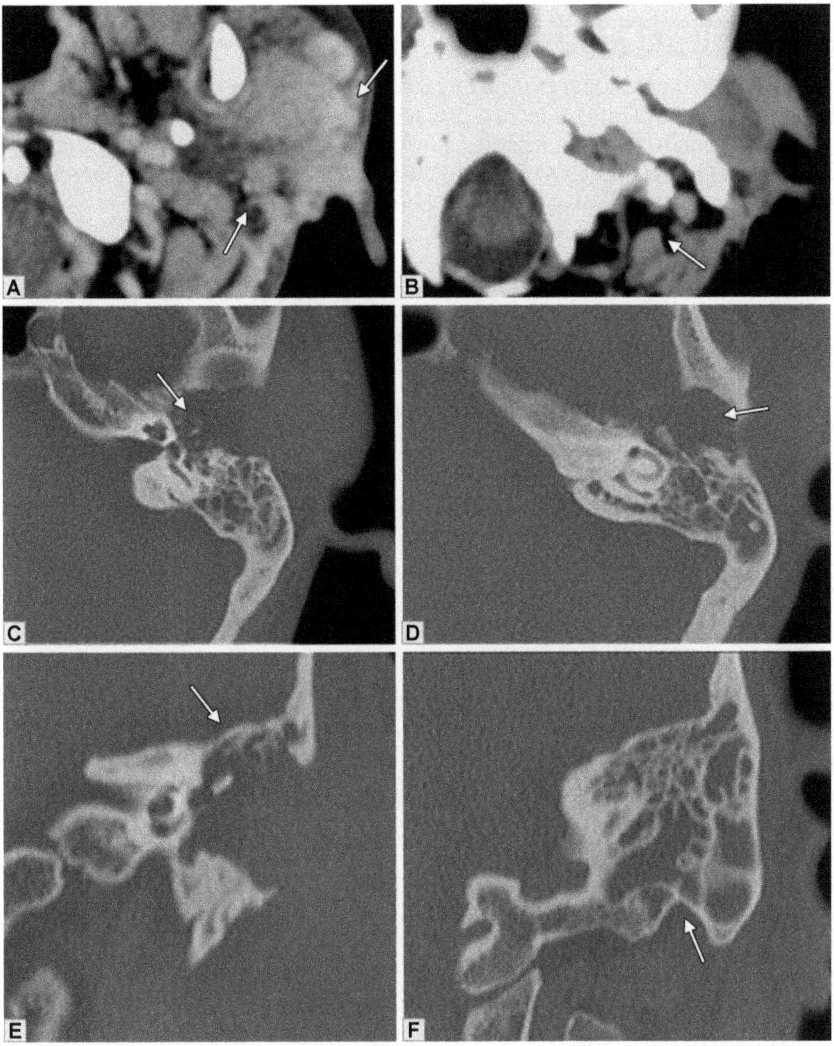

FIGS. 3A TO F: Malignant left external auditory meatus mass; Stage 4 (T4N1Mx). (A) Large heterogeneously enhancing EAC mass (thin arrow). (B) Left Level V lymph nodes (thick arrow in A and B). (C) Ossicle erosion (arrow). (D) Middle ear extension (arrow). (E) Intact tegmen tympani (arrow). (F) Opacified mastoid air cells (arrow).

Impression

Mass lesion left external auditory meatus likely malignant.

Staging

Stage 4 (T4N1Mx).

CASE 4 (FIGS. 4A TO F)

For tumor extent of biopsy proven facial schwannoma in a 25-year-old male who had presented with right-sided ear obstruction.

Mass lesion in the right middle ear cavity which is isointense (to gray matter) on T1WI (**Fig. 4A**) and T2WI (**Fig. 4C**) with few cystic areas and heterogeneous enhancement and extent as described below.

	Right	*Left*
• External ear:		
○ EAC wall bony erosion (Absent/Partial/Complete)	A	A
○ Soft tissue involvement (Absent/<5 mm/>5 mm)	A	A
• Middle ear (**Figs. 4C** and **D**):		
○ Soft tissue density (Present/Absent)	***P***	A
○ Ear ossicles (Intact/Eroded)	I	I
○ Bone erosion:		
– Tegmen tympani	*E*	I
– Sigmoid plate	I	I
– Facial nerve canal	*E*	I
• Inner ear (**Fig. 4B**):		
○ Internal auditory canal (Normal/Enlarged)	N	N
○ Cochlea (Normal/Eroded)	N	N
○ Vestibule (Normal/Eroded)	N	N
• Mastoid air cells (Normal/Opacified/Sclerotic)	***Op***	N
• Petrous apex (Normal/Eroded)	N	N
• Clivus (Normal/Eroded)	N	N
• Jugular foramen (Normal/Eroded/Enlarged)	N	N
• Carotid canal (Normal/Eroded)	N	N
• Foramen lacerum (Normal/Eroded)	N	N
• Cavernous sinus extension (Present/Absent)	A	A
• Intracranial extension (Present/Absent) (**Figs. 4E** and **F**)	***P***	***P***
• Dural extension (**Fig. 4E**)		
• Extradural (Absent/<2 cm/>2 cm)	***<2 cm***	A
• Intradural (A/<2 cm/2–4cm/>4 cm)	A	A
• Infratemporal fossa extension (Present/Absent)	A	A
• Lymph nodes (mention SAD if involved and U/L or B/L):	A	A
○ Level I		
○ Level II		
○ Level III		
○ Level IV		
○ Level V		
○ Level VI		
• Metastases (mention site)	A	A

Any Other Finding

Extension into the parotid gland (**Fig. 4C**) and intracranial extradural location is seen. Another similar heterogeneously enhancing mass lesion seen in the retroantral location (**Fig. 4F**).

Key: A: Absent; C: Complete; E: Eroded; En: Enlarged; I: Intact; N: Normal; Op: Opacified; P: Present; Pa: Partial; Pn: Pneumatized; Sc: Sclerotic

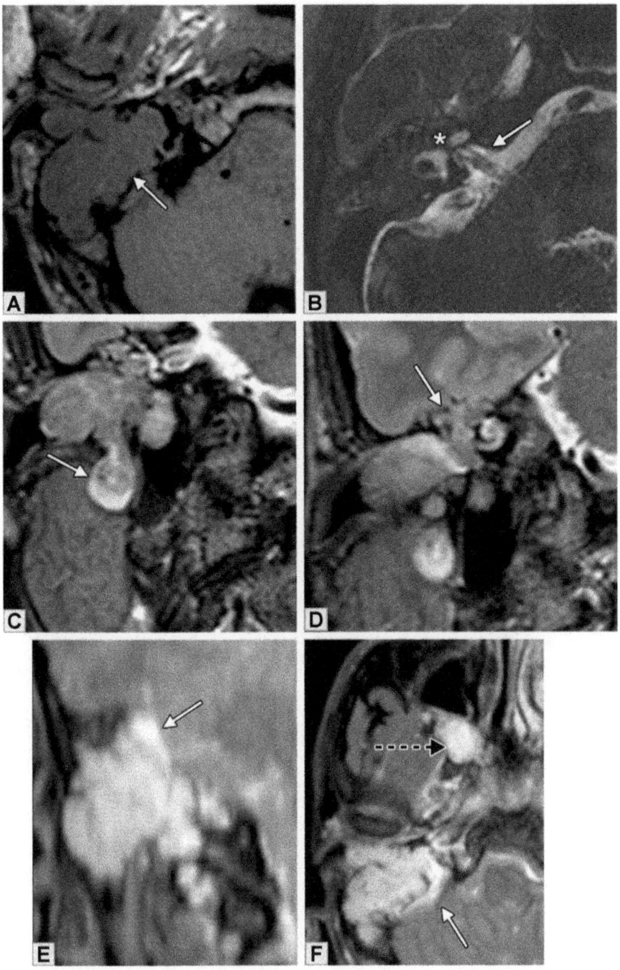

FIGS. 4A TO F: Right facial nerve schwannoma. (A) Isointense mass lesion in right middle ear cavity (arrow) on T1 WI. (B) Axial 3D heavily T2 WI (FIESTA). Hypointense mass along the first genu (*) and tympanic segment. Normal cisternal segment (arrow). (C) Coronal T2FS shows intraparotid extension (arrow). (D) Coronal T2FS shows extradural extension (arrow). (E) Coronal Post gad T1 WI shows heterogeneously enhancing mass with extradural extension (arrow). (F) Axial Post gad T1 WI shows another similar heterogeneously enhancing mass lesion (dashed arrow) in the retroantral location (mandibular nerve schwannoma).

Impression

Right facial nerve schwannoma with extension into locations as described above (mastoids, middle ear, external ear, parotid gland, and intracranial extradural) with small right mandibular nerve schwannoma.

6
SECTION

Location Based Approach

19

Approach to External Ear, Middle Ear, and Lateral Skull Base

Smita Manchanda, Ashu Seith Bhalla

This section deals with the common pathologies affecting the external ear, middle ear, and lateral skull base, and imaging based approach.

APPROACH TO EXTERNAL EAR ABNORMALITIES

The external ear includes external auditory canal (EAC) and pinna.

External Auditory Canal

The EAC can be involved by lesions which commonly present as soft tissue or bony involvement.[1] The common pathologies of the EAC are enlisted in **Box 1**, and the approach to the same is described in **Flowchart 1**.

- The EAC should be evaluated for the caliber, presence of soft tissue, and the status of bony walls.
- Soft tissue within the EAC can be associated with canal atresia (**Figs. 1A** and **B**) or bone involvement in the form of bone erosion or expansion. The approach to EAC pathologies is shown in **Figures 2** and **3**.
- Impacted wax (cerumen) is a common cause of soft tissue in the EAC. The classical imaging feature of cerumen is soft tissue with fat attenuation and a rim of air. There is no bone expansion/bone erosion.

BOX 1 Common pathologies affecting the external auditory canal (EAC).

- Congenital:
  - EAC atresia or stenosis
  - Dehiscent jugular vein
- Inflammatory/infections:
  - Malignant otitis externa
  - Keratosis obturans
  - Cholesteatoma
- Tumors and tumor-like conditions:
  - Carcinoma
  - Lymphoma
  - Contiguous involvement by tumors
  - Osteoma
- Trauma:
  - Fractures
  - Foreign body
  - Post-traumatic EAC stenosis
- Miscellaneous:
  - Vascular malformations
  - Osteoradionecrosis

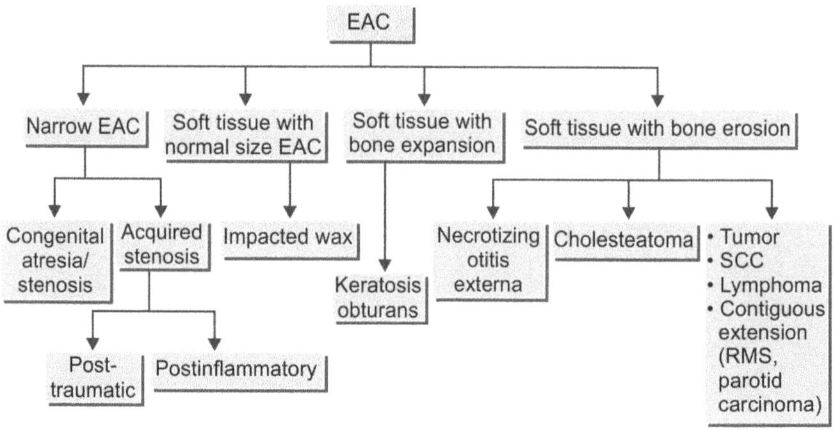

FLOWCHART 1: Algorithmic approach to pathologies of the EAC.

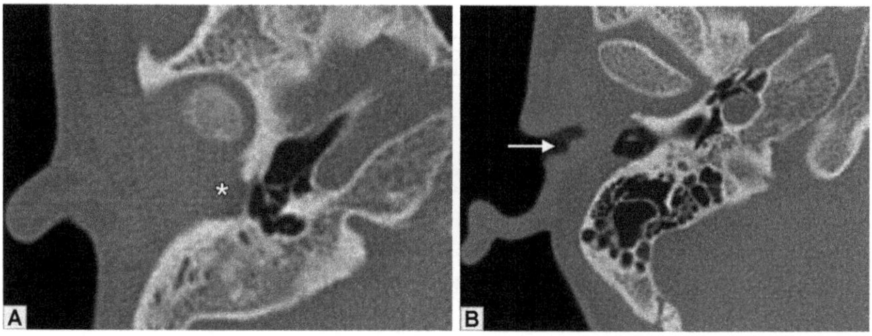

FIGS. 1A AND B: Atresia of external auditory canal: (A) Congenital atresia (asterisk) of bony and cartilaginous part; (B) Post-traumatic atresia of cartilaginous part (arrow).

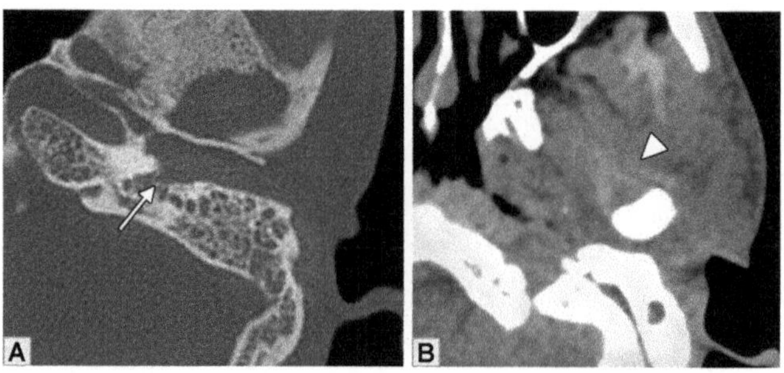

FIGS. 2A TO D: *Continued*

Continued

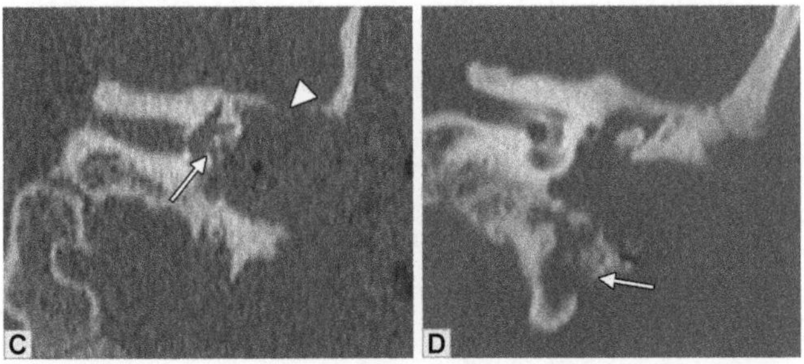

FIGS. 2A TO D: Soft tissue in external auditory canal (EAC) with bone erosion: (A and B) Malignant otitis externa: Soft tissue in EAC with bone erosion (arrow in A) and ill-defined soft tissue in masticator space (arrowhead); (C) Cholesteatoma: Soft tissue with erosion of tegmen tympani (arrowhead) and labyrinthine fistula (arrow); (D) Squamous cell carcinoma: Large soft tissue in EAC with permeative bone destruction (arrow).

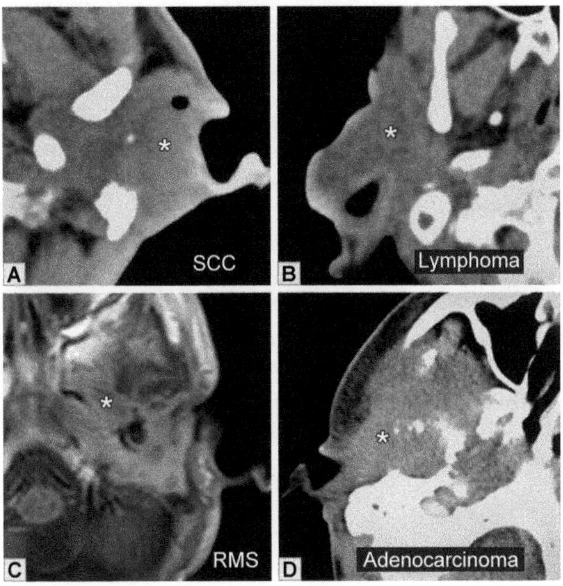

FIGS. 3A TO D: Soft tissue with bone erosion in external auditory canal (EAC): Tumors: (A) Squamous cell carcinoma (asterisk); (B) Lymphoma (asterisk); (C) Rhabdomyosarcoma (RMS) (secondary involvement by masticator space RMS) (asterisk); (D) Adenocarcinoma (secondary involvement by parotid adenocarcinoma) (asterisk).

- It is also important to differentiate between keratosis obturans (KO) and external ear cholesteatoma when soft tissue is seen in the EAC (**Figs. 4A** to **D**) (**Table 1**).

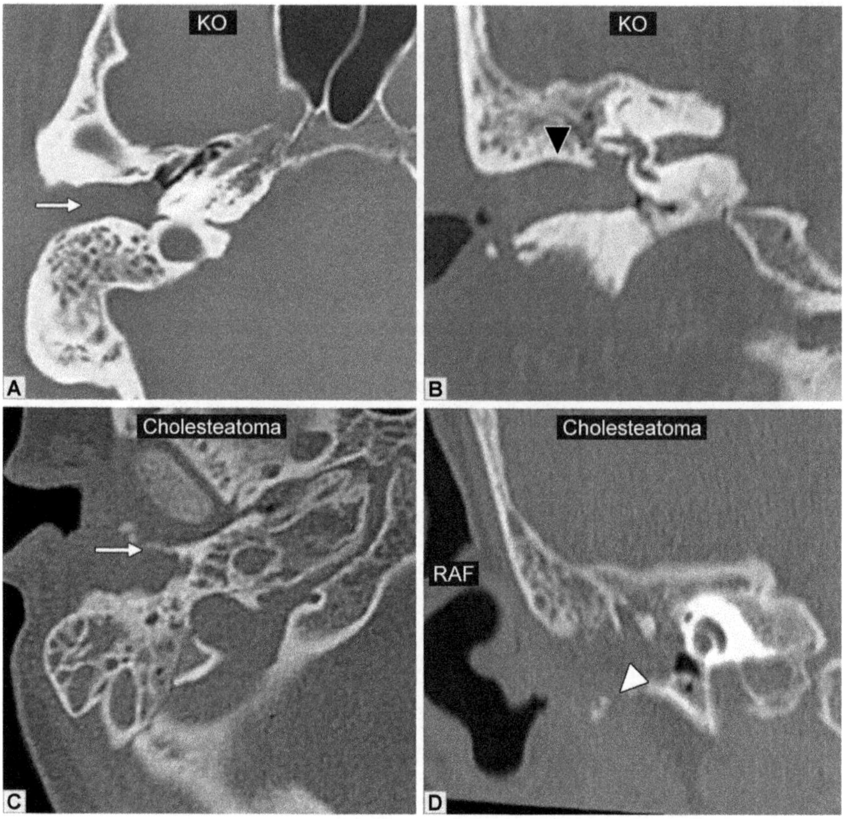

FIGS. 4A TO D: Keratosis obturans (KO) versus cholesteatoma: (A and B) Keratosis obturans: Soft tissue mass (arrow) with expansion and smooth widening of the bony canal (arrowhead); (C and D) External ear cholesteatoma: Soft tissue mass which erodes the inferior (arrowhead) and anterior (arrow) walls of external auditory canal (EAC) and extends into the mastoid cavity.

TABLE 1 Clinicoradiological features to differentiate between keratosis obturans (KO) and external ear cholesteatoma.

Feature	Keratosis obturans	External ear cholesteatoma
Age group	Younger	Older
Laterality	Frequently bilateral	Unilateral
Clinical presentation	Acute onset, otalgia	Chronic onset, otorrhoea
HRCT	Soft tissue mass with expansion or smooth widening of the bony canal	Soft tissue mass which erodes the inferior and posterior walls of EAC and extends into the mastoid cavity

Pinna

- The pinna lesions are clinically diagnosed and infrequently require radiological evaluation.[2]
- The common pathologies which are evaluated on imaging include congenital lesions, arteriovenous malformation, calcification, and malignancy [squamous cell carcinoma (SCC)] (**Figs. 5A** to **D**).
- Congenital lesions include microtia, preauricular sinus, and type 1 branchial fistula. In microtia, pinna is not only small and malformed but also often low lying.
- Calcification of the auricular cartilage may arise from a number of causes, including hyperparathyroidism, relapsing polychondritis, gout and pseudogout, ochronosis, trauma, frostbite, and diabetes mellitus.

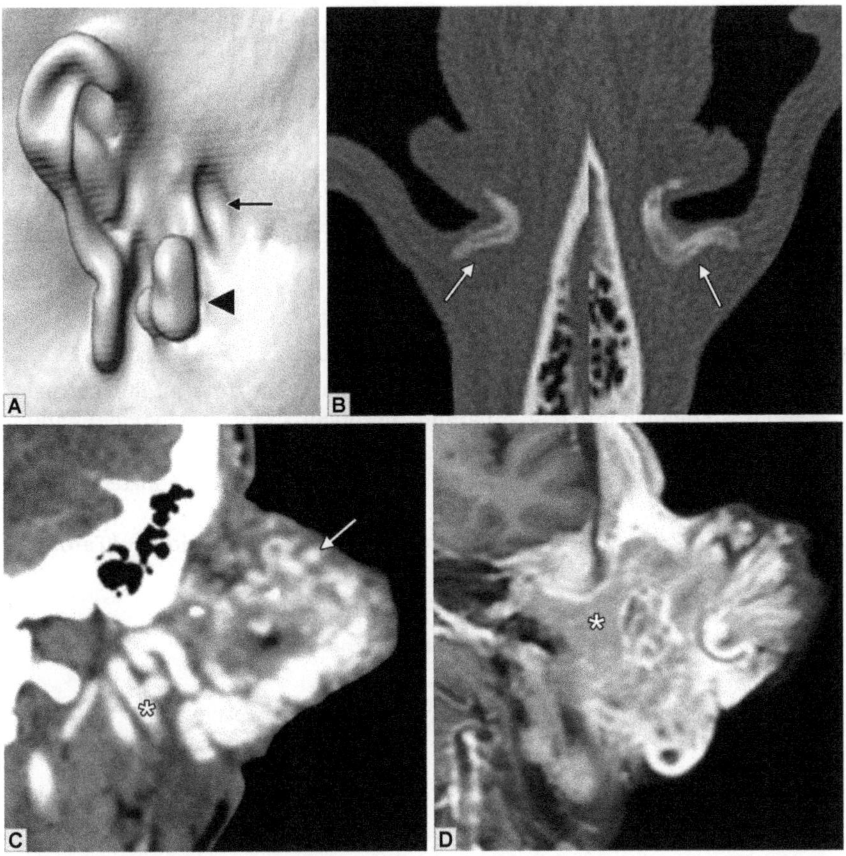

FIGS. 5A TO D: Pinna abnormalities: (A) Grade I microtia with preauricular tag (arrowhead) and pit (arrow); (B) Bilateral pinna calcification (arrows) in a case of diabetes mellitus; (C) Arteriovenous malformation pinna with arterial feeders (arrow) and early draining veins (asterisk); (D) Squamous cell carcinoma. Heterogenously enhancing mass in pinna and external auditory canal (EAC) (asterisk).

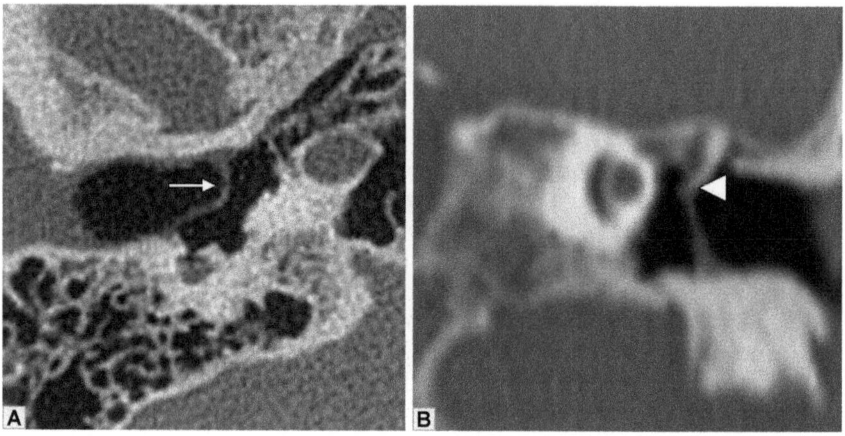

FIGS. 6A AND B: Tympanic membrane (TM) abnormalities: (A) Thickened and retracted TM (arrow) in a case of cholesteatomatous chronic suppurative otitis media (CSOM); (B) Handle of malleus (arrowhead) bulging through a perforated TM.

Tympanic Membrane

- It is a thin membrane that separates the external ear from the middle ear.
- Tympanic membrane (TM) can be absent in aural atresia, thickened, and retracted or perforated in chronic suppurative otitis media (CSOM) (**Figs. 6A** and **B**).

MIDDLE EAR CAVITY

- The middle ear cavity (tympanic cavity) contains the three auditory ossicles and is subdivided into epitympanum, mesotympanum, and hypotympanum (in relation to the planes of the TM).
- The common pathologies affecting the middle ear cavity are enlisted in **Box 2** and **Figs. 7** to **9**.
- The location of soft tissue[3] can provide a clue to the likely etiology (**Table 2**).

BOX 2 Common pathologies affecting the middle ear.

- Congenital:
  - Small size (as part) of microtia spectrum
  - Cholesteatoma
- Infections/inflammatory:
  - Secretory OM
  - Acute OM (rarely imaged unless complicated)
  - Chronic OM +/– cholesteatoma
  - Postinflammatory changes
- Tumors:
  - Glomus tympanicum/jugulotympanicum
  - LCH
- Rare miscellaneous lesions:
  - Cholesterol granuloma
  - Extramedullary hematopoiesis

(OM: otitis media; LCH: Langerhans cell histiocytosis)

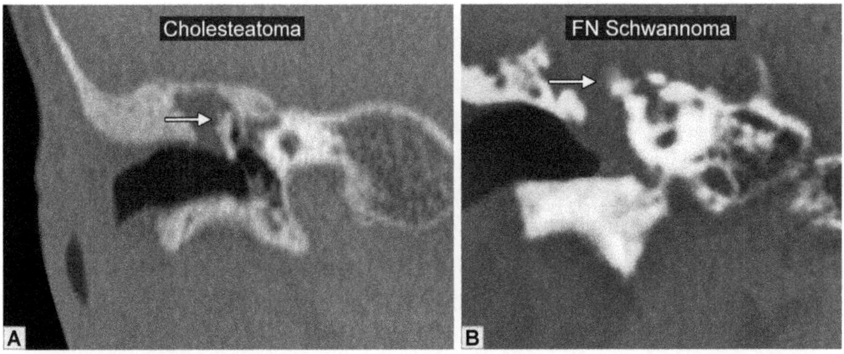

FIGS. 7A AND B: Location of soft tissue: Epitympanum and mesotympanum: (A) Cholesteatoma: Soft tissue with erosion of ossicles (arrow); (B) Facial nerve schwannoma: Soft tissue with widening of first genu (arrow) and bone expansion.

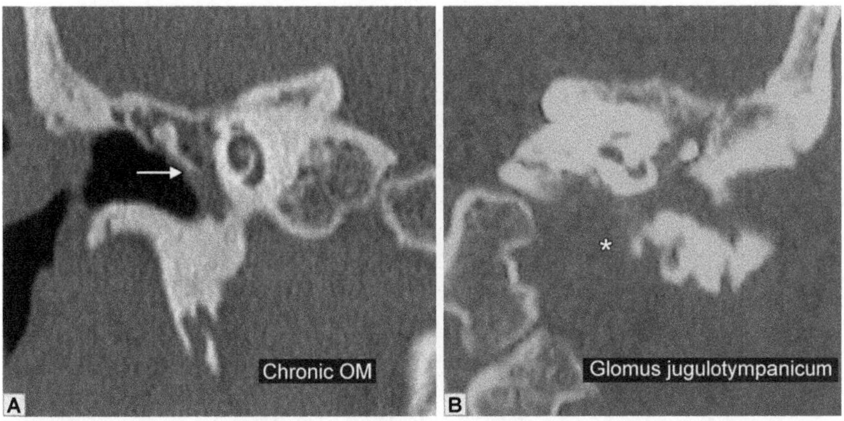

FIGS. 8A AND B: Location of soft tissue: Mesotympanum and hypotympanum: (A) Chronic otitis media: Soft tissue in mesotympanum and hypotympanum (arrow); (B) Glomus jugulotympanicum: Soft tissue in tympanic cavity and jugular foramen (asterisk).

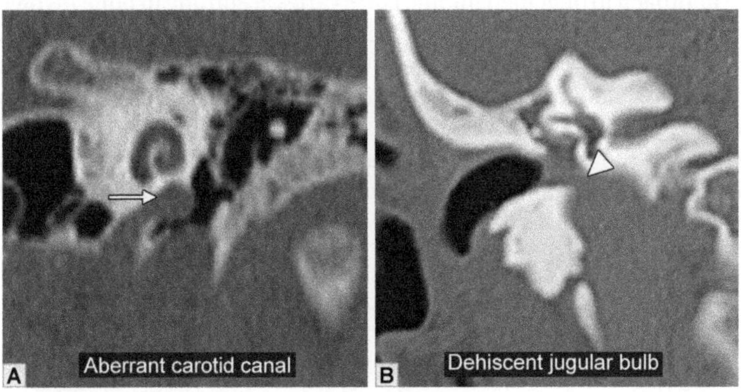

FIGS. 9A AND B: Soft tissue in hypotympanum: Vascular causes: (A) Aberrant carotid artery (arrow); (B) Dehiscent jugular bulb (arrowhead).

TABLE 2 **Location of soft tissue in middle ear and the likely etiologies.**

Location	Diseases/Etiologies
Epitympanum and mesotympanum (**Figs. 7A** and **B**)	• Cholesteatoma • Facial nerve schwannoma
Mesotympanum and hypotympanum (**Figs. 8A** and **B**)	• Cholesteatoma • Glomus tympanicum (mesotympanum) • Glomus jugulotympanicum (hypotympanum)
Hypotympanum (**Figs. 9A** and **B**)	• Glomus jugulotympanicum • Cholesteatoma • Aberrant carotid artery • Dehiscent jugular bulb

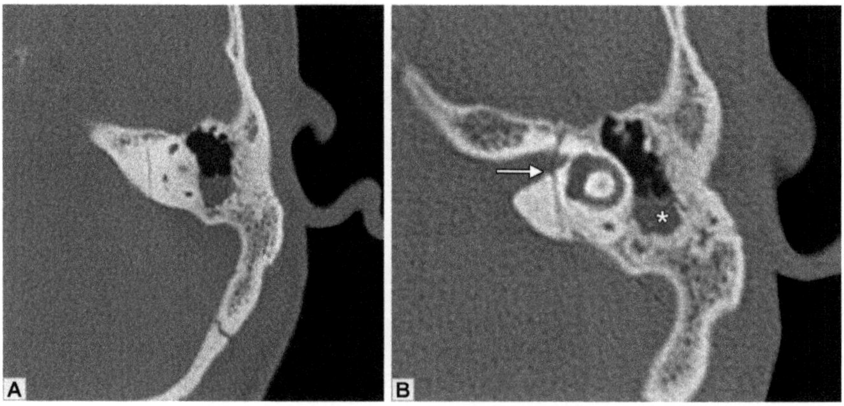

FIGS. 10A AND B: Traumatic middle ear opacification: Hemotympanum (asterisk) with transverse fracture extending into internal auditory canal (arrow).

- The approach to opacified middle ear[1,3] varies according to bone involvement (no bony involvement/bone erosion, bone expansion). Hemotympanum (**Figs. 10A** and **B**) is seen in cases of trauma and may be associated with fracture/ossicle dislocation. These are summarized in **Flowcharts 2** and **3** and illustrated in **Figures 11** to **14**.
- Ossicles of the middle ear can be affected by varied lesions. The diseases affecting ossicles in different patterns are summarized in **Table 3** and illustrated in **Figures 15** to **19**.

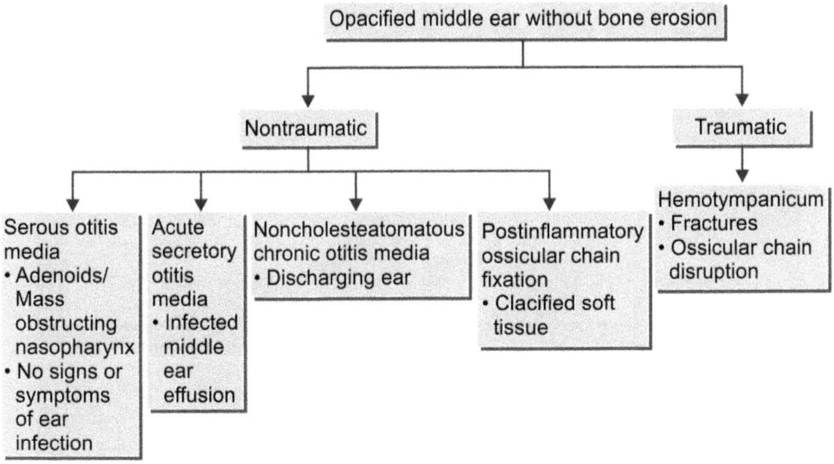

FLOWCHART 2: Approach to opacified middle ear without bone erosion.

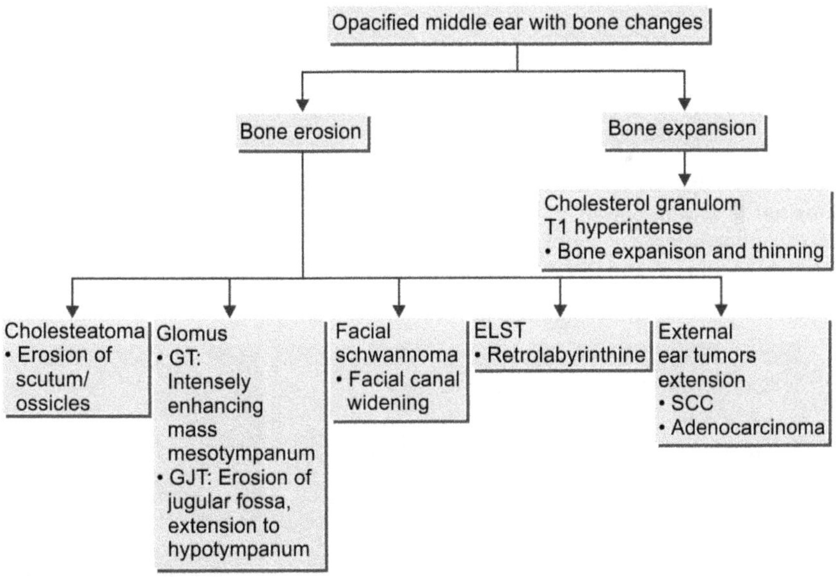

FLOWCHART 3: Approach to opacified middle ear with bone erosion/expansion.

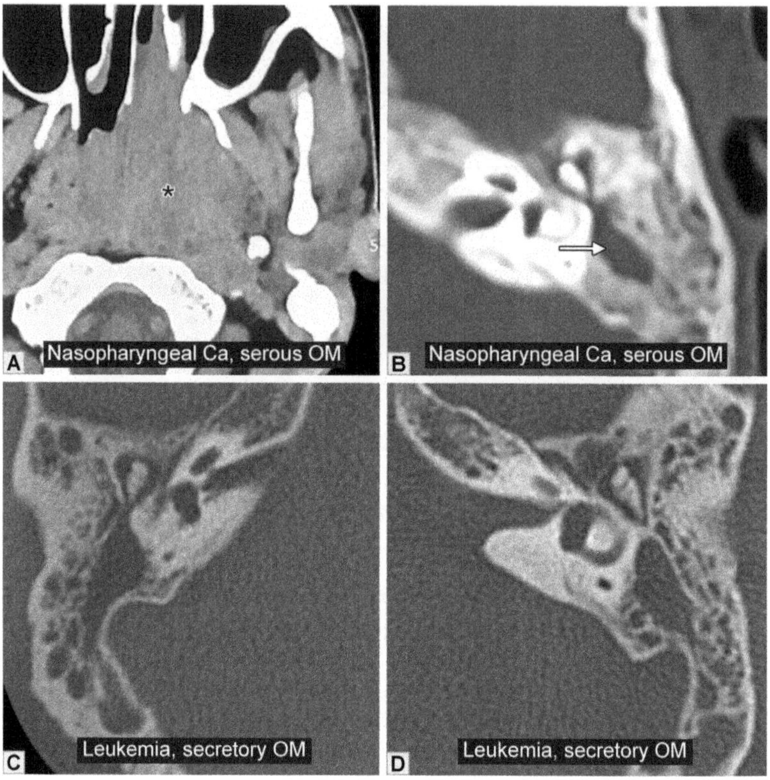

FIGS. 11A TO D: Nontraumatic middle ear opacification with no bone erosion: (A and B) Serous otitis media (OM): Large mass in nasopharynx in a case of nasopharyngeal carcinoma (asterisk) with serous OM (arrow) due to blocked Eustachian tube; (C and D) Acute secretory OM in a case of leukemia.

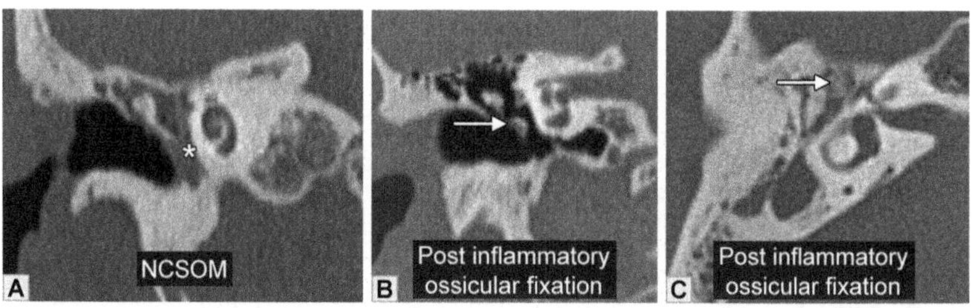

FIGS. 12A TO C: Nontraumatic middle ear opacification with no bone erosion: (A) Noncholesteatomatous chronic otitis media (asterisk). Soft tissue in mesotympanum and hypotympanum (asterisk) with intact ossicles (arrow); (B and C) Postinflammatory ossicular chain fixation: Calcification along tympanic membrane (arrow in B). Calcified soft tissue in tympanic cavity (arrow in C).

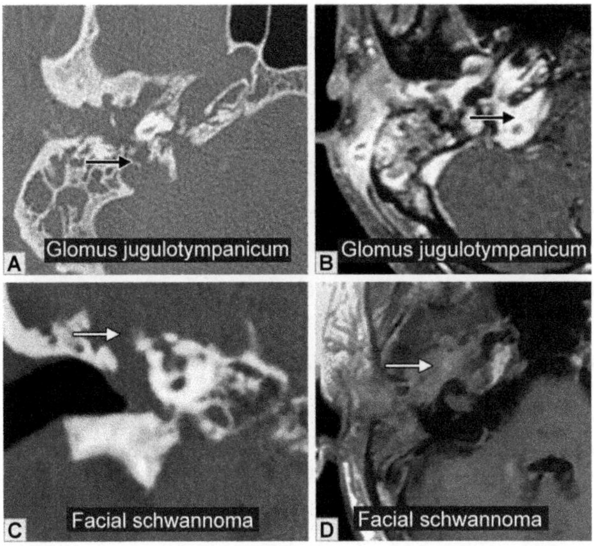

FIGS. 13A TO D: Nontraumatic middle ear opacification with bone erosion (extension of tumors): (A) Glomus jugulotympanicum *(CT)*: Erosion of walls of mastoid and jugular foramen (arrow); (B) Glomus jugulotympanicum (MRI): Intensely enhancing mass in middle ear cavity and jugular fossa (arrow); (C) Facial schwannoma (CT): Soft tissue along first genu (arrow) and middle ear cavity; (D) Facial schwannoma (MRI): Intermediate enhancement of the soft tissue mass (arrow).

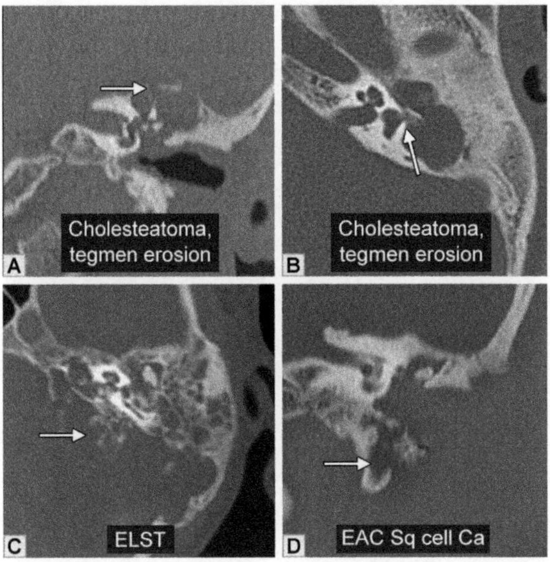

FIGS. 14A TO D: Nontraumatic middle ear opacification with bone erosion: (A) Cholesteatoma with erosion of tegmen tympani (arrow); (B) Cholesteatoma with labyrinthine fistula (arrow); (C) Endolymphatic sac tumor with permeative bone destruction (arrow); (D) External auditory canal squamous cell carcinoma with erosion of mastoid (arrow).

TABLE 3 **Pattern of ossicle involvement and underlying etiologies.**

Pattern	Diseases/Etiologies
Dysplastic (**Figs. 15A** to **D**)	• Microtia spectrum • Isolated middle ear anomaly
Fixation (**Figs. 16A** and **B**)	• Congenital ossicular fixation • Postinflammatory ossicular fixation
Erosion (**Figs. 17A** to **D**)	• Cholesteatomatous CSOM • Tumor (glomus, facial schwannoma, ELST)
Disruption (**Figs. 18A** and **B**)	• Trauma
Nonvisualization (**Figs. 19A** and **B**)	• Postoperative • Past history of CSOM (automastoidectomy)

(CSOM: chronic suppurative otitis media; ELST: endolymphatic sac tumor)

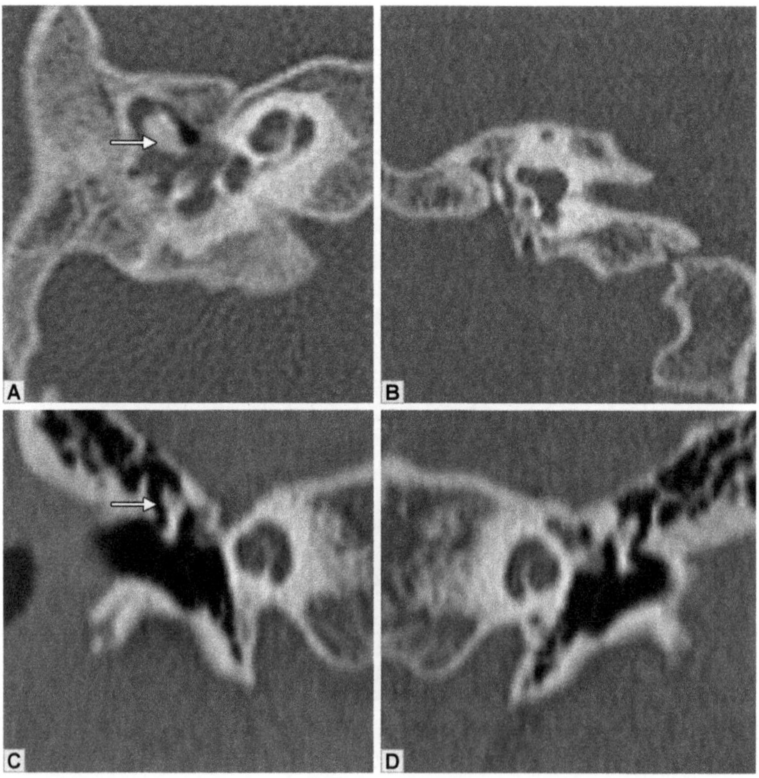

FIGS. 15A TO D: Dysplastic ossicles: (A and B) Microtia with congenital dysplastic ossicles (arrow); (C and D) Isolated middle ear anomaly: Normal size of external ear and middle ear cavity with dysplastic malleus (arrow).

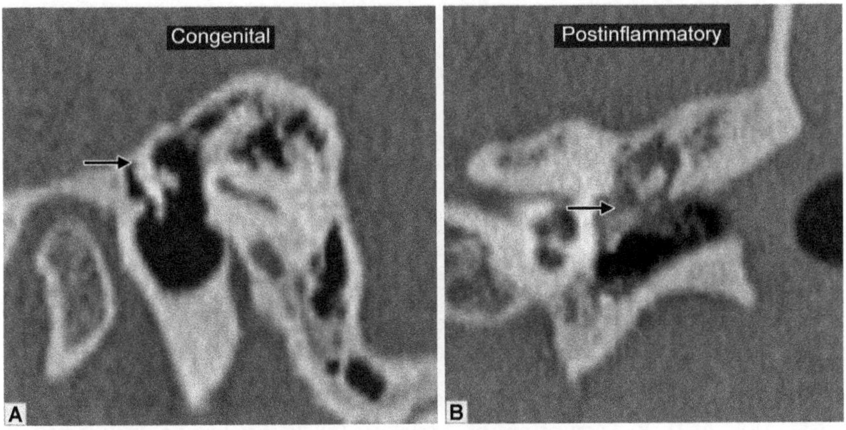

FIGS. 16A AND B: Ossicle fixation: (A) Congenital IM fixation: Malleus head abutting tegmen tympani (arrow); (B) Postinflammatory ossicular fixation: Calcified soft tissue in middle ear cavity (arrow) with ossicular erosion and fixation.

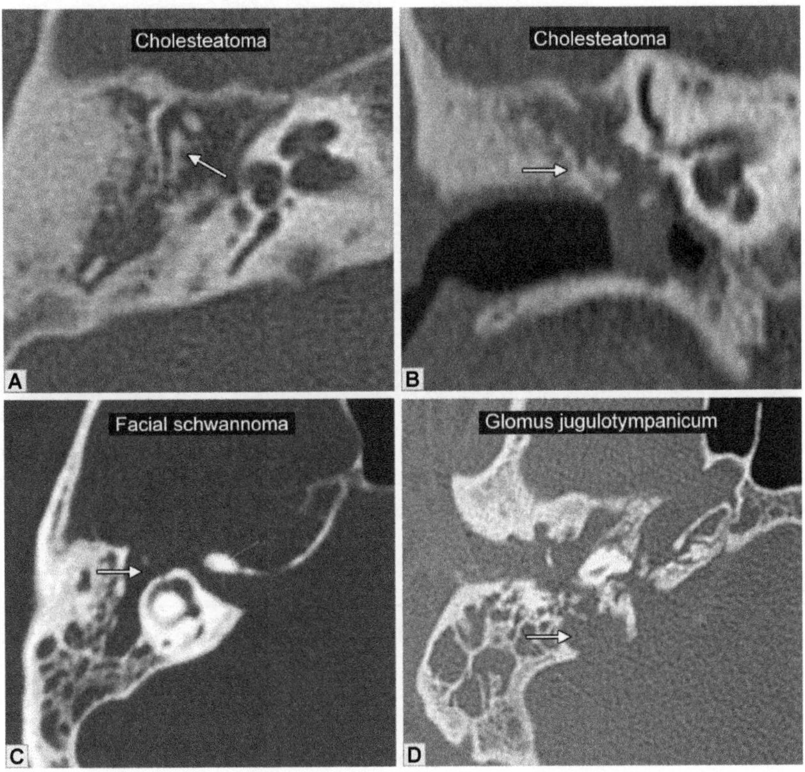

FIGS. 17A TO D: Erosion of ossicles: (A and B) Cholesteatoma: Soft tissue in middle ear cavity with ossicular erosion (arrow); (C) Facial schwannoma: Expansile soft tissue along first genu (arrow); (D) Glomus jugulotympanicum: Soft tissue with erosion of jugular foramen (arrow) and ossicles.

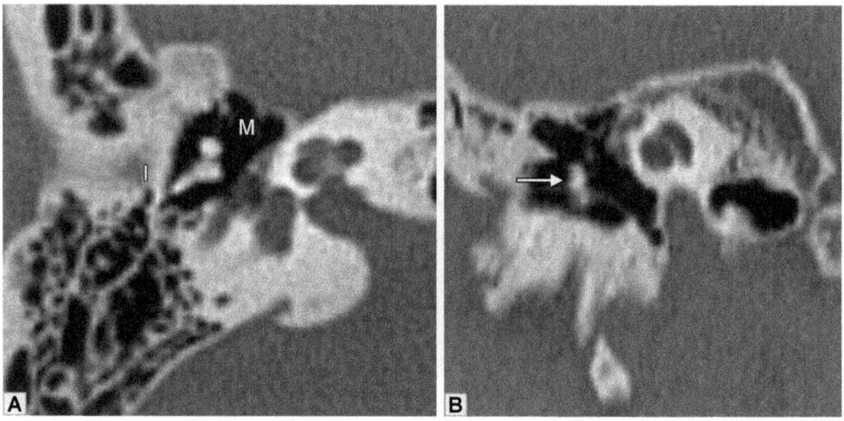

FIGS. 18A AND B: Disruption of ossicles: (A) Post-traumatic incudomalleal dislocation; (B) Post-traumatic dislocation (arrow) of incus (I) and malleus (M) (lying in the mesotympanum).

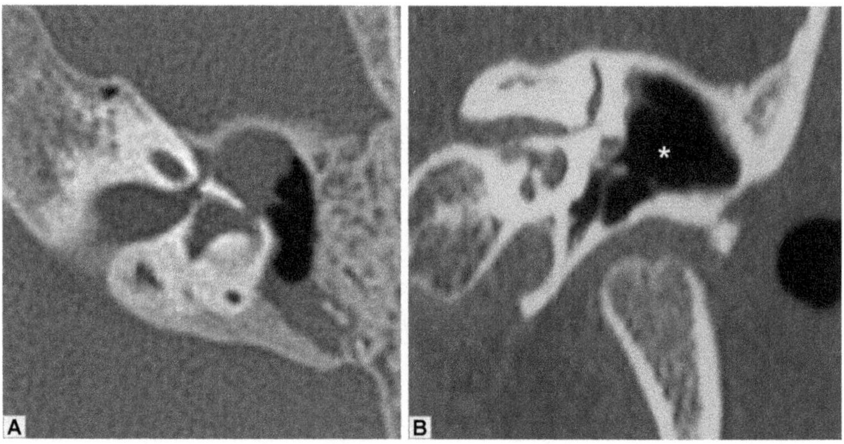

FIGS. 19A AND B: Ossicles not visualized: (A) Postoperative cavity with ossicles not visualized; (B) Automastoidectomy: No history of surgery; however, cavity with no ossicles (asterisk).

LATERAL SKULL BASE

- This includes the region from posterior wall of orbit to the petrous temporal bone (including the infratemporal fossa and pterygopalatine fossa), the posterior segment of middle cranial fossa, and part of the posterior cranial fossa.[4]
- The important structures in this region include the external/middle/inner ear, the 7th/8th nerve complex, maxillary (V2), and mandibulary (V3) divisions of

the trigeminal nerve, vagus, glossopharyngeal, spinal accessory, hypoglossal nerves, the internal carotid artery, internal jugular vein, lateral and sigmoid sinus, cerebellopontine angle, and related vascular bundles and temporomandibular joint.

- Pathology in this region includes tumors, cholesteatomas, infections, vascular lesions, and meningoencephaloceles.[5]
- The common tumors can be subdivided depending on the main site of origin (**Table 4**).
- The common tumors include schwannoma of the 5th and 7th nerve (**Figs. 20A** to **C**), meningiomas, chordoma of the clivus, jugular and tympanic paraganglioma, tumors of the nasopharynx, and SCCs or basal cell cancers of the scalp and ear.
- Tumors of the tympanomastoid region are described in **Figures 21** to **23**; and central skull base tumor extension in **Figure 24**. These are also covered in Chapters 16 and 22.

TABLE 4 **Tumors and tumor-like conditions of the lateral skull base.**

Region	Common tumors
Tympanomastoid region	• Chondrosarcoma • Giant cell tumor • Chondrobalstoma • ABC • Osteoblastoma • FD • LCH
Central skull base tumor extension	• Meningioma • Chondrosarcoma • Metastases • Chordoma • Rhabdomyosarcoma • Nasopharyngeal CA
External, middle, and inner ear tumors	• Malignant tumor of EAC • Cholesteatoma • Schwannoma • Meningioma • Paraganglioma • Endolymphatic sac tumor
Petrous apex tumors	• Petroclival fissure chondrosarcoma • Petroclival meningioma • Schwannoma • Metastases

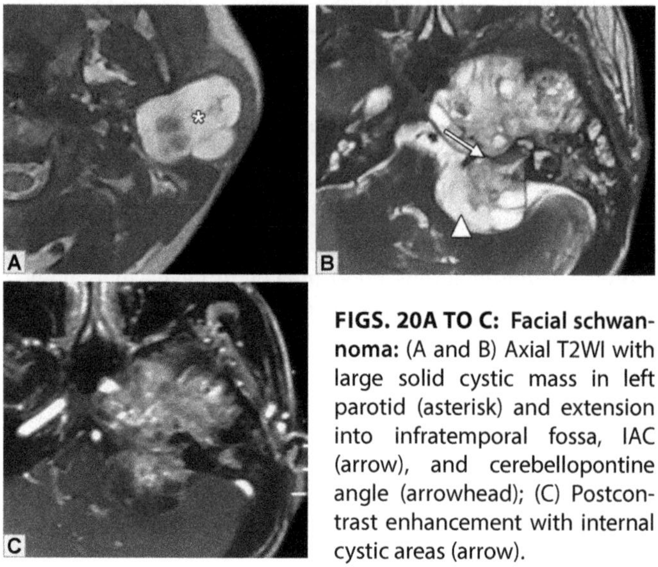

FIGS. 20A TO C: Facial schwannoma: (A and B) Axial T2WI with large solid cystic mass in left parotid (asterisk) and extension into infratemporal fossa, IAC (arrow), and cerebellopontine angle (arrowhead); (C) Postcontrast enhancement with internal cystic areas (arrow).

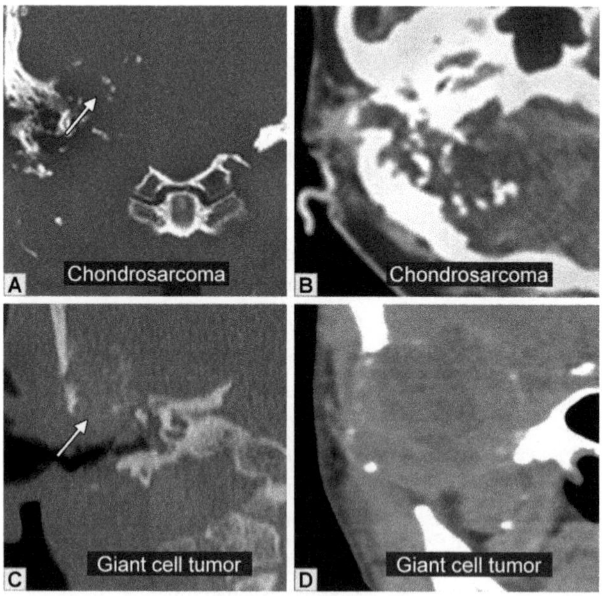

FIGS. 21A TO D: Tumors of tympanomastoid region: (A and B) Chondrosarcoma: Expansile mass right temporal bone with ring and arc pattern of calcification (arrow); (C and D) Giant cell tumor: Expansile mass right temporal bone with permeative bone destruction (arrow).

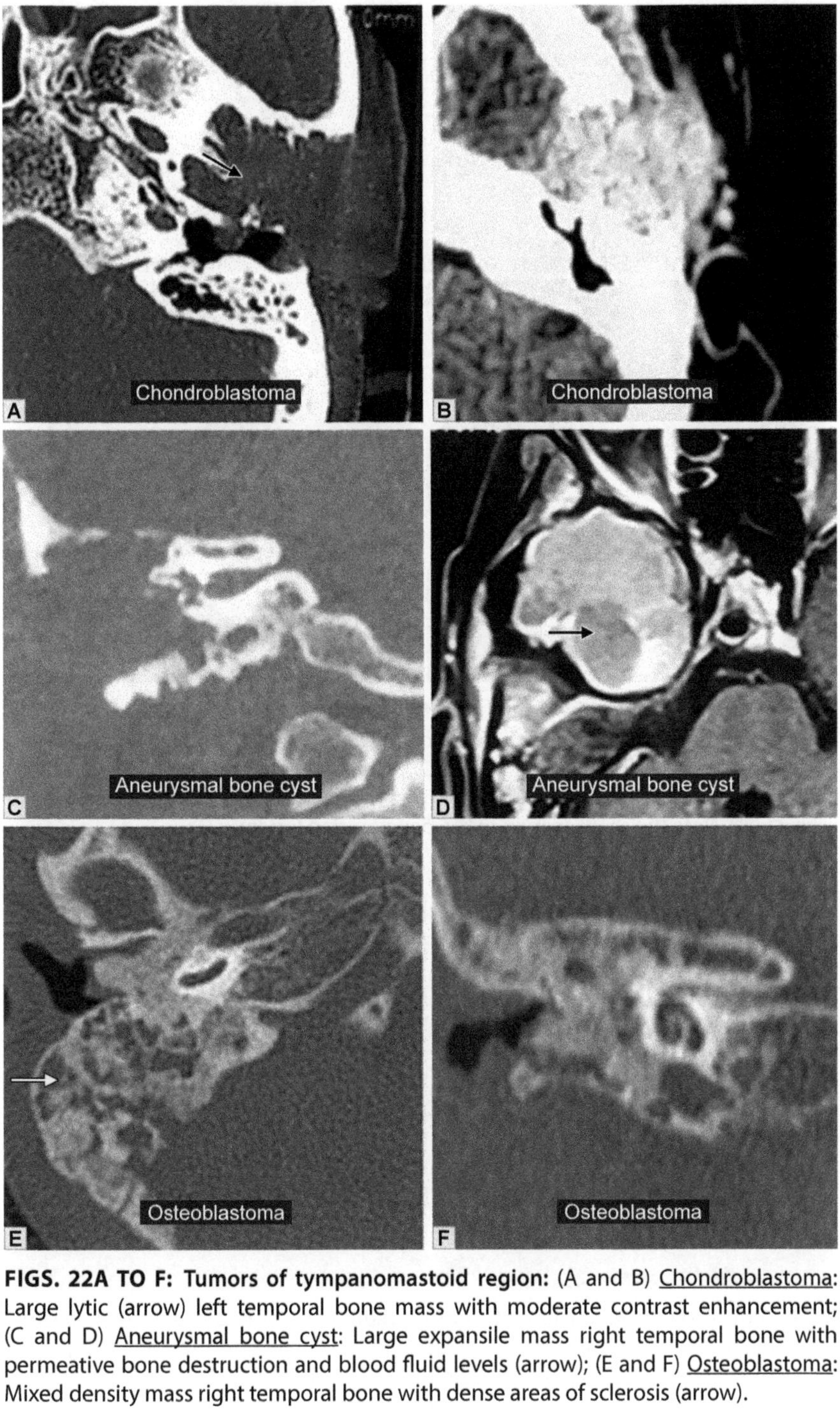

FIGS. 22A TO F: Tumors of tympanomastoid region: (A and B) Chondroblastoma: Large lytic (arrow) left temporal bone mass with moderate contrast enhancement; (C and D) Aneurysmal bone cyst: Large expansile mass right temporal bone with permeative bone destruction and blood fluid levels (arrow); (E and F) Osteoblastoma: Mixed density mass right temporal bone with dense areas of sclerosis (arrow).

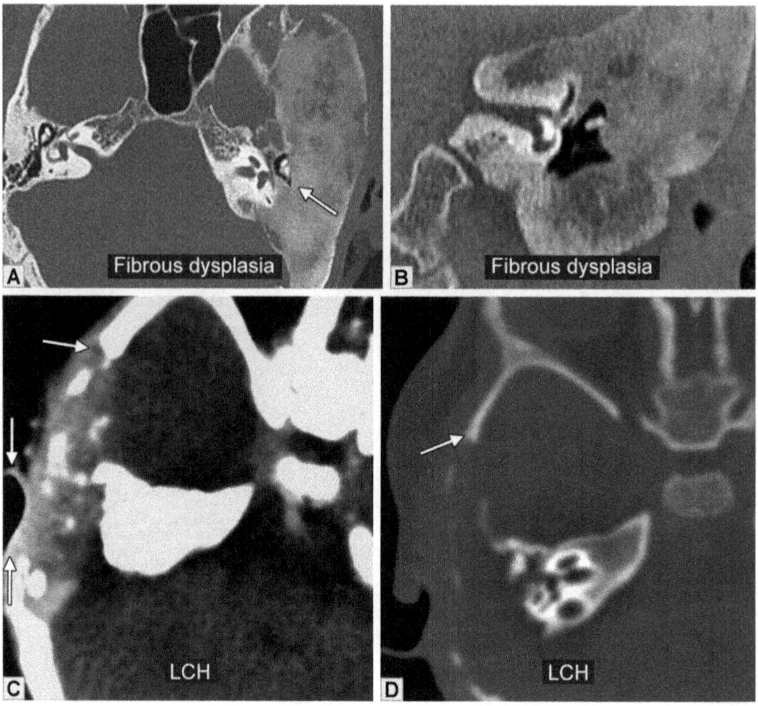

FIGS. 23A TO D: Tumor-like conditions of tympanomastoid region: (A and B) Fibrous dysplasia: Ground glass density expansion of left temporal bone with narrowing of middle ear cavity (arrow in A); (C and D) Langerhans cell histiocytosis: Lytic lesion involving right squamous and mastoid temporal bone with small soft tissue component (arrow in C). Note the sharp margin of the bone erosion (arrow in D).

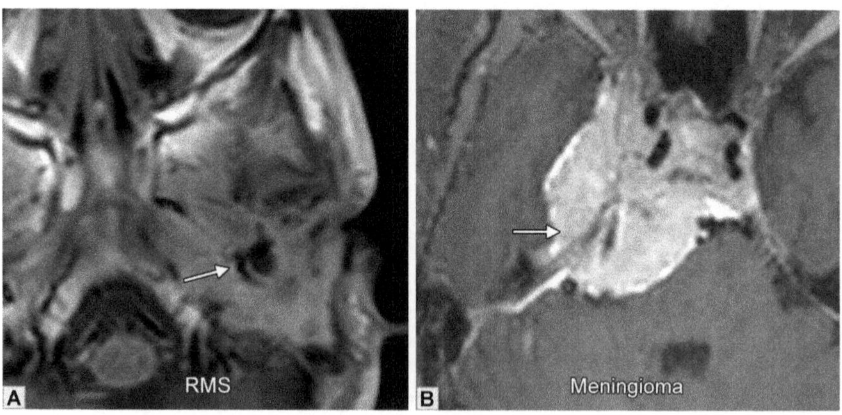

FIGS. 24A AND B: Extension of central skull base and petrous apex lesions into lateral skull base: (A) Rhabdomyosarcoma: Heterogenously enhancing mass extending into the infratemporal fossa, middle ear, and inner ear (arrow); (B) Petroclival meningioma: Heterogenously enhancing mass involving clivus, petrous apex (arrow), and with extraxial mass effect over the brainstem.

In conclusion, pathologies of the external and middle ear encompass a wide spectrum of diseases. The approach to these entities should include clinical assessment along with a systematic evaluation of the key structures within the temporal bone and surrounding bones and soft tissue.

REFERENCES

1. Trojanowska A, Drop A, Trojanowski P, Rosińska-Bogusiewicz K, Klatka J, Bobek-Billewicz B. External and middle ear diseases: radiological diagnosis based on clinical signs and symptoms. Insights Imaging. 2012;3(1):33-48.
2. Harnsberger HR. The temporal bone: external, middle and inner ear segments. In: Gay SM (Ed). Handbook of Head and Neck Imaging. Mosby, St.: Louis; 1995. pp. 426-58.
3. Anabarsu A, Chandrasekaran K, Balakrishnan S. Soft tissue attenuation in middle ear on HRCT: Pictorial review. Indian J Radiol Imaging. 2012;22(4):298-304.
4. Irish JC, Gullane PJ, Gentili F, Freeman J, Boyd JB, Brown D, et al. Tumors of the skull base: outcome and survival analysis of 77 cases. Head Neck. 1994;16:3-10.
5. Thurnher D, Novak CB, Neligan PC, Gullane PJ. Reconstruction of lateral skull base defects after tumor ablation. Skull Base. 2007;17(1):79-88.

20

Imaging of the Labyrinth

Ashu Seith Bhalla, Smita Manchanda

- Pathologies of Membranous Labyrinth
- Pathologies of Osseous Labyrinth

The labyrinth of the inner ear is the combined sensory organ of hearing and equilibrium. It consists of the bony labyrinth and the membranous labyrinth (**Fig. 1**) and perilymph flows within the intervening space between the osseous and membranous labyrinths.

- *Osseous labyrinth*:
  - It surrounds the membranous labyrinth.
  - The bony labyrinth comprises of the vestibule (that contains utricle and saccule), semicircular canals (SCCs) (that contains semicircular ducts), and the cochlea.
- *Membranous labyrinth*: Membranous labyrinth consists of utricle, saccule, semicircular ducts, cochlear duct, and endolymphatic duct and sac. These structures contain endolymph.
- The endolymphatic space is the smallest compartment of the inner ear fluid containing structures and is contained within the membranous labyrinth.
- This space is surrounded by the perilymphatic space which lies between the outer wall of the membranous labyrinth and the wall of the bony labyrinth. The structures which contain endolymph and perilymph are detailed in **Table 1**.
- The anatomy has been further detailed in Chapter 3.

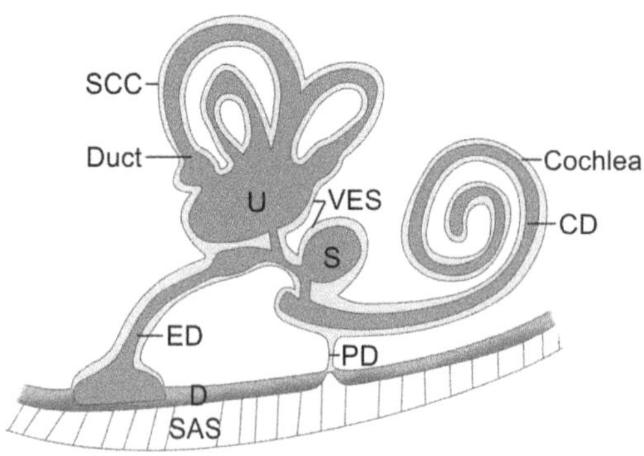

FIG. 1: Anatomy of osseous and membranous labyrinth: Osseous labyrinth: Vestibule (VES), semicircular canals (SCCs), and cochlea; Membranous labyrinth: Utricle (U) and saccule (S), semicircular ducts, cochlear duct (CD), and endolymphatic duct (ED). Perilymph: In light gray; Endolymph: In dark gray.

TABLE 1 Endolymph and perilymph in the inner ear structures.

	Structure within the cochlea	Structure within the vestibule	Composition
Endolymph	Cochlear duct (scala media)	Saccule and utricle	Very high potassium, low sodium, and negligible calcium
Perilymph	Scala vestibuli and scala tympani	Bony labyrinth of the vestibule	Similar to extracellular fluid

PATHOLOGIES OF THE LABYRINTH

The pathologies of the vestibulocochlear system can involve either the bony labyrinth or the membranous labyrinth. These will overlap but can be classified depending on the predominant system involved.

Pathologies of the Membranous Labyrinth

These are further classified as summarized in **Box 1**.

BOX 1 Pathologies of the membranous labyrinth.

- Congenital anomalies:
  - Vestibular aqueduct dilatation
  - Semicircular canal dysplasias
  - Inner ear malformations
- Labyrinthine hemorrhage:
  - Systemic causes
  - Trauma
  - Postoperative
- Labyrinthitis:
  - Infections (bacterial/viral)
  - Inflammatory
  - Autoimmune
- Perilymphatic fistulas
- Endolymphatic hydrops:
  - Ménière's disease
  - Pseudo Ménière's
- Tumors:
  - Labyrinthine schwannoma
  - Lipoma
  - Labyrinthine metastases
  - Endolymphatic sac tumors
  - Invaded by adjacent tumor (cholesteatoma of the middle ear/cholesterol granuloma of the petrous apex)

Congenital Anomalies

- The congenital anomalies of the labyrinth can be isolated or syndromic. These can include a dilated or hypoplastic segment.
- The inner ear malformations can vary from Michel's aplasia to single cochlear cavity to Mondini syndrome and have been covered in detail in Chapter 11.
- The dilatation of the vestibular aqueduct and the SCC dysplasias have also been described in Chapter 11.

Labyrinthine Hemorrhages

- The etiology of hemorrhage[1] within the labyrinth can be:
  - *Clinical predisposition*: Blood dyscrasias, leukemia, patients with systemic disease like Takayasu arteritis or patients on anticoagulants.
  - Trauma with or without a fracture
  - Postoperatively
  - Secondary to fistulation by cholesterol granuloma (a lesion often associated with hemotympanum, i.e., blood in middle ear).
- Imaging:
  - *High-resolution CT (HRCT)*: Hemorrhage is not visible in CT, though associated fracture if any can be seen.
  - *MRI*: On MRI, it appears as spontaneous T1 hyperintensity. This has medicolegal significance in inner ear trauma leading to labyrinthine destruction without obvious fracture in CT.

Labyrinthitis

- Labyrinthitis is the inflammation of the labyrinth.
- *Etiology*: The etiology can be infectious (bacterial and viral), inflammatory, or autoimmune.[2]
  - *Infectious labyrinthitis*: The pattern of spread of disease can be contiguously through the middle ear, cerebrospinal fluid, and meninges or hematogenous. This can occur either via spread from the middle ear through the oval window or the round window or as extension from the meninges passing through cochlea aqueduct/internal auditory canal (IAC). The scar of granuloma can calcify and narrow the cochlear canal with basal turn ossification and hyperostosis at the round window. Labyrinthitis secondary to bacterial meningitis is a cause of severe sensorineural hearing loss (SNHL) and a common indication of cochlear implant (CI) (**Figs. 2A** to **D**). It can also be associated with viral meningitis/arachnoiditis (**Figs. 3A** to **D**).
  - *Autoimmune or secondary to systemic labyrinthitis:* This is suspected in cases where patient does not have bacterial/viral infection and has been associated with granulomatous polyangitis or sarcoidosis. Cogan syndrome is autoimmune labyrinthitis with uveitis. In these cases, it is essential to start corticosteroid therapy early to preserve the sensory functions, and attempt to preserve the impermeability of the labyrinth (for later cochlear implant placement).
- *Stages*: Labyrinthitis[1,2] can progress from acute inflammatory stage to fibrous and the osseous stage (**Table 2**).

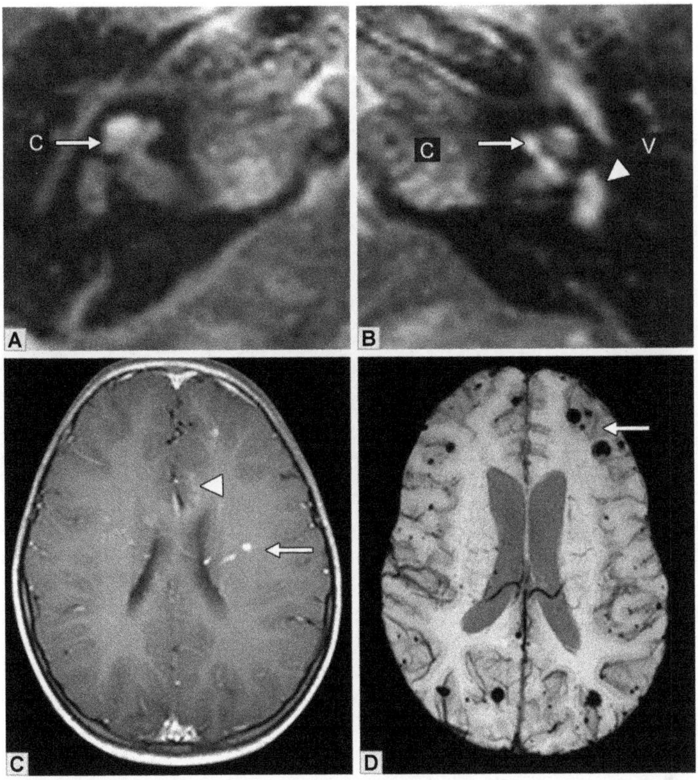

FIGS. 2A TO D: Acute labyrinthitis in a case of staphylococcal meningoencephalitis: Axial T1W postcontrast images of right (A) and left (B) side: Enhancement of cochlea (arrows) and vestibule (arrowhead); (C) Axial T1W postcontrast image of brain: Nodular parenchymal (arrow) and meningeal (arrowhead) enhancement; (D) Multiple areas of blooming (arrow) on gradient-echo (GRE) image suggestive of focal bleeds.

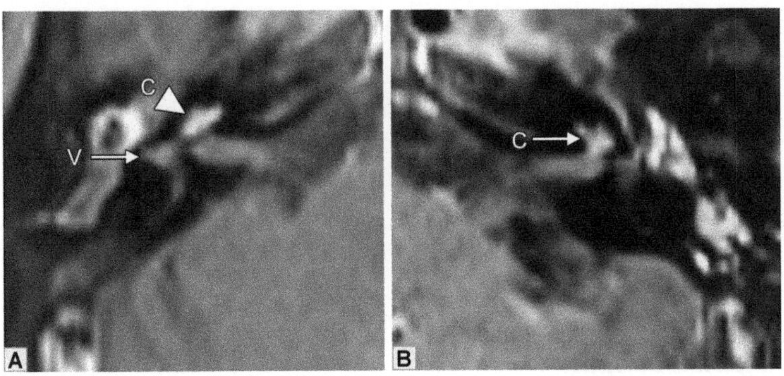

FIGS. 3A TO D: *Continued*

Continued

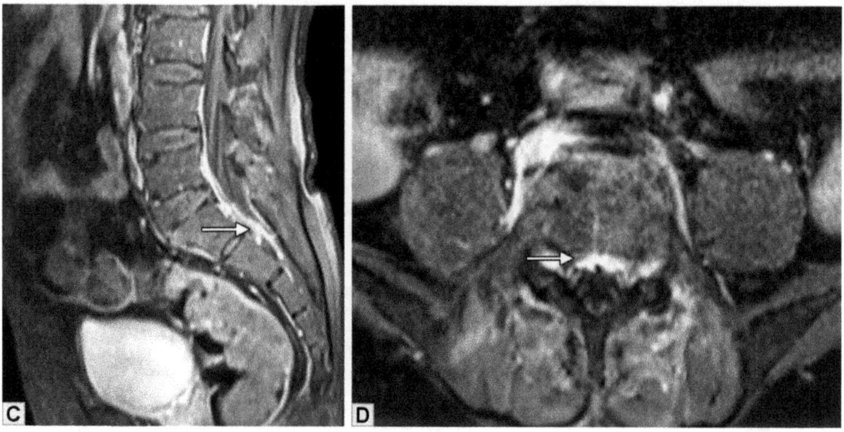

FIGS. 3A TO D: Acute labyrinthitis in a case of viral spinal meningitis: (A) Axial postcontrast T1-weighted image (T1WI) (right) shows enhancement of vestibule (V) (arrow) and apical and middle turn of cochlea (C) (arrowhead); (B) Axial postcontrast T1WI (left) shows enhancement of middle turn of cochlea (arrow); (C and D) Sagittal and axial postcontrast T1WI LS spine shows enhancement of anterior nerve roots of the cauda equina (arrows in C and D).

TABLE 2 Stages of labyrinthitis.

Stage	Pathogenesis	Reversibility	Imaging features
Acute inflammation (**Figs. 2** and **3**)	Perilymphatic space filled with inflammatory cells	Reversible	• *MRI*: Labyrinthine enhancement • High T1 signal intensity (high protein content of inflammatory tissue)
Fibrous (**Figs. 4A** and **B**)	Fibroblastic proliferation	Irreversible	• *MRI*: Diffuse/patchy/multifocal enhancement • Signal loss on 3D T2-weighted image (T2WI) • *CT*: Slight increased density
Osseous (**Figs. 5A** and **B**)	Bone formation	Irreversible	• *MRI*: Signal loss on 3D T2WI • Enhancement rarely • *CT*: Bony obliteration maybe seen

Perilabyrinthine Fistulas

- Perilabyrinthine fistula is due to an abnormal communication between the inner ear and the middle ear (via the oval or round window) (**Figs. 6A** and **B**). This results in leak of perilymphatic fluid into the middle ear.[1] An abnormal

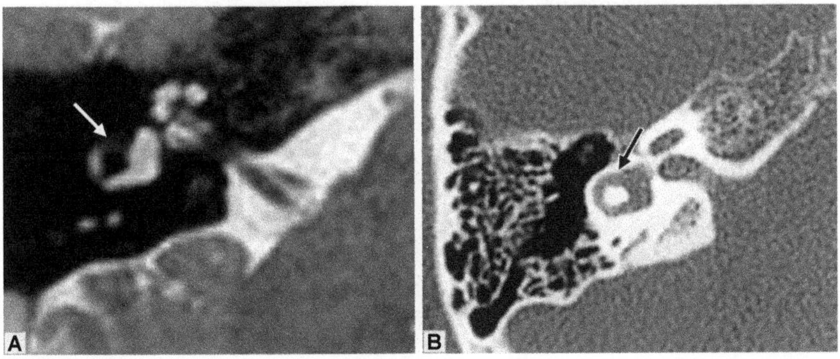

FIGS. 4A AND B: Labyrinthitis (fibrotic stage): (A) Axial CISS MRI of right (A) side shows focal loss of T2-hyperintense signal in lateral SCC (arrow); (B) Axial HRCT at same level shows normal attenuation of right lateral SCC (arrow).

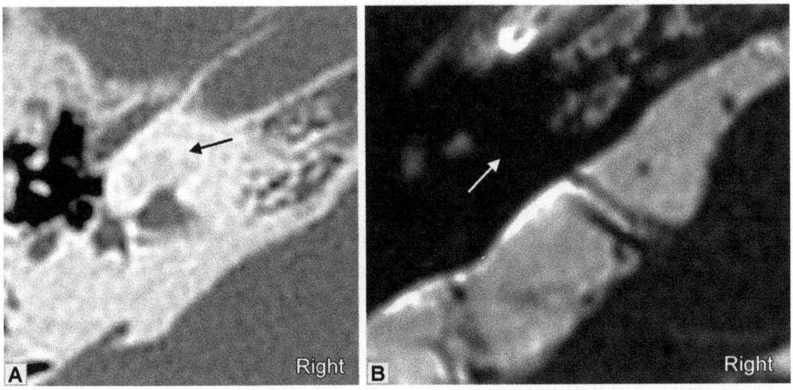

FIG. 5A AND B: Labyrinthitis (Osseous Stage)/Labyrinthitis ossificans: Axial HRCT (Right) shows a completely ossified cochlea. No residual fluid-filled lumen is seen and only the outline of the cochlear contour is faintly visible (arrow). Axial CISS of the right inner ear (B) shows loss of the normal labyrinthine signal intensity (arrow).

communication of the inner ear with the subarachnoid spaces through a large modiolus may result in the "gusher syndrome".

- It is a cause of the so called "third window" phenomenon and has been covered in Chapter 21.

Endolymphatic Hydrops

- Endolymphatic hydrops (EH) is an increase in the endolymphatic fluid pressure. This occurs because there is distension of structures which contain endolymph in an enclosed fluid space. The membranous labyrinth has the structures which contain this endolymph (cochlear duct, saccule, and utricle). It is believed that EH is the underlying pathologic mechanism of Ménière's disease (MD); however, the cause/effect relationship is not clear.

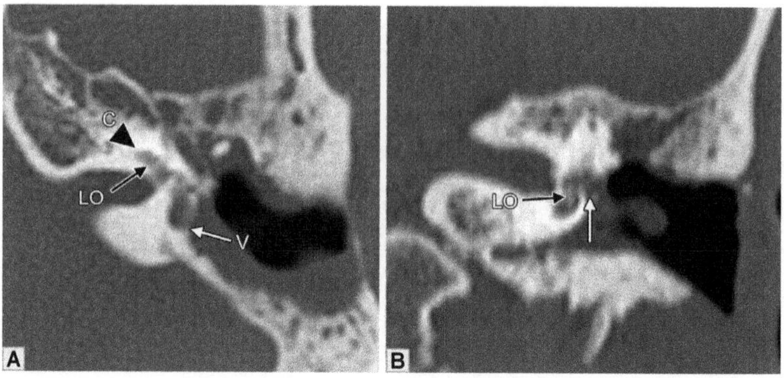

FIGS. 6A AND B: Perilabyrinthine fistula [vestibule (V)]: (A) Axial image shows abnormal opening in the lateral wall of vestibule (white arrow) in a postoperative case of left MRM. Increased density (black arrow) in cochlea (C) (arrowhead) is suggestive of labyrinthitis ossificans (LO); (B) Coronal image shows soft tissue in the middle ear and external ear with fistulous communication with the vestibule at the oval window (arrow). Increased density in vestibule (black arrow) is suggestive of LO.

- *Ménière's disease:*
  - Ménière's disease is a chronic disease characterised by spontaneous episodic attacks of vertigo, fluctuating hearing loss (HL) at low frequencies, tinnitus, aural fullness, and pressure with a progressive loss of the audiovestibular functions. It is commonly seen in the 40–60-year-old age group with slight preponderance in females and in whites.[3]
  - There is associated EH and this accumulation of endolymph can result in damage to the ganglion cells.
  - However, it is important to note that not all EH have MD and vice versa.[3]
  - Endolymphatic hydrops can be either vestibular or cochlear and it has been seen that vestibular hydrops is more common in patients with definite MD than cochlear hydrops.
  - *Diagnostic criteria*:
    - For a diagnosis of MD, a combination of the patient's symptoms along with the clinical examination and functional tests are all taken into account. In 2015, the classification committee of the Bárány Society formulated simplified diagnostic criteria for MD.[4] It now includes two categories: (1) Definite; and (2) Probable MD.
    - The criteria for *definite MD* include two or more spontaneous episodes of vertigo (duration from 20 min to 12 h); documented low to midfrequency SNHL in one ear, defining the affected ear on more than one occasion before, during, or after one of the vertigo episodes; fluctuating aural symptoms (hearing, fullness, or tinnitus) in the affected ear and these symptoms are not accounted for by any other vestibular diagnosis.
    - The criteria for *probable MD* is defined by episodic vestibular symptoms like vertigo or dizziness in association with fluctuating aural symptoms occurring in a duration from 20 minutes to 24 hours.

- *Role of MRI*:
  - Recent advances in MRI techniques enable us to demonstrate EH.
  - The role of MRI is primarily in discriminating the affected ear in patients with MD. Also, imaging is helpful in the evaluation of EH when conservative treatment fails and in assessing possible bilateral disease with unilateral symptoms.
  - *Principle*: Contrast can cross the blood-perilymph barrier and penetrate the perilymph compartment and this creates a negative contrast with the nonenhancing endolymphatic spaces.
  - *Types of techniques*: This includes both noncontrast and contrast-enhanced techniques and are summarized in **Box 2**.
- *Noncontrast MRI technique*:
  - This is based on the principle that fluid-containing structures are well visualized on heavily T2-weighted sequence (**Figs. 7** and **8**). EH causes an increase in the height and width of the saccule and this distended saccule can be seen as an *oval, hypointense structure* in the fluid-filled vestibule on a coronal multiplanar reconstruction (MPR). The normal height of the saccule is 1.6 mm on the coronal reconstruction of 3D constructive interference in steady state (CISS). In MD, the height is >1.6 mm.
  - *Advantages*: No contrast administration
  - *Disadvantages*: Due to low sensitivity of this technique, it cannot evaluate cochlear hydrops and there is a poor reproducibility in measuring such small anatomic structures.

BOX 2 Modifications in MRI techniques to evaluate Ménière's disease.

- Noncontrast technique: Heavily T2-weighted sequence
- Contrast-enhanced techniques:
  - Intratympanically administrated gadolinium
  - Delayed imaging after intravenously administrated gadolinium

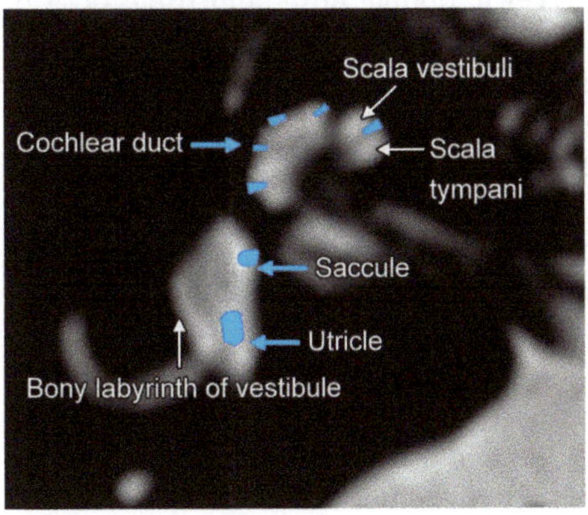

FIG. 7: Schematic illustration on T2-weighted CISS image to show normal endolymph and perilymph. Endolymph (in blue): Cochlear Duct, Saccule and Utricle. Perilymph: Scala vestibuli, Scala tympani Bony labyrinth of the vestibule.

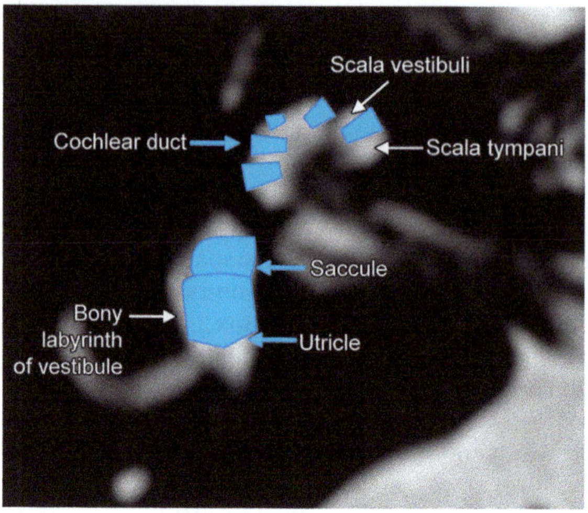

FIG. 8: Schematic illustration on T2-weighted CISS image to show endolymphatic hydrops.
- Vestibular endolymphatic Space/vestibule ratio is >50%.
- Endolymphatic compartment (Cochlear duct) exceeds the area of the scala vestibuli.

- *Contrast-enhanced MRI techniques*:
  - *Intratympanically administrated gadolinium*:
    - Gadolinium is administered in variable dilution (5–16-fold in literature) by puncturing the tympanic membrane and is likely absorbed through the round window membrane.
    - Gadolinium gets distributed in the perilymph space as the endolymphatic compartment is impermeable. The scala media (cochlear duct, endolymphatic space) is visualized as a filling defect on the 3D fluid-attenuated inversion recovery (FLAIR) sequence.
    - Although a useful technique, it has not gained popularity due to its invasive nature.
  - *Intravenously administrated gadolinium*:
    - Contrast-enhanced MRI with intravenous gadolinium is currently the imaging technique of choice for evaluation of MD.
    - *Method*: Single dose [0.2 mL/kg of gadolinium diethylenetriamine penta-acetic acid (Gd-DTPA)], double dose, and triple dose of gadolinium can be used followed by scan acquisition at 4 hours. Sequence acquired can be either an optimized 3D FLAIR sequence (turbo spin echo) or heavily T2-weighted 3D FLAIR sequence. The inversion time of the 3D FLAIR sequences is varied and *positive perilymph* or *positive endolymph* images can be acquired.
    - *Advantages*: It can evaluate and compare both ears, absorption is not dependent on oval or round window permeability and it allows an assessment of the blood-perilymph barrier.
  - *MRI appearance*:
    - Accumulation of intravenously injected gadolinium is seen in the perilymphatic space (**Fig. 9**), the subarachnoid space around the optic nerve, fluid in anterior portion of eyes, Meckel's cave, and fundus of internal acoustic canal.

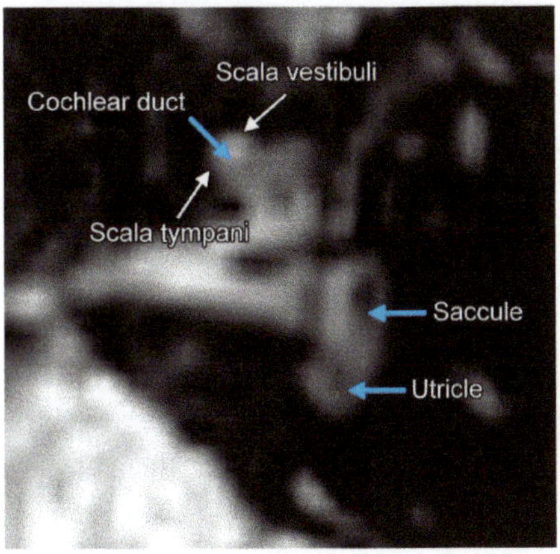

FIG. 9: Normal Labyrinth on axial delayed gadolinium enhanced 3D-FLAIR MR imaging.
- Scala vestibuli and scala tympani: Enhancing.
- Cochlear duct or scala media: Non enhancing thin, hypointense line.
- Saccule and utricle: Non enhancing

TABLE 3 **MRI appearance of endolymphatic hydrops (Ménière's disease) on a delayed postcontrast scan.**

	Cochlea	Vestibule
Normal	Barely visible nonenhancing cochlear duct seen in enhancing scala vestibuli and scala tympani	• Nonenhancing saccule and utricle seen in the enhancing vestibule • *Saccule*: The smallest structure and located anterior, medial, and inferior in the vestibule
Grade I hydrops	• Mild dilation of nonenhancing cochlear duct • Parts of enhancing perilymph of scala vestibuli are spared	• Distention of endolymph space of saccule or utricle or both • Perilymphatic space still visible along periphery of bony vestibule
Grade II hydrops	• Maximally distended cochlear duct • scala vestibuli is uniformly obstructed	• Markedly dilated endolymphatic spaces • No visible surrounding enhancing perilymphatic space

    - Barath and colleagues[5] have described the normal appearances on a delayed scan and graded the EH as detailed in **Table 3**.
  - Although the current clinical diagnostic criteria of MD do not include MRI grading of EH, it is likely that further advances in technology and validation of this technique will result in it becoming a useful diagnostic tool with therapeutic implications.
- *Pseudo Ménière's*: This term is used for conditions which clinically mimic the diagnosis of Ménière's disease; and includes focal anomalies of membranous labyrinth, any meningeal anomaly with respect to the opening of endolymphatic sac or cochlear aqueduct and stenosis of basilar artery.

Tumors

- The clinical presentation of labyrinthine tumors is similar to MD. However, they can also present with conductive HL (bulge into the middle ear through the oval window with stapedial dysfunction).

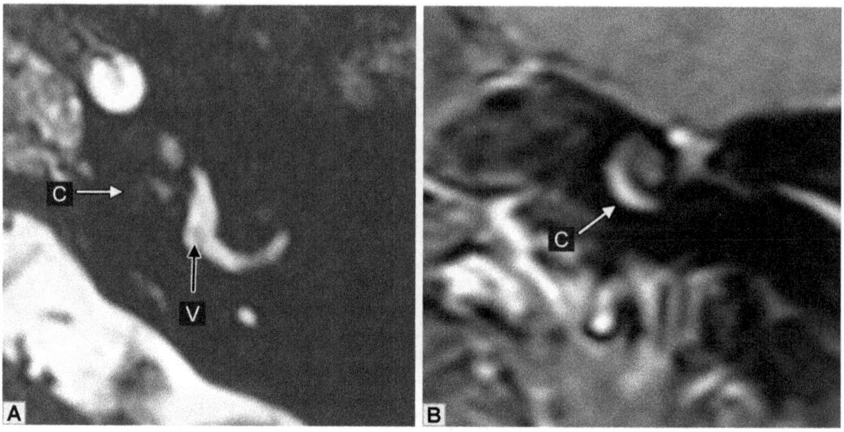

FIGS. 10A AND B: Labyrinthine (cochlear) schwannoma: (A) Axial CISS shows focal loss of T2-hyperintense signal in basal turn of cochlea (C) (white arrow); vestibule (V) (black arrow) is normal; (B) Coronal postcontrast T1WI shows diffuse enhancement in the area of T2 hypointensity (arrow).

- Labyrinthine schwannomas are the most common of these tumors.[1] These can be extension of the IAC schwannomas or rarely be isolated within the labyrinth (see Chapter 12). On MRI, there is characteristic loss of T2-hyperintense signal of the labyrinth with mild expansion. Postcontrast T1-weighted images reveal focal enhancement in the zone of T2 hypointensity (**Figs. 10A** and **B**).
- The other labyrinthine tumors are very rare, and include lipomas and labyrinthine metastases (which have extended to the cochlea/vestibule by the perineural route)
- Endolymphatic sac tumors have been covered in Chapter 16.

PATHOLOGIES OF THE OSSEOUS LABYRINTH

The pathologies of the osseous labyrinth include fractures, otosclerosis, and bone dysplasias (**Box 3**).

Congenital Anomalies

The inner ear malformations (detailed in Chapter 11) involve both the osseous and membranous labyrinth.

Trauma (Labyrinth Fractures)

- High-resolution CT is the investigation of choice for detecting a fracture line passing through the labyrinth. A fracture line passing through the windows of the labyrinth (**Figs. 11A** and **B**) can bring the middle ear and inner ear into communication with resultant perilymphatic fistulas. These are detailed in Chapter 23.
- Presence of pneumolabyrinth confirms the communication between the middle ear and the inner ear and it can be further complicated by communication with the subarachnoid spaces.

BOX 3 Pathologies of the osseous labyrinth.

- Congenital anomalies
- Trauma
- Labyrinthitis ossificans
- Otosclerosis
- Bone dysplasias

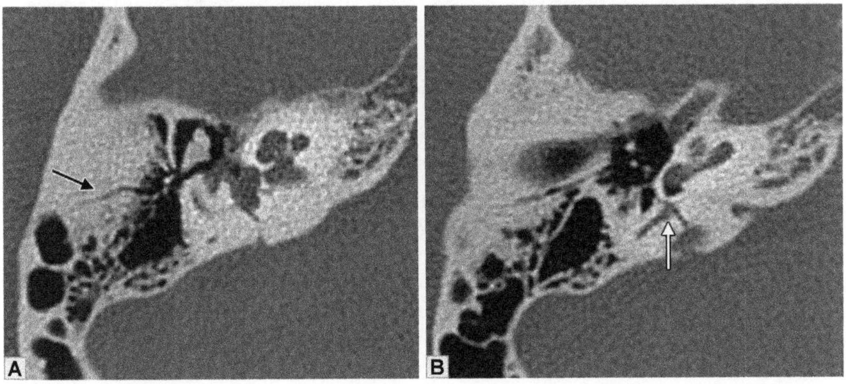

FIGS. 11A AND B: Fracture involving bony labyrinth: (A and B) Mixed temporal bone fracture pattern with longitudinal (black arrow) and transverse fracture (white arrow). Transverse fracture involves the vestibule (arrow in A) and posterior SCC (arrow in B).

Labyrinthitis Ossificans

- Labyrinthitis ossificans (LO) refers to pathological ossification of the membranous labyrinth as a consequence of insult to the inner ear. Cochlea and SCCs (especially lateral SCC) are mostly affected; vestibular ossification is seen much less commonly.
- Increased density of cochlea is seen in early stages followed by irregularity, sclerosis, and eventually obliteration of cochlear lumen on CT (**Figs. 12A** and **B**). Loss of T2-hyperintense signal on CISS sequence is typical.

Otosclerosis

- Also known as *otospongiosis*, it is a multifactorial bone disorder (also covered in Chapter 21). There is abnormal bone reabsorption and remodeling along with new bone formation and vascular proliferation. It is classified as tumor of otic capsule origin under the WHO classification (2017) of tumors of the ear.
- *There are two types of otosclerosis*: (1) Fenestral; and (2) Cochlear otosclerosis.[6]
- *Fenestral otosclerosis*: Fissula ante fenestram is the area anteromedial to the oval window. Early disease is seen as demineralization at this site (as the spongiotic bone replaces the normal dense bone). The cochlear promontory, round window niche, and facial nerve canal can also be involved (also see Chapter 21).

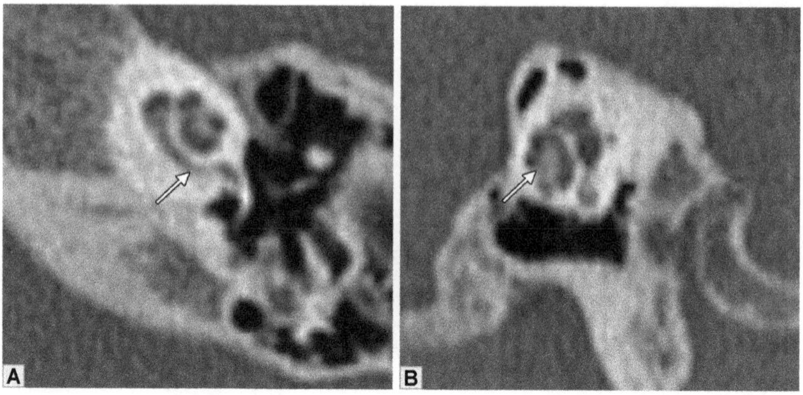

FIGS. 12A AND B: Labyrinthitis ossificans: (A) Axial HRCT: Ossification in the basal turn of cochlea (arrow); (B) Sagittal oblique: Ossification involving the apical and middle turns also (arrow).

- *Cochlear (retrofenestral or labyrinthine) otosclerosis*: It is less common and usually seen along with fenestral otosclerosis. Extensive demineralization is seen around the cochlea in a ring-like fashion, referred to as the "double ring" (**Figs. 13A** and **B**). It can be adjacent to the lumen of the labyrinth or be separated by normal or sclerotic bone. On MRI, the ring of pericochlear and perilabyrinthine abnormality is seen as intermediate signal on T1- and T2-weighted images with postcontrast enhancement in the active phase (because of the pooling of contrast in the blood vessels found in this active otospongiotic foci). MRI is especially useful in areas which are a diagnostic challenge on CT (e.g., the lateral wall of the labyrinth because of partial volume averaging). The grading system (on CT) as described by Symons and Fanning[6] is summarized in **Table 4.**

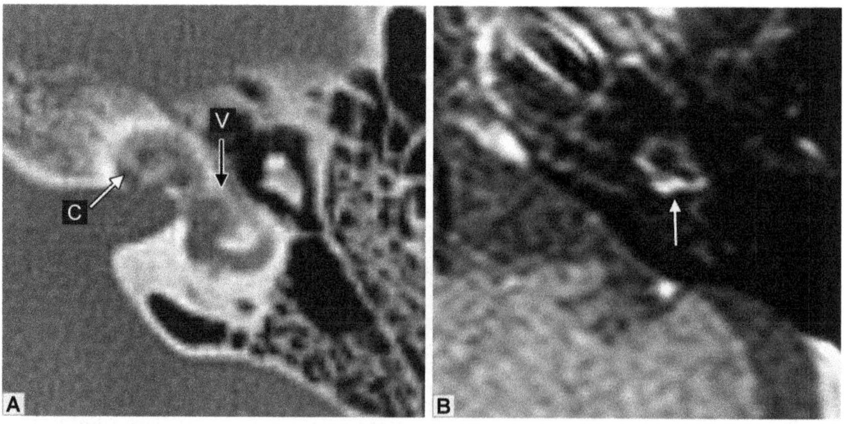

(C: cochlea; V: vestibule)

FIGS. 13A AND B: Cochlear otosclerosis: (A) Axial HRCT shows "Double-Ring/Halo sign" in cochlea (arrows) with vestibular involvement (black arrow); (B) Axial postcontrast T1WI shows perilabyrinthine enhancement along the cochlea (arrow).

TABLE 4 **CT grading of otosclerosis.**

Grade	Extent of disease
Grade 1	Only fenestral with either spongiotic or sclerotic lesion
Grade 2	Patchy localized cochlear disease (with or without fenestral involvement)
Grade 2A	Limited to basal cochlear turn
Grade 2B	Limited to middle/apical cochlear turns
Grade 2C	Involvement of both (patchy)
Grade 3	Diffuse confluent cochlear involvement

Bone Dysplasia

Temporal bone may also be involved in other dysplasias like fibrous dysplasia, Paget's disease, osteopetrosis (**Figs. 14A** and **B**), and osteogenesis imperfecta. HRCT shows the involvement of osseous labyrinth whereas MRI is required for the evaluation of involvement of membranous labyrinth.

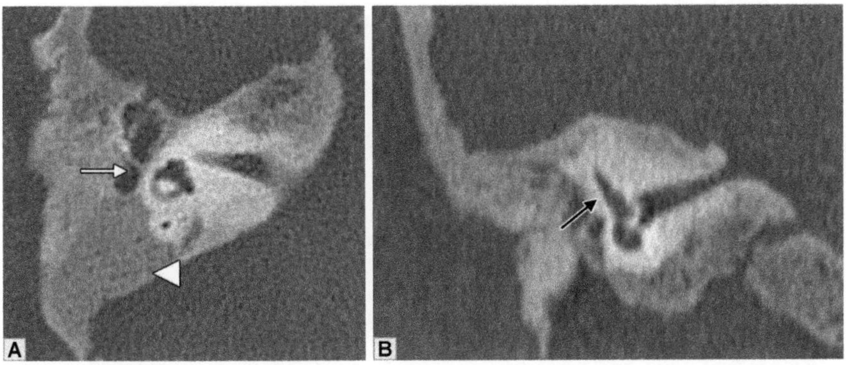

FIGS. 14A AND B: Osteopetrosis involving skull bones: Axial (A) and Coronal (B) HRCT images demonstrate diffusely increased bone density with poor formation of the right mastoid air cells (arrowhead) and narrowed tympanic cavity (arrow). Narrowing of IAC with sclerotic changes in the bony labyrinth (black arrow).

In conclusion, vestibulocochlear system pathologies can involve either the bony labyrinth or the membranous labyrinth. Postcontrast MRI along with heavily T2-weighted sequences play a key role in the evaluation of these disorders, with HRCT having a complimentary role.

REFERENCES

1. Marsot-Dupuch K, Gayet-Delacroix M. Imaging of the Cochleo-vestibular system. J Radiol. 1999;80: 351-62.

2. Verbist BM. Imaging of sensorineural hearing loss: a pattern-based approach to diseases of the inner ear and cerebellopontine angle. Insights Imaging. 2012;3:139-53.
3. Bernaerts A, Foer BD. Imaging of Ménière's Disease. Neuroimag Clin N Am. 2019;29:19-28.
4. Goebel JA. 2015 equilibrium committee amendment to the 1995 AAO-HNS guidelines for the definition of Ménière's disease. Otolaryngol Head Neck Surg. 2016;154(3):403-4.
5. Baráth K, Schuknecht B, Naldi AM, Schrepfer T, Bockisch CJ, Hegemann SCA. Detection and grading of endolymphatic hydrops in Menière disease using MR imaging. AJNR Am J Neuroradiol. 2014;35(7): 1387-92.
6. Lee TC, Aviv RI, Chen JM, Nedzelski JM, Fox AJ, Symons SP, et al. CT grading otosclerosis. AJNR Am J Neuroradiol. 2009;30(7):1435-9.

21

Windows of the Ear: Imaging

Surabhi Vyas, Ashu Seith Bhalla, Gh Mohammad Wani

- Windows of the ear are important structures which help in transmission of sound waves from external environment to the sensory system of the hearing pathways. They are normal communications *connecting middle and inner ear*.
- There are two normal windows, the oval and the round windows (RWs). Both the windows are involved in sound transmission (**Figs. 1A** and **B**).
- The sound waves travel to the tympanic membrane (TM) and thence to the ossicular chain as vibrations. These vibrations cause stapes to pulse against the membrane of the oval window, transmitting them to the adjacent perilymph. The perilymph continues the transmission of the waves to the scala vestibuli, scala tympani which then exit through the RW pushing its membrane outwards (**Fig. 2**).
- Third window on the other hand is a pathological communication between inner ear and the cerebrospinal fluid (CSF), at an abnormal site (e.g., endolymphatic duct dilatation).
- The normal connections between inner ear and CSF are vestibular aqueduct, cochlear aqueduct, and foramina for vessels and nerves.
- *Windows of the inner ear*: These refer to openings between inner ear and CSF space (e.g., petromastoid canal and singular canal).

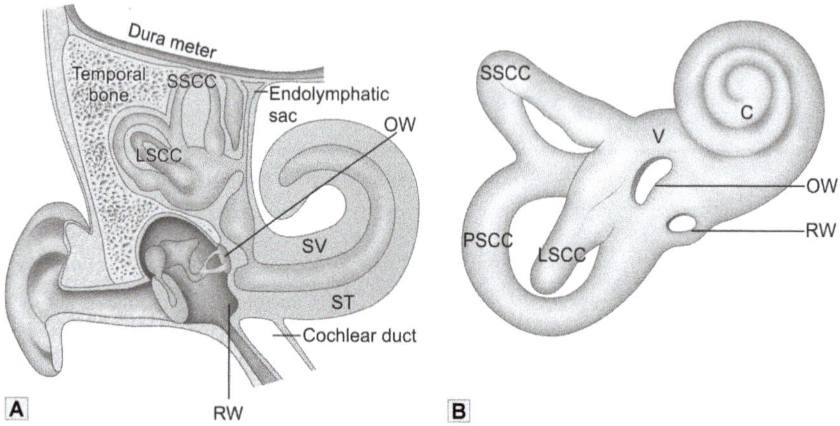

(C: cochlea; LSCC: lateral semicircular canal; OW: oval window; PSCC: posterior semicircular canal; RW: round window; SSCC: superior semicircular canal; ST: scala tympani; SV: scala vestibuli; V: vestibule)

FIGS. 1A AND B: Windows of the ear: (A) Line diagrams showing the windows of the ear. (B) External view of the oval and round windows.

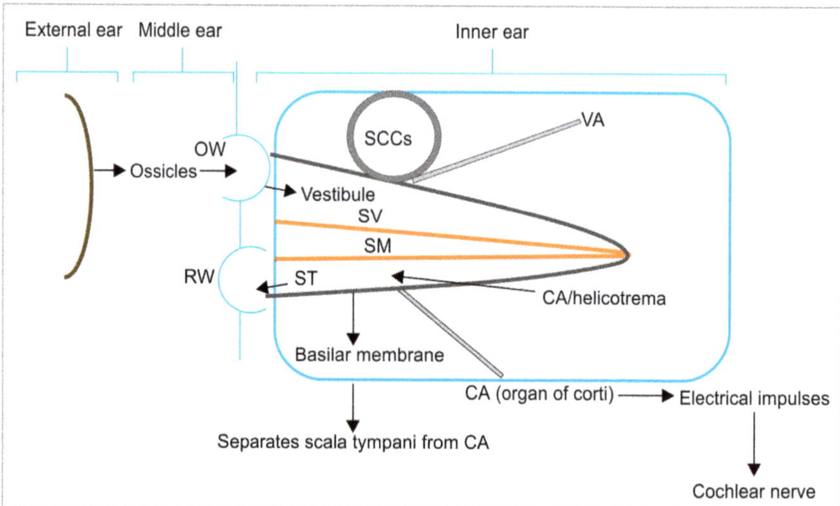

(CA: cochlear aqueduct; OW: oval window; RW: round window; SCC: semicircular canals; SM: scala media; ST: scala tympani; SV: scala vestibuli; VA: vestibular aqueduct)

FIG. 2: Pathways and mechanism of sound transmission at the oval and round windows. Inward movement occurs at oval window, and outward movement at round window. Perilymph is incompressible. Vibration creates a pressure gradient across basilar membrane which activates the hairy cells.

OVAL WINDOW

Synonyms: First window, fenestra ovalis, and fenestra vestibuli.

Normal Anatomy

- Oval window (OW) is a bean-shaped opening along the medial wall of the mesotympanum and communicates with the vestibule. It is covered by a membrane (**Figs. 3A** and **B**). The annular ligament along its rim provides a rest to the footplate of stapes.
- Its size varies from 1.26 to 2.4 mm, such that the horizontal diameter ranges from 2.4 to 2.86 mm and vertical diameter ranges from 1.23 to 1.6 mm.[1]
- The OW and the facial canal are optimally evaluated on coronal CT images.

Pathologies

The pathologies affecting the OW are enumerated in **Table 1**; and the common specific entities are discussed subsequently.

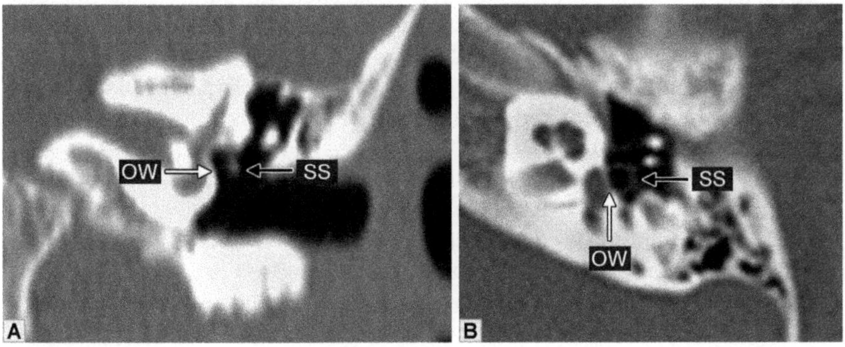

(OW: oval window; SS: stapes superstructure; V: vestibule)

FIGS. 3A AND B: Normal oval window: (A) Coronal and (B) axial CT images show normal oval window and stapes superstructure.

TABLE 1 Pathologies affecting the oval window (OW).

Anatomical variations	• Persistent stapedial artery • Aberrant internal carotid artery (ICA) • Overhanging of the OW recess by tympanic part of facial canal
Congenital abnormalities	• OW stenosis • OW atresia
Infective abnormalities	• Chronic suppurative otitis media (CSOM) with cholesteatoma • Tympanosclerosis
Trauma	• Fracture
Miscellaneous abnormalities	• Otosclerosis

Anatomical Variants Affecting the Oval Window

- *Persistent stapedial artery (PSA)*: It is a rare congenital variant, presenting with hearing loss, pulsatile tinnitus; wherein the artery connecting the internal carotid artery (ICA) to middle meningeal (MMA) and external carotid artery (ECA) in fetal life fails to regress. It is also associated with aberrant ICA, absent foramen spinosum, and thickening of the tympanic part of facial canal. On imaging, the aberrant artery is visualized traversing between stapes crura and over the OW.
- *Aberrant ICA*: It results from agenesis of the first segment of the embryonic ICA, and is replaced by a prominent inferior tympanic artery. The latter enters the middle ear cleft through an enlarged inferior tympanic canal and the takes a sharp inferior turn to pass inferior to the promontory and then into the horizontal part of the petrous carotid canal.
- *Overhanging of the OW recess* by tympanic part of facial nerve (FN) canal: The FN canal may be dehiscent with bare FN, which increases the chances of surgical trauma and consequent FN palsy (**Figs. 4A** and **B**).

Oval Window Stenosis/Atresia

- Oval window stenosis or atresia may be associated with aural atresia, microtia, or can be isolated. OW atresia occurring in isolation, is considered as a minor middle ear anomaly (**Figs. 5A** and **B**).
- It is a rare condition with absence of OW, instead there is a bony plate located between the middle ear and vestibule.[2] The condition is more often unilateral but may also be bilateral.
- *Embryology*: Oval window atresia results from the failure of fusion of the primitive vestibule with primitive stapes.
- Clinical presentation is of conductive hearing loss, without evidence of either middle ear or external auditory canal anomalies.
- It is often associated with malposition of the FN canal and malformation of stapes. It may also be associated with aural atresia and CHARGE syndrome.

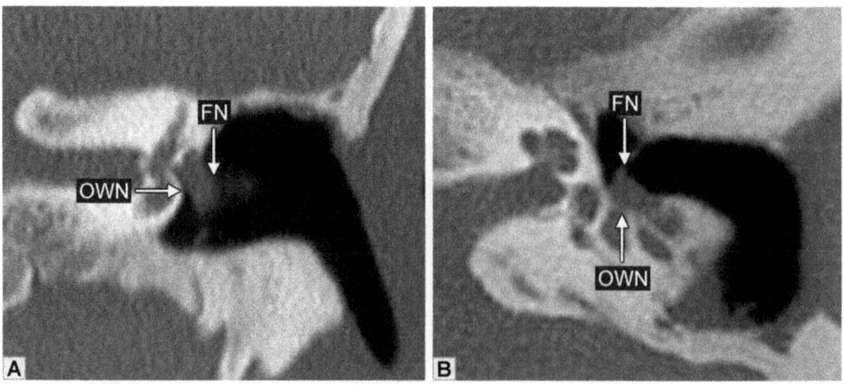

FIGS. 4A AND B: Overhanging facial nerve: (A) Coronal and (B) axial images showing overhanging tympanic part of facial nerve (FN, arrow) on the oval window niche (OWN) with dehiscence of the bony facial nerve canal.

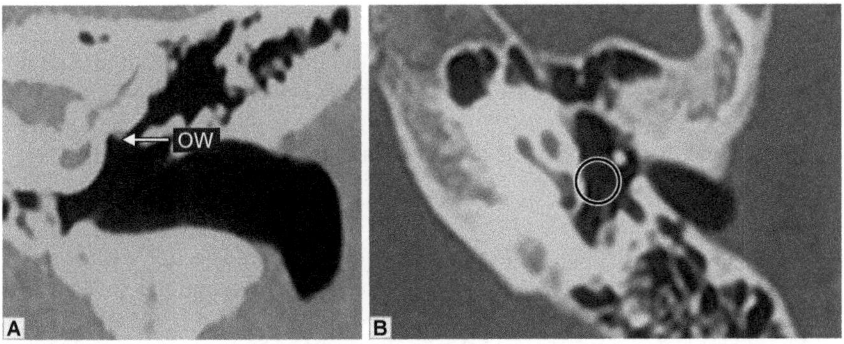

FIGS. 5A AND B: Oval window (OW) atresia—isolated: (A) Coronal HRCT images showing shallow OW and absence of its normal rectangular shape. (B) Axial image at the level of mesotympanum shows nonvisualization of the OW and stapes footplate, location marked.

- *Imaging*:
  - Obliteration or narrowing of the OW niche; this can be concentric along medial tympanic wall or osseous in nature, due to a thick bony plate.
  - Associated ossicular abnormalities are visualized best on axial images as malformation of stapes in the form of displacement from the OW, inability to identify the crura, absent or posteriorly fixed stapes, or malformed or absent lenticular process of incus (less commonly) (**Figs. 6A** and **B**). On coronal images, there is increased thickness (>0.7 mm) of the footplate.
  - Aberrant inferior course of tympanic segment of fascial nerve and dehiscent bony fascial canal.[3]
  - These are best visualized on CT.
- *Treatment*: Surgical correction

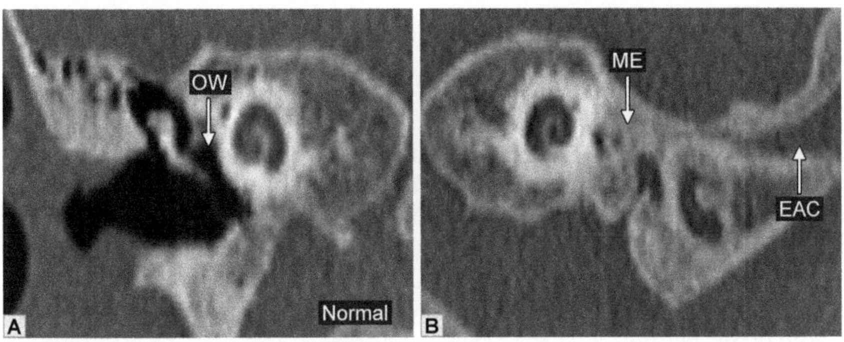

(EAC: external auditory canal; ME: middle ear)

FIGS. 6A AND B: Atretic oval window (OW) in a case of microtia: (A) Coronal HRCT of normal right external, middle ear and stapes foot plate and OW (arrow). (B) Coronal HRCT of affected left side with microtia shows atresia of the external auditory canal and dysplastic middle ear cavity. Stapes is aplastic.

- *Differentials*:
  - Congenital stapes fixation where stapes development is normal without the development of the annular ligament, which leads to foot plate ankylosis.
  - Otosclerosis which will be discussed later in the chapter.

Cholesteatoma

- Cholesteatoma is a congenital or acquired condition [associated with chronic suppurative otitis media (CSOM)], which may uncommonly involve the temporal bone windows.
- The disease causes erosions of the malleus and incus more than the stapes. However, the involvement of the latter may be accompanied by involvement of the OW (**Figs. 7A** and **B**).

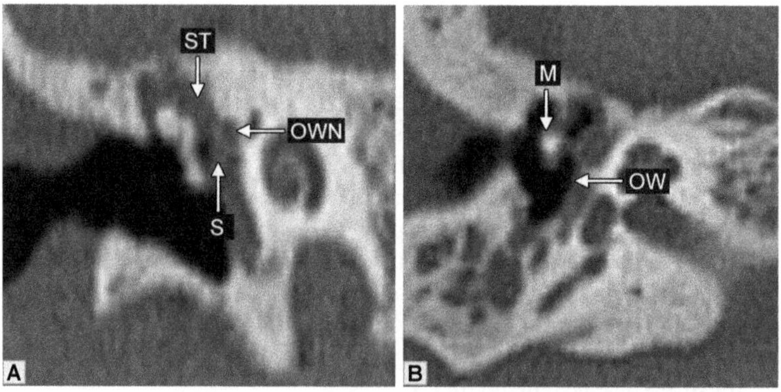

FIGS. 7A AND B: Cholesteatoma involving the right oval window (OW): (A) Coronal and (B) axial HRCT images showing hypodense soft tissue (ST) in the epitympanum, oval window niche (OWN). Bony erosion of the malleus (M) and stapes (S).

Tympanosclerosis

- Tympanosclerosis involves dense/calcific connective tissue in the middle ear cavity.
- Etiology is uncertain, however, it is postulated to be a sequel of inflammatory process like chronic otitis media or trauma.
- It involves most commonly the TM (myringosclerosis) and to lesser extent the ossicles and OW.
- When it involves the stapes, it affects the crura which shows increased density in contrast to otosclerosis which affects the footplate (thickened, hazy, and increased density).

Trauma

- Physical trauma causing fracture involving the region of the windows present with hearing loss and/or CSF fistula (**Figs. 8** and **9**).
- Treatment is conservative or surgical exploration.

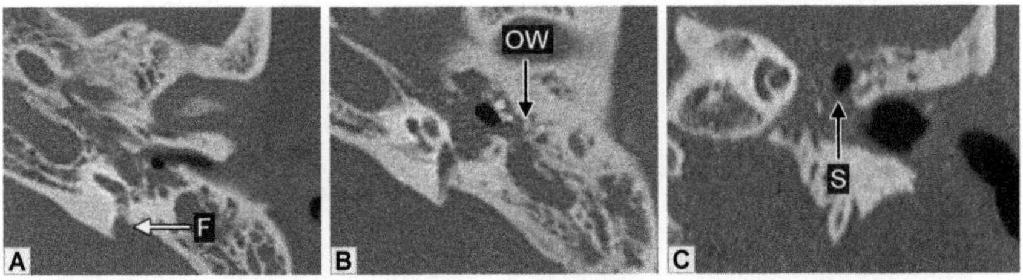

FIGS. 8A TO C: Traumatic involvement of the left oval window (OW): (A and B) Axial and (C) coronal HRCT images showing transverse fracture (F) of the left petrous temporum (arrow, A) involving the OW (arrow, B). There is inferolateral displacement of the left stapes (S).

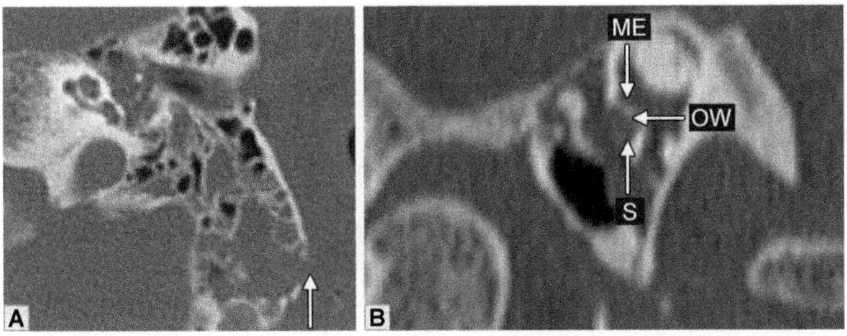

FIGS. 9A AND B: Traumatic involvement of the left oval window (OW)—blast victim: (A) Axial HRCT and (B) coronal images showing bony discontinuity of the mastoid (arrow, A), medial wall of the middle ear (ME), OW with displaced stapes foot plate (S).

Otosclerosis

- *Synonym*: Otospongiosis. Also see Chapter 25.
- It is an autosomal dominant disease and is characterized by replacement of the mature lamellar bone of the otic capsule by spongiotic bone.
- *Clinical features*: Hearing loss which may be conductive, sensorineural, or mixed depending on the pattern of involvement.
- Types and patterns of involvement include:
  - Fenestral otosclerosis is the most common pattern and the most common site of involvement is fissula ante fenestram (anterior to OW). Here, stapes footplate is abnormally thickened to >0.6 mm (normal thickness is 0.3–0.5 mm) (**Figs. 10A** and **B**). Less common is fenestral otosclerosis of the RW.
  - Less common form is pericochlear or internal auditory canal (IAC) disease.
  - Treatment is surgical, stapedectomy/stapes prosthesis.

Surgical Prosthesis

Ossicular chain disruption, erosions or fixation can be treated with partial or complete prosthetic replacement. The replacement normalizes sound wave

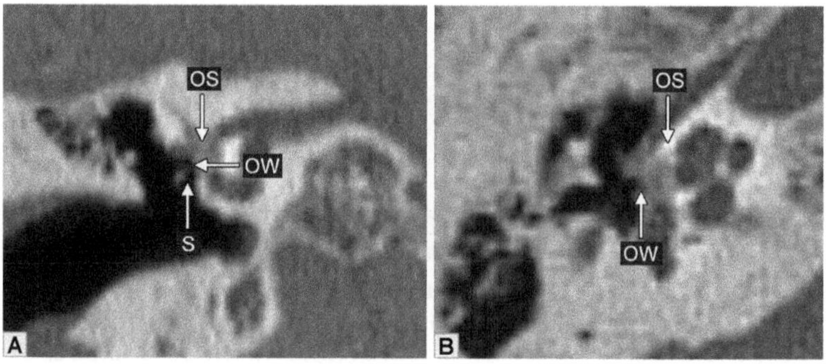

FIGS. 10A AND B: Right otosclerosis (fenestral type): (A) Coronal and (B) axial images showing lucent bony density anterior to the right oval window (OW) (fissula ante fenestram). The stapes is thickened.

transmission from the TM to the inner ear structures. The prostheses are categorized depending on the structures they replace:

- Stapes prosthesis is used in otosclerosis which causes stapes footplate fixity to OW.
- Partial ossicular replacement prosthesis (PORP) extends from TM to head of stapes.
- Total ossicular replacement prosthesis (TORP) extends from TM to the footplate of stapes and replaces entire ossicular chain.
- A preoperative CT is an essential prerequisite for assessment of variant anatomy, if any, and for surgical/implant planning.
- Complications of the surgical prosthesis include dislocation, subluxation, distortion, breakage and extrusion of the prosthesis as well as formation of perilymphatic fistula, granulomas, and fibrotic tissue (**Figs. 11** and **12**).

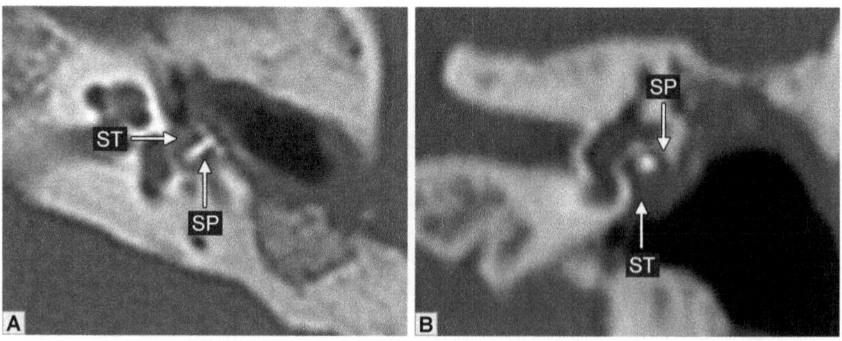

FIGS. 11A AND B: Complication of stapes prosthesis: (A) Axial and (B) coronal (B) images showing the stapes prosthesis (SP) in situ, with surrounding soft tissue (ST) suggestive of granuloma and fibrotic tissue.

Courtesy: Dr Aparna Shyamkumar, Dr Geethu Punnen, CMC, Vellore.

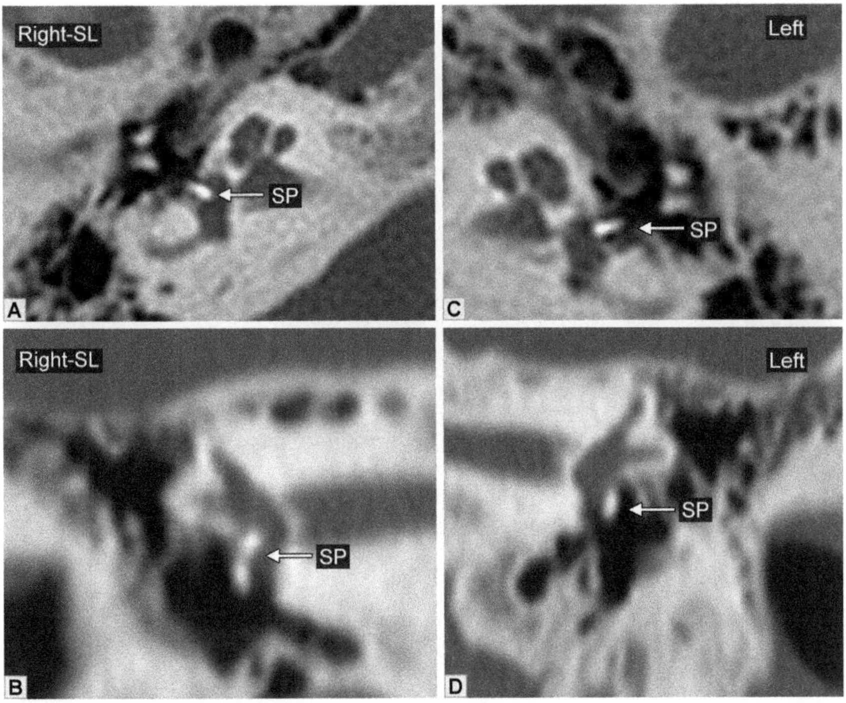

(SL: subluxation; SP: stapes prosthesis)

FIGS. 12A TO D: Stapes prosthesis subluxation: (A and B) Subluxated right stapes prosthesis; and (C and D) Normal left stapes prosthesis. The left prosthesis is in situ, the right prosthesis is subluxated into the oval window.

Courtesy: Dr Aparna Shyamkumar, Dr Geethu Punnen, CMC, Vellore.

ROUND WINDOW

Synonym: Second window.[4]

Normal Anatomy

- Round window is an opening between the basal turn of cochlea and the inner ear.
- Round window unlike its name is not round but has ovoid shape and should be assessed in all three planes.
- The actual opening on the side of the middle ear is a pouch-shaped structure referred to as the round window niche (RWN), which is guarded by a membrane (**Figs. 13A** and **B**).
- Round window pathologies result in conduction hearing loss.
- The size of a normal window in horizontal plane is 1.5–2.1 mm, in vertical plane is 1.9 mm, while the anteroposterior/thickness is 0.65 mm.
- Round window niche: The width of the RWN opening varies from 0.5 to 3 mm. Its boundary is defined by an overhanging part of the cochlear promontory. Variations in this can obscure the RWN presenting difficulties during CT.

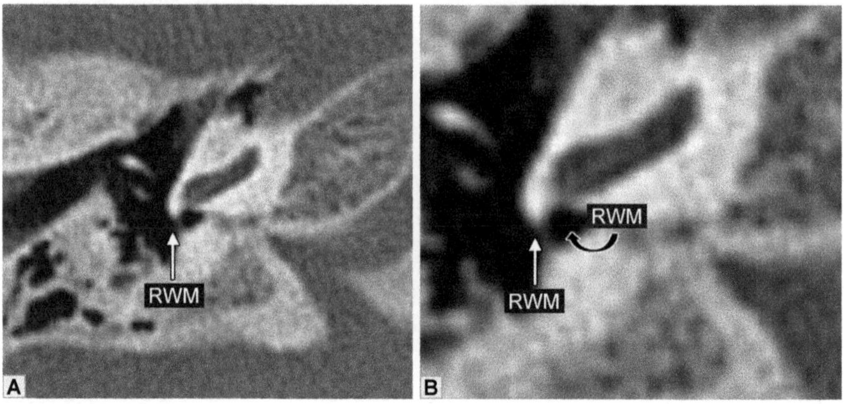

FIGS. 13A AND B: Round window (RW): Normal appearance: (A) Axial HRCT image and (B) magnified image showing the normal anatomy of the RW membrane (RWM, arrow), and air-containing round window niche (RWN) (curved arrow).

Pathologies

Pathologies affecting the RW are enumerated in **Table 2**, and important conditions are discussed subsequently.

Round Window Stenosis/Atresia

- Round window atresia is rare, while stenosis is commoner; the criteria for stenosis is a diameter <1.5 mm.

TABLE 2 Pathologies affecting the round window (RW).

Developmental anomalies	• RW stenosis • RW atresia • Jugular bulb dehiscence and diverticula
Infective	• Otitis media • Obscured RW or RWN due to inflammation secondary to otitis media
Trauma	• Ruptured RW membrane due to barotrauma • Fracture through RW
Miscellaneous abnormalities	• Labyrinthitis ossificans • Otosclerosis • Paget disease • Fibrous dysplasia • Otosyphilis • Osteogenesis imperfecta • Neoplasms (metastasis and primary soft tissue and bone tumors centered in the RW)

(RWN: round window niche)

- These result in conductive/mixed hearing loss.
- These may be syndromic or nonsyndromic. The associated syndromes or anomalies include:
  - CHARGE syndrome: Coloboma (C), Cardiac/Heart defects (H), choanal atresia (AR), genitourinary anomalies (G) and Ear anomalies mostly aural atresia (E)
  - Aural atresia/microtia
  - Inner ear anomalies involving incomplete partition (IP)
  - Mandibular anomalies

Inflammatory Conditions

- In *otitis media*, effusion and mucosal thickening can cover the RW; however, involvement of RW or RWN by cholesteatoma is rare.
- In *labyrinthitis ossificans* (LO), basal turn of the cochlea and RW are early sites of involvement. RW is in fact the route of spread of OM to cochlea.
  - On CT, thickening or high density is present involving the RW membrane (**Fig. 14**). For LO content in hearing loss, refer Chapter 25.
- The pattern/preferential site of involvement may vary according to the cause of LO, although it is not possible to predict the underlying cause simply based on the site of involvement.
- For instance, in basal meningitis, the infection extends through the cochlear aqueduct to the scala tympani involving basal turn first. The spread however may also less frequently come through IAC and modiolus.
- In OM, spread can occur through RW into scala tympani, hence RW is involved early.
- Labyrinthitis ossificans results in development of sensorineural hearing loss (SNHL). Cochlear implant (CI) is challenging and if involvement is extensive, CI is contraindicated.

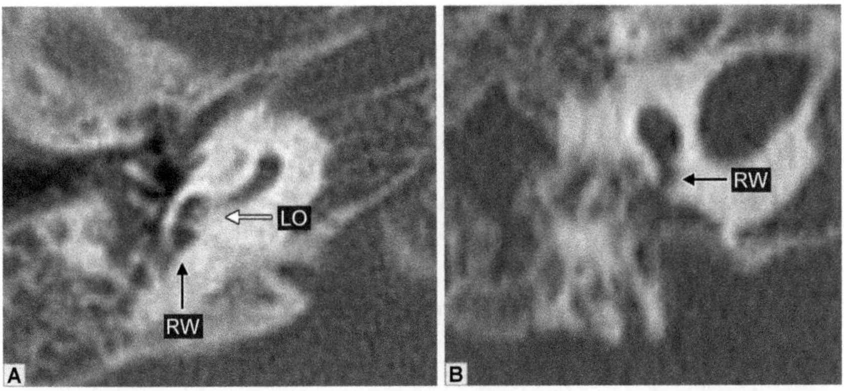

FIGS. 14A AND B: Round window (RW) stenosis in a case of labyrinthitis ossificans (LO): (A) Axial and (B) coronal HRCT images showing narrowing of the RW (black arrows) with hazy increased density in the basal turns of cochlea and RW (white arrow).

Jugular Bulb Dehiscence and Diverticulum

- This variant is present in up to 15% population and progresses over time.
- The dehiscence may be mimic a vascular middle ear mass, which may be catastrophic if sampled.
- If the dehiscence is into RWN, it presents with conductive hearing loss and if it is in to the inner ear, it presents with venous pulsatile tinnitus and hearing loss.

Trauma

- Traumatic fracture can affect the region of the RW similar to OW.
- *Barotrauma* can cause damage to the membranes due to nonequalization/ rapid equalization of the pressure gradients across the membranes. This may in turn lead to perilymphatic fistula which may or may not be accompanied by pneumolabyrinth. CT shows changes of RW membrane rupture in the form of replacement of the normal air density at the RWN by fluid density.

Otosclerosis

- The fenestral otosclerosis of the RW is a less common variant of otosclerosis, and is associated with poor surgical outcome.

THIRD WINDOW

- Third window is a pathological communication between inner ear and the CSF, at an abnormal site.
- Third window abnormalities present with:
  - Vertigo
  - Hearing loss
  - Pulsatile nystagmus
  - *Tullio sign*—vertigo and nystagmus precipitated by loud sounds
  - *Hennebert sign*—nystagmus caused by increase or decrease in external auditory canal pressure.
  - Autophony (loud hearing of owns voice)
  - Oscillopsia (false sensation of constant motion of the surroundings)
- Due to creation of an additional window there is shunting of the acoustic energy from the OW with further decrease in transmission to RW. Further, the third window can induce motion in endolymph in addition to the round and OWs.
- Third window abnormalities are enumerated in **Box 1**.

BOX 1 Causes of third window abnormalities.

- Bony dehiscence of semicircular canals
- Enlarged opening of the vestibular aqueduct
- Dehiscence of the scala vestibuli side of the cochlea
- Thinning of the bony plate between the cochlea and vascular channels

Bony Dehiscence of Semicircular Canals

- Bony dehiscence of semicircular canal (SCC) refers to focal bony discontinuity in the wall of canal.[5]
- Superior SCC is the most frequently involved; either in isolation or along with posterior SCC. Involvement of the posterior SCC is rare.
- A rare subset of superior SCC dehiscence may cause continuity into superior petrosal sinus.
- It is usually idiopathic, however few risk factors include:
  - Congenital bony underdevelopment
  - Trauma causing shear stress
  - Valsalva maneuver causing increased pressure
  - Vascular pulsations causing slow bony erosion
- *Imaging*:
  - High-resolution CT is the imaging modality of choice to demonstrate the bony discontinuity (**Figs. 15A** and **B**).
  - In addition to coronal planes, multiplanar reformats reconstruction (MPR) parallel to Pöschl plane (plane perpendicular to the long axis of temporal bone, so that temporal bone is evaluated from anteromedial to posterolateral aspect) and perpendicular to Stenver's plane (oblique coronal plane) are employed for imaging assessment.

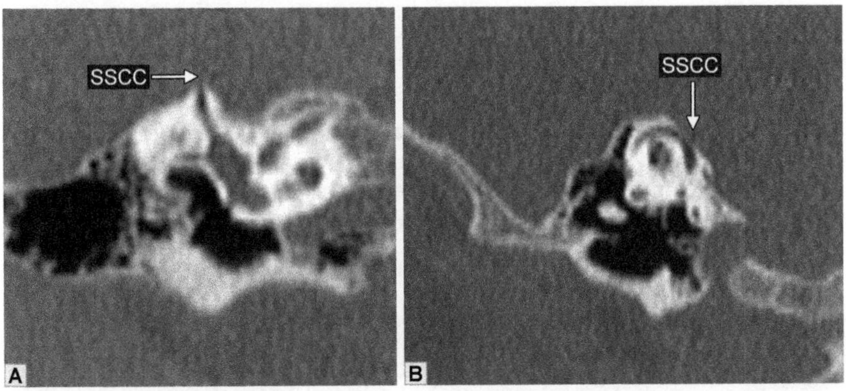

FIGS. 15A AND B: Superior semicircular canal (SSCC) dehiscence: (A) HRCT coronal oblique and (B) sagittal oblique planes show a focal bony dehiscence of SSCC (arrow). The defect is subtle and may not be apparent on routine orthogonal reformatting planes. This highlights the importance of oblique reformatting planes to detect the abnormality.

Perilabyrinthine Fistula

- Destructive processes of middle ear causing thinning and destruction of the otic capsule result in communication with SCCs, vestibule, scala vestibuli of cochlea, and features of third window phenomenon follow. These are referred to as perilabyrinthine fistula (PLF).

- *Causes* of PLF include chronic infection like cholesteatoma, otitis media, trauma (transverse fractures of the temporal bone), iatrogenic (postsurgical following mastoidectomy, stapedectomy, and fenestration) (**Figs. 16A** and **B**).
- As the lateral SCC is located adjacent to the middle ear, it is the most frequently involved (**Figs. 17A** to **C**).
- Cochlear-carotid dehiscence occurs rarely with loss of the intervening bony septum.
- *Clinical features*:
  - Patients present with dizziness and hearing loss; the latter being fluctuating in nature. The symptoms can be replicated by activities which

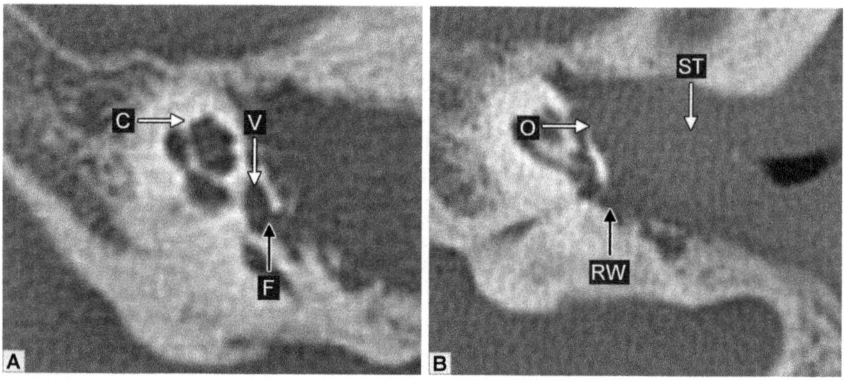

(C: cochlea; F: fistula; O: ossicles; RW: round window; ST: soft tissue; V: vestibule)

FIGS. 16A AND B: Perilabyrinthine fistula—vestibule: (A) Axial image showing abnormal opening in the lateral wall of vestibule in a postoperative case (left MRM). (B) Axial image showing soft tissue in the middle ear and external ear. The ossicular chain is disorganized. Note also made of fluid in the RW (black arrow, B).

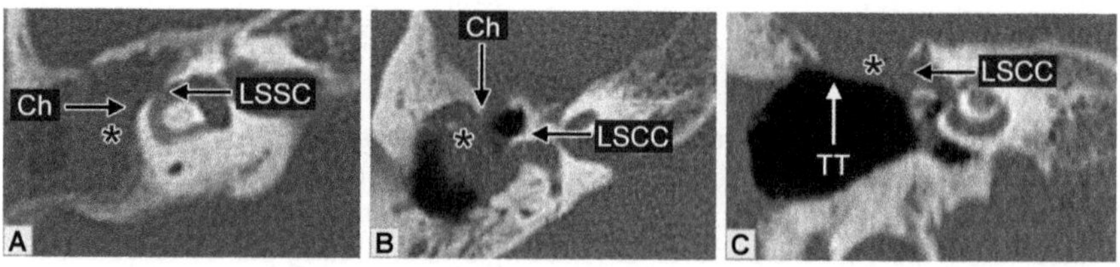

(Ch: cholesteatoma; LSCC: lateral semicircular canal; TT: tegmen tympani)

FIGS. 17A TO C: Perilabyrinthine fistula-dehiscent lateral semicircular canal (LSCC): (A) Axial image showing a focal bony defect in the LSCC with a cholesteatomatous soft tissue. (B) Axial and (C) coronal images of different patient showing cholesteatomata (asterisk) in the middle ear with large erosion of the right LSCC (arrows). Note is also made of erosion of the tegmen tympani (white arrow).

bring about change in atmospheric pressure like mountaineering and scuba diving (pressure sensitivity).
  - Geyser or gusher syndrome can accompany, with CSF leakage from the ear.
- *Imaging*:
  - Computed tomography shows abnormal bulge of membranes at the oval or RWs, which may be accompanied by middle ear fluid, especially the tympanic recess. Air within the labyrinth (pneumolabyrinth) is a direct sign of the fistula.
  - Another finding is disorientation of stapes footplate, which is normally oriented parallel to the long axis of vestibule and medial vestibular wall. Rarely, CT can be normal.
  - Magnetic resonance imaging may show enhancement of the labyrinth, due to resultant labyrinthitis.

Enlarged Vestibular Aqueduct (EVA)

- It is a congenital anomaly, causing enlargement of the vestibular aqueduct at the level of endolymphatic duct. It is covered in detail in Chapter 11.
- *Normal anatomy*: Vestibular aqueduct is a narrow bony canal extending from the medial wall of vestibule to the posterior surface of the petrous temporum. In the Pöschl projection, its diameter ranges from 0.3 to 0.9 mm with a mean of 0.5 mm.
- *Causes*: Congenital causes (associated with Pendred syndrome, CHARGE syndrome, branchio-oto-renal syndrome) or in isolation.
- *Clinical features*: Complex patterns of hearing loss are present.
- *Imaging*: CT findings are frequently seen bilaterally. *CT criteria* of EVA are as follows:
  - Visual evaluation—dilatation compared to the posterior SCC.
  - Valvassori criterion—transverse diameter of vestibular aqueduct at its midpoint ≥1.5 mm (**Fig. 18**).
  - Cincinnati criteria—diameter at midpoint ≥1 mm or at operculum ≥2 mm.
  - Pöschl (45° oblique) projection—more than the normal range of 0.3–0.9 mm.

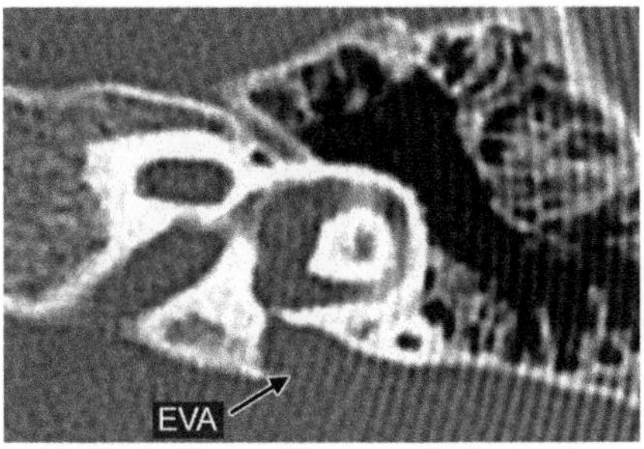

FIG. 18: Enlarged vestibular aqueduct (EVA): Axial CT image showing EVA measuring >1.5 mm at its mid point (arrow).

CONCLUSION

In conclusion, oval and RWs are structures of paramount importance in the hearing pathway and are affected by a variety of disorders, leading to hearing impairment, nystagmus, and pressure symptoms. Third window, on the other hand, is an abnormal communication between the inner ear and CSF. Radiological evaluation of these windows forms the backbone of evaluation and thus familiarity with normal anatomy, anatomical variants, and abnormalities help in achieving correct diagnosis and optimum management.

REFERENCES

1. Zdilla MJ, Skrzat J, Kozerska M, Leszczynski B, Tarasiuk J, Wro ski S. Oval window size and shape: a Micro-CT anatomical study with considerations for stapes surgery. Otol Neurotol. 2018;39(5):558-64.
2. Zeifer B, Sabini P, Sonne J. Congenital absence of the oval window: radiologic diagnosis and associated anomalies. AJNR Am J Neuroradiol. 2000;21(2):322-7.
3. Huang TS. Anomalously coursing facial nerves above and below the oval window: three case reports. Otolaryngol Head Neck Surg. 1997;116(4):438-41.
4. Benson JC, Diehn F, Passe T, Guerin J, Silvera VM, Carlson ML, et al. The Forgotten Second Window: A Pictorial Review of Round Window Pathologies. AJNR Am J Neuroradiol. 2020;41(2):192-9.
5. Ho ML, Moonis G, Halpin CF, Curtin HD. Spectrum of third window abnormalities: semicircular canal dehiscence and beyond. AJNR Am J Neuroradiol. 2017;38(1):2-9.

22

Petrous Apex Lesions: Imaging

Priyanka Naranje, Ajay Garg, Ankur Goyal

- Classification
  - Pseudolesions
  - Congenital Lesions
  - Infective/Inflammatory Lesions
  - Neoplasms—Primary and Metastatic
  - Vascular Lesions
  - Diffuse Bone Diseases
  - Extension from Adjacent Diseases
- Imaging Approach

- The petrous apex (PA) of temporal bone is situated anterior and medial to the inner ear in the angular space between greater wing of sphenoid anteriorly and occipital bone posteriorly. PA is bounded by petrosphenoidal fissure anteromedially and middle cranial fossa laterally. Medially, it is flanked by petroclival fissure while posteriorly it is related to posterior cranial fossa (**Fig. 1**).
- It is related to Meckel's cave superomedially (in which lies the trigeminal ganglion) and Dorello's canal in the petrosphenoidal ligament (which contains 6th cranial nerve); thus these structures may be involved in PA

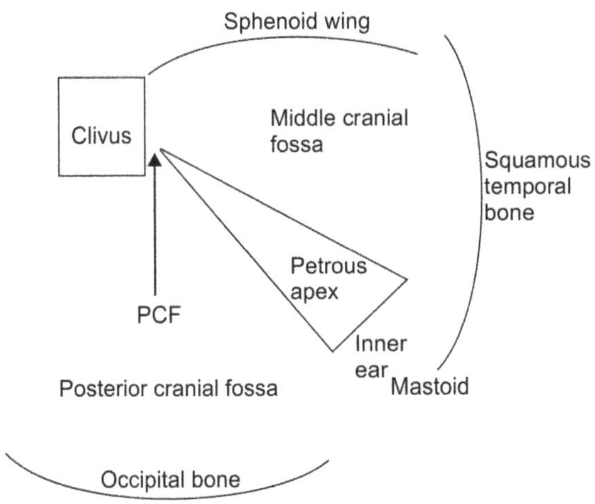

(PCF: petroclival fissure)

FIG. 1: Schematic diagram showing relations of petrous apex.

lesions. The internal auditory canal (IAC) separates the PA into an anterior part (which contains bony marrow) and a small dense posterior part (derived from otic capsule).

- The proximity of neural and vascular structures makes PA lesions important as these may present with severe clinical sequelae. CT and MRI play an important role in diagnosis and characterization of various PA lesions.[1]

CLASSIFICATION

The PA lesions are classified as follows.[2]

- *Pseudolesions*:
  - Pneumatized PA
  - Asymmetric marrow
  - Apical cephalocele/meningocele
- *Congenital lesions*:
  - Congenital cholesteatoma
- *Infective/inflammatory lesions*:
  - Effusion/trapped fluid
  - Mucocele
  - Cholesterol granuloma
  - Apical petrositis/osteomyelitis
- *Neoplasms*: Primary and metastatic
- *Vascular lesions*:
  - Internal carotid artery (ICA) aneurysm
- *Diffuse bone disease:*
  - Sclerosing diseases like fibrous dysplasia, Paget's disease
  - Metabolic bone disease
- Extension from adjacent diseases

Pseudolesions

These are usually detected incidentally in patients undergoing imaging evaluation and do not require any treatment.

Pneumatized Petrous Apex

Petrous apex may show pneumatization in about one-third of the population and this normal variation should not be taken as abnormal (**Fig. 2**). Air cells of pneumatized PA are susceptible to similar diseases that occur in the mastoid (inflammation and obstruction).

Asymmetric Marrow

- This is a rare incidental finding. If one side is pneumatized and other is not, then nonpneumatized marrow may be mistaken for a mass lesion.
- On MRI, it shows signal intensity of normal fatty marrow on T1-weighted (T1W) images.

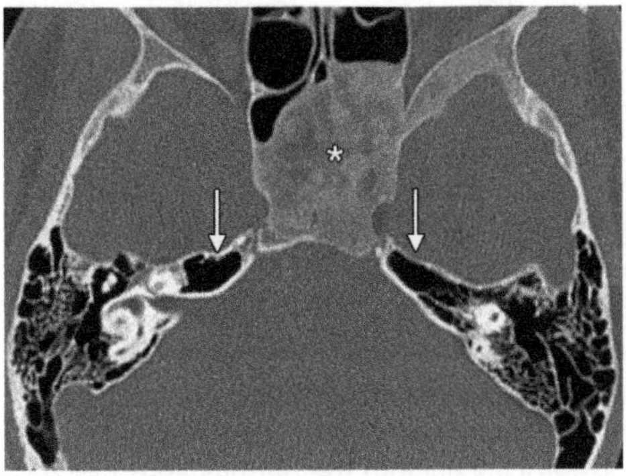

FIG. 2: Pneumatized petrous apices: Axial CT image bone window shows that bilateral (B/L) petrous apices are pneumatized. Note made of expansion and ground glass appearance involving sphenoid bone (asterisk), indicative of fibrous dysplasia.

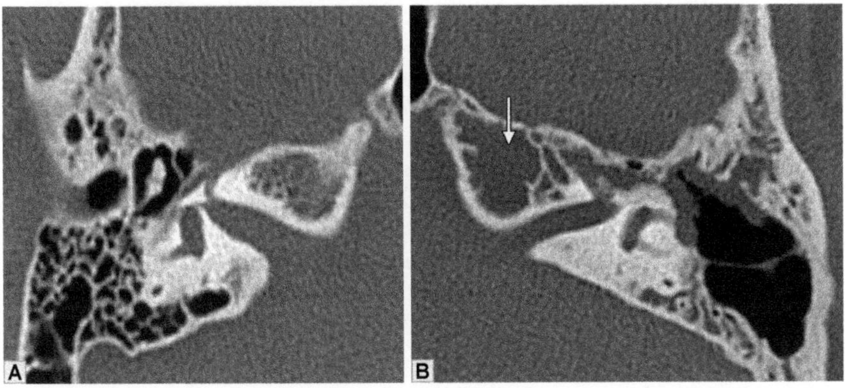

FIGS. 3A AND B: Asymmetrically pneumatized left petrous apex (PA) in a case of recurrent left otomastoiditis (with history of surgery). (A) Right PA is not pneumatized. (B) Opacification of pneumatized left PA (arrow) with postoperative changes in middle ear cavity.

- Asymmetrically nonpneumatized PA may appear very bright on T1W images, thus mimicking cholesterol granuloma. However, it may be distinguished by its loss of signal on fat-suppressed images and normal bone morphology and attenuation on CT (**Figs. 3A** and **B**).
- Absence of any bony expansion and enhancement help to diagnose this pseudolesion.

Apical Cephalocele/Meningocele or Arachnoid Cyst of Petrous Apex

- Apical cephalocele or meningocele represents the herniation of CSF in the Meckel's cave posterolaterally into the PA.
- It may be congenital or acquired.
- Usually the involvement is unilateral, but bilateral findings may be seen in raised intracranial pressure (as in pseudotumor cerebri).

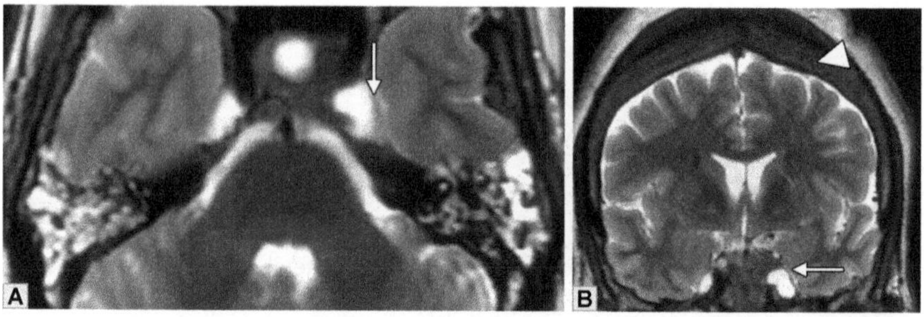

FIGS. 4A AND B: Apical meningocele in a patient of acromegaly: (A) Axial and (B) coronal T2-weighted (T2W) MR images demonstrate there is herniation of cerebrospinal fluid (CSF) from the left Meckel's cave posterolaterally into the petrous apex (arrows). Note made of bilateral otomastoiditis in (A) and diffuse calvarial thickening in (B) (arrowhead).

- Expansile PA lesion on CT with enlarged porus trigeminus notch (trigeminal notch is a smooth impression on the PA that encloses the posterior portion of Meckel's cave) and scalloped margins.
- Magnetic resonance imaging shows CSF signal intensity ovoid lesion (**Figs. 4A** and **B**). Communication with CSF of Meckel's cave is best demonstrated on coronal T2WI.
- It is a "no-touch lesion" and rarely may need treatment in case of spontaneous/traumatic communication between apical cephalocele and petrous air cells.

Congenital Cholesteatoma/Epidermoid Cyst

- Congenital cholesteatomas occur due to aberrant stratified squamous epithelial rests trapped during embryogenesis. It makes up 4–9% of PA lesions.[2]
- These usually present in middle age group (30–40 years), may also be seen in children and presents with unilateral sensorineural hearing loss (SNHL).
- These are slow-growing lesions and pathologically, consist of cysts lined with stratified squamous epithelium and filled with keratinous debris.
- *CT*: Expansile lobulated mass with no enhancement, and variable bone destruction.
- *MRI*: Hypo- on T1W, hyper-/intermediate signal on T2W and no enhancement or minimal rim enhancement/delayed enhancement. There is incomplete suppression of signal on FLAIR (fluid-attenuated inversion recovery) (**Figs. 5A** to **D**).
- Presence of *diffusion restriction on diffusion-weighted imaging (DWI) is hallmark.*
- These lesions may extend beyond PA to involve IAC, inner ear structures, facial nerve canal, medial mastoid, or horizontal carotid canal.
- Treatment is surgical resection.

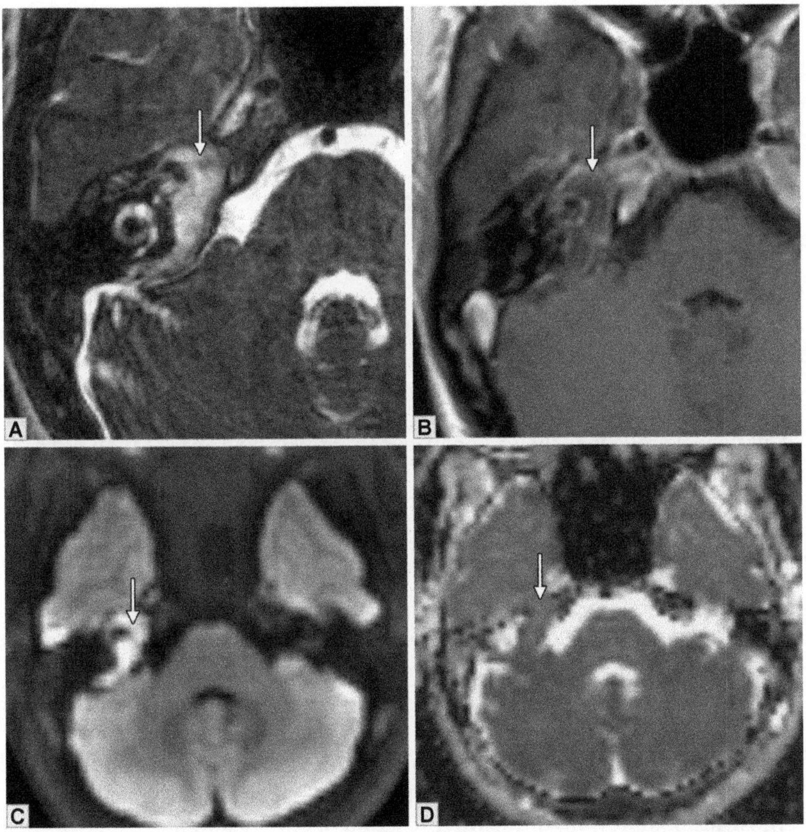

FIGS. 5A TO D: Congenital cholesteatoma of petrous apex (PA) (arrows): (A) T2WI shows intermediate signal intensity (SI) lobulated lesion in the PA. (B) No enhancement seen on postgadolinium image. (C and D) Diffusion restriction seen within the lesion (hallmark of epidermoid cyst).

Infective/Inflammatory Lesions

Effusion/Trapped Fluid

- It represents the sterile fluid collection in pneumatized PA, which persists even after the treatment of remote otomastoiditis. These are usually detected incidentally.
- *CT*: Opacification of pneumatized PA. There is no expansion or bone erosions and absence of concurrent otomastoiditis (**Fig. 6**).
- *MRI*: Variable signal on T1W, T2W hyperintense, no enhancement. Retained secretions may parallel the signal intensity of cholesterol granuloma on noncontrast MRI.
- No treatment is required.
- May pose diagnostic dilemma if hyperintense on T1, but other T1 hyperintense lesions (cholesterol granuloma and mucocele) cause cortical expansion.

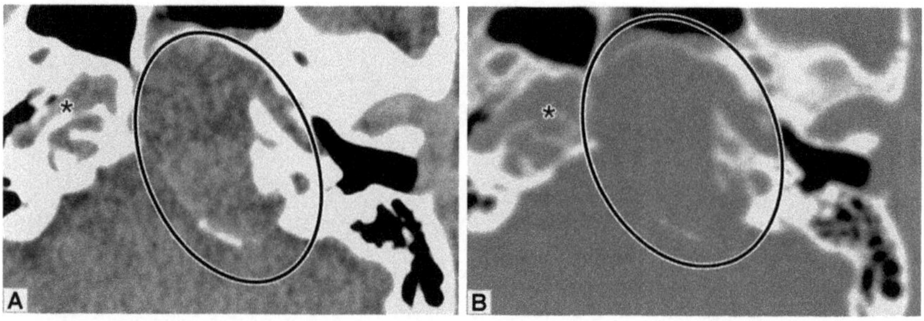

FIGS. 6A AND B: Pneumatized bilateral petrous apices with right petrous apex effusion and left petrous apex mucocele.

- Opacification of right petrous apex with fluid attenuation, suggesting effusion (black asterisk).
- Left sided petrous apex shows smooth expansion with fluid opacification, indicating mucocele formation (encircled).

Mucocele

- Petrous apex mucoceles are uncommon lesions and occurs due to obstructed drainage of pneumatized PA air cells. Patients present with headache or these lesions are incidentally detected.
- *CT*: Opacification of pneumatized PA with smooth expansion of cortical margins (**Fig. 6**).
- *MRI*: Usually hypointense on T1 (proteinaceous contents may occasionally give rise to T1 hyperintensity) and hyperintense on T2WI (**Figs. 7A** and **B**). These lesions show no diffusion restriction or enhancement.
- Surgery is needed if the lesion enlarges on follow-up.
- It may mimic cholesterol granuloma if lesion shows hyperintense signal on T1WI.

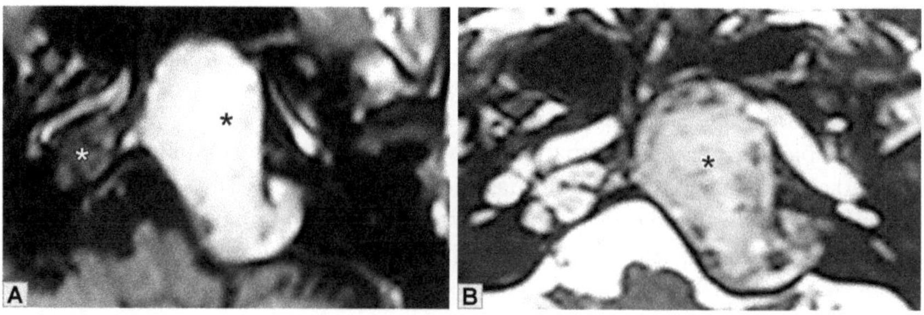

FIGS. 7A AND B: Bilateral petrous apex mucoceles.

- Axial T1W (a) and T2W (b) MR images show expansion of both petrous apices with hyperintensity on T2W sequence.
- Right sided mucocele is hypointense on T1W (white asterisk) while on left is hyperintense (black asterisk), due to proteinaceous contents.

Cholesterol Granuloma

- Patients present with SNHL, tinnitus (when IAC is involved) or may be asymptomatic.
- It results from foreign body giant cell and hemorrhagic reaction to cholesterol crystals.
- A pneumatized PA is a common site for the cholesterol granuloma to develop, after middle ear.
- *CT*: Well-demarcated expansile lesion with smooth margins, central soft tissue attenuation and no calcification. Cortical thinning with bony dehiscence may occur.
- *MRI*: High T1 signal, high T2 signal, may have peripheral hypointense (hemosiderin) rim (**Figs. 8A** and **B**). T1 hyperintensity is due to presence of hemorrhage, breakdown of blood products, and cholesterol crystals. Not suppressed on FLAIR. May show no enhancement or subtle peripheral enhancement. This is in contrast to granulation tissue of inflammatory conditions which is highly vascular and shows intense postcontrast enhancement.
- Treatment is surgical drainage in symptomatic patients.

Apical Petrositis/Petrous Apicitis

- Petrous apicitis occurs due to extension of otomastoiditis into a pneumatized PA with suppurative inflammation. Occasionally nonpneumatized PA may also be involved.
- Petrous apex may also be involved as a part of advanced disease in cases of skull base osteomyelitis.
- *Gradenigo syndrome* is a clinical triad associated with petrous apicitis—consists of retro-orbital pain and otorrhea (due to apical petrositis and otomastoiditis), deep facial pain (CN V), and lateral rectus palsy with diplopia (CN VI) (**Table 1**).

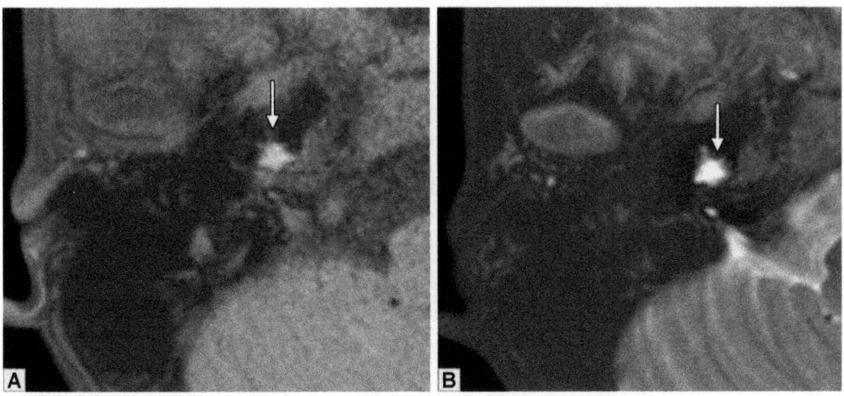

FIGS. 8A AND B: Cholesterol granuloma: (A) Axial T1W (fat-suppressed) image and (B) T2W MR image show an incidentally detected subcentimetric well-defined lesion in the right petrous apex, hyperintense on both sequences (arrows). T2 hypointense rim is noted around the lesion.

TABLE 1 Triad of Gradenigo syndrome.

Clinical presentation	Level of anatomical involvement
Otomastoiditis	Middle ear, mastoid
Horizontal diplopia and abducens palsy	Dorello's canal (below the superior sphenopetrosal ligament) carrying 6th cranial nerve to the cavernous sinus
Facial and retro-orbital pain	Meckel's cave carrying the 5th cranial nerve

- *CT*:
  - *Initial stages*: Fluid collection in PA (**Figs. 9A** and **B**).
  - *Later stages*: Opacification of PA air cells with expansion, permeative bone destruction with trabecular breakdown and erosions, with concurrent otomastoiditis (**Figs. 10A** and **B**). There may be associated cavernous sinus thrombosis/phlegmon, meningitis, and epidural abscess.

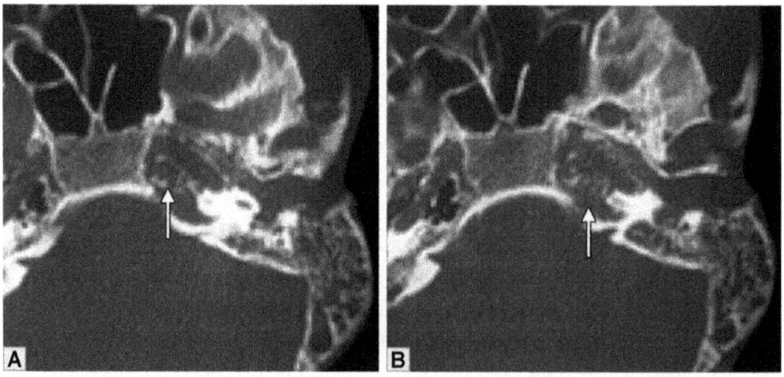

FIGS. 9A AND B: Tubercular otomastoiditis extending into a pneumatized petrous apex (PA): Fluid collection with mild expansion of PA air cells (arrows). Opacification of middle ear cavity and mastoid air cells is noted on left side. The patient responded to antitubercular treatment.

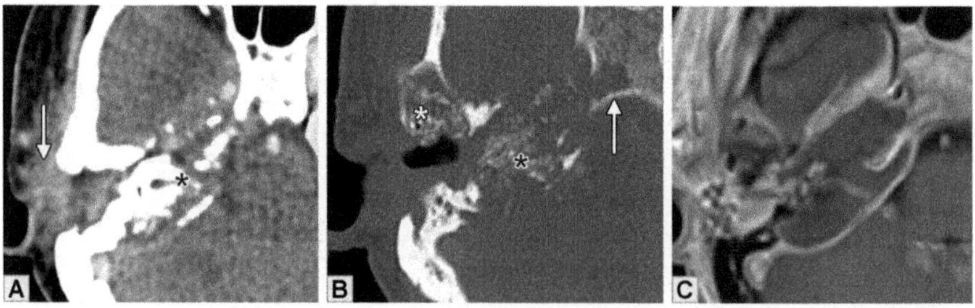

FIGS. 10A TO C: Osteomyelitis involving right temporal bone with involvement of PA: Axial CECT image soft tissue (A) and bone window (B) show aggressive destructive lytic lesion involving petrous (black asterisk) and squamous parts (white asterisk) of right temporal bone and right temporomandibular joint with enhancing soft tissue (arrow in A). There is permeative involvement of petrous bone with lysis, extending upto basisphenoid (arrow in B). Postcontrast MR image (C) shows peripheral enhancement.

- *MRI*:
  - *Initial stages*: T2/STIR hyperintensity and diffuse enhancement on postcontrast images.
  - *Later stages*: Areas of abscess formation show high T2 signal and peripheral rim/internal heterogeneous enhancement with restricted diffusion (**Fig. 10C**). Adjacent meningeal/cranial nerve enhancement may also be present.
  - It may further extend to the skull base leading to multiple cranial nerve palsies (Vernet' syndrome, 9th to 11th nerve) with resultant cranial nerve enhancement.
- Nonaerated PA may be rarely involved by spread from vascular route/adjacent osteomyelitic bone. This usually occurs in diabetic patients and *Pseudomonas* is the most common causative organism.
- Chronic osteomyelitis may have mixed lytic-sclerotic involvement of the involved bones.
- *Treatment*: Antibiotics; surgery (infracochlear) in severe cases, usually reserved for abscess formation. Hence, it is important on imaging to specify the formation of abscess.

Neoplasms

Primary Neoplasms

- *Petroclival fissure chondrosarcoma*: It presents as an ill-defined expansile lobulated destructive mass lesion in paramidline region showing heterogeneous enhancement involving PA and basisphenoid. It arises from petro-occipital synchondrosis. Chondroid matrix calcification in the form of arcs and whorls is seen in about half the patients. T2 hyperintensity on MRI is characteristic (**Figs. 11A** to **C**).
- *Petroclival meningioma*: It is seen as dural-based hyperdense mass lesion which shows intense homogeneous enhancement. These lesions usually cause hyperostosis of adjacent PA but sometimes may be intraosseous.

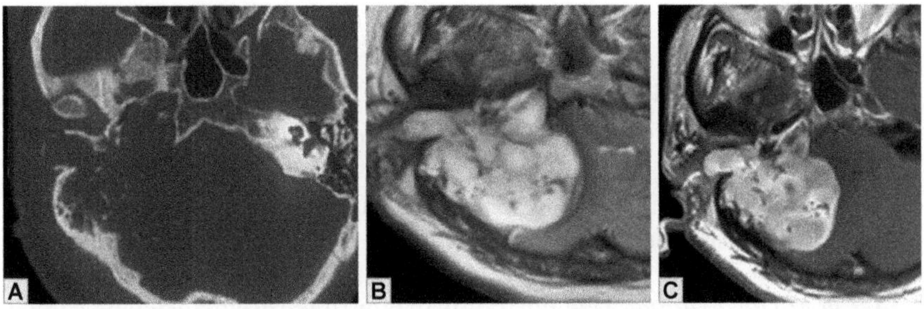

FIGS. 11A TO C: Petrous apex chondrosarcoma: (A) CT image shows expansile, destructive lytic lesion involving petrous part of right temporal bone (including apex) with foci of chondroid calcification. (B and C) Hyperintensity on T2WI and postcontrast enhancement with extradural extension in posterior cranial fossa is also noted.

- *Schwannoma*: Schwannomas arising from distal cisternal segment of the trigeminal nerve or in the region of Meckel's cave, involve the PA. In addition, large facial nerve/first genu or 8th nerve schwannomas can extend medially into PA. Schwannomas are hyperintense on T2W, show avid enhancement and may have cystic components. These lesions may also show hemorrhage.

Metastases

- Skull base is commonly involved in hematogenously disseminated metastases.
- Most common primary malignancy is adenocarcinoma from breast (**Fig. 12A**), lung, prostate, melanoma, neuroblastoma, and renal cell carcinoma.
- These appear as permeative, destructive purely lytic, or mixed lytic-sclerotic lesion on CT.
- Multiple myeloma deposits and sometimes metastases may be well-demarcated expansile lytic lesions, but show enhancing soft tissue.

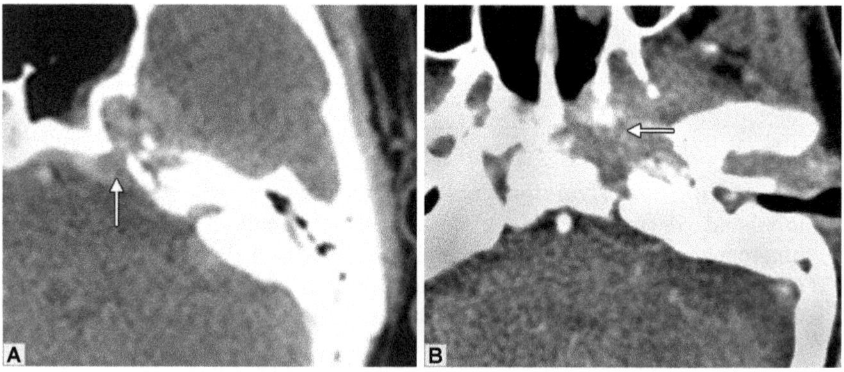

FIGS. 12A AND B: Malignant involvement of petrous apex (PA): (A) A 50-year-old female patient with breast carcinoma shows aggressive lytic lesion in left PA with enhancing soft tissue (arrow), suggestive of metastasis. Similar other lesions were seen in the cranial vault. (B) A 35-year-old male patient shows contiguous extension of nasopharyngeal carcinoma to involve left PA (arrow).

Vascular Lesions

Petrous Internal Carotid Artery Aneurysm

- It may present as incidental detection or there may be SNHL, pulsatile tinnitus, or stroke.
- *CT*: Ovoid enlargement of horizontal petrous ICA canal (**Figs. 13A** to **C**). Curvilinear calcification may be seen in the wall of aneurysm. Margins are usually smooth and scalloped.
- *CT or MR angiography*: Demonstration of flow (intense enhancement similar to vessel) within the lesion and continuity with ICA is diagnostic.[3]
- *Complex signal intensity on T1*: Bright due to clot and sluggish flow, dark due to fast flow and calcification. Complex signal on T2, hemosiderin and pulsation artifact in phase-encoding direction.

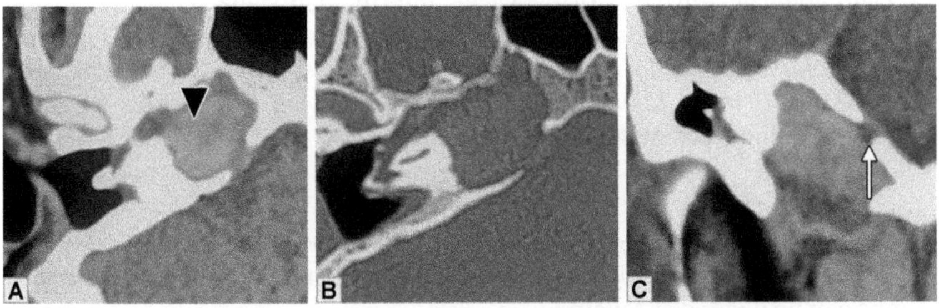

FIGS. 13A TO C: Petrous ICA aneurysm: Noncontrast CT images of a 23-year-old male shows expansile, hyperdense lesion centered in PA (arrowhead). The posterior wall of carotid canal is dehiscent and there is scalloping of adjacent bony margins. Peripheral hypodensity is noted within the lesion which represents thrombus (arrow).

- In a pulsatile aneurysm, intralesional flow may be suggested by motion artifact on MRI, most commonly on contrast-enhanced T1WI sequence. It occurs in the phase-encoding direction.
- Differentials include cholesterol granuloma, aberrant ICA (artery enters middle ear posterolateral to normal entry site), and jugular bulb dehiscence (due to absence of sigmoid plate of bone).
- Treatment is endovascular coiling in symptomatic cases.

Diffuse Bone Diseases

- *Fibrous dysplasia* commonly involves skull base and is characterized by osseous expansion and ground glass internal appearance on CT. Though rare, PA involvement can occur and can result in narrowing of neural/vascular foramina.
- *Paget's disease* usually involves the skull vault and otic capsule involvement is rarely described. Other than these sclerosing diseases, metabolic bone disease can also involve the PA along with other skull bones.

Extension from Adjacent Diseases

- Petrous apex may get secondarily involved from adjacent disorders such as in skull base osteomyelitis, clival chordoma, and jugular paraganglioma.
- Invasive "downgoing" intracranial processes may involve the PA.
- Invasive "upgoing" infiltrating lesions like nasopharyngeal or sinonasal malignancies (**Fig. 12B**), rhabdomyosarcoma, and fungal infections.

Miscellaneous Lesions

- *Granulomatosis with polyangiitis (GPA)* may present with mass lesions in sinonasal region as well as PA.
- *Inflammatory pseudotumor*: Though temporal bone is a rare site of involvement, but when involved, commonly affects the PA.[4]

- *Lymphoma* of skull base can involve PA. Intermediate signal on T2W, diffusion restriction and permeative bone involvement are usually seen.
- *Langerhans cell histiocytosis* usually involves mastoid and squamous parts of temporal bone, however may involve PA as well. The lesions are well-circumscribed, osteolytic soft tissue masses.

IMAGING APPROACH

Imaging-based approach is illustrated in **Flowchart 1**. The basic patterns of lesions can be divided as follows:

- *Nonexpansile PA lesions*: Effusion, pneumatized PA, and asymmetric PA marrow.
- *Aggressive lesions with bone erosion*: These cause permeative involvement and destruction. Include apical petrositis, Langerhans cell histiocytosis, metastases, and plasmacytoma.
- *Expansile PA lesions*: Benign lesions which cause smooth scalloping.
  - Cholesteatoma—diffusion restriction
  - Cholesterol granuloma—T1 hyperintense
  - Mucocele—fluid signal with free diffusion
  - Petrous ICA aneurysm—CT/MR angiography and pulsation artifacts
  - PA cephalocele—fluid signal continuous with Meckel's cave

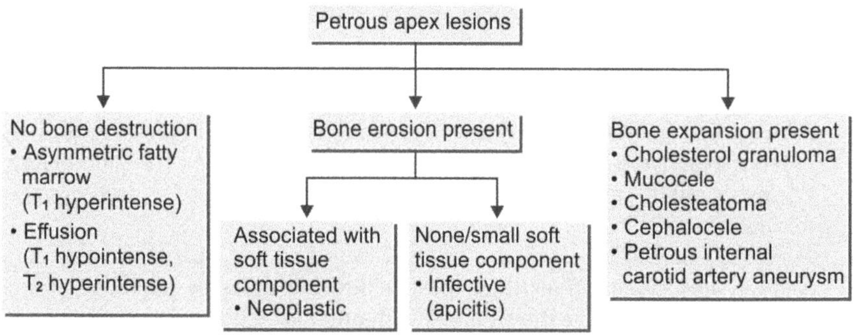

FLOWCHART 1: Pattern approach based on osseous changes.

REFERENCES

1. Chapman PR, Shah R, Curé JK, Bag AK. Petrous apex lesions: pictorial review. AJR Am J Roentgenol. 2011;196 (3 Suppl):WS26-37 Quiz S40-3.
2. Razek AA, Huang BY. Lesions of the petrous apex: classification and findings at CT and MR imaging. Radiographics. 2012;32(1):151-73.
3. Harnberger HR, Glastonbury CM, Michel MA, Koch BL. Diagnostic Imaging - Head and neck (second edition). Amirsys. Section 5 Petrous apex.
4. Campion T, Taranath A, Pinelli L, Ugga L, Nash R, Talenti G, et al. Imaging of temporal bone inflammations in children: a pictorial review. Neuroradiology. 2019;61:959-70.

7
SECTION

Miscellaneous

23

Temporal Bone Trauma

Atin Kumar, Shivanand Gamanagatti

- Classification
- Specific Types of Fractures
- Normal Variants Mimicking Fractures
- Specific Situations
- Teaching Points

- Temporal bone fractures are usually a result of blunt head injury (high impact).
- Up to 14–22% of patients with skull fractures have temporal bone fracture.[1]
- These are often associated with other intracranial injuries. Hence symptom recognition for temporal bone injury might be delayed.
- Acute clinical presentations of temporal bone fracture may be bleeding from the ear or acute facial nerve paralysis.
- Multidetector CT is the investigation of choice.[2]

CLASSIFICATION

Various classification systems exist. Classification helps to understand the trauma-associated complications and prognosticate.

Ulrich Classification[3]

- This classification of temporal bone fractures is based on the relationship of the fracture line with the long axis of the petrous temporal bone (**Figs. 1A** and **B**).
- In majority (70–90%), fracture line is oriented along the long axis, and is termed as longitudinal fracture (**Figs. 2A** and **B**). It usually occurs secondary to lateral impact to the skull.
- In 10–30% cases, the fracture line is transversely oriented, perpendicular to the axis of the petrous temporal bone, and is called transverse fracture (**Figs. 3A** and **B**). It occurs secondary to frontal or occipital impact to the skull.
- When both longitudinal and transverse components coexist, it is termed as mixed temporal bone fracture (**Figs. 4A** to **C**).

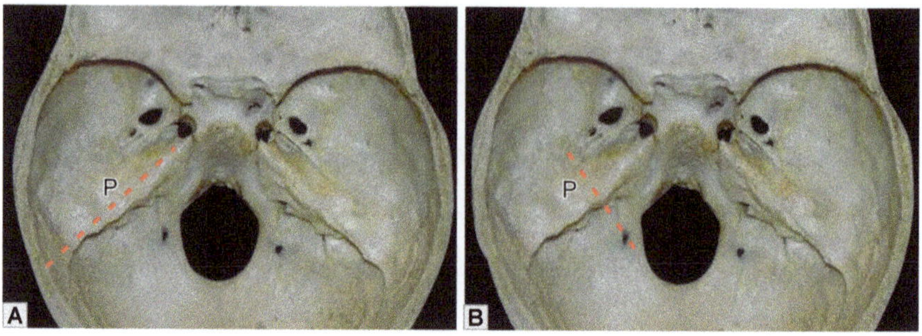

FIGS. 1A AND B: Fractures of the temporal bone: Images of the base of skull showing the axis (broken line) of the longitudinal fracture (A) and transverse fracture (B) of petrous temporal bone (P).

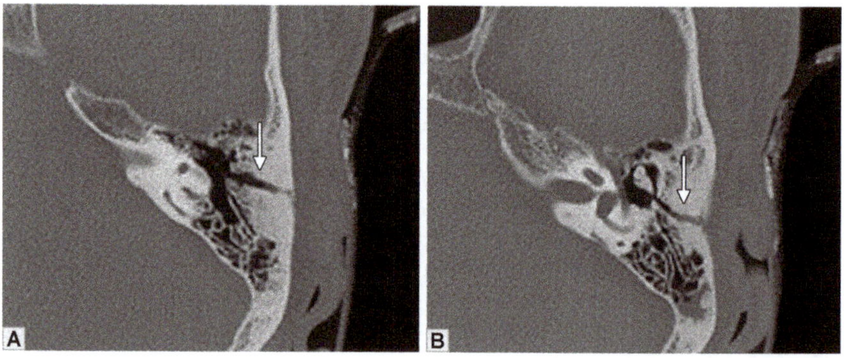

FIGS. 2A AND B: Longitudinal fracture: Axial HRCT images show a longitudinal fracture of left temporal bone (arrows) extending medially till the middle ear cavity. The ossicles appear normal.

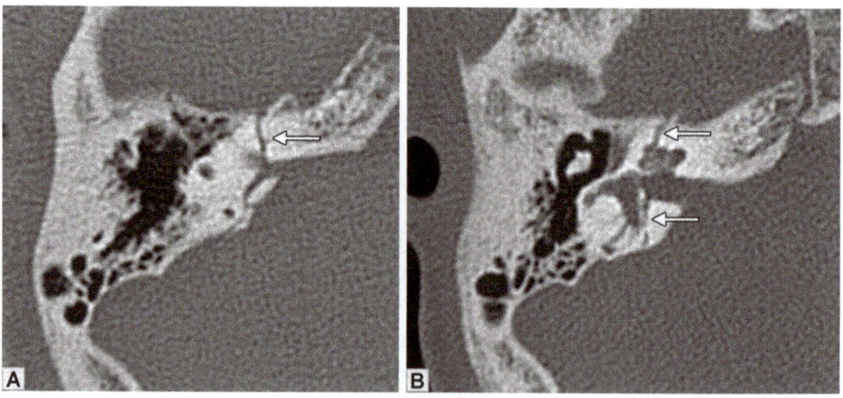

FIGS. 3A AND B: Transverse fracture: Axial HRCT images show a transverse fracture of right temporal bone (arrows) perpendicular to its long axis. The fracture line is running across the labyrinth.

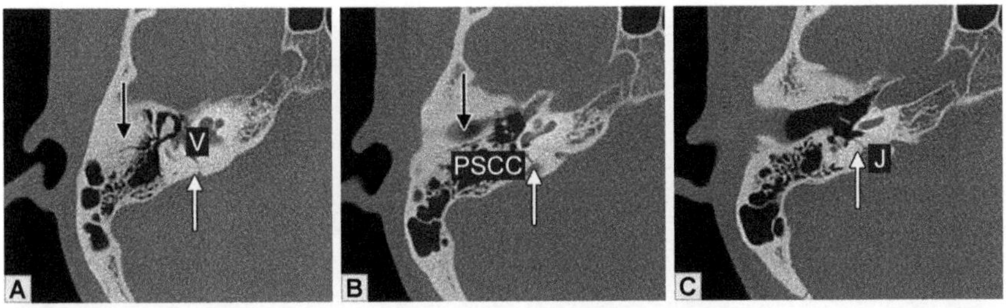

FIGS. 4A TO C: Mixed temporal bone fracture: Axial HRCT images from cranial to caudal direction show mixed temporal bone fracture pattern—both longitudinal (black arrows) and transverse fractures (white arrows) are seen. The longitudinal fracture extends into the middle ear cavity while the transverse fracture involves the vestibule (V in A), posterior semicircular canal (PSCC in B), and extends into jugular foramen (J in C) inferiorly.

Brodie's Classification[1]

- This classification divides the fractures based on the relationship of the fracture line with the otic capsule. This is a more practical classification for predicting the patient outcome and sequelae of injury.
- If the otic capsule is traversed by fracture line, it is termed "otic capsule-violating (OCV) fracture." If the otic capsule is left intact, it is called "otic capsule-sparing (OCS) fracture" (**Figs. 5** to **7**).

Ishman and Friedland Classification[4]

This classification divides the temporal bone fractures into petrous and nonpetrous based on involvement or sparing of petrous apex.

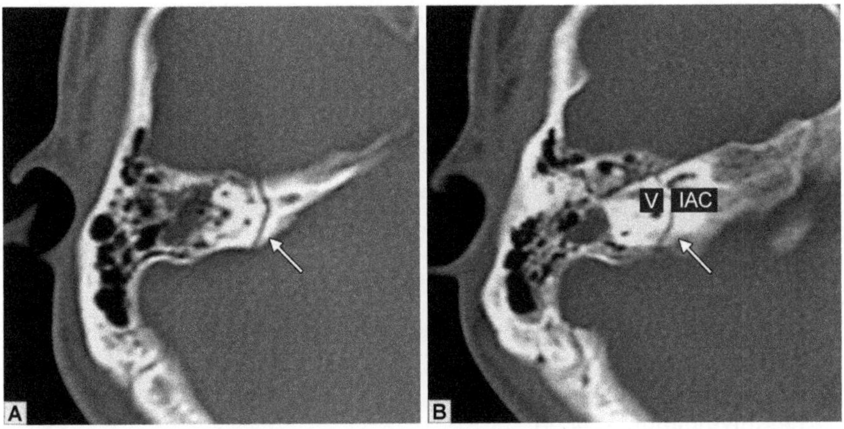

FIGS. 5A AND B: Otic capsule-violating (OCV) fracture: Axial HRCT serial images show a transverse OCV fracture (arrows) of the right temporal bone running between the internal auditory canal (IAC) and vestibule (V).

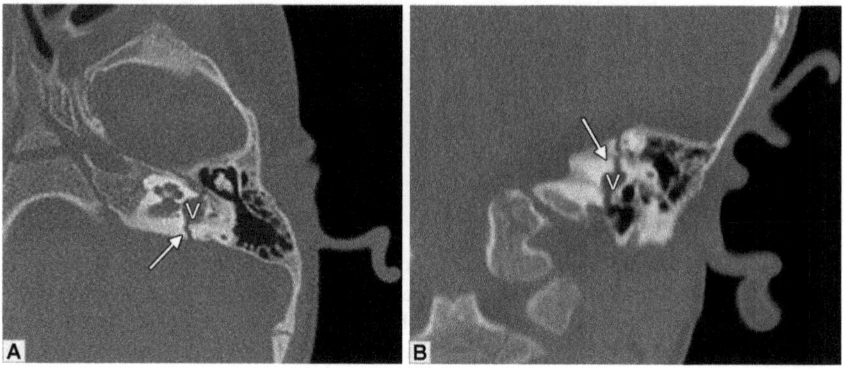

FIGS. 6A AND B: Otic capsule-violating (OCV) fracture: (A) Axial HRCT image and (B) coronal reformatted image show a transverse OCV fracture (arrows) involving the vestibule (V).

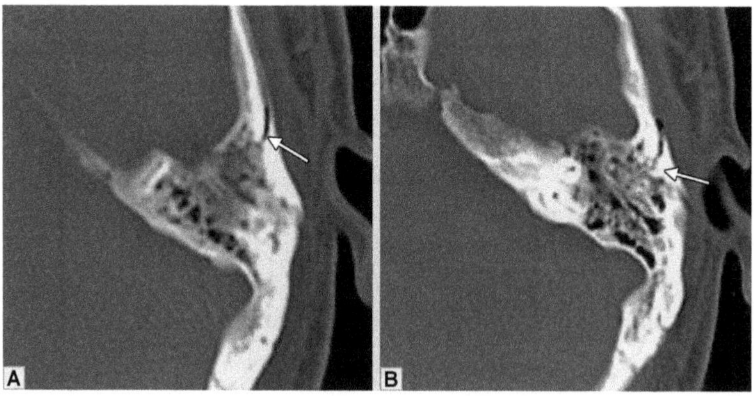

FIGS. 7A AND B: Otic capsule-sparing (OCS) fracture: Axial HRCT images show a transverse fracture of left temporal bone involving squamous part (arrow in A) and extending till mastoid air cells (arrow in B) but sparing the otic capsule.

SPECIFIC TYPES OF FRACTURES

Longitudinal Fractures (Ulrich)

- Fracture line is parallel to the long axis of the petrous temporal bone (**Figs. 2A** and **B**).
- Longitudinal fractures occur secondary to lateral impact to the skull.
- These lead to conductive hearing loss (CHL), the causes of which may be ossicular injury (**Fig. 8A** and **B**), tympanic membrane rupture or hemotympanum (**Fig. 9**).
- Otic capsule (labyrinth) involvement is uncommon.
- These are further classified into anterior and posterior subtype.

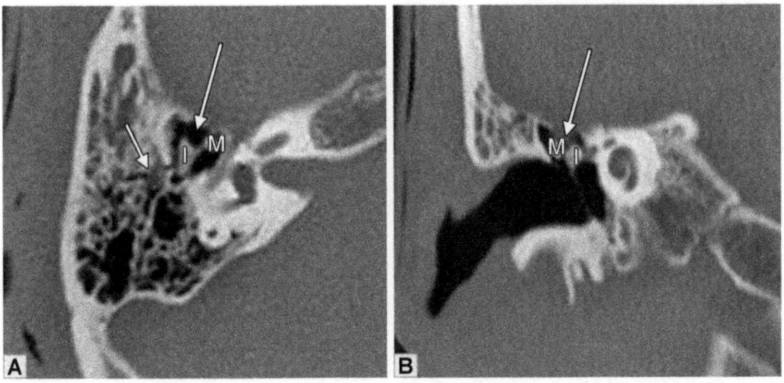

FIGS. 8A AND B: Ossicular disruption: (A) Axial and (B) coronal reformatted HRCT images show a longitudinal fracture of right temporal bone (small arrow) extending into the middle ear cavity. The ice-cream cone appearance of the malleus (M) and incus (I) is disrupted (long arrows) signifying ossicular injury.

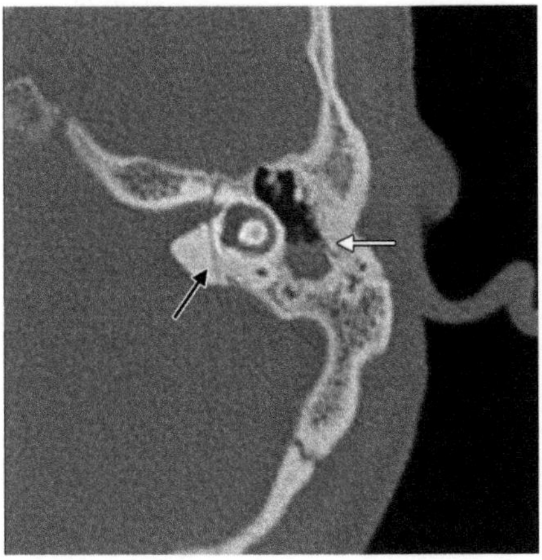

FIG. 9: Hemotympanum: Axial HRCT image shows a transverse fracture (black arrow) running through internal auditory canal (IAC). There is a fluid level in the middle ear cavity signifying hemotympanum (white arrows). A small longitudinal fracture was seen in inferior sections (not shown) extending into middle ear cavity.

Anterior Subtype

- This is the commoner variant wherein the fracture line traverses through the anterior and/or middle part of the squamous temporal bone **(Fig. 10)**.
- The facture line violates the anterior wall of the external auditory canal (EAC), tegmen tympani, and genu of facial nerve canal.

Posterior Subtype (Figs. 11)

- This is less commonly seen.
- The bony structures violated by the fracture line are the posterior wall of EAC, second genu of facial nerve canal, mastoid (descending) part of facial nerve canal, squamous temporal bone, and mastoid process.
- Foramen lacerum and seldom the jugular foramen may be involved.

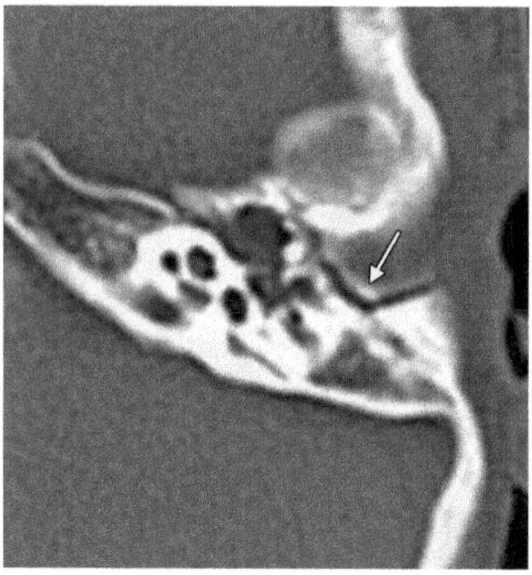

FIG. 10: Anterior subtype of longitudinal fracture: Axial HRCT image (cranial to caudal) shows a longitudinal fracture (arrow) of the left temporal bone running anteriorly to extend into middle ear cavity and mastoid air cells.

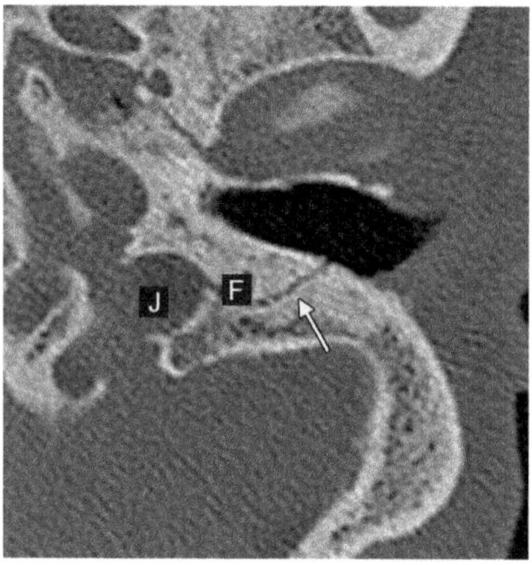

FIG. 11: Posterior subtype of longitudinal fracture: Axial HRCT image shows a longitudinal fracture (arrow) of the left temporal bone running posteriorly from posterior wall of EAC to extend across the mastoid segment of the facial nerve (F) and jugular fossa (J).

Transverse Fracture (Ulrich)

- Fracture line is perpendicular to the long axis of the petrous temporal bone (**Figs. 3** and **5** to **7**).
- Transverse fracture occurs secondary to frontal or occipital impact to the skull.
- This may lead to sensorineural hearing loss (SNHL) because of injury to the labyrinth and cochlear nerve injury[5] (**Figs. 9A** and **B**).
- Complication of facial nerve paralysis is more commonly seen compared to longitudinal fractures. The paralysis may be complete and present immediately.
- Perilymphatic fistula can occur secondary to oval window/stapedial footplate disruption.

Otic Capsule-violating Fracture (Brodie)

- Fracture line traverses the inner ear structures [cochlea, vestibule, and semicircular canals (SCCs)] (**Figs. 5** and **6**) and often through the jugular foramen and internal auditory canal (IAC).

- *Complications*: SNHL, cerebrospinal fluid (CSF) otorrhea (**Figs. 12A** to **C**), and facial nerve injury (**Figs. 13A** and **B**) (much higher incidence compared to OCS fracture patients)

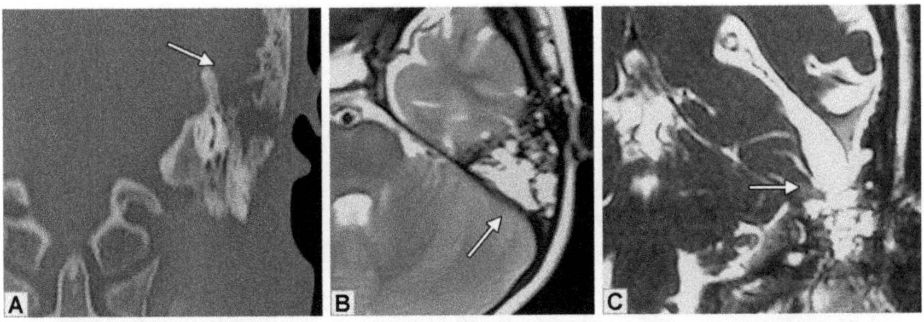

FIGS. 12A TO C: Post-traumatic CSF otorrhea: (A) Coronal reformatted HRCT image shows a fracture of roof of the left temporal bone with opacification of left mastoid air cells (arrow); (B) Turbo spin-echo (TSE) T2-weighted MRI axial image also shows opacification of left mastoid air cells with fluid (arrow). (C) Coronal 3D CISS MR image shows the communication of the intracranial CSF with the mastoid air cells through the fracture (arrow).

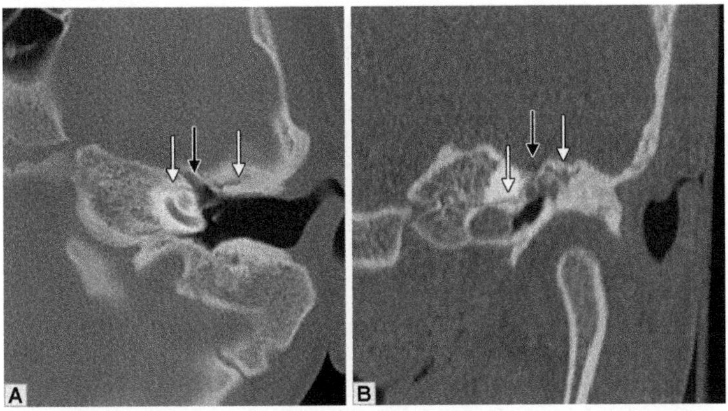

FIGS. 13A AND B: Facial nerve involvement in fracture: (A) Axial and (B) coronal reformatted HRCT images show fracture of right temporal bone (white arrows) involving the horizontal part of the facial nerve (black arrows).

Otic Capsule-sparing Fracture (Brodie)

- Fracture line spares the inner ear structures (**Figs. 7A** and **B**) and typically involve the mastoid air cells, EAC, middle ear, and tegmen tympani.
- *Complications:* CHL, intracranial injuries maybe associated (e.g., epidural hematomas and subarachnoid hemorrhage).

Petrous Fracture (Ishman and Friedland)

- Fracture line extends to the petrous apex or the labyrinth/otic capsule.
- *Complication*: CSF otorrhea, facial nerve injury.

Nonpetrous Fracture (Ishman and Friedland)

- Fracture line may involve the middle ear and mastoid.
- *Complication*: CHL
- Petrous apex or labyrinth/otic capsule are not involved.
- Multiple fractures may also be seen on the same side (**Figs. 14A** and **B**).

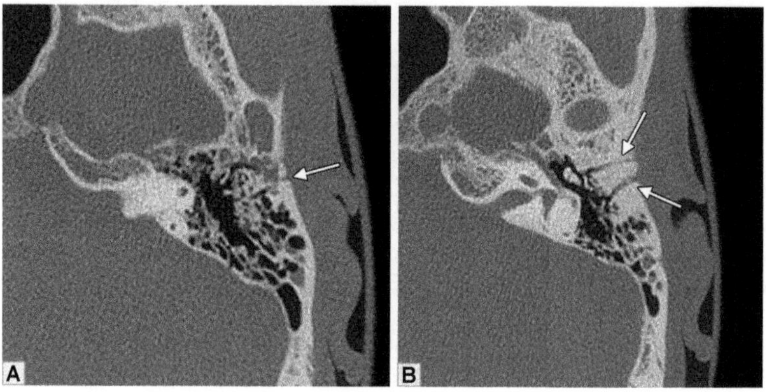

FIGS. 14A AND B: Multiple fractures: Serial axial HRCT images shows two transverse fractures of left temporal bone. The fractures start at a common external point (arrow in A) and bifurcate into two separate transverse lines inferiorly (arrows in B). Both the fractures reach up to the middle ear cavity.

NORMAL VARIANTS MIMICKING FRACTURES

Several normal structures can mimic fractures, and for obvious reasons it is important to make the distinction.

Cochlear Cleft

- It is a narrow curvilinear structure extending from the cochlea toward the promontory (**Fig. 15**).
- It is commonly seen in infants and children and is less frequently seen in adults.[5]
- It may mimic a fracture line or rarified bone in otosclerosis.

Petromastoid Canal (Fig. 16)

- *Synonym*: Subarcuate canal
- This canal connects the mastoid antrum with the cranial cavity
- *Contents*: Subarcuate artery and vein.
- It is seen in superior sections on axial CT scans and lies between anterior and posterior limbs of superior SCC.
- Its diameter is around 0.5 mm.

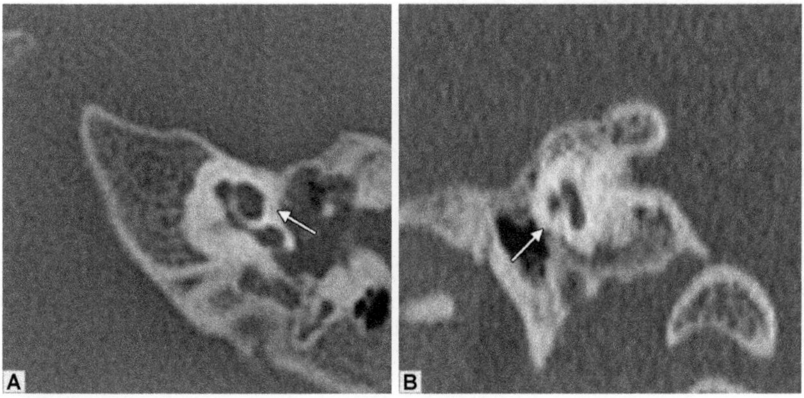

FIGS. 15A AND B: Cochlear cleft: (A) Axial and (B) oblique sagittal HRCT images reveal a thin linear lucency (arrow) extending from the apical turn of cochlea. This can mimic fracture lines.

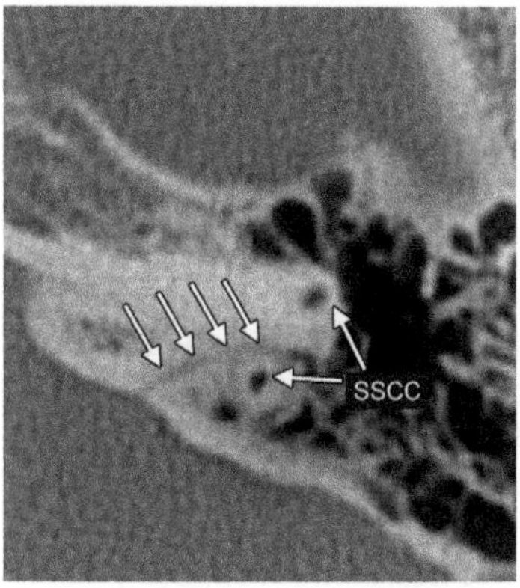

FIG. 16: Petromastoid canal: Axial HRCT image shows petromastoid canal (arrows) on left side mimicking a fracture.

Cochlear Aqueduct (Fig. 17)

- It is a narrow bony canal which runs in the same direction as the inner auditory canal and connects the perilymph with the subarachnoid space.
- It is seen in sections more caudal than the IAC.
- It can be a potential route of spread of infection from CSF to the inner ear and vice versa.
- Postmeningitic labyrinthitis ossificans is a complication of such spread of infection.

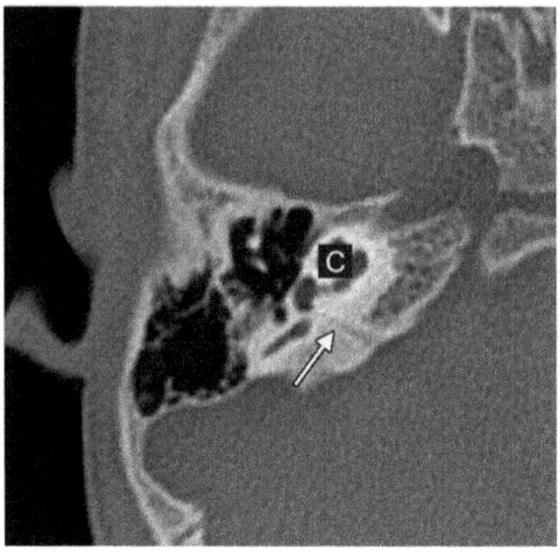

FIG. 17: Cochlear aqueduct: Axial HRCT image shows cochlear (C) aqueduct on right side (arrow) mimicking a fracture.

SPECIFIC SITUATIONS

External Auditory Canal Trauma

Fractures of anterior wall of the EAC are a result of impaction injury by the mandibular condyle into the posterior wall of the temporomandibular joint. Complications include EAC stenosis, if untreated.

Ossicular Injuries

- Fracture is less common than dislocation or subluxations of ossicles.
- It is seen more often associated with longitudinal fractures.
- *Complication*: CHL
- Ossicular injuries should be suspected in CHL persisting >2 months after trauma.
- *Types of dislocation*: Incudomalleolar joint separation (seen as "ice cream" fallen off "cone"), incudostapedial joint separation (most common), dislocation of the incus, dislocation of the malleoincudal complex, and stapediovestibular dislocation.
- The incus is most prone to fracture, as it has less ligamentous support.

Facial Nerve Injury

- The facial nerve is injured in 7% of patients with a temporal bone fracture.[1,6]
- It is more commonly associated with transverse fractures (up to 50%) compared to longitudinal fractures (10–20%).
- Most injuries occur in the labyrinthine segment, in the region of the geniculate ganglion (**Figs. 12A** and **B**). Involvement of the tympanic or mastoid segments is less frequent.
- Manifest as immediate complete paralysis (often secondary to partial or complete nerve transection, compression by bony fragments) or delayed paralysis (secondary to contusion/edema of the nerve or hematoma in the canal).
- Radiological detection of bony spicules impinging upon the facial nerve canal is an indication for urgent decompressive surgery.

Cochlear Injury

- Trauma to cochlea is complicated by SNHL.
- Cochlear concussion is a form of injury where cochlear injury might result in SNHL without any obvious temporal bone fracture.
- Oblique multiplanar reformats (MPR) images in a plane parallel to the long and short axis of petrous temporal are essential adjuncts to routine axial images.

Vestibular Injury

- Main manifestations of injury to vestibule, vestibular nerve, and vestibular aqueduct is vertigo.
- Similar to cochlear concussion, vestibular concussion may cause vertigo even in those fractures which are OCS.
- Vestibular concussion and perilymphatic fistula are the causes of post-traumatic vertigo without any evident bony injury.

Semicircular Canals Trauma

- Semicircular canals trauma also results in vertigo.
- All three SCCs should be evaluated individually by reformatted images in oblique coronal and sagittal planes in addition to routine axial images.

TEACHING POINTS

- Multidetector CT is useful in identifying injury to crucial structures and predicting possible complications.
- Complications of temporal bone injury include hearing loss (sensorineural or conductive), vertigo, perilymph fistula, facial nerve palsy, vascular injury, and CSF otorrhea.
- While interpreting CT images, a more meticulous assessment of all critical structures is advisable, instead of subclassification into transverse or longitudinal.
- Computed tomography findings suggestive of concealed temporal bone fracture include soft tissue density in the EAC, middle ear, or mastoid; air-fluid level in sphenoid sinus; and pneumocephalus adjacent to the temporal bone.
- In head injury, soft tissue opacification of mastoid air cells on CT should be considered as an indicator of a temporal bone fracture.

REFERENCES

1. Brodie HA, Thompson TC. Management of complications from 820 temporal bone fractures. Am J Otol. 1997;18(2):188-97.

2. Zayas JO, Feliciano YZ, Hadley CR, Gomez AA, Vidal JA. Temporal Bone Trauma and the Role of Multidetector CT in the Emergency Department. Radiographics. 2011;31:1741-55.
3. Ulrich K. Verletzungen des Gehorlorgansbel Schadel basis frakturen (Ein Histologisch und Klinissche Studie). Acta Otolaryngol Suppl. 1926;6:1-150.
4. Ishman SL, Friedland DR. Temporal bone fractures: traditional classification and clinical relevance. Laryngoscope. 2004;114(10):1734-41.
5. Kurihara YY, Fujikawa A, Tachizawa N, Takaya M, Ikeda H, Starkey J. Temporal bone trauma: typical CT and MRI appearances and important points for evaluation. Radiographics 2020;40(4):1148-62.
6. Lantos JE, Leeman K, Weidman EK, Dean KE, Peng T, Pearlman AN. Imaging of Temporal Bone Trauma: A Clinicoradiologic Perspective. Neuroimaging Clin N Am. 2019;29(1):129-43.

24 Reporting Template with Illustrative Cases

(Trauma and Fibrous Dysplasia)

Smita Manchanda

REPORTING TEMPLATE

Right *Left*

- External ear:
  - Bony canal
  - Tympanic membrane (TM)
  - Soft tissue/fluid
- Middle ear:
  - Soft tissue/fluid/hemotympanum
  - Ossicles:
    - Malleus
    - Incus
    - Stapes
  - Incudomalleal articulation
  - Incudostapedial articulation
  - Stapediovestibular articulation
- Facial nerve canal:
  - Labyrinthine segment
  - Tympanic segment
  - Mastoid segment
- Semicircular canal (SCC):
  - Lateral SCC
  - Superior SCC
  - Posterior SCC
- Vestibule
- Cochlea
- Internal auditory canal (IAC)
- *Mastoids*: Soft tissue/fluid/hemomastoid
- Squamous temporal
- Petrous apex
- Sphenoid sinus
- Any other finding

Key: A: Absent; CF: Comminuted fracture; D: Dislocation; Di: Disruption; F: Fluid; HM: Hemomastoid; HT: Hemotympanum; I: Intact; LF: Linear fracture; N: Normal; OF: Oblique fracture; P: Present; ST: Soft tissue; TF: Transverse fracture

IMPRESSION

Classify fractures as (see Chapter 19):

- Longitudinal/Transverse/Mixed
- Otic capsule-violating/Otic capsule-sparing
- Petrous/Nonpetrous

CASE 1 (FIGS. 1A TO F)

An 8-year-old female with left-sided ear pain post-trauma.

Longitudinal fracture of left temporal bone reaching lateral wall of middle ear cavity (**Fig. 1B**).

	Right	*Left*
• External ear:		
○ Bony canal	N	N
○ TM	N	N
○ Soft tissue/fluid	–	–
• Middle ear:		
○ Soft tissue/fluid/hemotympanum	N	N
○ Ossicles:		
– Malleus	I	I
– Incus	I	I
– Stapes	I	I
○ Incudomalleal articulation	I	I
○ Incudostapedial articulation	I	I
○ Stapediovestibular articulation	I	I
• Facial nerve canal:		
○ Labyrinthine segment	I	I
○ Tympanic segment	I	I
○ Mastoid segment	I	I
• SCC:		
○ Lateral SCC	I	I
○ Superior SCC	I	I
○ Posterior SCC	I	I
• Vestibule	I	I
• Cochlea	I	I
• IAC	N	N
• Mastoids:		
○ Soft tissue/fluid/hemomastoid	N	N
• Squamous temporal (**Figs. 1C** and **D**)	N	LF
• Petrous apex	N	N
• Sphenoid sinus	N	N

Key: A: Absent; CF: Comminuted fracture; D: Dislocation; Di: Disruption; F: Fluid; HM: Hemomastoid; HT: Hemotympanum; I: Intact; LF: Linear fracture; N: Normal; OF: Oblique fracture; P: Present; ST: Soft tissue; TF: Transverse fracture

Impression

Left longitudinal and otic capsule-sparing, nonpetrous fracture of the temporal bone.

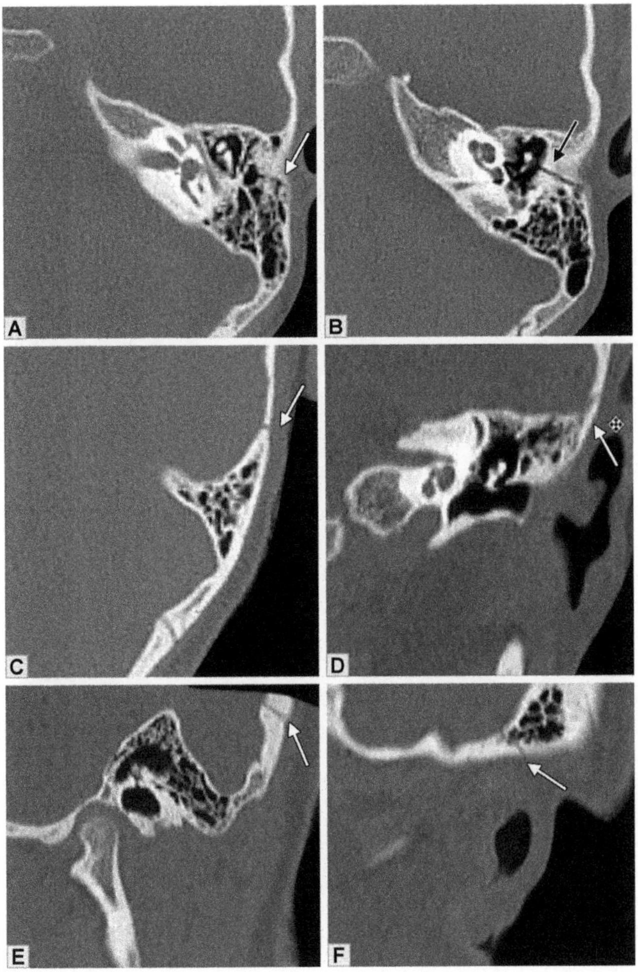

FIGS. 1A TO F: HRCT: (A to C) Axial (superior to inferior); (D) Coronal; (E and F) Left sagittal.

CASE 2 (FIGS. 2A TO F)

A 20-year-old male with right facial nerve palsy post-trauma.

Right transverse fracture involving facial nerve canal, left longitudinal fracture (**Figs. 2A** and **B**) and fracture of lateral wall of sphenoid sinus. Bilateral hemisphenoid and hemiethmoid, right concha bullosa and left deviated nasal septum with left bony spur (**Figs. 2E** and **F**).

	Right	*Left*
• External ear:		
○ Bony canal	CF anteromed wall (**Fig. 2C**)	OF anteromed wall (**Fig. 2D**)
○ TM	N	N
○ Soft tissue/fluid	ST	ST
• Middle ear (**Fig. 2A**):		
○ Soft tissue/fluid/hemotympanum	HT	HT
○ Ossicles:		
– Malleus	I	I
– Incus	I	I
– Stapes	I	I
○ Incudomalleal articulation	I	I
○ Incudostapedial articulation	I	I
○ Stapediovestibular articulation	I	I
• Facial nerve canal:		
○ Labyrinthine segment	Di	I
○ Tympanic segment	Di (**Fig. 2A**)	I
○ Mastoid segment	I	I
• SCC:		
○ Lateral SCC	I	I
○ Superior SCC	I	I
○ Posterior SCC	I	I
• Vestibule	I	I
• Cochlea	I	I
• IAC	N	N
• Mastoids (**Fig. 2B**):		
○ Soft tissue/fluid/hemomastoid	HM	HM
• Squamous temporal	LF	N
• Petrous apex (**Fig. 2A**)	TF	N
• Sphenoid sinus	N	TF lateral wall (**Fig. 2F**)

Key: A: Absent; CF: Comminuted fracture; D: Dislocation; Di: Disruption; F: Fluid; HM: Hemomastoid; HT: Hemotympanum; I: Intact; LF: Linear fracture; N: Normal; OF: Oblique fracture; P: Present; ST: Soft tissue; TF: Transverse fracture

Impression

- Right transverse and otic capsule-violating petrous fracture involving facial nerve canal.
- Left longitudinal and otic capsule-sparing, nonpetrous fracture of the temporal bone.
- Fracture lateral wall of sphenoid sinus with fractures bilateral external auditory canals.

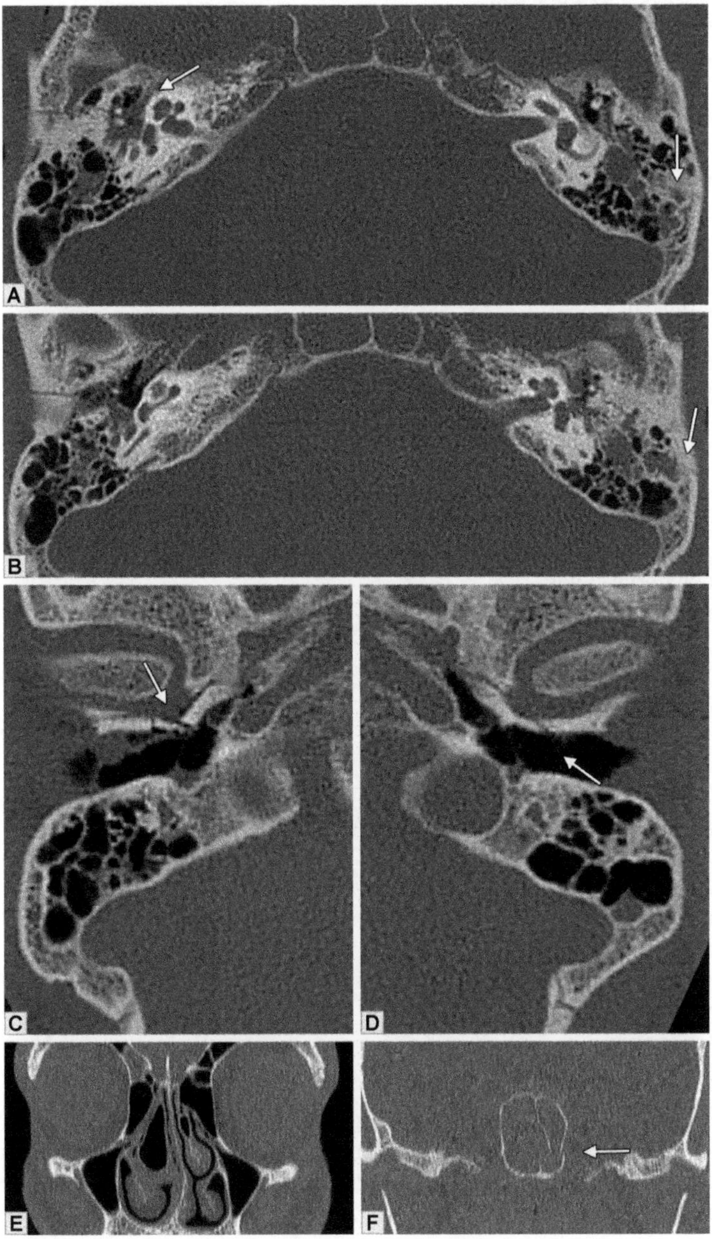

FIGS. 2A TO F: HRCT: (A and B) Axial (superior to inferior); (C and D) Axial magnified; (C) right and (D) left; (E and F) Coronal (anterior to posterior).

CASE 3 (FIGS. 3A TO F)

A 28-year-old male with right-sided hearing loss and history of trauma 1 year back.
Right labyrinthitis ossificans.

	Right	*Left*
• External ear:		
○ Bony canal	N	N
○ TM	N	N
○ Soft tissue/fluid	–	–
• Middle ear:		
○ Soft tissue/fluid/hemotympanum	N	N
○ Ossicles (**Figs. 3A, E** and **F**):		
– Malleus	D	I
– Incus	D	I
– Stapes	D	I
○ Incudomalleal articulation	Di	I
○ Incudostapedial articulation	Di	I
○ Stapediovestibular articulation	Di	I
• Facial nerve canal:		
○ Labyrinthine segment	I	I
○ Tympanic segment	I	I
○ Mastoid segment	I	I
• SCC (**Figs. 3C** and **D**):		
○ Lateral SCC	Di	I
○ Superior SCC	Di	I
○ Posterior SCC	Di	I
• Vestibule (**Figs. 3B** to **D**)	Hyperdense contents	I
• Cochlea	I	I
• IAC	N	N
• Mastoids:		
○ Soft tissue/fluid/hemomastoid	N	N
• Squamous temporal	N	N
• Petrous apex	N	N
• Sphenoid sinus	N	N

Key: A: Absent; CF: Comminuted fracture; D: Dislocation: Di: Disruption; F: Fluid; HM: Hemomastoid; HT: Hemotympanum; I: Intact; LF: Linear fracture; N: Normal; OF: Oblique fracture; P: Present; ST: Soft tissue; TF: Transverse fracture

Impression

Post-traumatic disruption of right middle ear ossicles, SCCs, and vestibule with labyrinthitis ossificans.

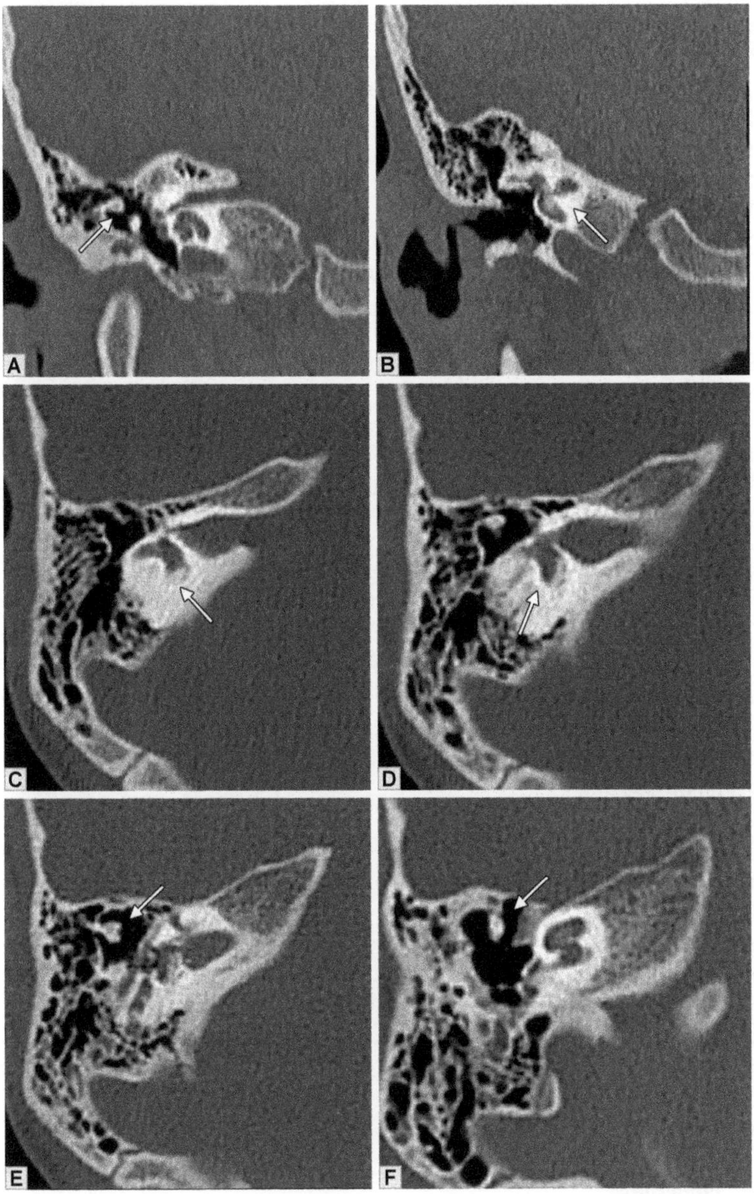

FIGS. 3A TO F: HRCT: (A and B) Coronal (anterior to posterior); (C to F) Axial (superior to inferior).

CASE 4 (FIGS. 4A TO E)

A 11-year-old girl presenting with swelling of the face since 1 year.

- Expansion and ground glass density of bilateral temporal, left sphenoid, zygomatic, maxillary bones; right hemimandible, clivus, and bilateral occipital condyles.
- Narrowing of right pterygomaxillary fissure, inferior orbital fissure, foramen ovale, foramen spinosum, and vidian nerve canal.
- Complete obliteration of the right maxillary and bilateral sphenoid sinuses (**Figs. 4D** and **E**).

	Right	*Left*
• External ear:		
○ Bony canal	N	N
○ TM	N	N
○ Soft tissue/fluid	N	N
• *Middle ear*: Narrowed by the expanding bone on right side (**Figs. 4A** and **B**)		
○ Soft tissue/fluid/hemotympanum	N	N
○ Ossicles:		
– Malleus	N	I
– Incus	N	I
– Stapes	N	I
○ Incudomalleal articulation	N	I
○ Incudostapedial articulation	N	I
○ Stapediovestibular articulation	N	I
• Facial nerve canal:		
○ Labyrinthine segment	I	I
○ Tympanic segment	I	I
○ Mastoid segment	I	I
• SCC:		
○ Lateral SCC	I	I
○ Superior SCC	I	I
○ Posterior SCC	I	I
• Vestibule	I	I
• Cochlea	I	I
• IAC	N	N
• Mastoids (**Fig. 4C**):		
○ Soft tissue/fluid/hemomastoid	***Ground glass bilaterally***	

Key: A: Absent; CF: Comminuted fracture; D: Dislocation; Di: Disruption; F: Fluid; HM: Hemomastoid; HT: Hemotympanum; I: Intact; LF: Linear fracture; N: Normal; OF: Oblique fracture; P: Present; ST: Soft tissue; TF: Transverse fracture

Impression

Expansion and ground glass density involving the base of skull and facial bones predominantly on the right side with foraminal narrowing as described s/o fibrous dysplasia.

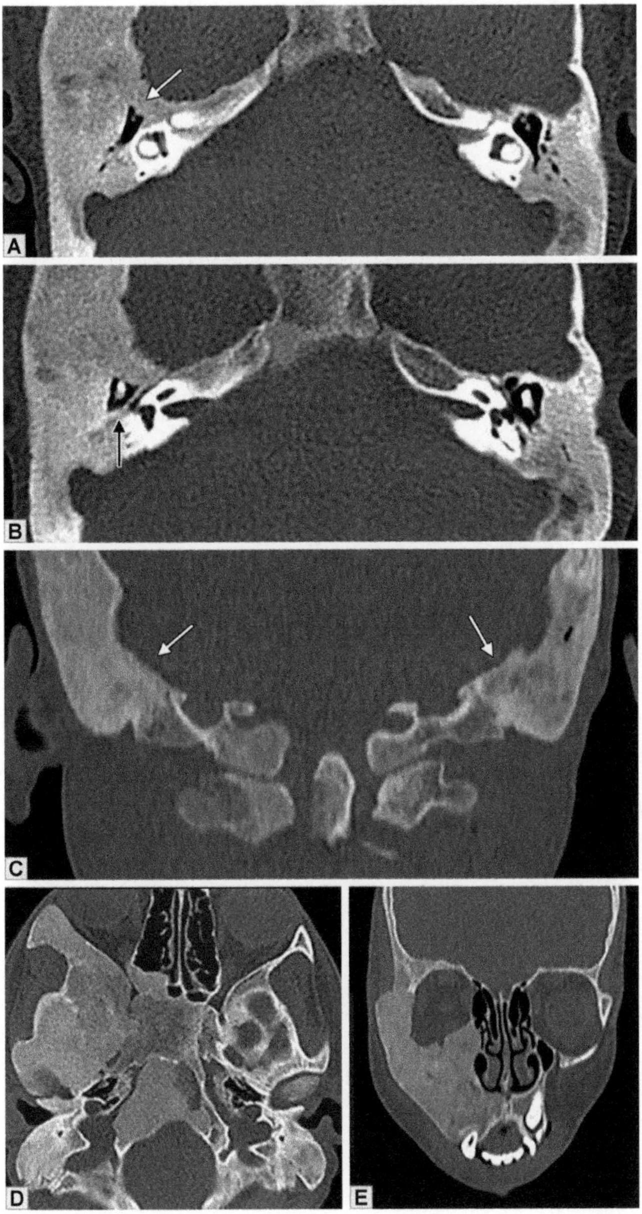

FIGS. 4A TO E: HRCT and noncontrast CT (NCCT): (A and B) Axial (superior to inferior) HRCT; (C) Coronal HRCT; (D) Axial NCCT; (E) Coronal NCCT.

8 SECTION

Clinico Radiological Approach

25

Approach to Hearing Loss

Hitesh Verma, Priyanka Naranje, Vinit Baliyan

- Hearing loss (HL) refers to reduced sensitivity for sound in speech frequencies which can normally be heard. The classification can be based on the type, degree, or pattern of HL.
- Hearing loss is the most common congenital sensory impairment with incidence of 6 in 1,000 children.[1] Diagnostic workup for HL includes a radiological assessment using computed tomography (CT) and magnetic resonance imaging (MRI) in addition to complete physical examination, laboratory testing, and genetic testing.

TYPES OF HEARING LOSS

Conductive Hearing Loss

- The pinna, external auditory canal, and middle ear transmit sound to inner ear. Any pathology in these parts will present as conductive hearing loss (CHL).
- This is a reversible type of HL and can be mostly corrected medically and/or surgically.
- The common causes of CHL are enumerated in **Table 1**.

TABLE 1 Causes of conductive hearing loss.

External ear causes	Middle ear causes
Waxs	Otitis media
Otitis externa	Middle ear mass (benign or malignant)
Malformation of pinna and external auditory canal (EAC)	Foreign body in middle ear
Mass/foreign body in EAC	Middle ear malformations
Tympanic membrane perforation	

Sensorineural Hearing Loss

- The cochlea converts sound energy into electrical signal and cochlear nerve transmits electrical signal to brain.
- Abnormality of cochlea and cochlear nerve will lead to sensorineural hearing loss (SNHL).
- This is mostly permanent and cannot be corrected medically and surgically.
- Causes of SNHL can be congenital or acquired (such as aging, trauma, ototoxicity, infection, and noise-induced) (**Figs. 1** and **2**).

Mixed Hearing Loss

- When a patient has a combination of CHL and SNHL, it is referred to as mixed HL.

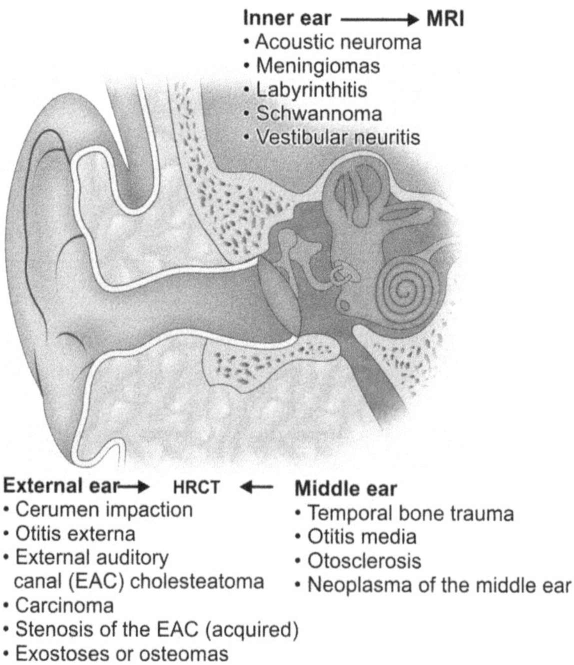

FIG. 1: Causes of hearing loss—causes in the ear.

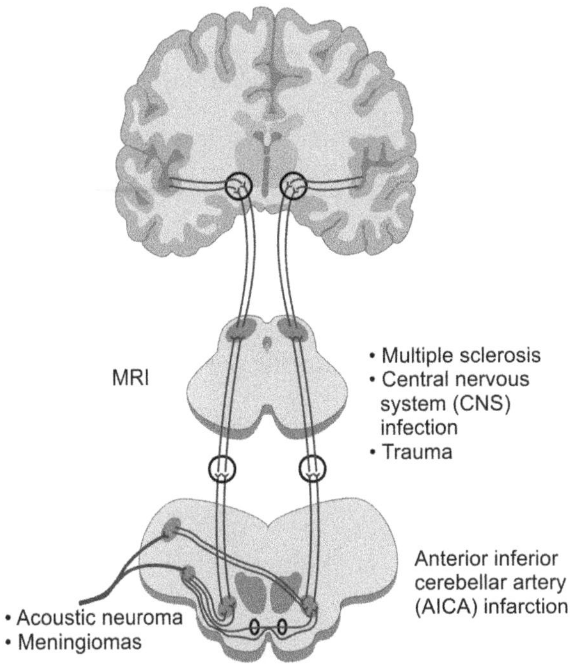

FIG. 2: Causes of hearing loss—central hearing pathway.

DEGREE OF HEARING LOSS

To document amount of HL, it is divided into various degrees; from mild to profound type based on *audiometry* (**Table 2**).

TABLE 2 **Degrees of hearing loss.**

Normal	Up to 25 dB
Mild	26–40 dB
Moderate	41–55 dB
Moderate-severe	56–70 dB
Severe	71–90 dB
Profound	>91 dB

(dB: decibel)

PATTERN OF HEARING LOSS

The graphic illustration of pattern of HL is an audiogram. If the HL lies in speech frequencies, it is known as low frequency HL. High frequency HL involves high tones.

DIAGNOSIS

- *History and examination*: It helps in establishing the diagnosis several times.
- *Hearing evaluation by clinical methods*: This can be done by various tests, e.g., finger rubbing test, speech test, and tuning fork tests.
- *Audiological tests*: These can be subjective or objective tests.

Subjective Tests

- *Pure tone audiometry*:
    - The pure tone is generated by electronic device (audiometer); and the results are plotted in form of graph called audiogram.
    - An audiogram helps in calculating degree, type, and pattern of HL (**Figs. 3A** to **C**).
- *Speech audiometry*: This test measures patient's capability to hear and understand speech.

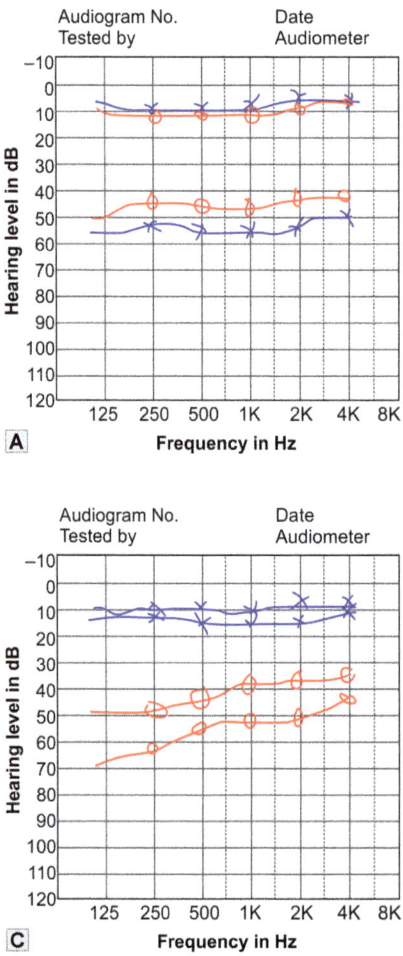

FIGS. 3A TO C: Pure tone audiometry: (A) The air conduction threshold is approximately 55 dB and bone conduction threshold is <25 dB on both side and AB gap is approximately 30 dB on both side (suggestive of bilateral CHL). Red color is for right and blue color is for left side; (B) Right side is normal as both air and bone conduction tracing is >25 dB. The air and bone conduction tracing is below 25 dB with <10 dB AB gap with sloping at higher frequencies (suggestive of left SNHL); (C) Left side (blue lines) normal hearing. Right side (red color) graph is showing dip in both air and bone conduction threshold with AB gap is >10 dB. The tracing shows dip more at low frequencies (suggestive of low frequency mixed hearing loss).

Objective Tests

- *Impedance audiometry*:
    - The compliance of middle ear at different pressure levels and position of tympanic membrane is assessed by amount of sound energy reflected back.
    - The hearing threshold, cochlear, and retrocochlear pathology can be assessed with acoustic reflex test.
- *Electrocochleography*: The electric activity of cochlea and cochlear nerve is recorded by placing electrode on promontory.
    - Brainstem evoked response audiometry (BERA): The electric activity of auditory pathway is elicited by auditory stimulation of inner ear.
    - Otoacoustic emission (OAE):
        - The sound generated by outer hair cells is checked by placing highly sensitive microphone in external auditory canal.
        - This test helps in assessing cochlear status.

IMAGING

- Imaging plays a crucial role in the diagnostic evaluation of patients with HL. The goals of imaging are:
    - Identify structural causes of HL
    - Identifying a potential surgical candidate
    - Report anatomic risk factors in the context of surgical planning
    - To check feasibility of cochlear implantation
    - Search for underlying syndromic features
- Computed tomography with high resolution and bone algorithm: Best utilized in HL related to following structures.
    - External auditory canal
    - Middle ear space including the ossicles
    - Mastoid and petrous air cell system, and the otic capsule
- *Magnetic resonance imaging*: Best utilized in HL related to following structures (retrocochlear pathology): internal auditory canal, cerebello-pontine angle, and brainstem. Gadolinium contrast should be utilized whenever there is suspicion of mass or infection.

Imaging of Conductive Hearing Loss (Tables 3 and 4)

- Conductive hearing loss is often obvious clinically and imaging studies are generally not required before intervention.
- Imaging can be valuable in cases in which the cause is uncertain.

Imaging of Sensorineural Hearing Loss (Tables 5 and 6)

- Sensorineural hearing loss may present as sudden HL and shows usually asymmetric involvement.
- When the cause is uncertain, MRI is the modality of choice. High-resolution CT (HRCT) has a complimentary role in assessment of inner ear pathology.

TABLE 3 Imaging findings in conductive hearing loss (external ear pathology).

Diseases causing conductive hearing loss	Imaging findings (HRCT)	Role of imaging
Impacted wax	• Isointense to soft tissue • No bony erosion	• Diagnosed clinically • May be detected incidentally
Otitis externa (OE)	• Thickening of the soft tissues • Bony erosion in necrotizing OE	Important role in necrotizing OE
External auditory canal (EAC) cholesteatoma	Localized soft tissue mass with bony erosion	• Difficult to distinguish from malignant neoplasm • Biopsy essential
Squamous cell carcinoma and basal cell carcinoma	• Soft tissue masses • Usually associated with bony erosion	• Extent of disease • Differential diagnosis: Necrotizing OE
Stenosis of the EAC (acquired)	Soft tissue narrowing within the EAC	• Medial extent of disease and middle ear involvement • Critical for planning of operative management
Exostoses or osteomas	Bony outgrowths within EAC	• Diagnosed clinically, imaging adjunctive • Exostoses: B/L, multiple and sessile • Osteomas: Single and pedunculated

TABLE 4 Imaging findings in conductive hearing loss (middle and internal ear pathology).

Diseases causing conductive hearing loss	Imaging findings (HRCT)	Role of imaging
Temporal bone trauma (longitudinal fractures)	Ossicular discontinuity or hemotympanum	Extent, associated facial nerve and intracranial injuries
Otosclerosis (discussed later in chapter)	Demineralization at the fissula ante fenestram	• Extent • Status of stapes
Acute otitis media	• Opacification of the middle ear (ME) and mastoid air cells • Fulminant infection causes coalescence of mastoid air cells	Only if complications suspected

Continued

Continued

Diseases causing conductive hearing loss	Imaging findings (HRCT)	Role of imaging
Chronic otitis media	Opacification of the ME erosions; specially scutum and ossicles	• Identification of erosions (cholesteatoma/unsafe disease) and complications on high-resolution CT • MRI can distinguish between fluid, thickened mucosa, and cholesteatoma
Neoplasms of the ME	• Soft tissue masses • Bone erosion may be present	Extent assessment
Glomus tympanicum	Smooth soft tissue density in the mesotympanum without involvement of the jugular foramen	
Glomus jugulare	• Erosive process at the jugular foramen, with permeative bony destruction • MRI—"salt and pepper" appearance	

TABLE 5 **Intratemporal causes of sensorineural hearing loss.**

Cause of SNHL	Imaging findings	Role of imaging
Infectious or autoimmune labyrinthitis	Diffuse enhancement of the membranous labyrinth	May progress to fibrosis or ossification—T2WI show reduction in fluid volume
Intracochlear or intralabyrinthine schwannoma	Intense and discrete enhancing mass lesion	Critical for diagnosis
Vestibular neuritis	VIIIth nerve enhancement in the absence of tumor	To confirm the diagnosis and rule out other possibilities
Cochlear otosclerosis	Discussed later in this chapter	HRCT for extent and status of stapes
Labyrinthitis ossificans (LO)	Discussed later in this chapter	
Ménière's disease/ idiopathic endolymphatic hydrops	• CT: Small or nonvisualization of vestibular aqueduct • MRI: Can show lack of a visible endolymphatic duct and sac	CT and MRI may identify the site of impaired endolymphatic flow
Cochlear nerve deficiency (CND)	Unilateral/bilateral, absent or hypoplastic cochlear nerve	Allows visualization of the cochlear nerve

TABLE 6 Intracranial causes of sensorineural hearing loss.

Intracranial extra-axial lesions		
Acoustic neuroma (85% of CPA masses)	• Enhancing extra-axial mass with IAC extension (Ice-Cream cone) • IAC may be enlarged • Bilateral schwannomas—neurofibromatosis type II	• Critical for diagnosis and extent • Surgical planning
Meningiomas	Enhancing extra-axial mass with dural attachment in the posterior fossa	Critical for diagnosis and differentiation from neuroma
Neurosarcoidosis	Nodular leptomeningitis may involve the IAC	Helps to rule out other causes of hearing loss
Superficial siderosis	Rim of hypointensity over the cerebellum and brainstem on T2-weighted images	Diagnosis of condition and underlying abnormality
Intracranial intra-axial lesions		
AICA infarction	Infarcts of the lateral pons	Indispensable for diagnosis
Multiple sclerosis	Demyelinating plaques of the pons or medulla	Imaging is crucial for diagnosis and disease progression and therapeutic response
CNS infections	Abscesses or granulomas within the central auditory pathway	
Trauma	• Otic capsule disruption • Perilymphatic fistula-increased signal adjacent to the oval window on T2-weighted image, air density within the labyrinth on CT	• High-resolution CT is critical in evaluation of otic capsule disruption • Clinical suspicion usually outweighs imaging for decision making in perilymphatic fistula

SPECIFIC CONDITIONS

Most conditions enlisted in the **Tables 3** to **6** have been discussed elsewhere in the book. Few miscellaneous conditions are detailed below.

Labyrinthitis Ossificans

- Labyrinthitis ossificans (LO) is the most common cause of acquired SNHL in children.[2]
- It refers to pathological ossification of the membranous labyrinth as a consequence of insult to the inner ear (also see Chapters 20 and 21).

- *Causes include:*
  - Infectious/inflammatory (bacterial meningitis, CSOM most common)
  - Trauma
  - Autoimmune
  - Leukemia, tumors, and vascular occlusion
- *High-resolution CT*:
  - Cochlea and semicircular canals (SCCs) (especially lateral SCC) are mostly affected; vestibular ossification is seen much less commonly.
  - In the cochlea, scala tympani of the basal turn is first to be involved; especially around the round window.
  - Increased density of cochlea in early stages.
  - Indistinctness of endosteum of basal turn of cochlea.
  - Subsequently, irregularity, sclerosis, and eventually obliteration of cochlear lumen are seen (**Figs. 4** and **5**).
  - Semicircular canals show similar changes (**Figs. 6A** and **B**).

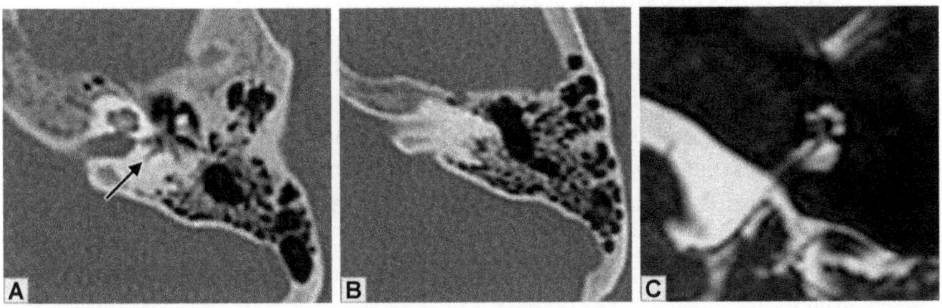

FIGS. 4A TO C: Labyrinthitis ossificans: A 26-year-old female with SNHL. (A to B) HRCT axial section inferior to superior and (C) axial MRI CISS sequence reveal normal cochlea with nonvisualized, sclerosed semicircular canals (SCCs) and vestibule. Only remnants of the SCCs and vestibule are seen on CT (arrows)—likely in fibrous stage, hence, not visualized on MRI.

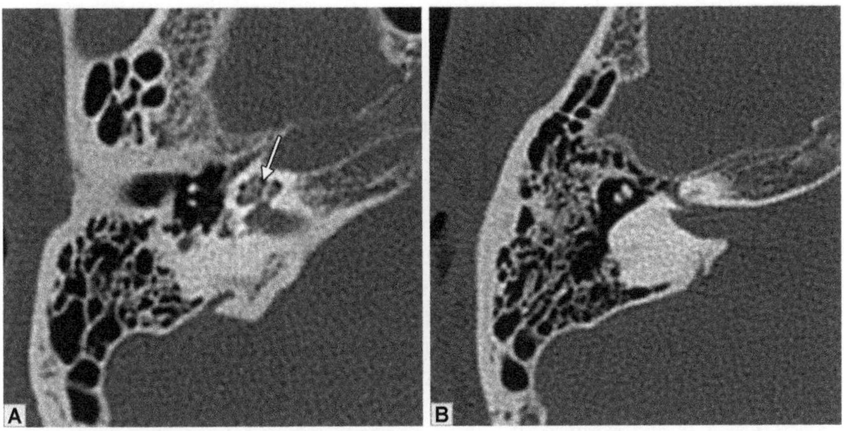

FIGS. 5A AND B: Labyrinthitis ossificans: A 26-year-old male; early ossification in the cochlea (white arrow) with obliterated semicircular canals (SCCs).

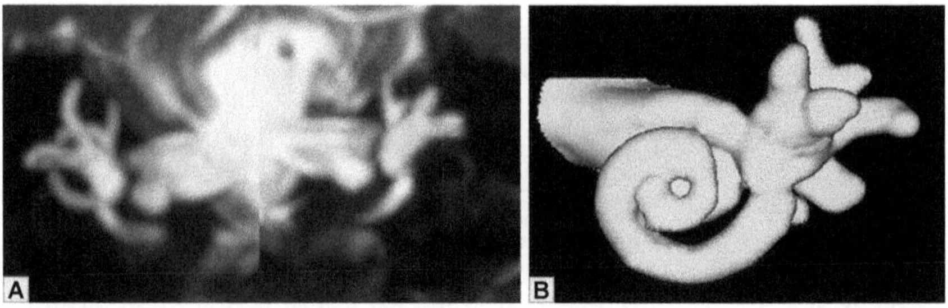

FIGS. 6A AND B: Labyrinthitis ossificans involving the semicircular canals (SCCs): (A) Coronal reconstructions and (B) 3D reconstruction of FIESTA sequence showing bilateral but asymmetric "truncated" appearance of the SCCs (left more severe than right).

- *Magnetic resonance imaging*:
  - More sensitive than CT as it detects the changes in the fibrous stages, even before onset of ossifying stages.
  - Bright fluid signal on T2-weighted imaging (T2WI) is absent in affected inner ear structures. It is best seen on CISS/FIESTA (constructive interference in steady state/fast imaging employing steady-state acquisition) sequence; although also apparent on FSE (fast spin-echo) T2WI.
- *Stages*: LO involves inflammation of the perilymphatic spaces with relative sparing of endolymphatic spaces. Pathologically, the evolution is divided in three stages:
  - First stage (acute): Purulent or serofibrinous exudates in perilymphatic space
  - Second stage (fibrous): Fibroblastic proliferation and fibrosis
  - Third stage: Osteoid deposition
- Labyrinthitis ossificans is a relative contraindication to cochlear implant.

Cochlear Otosclerosis

Synonym: Otospongiosis

- Cochlear otosclerosis (CO) represents idiopathic sclerosis of parts of the bony labyrinth.
- *Pathology:* It results from partial replacement of normal dense endochondral bone by spongy, vascular haversian bone (**Flowchart 1**).
- *Cause*: It is a multifactorial disorder of the bone, resulting due to abnormal bone reabsorption, new bone deposition, and vascular proliferation and implicated to have genetic and environmental causes.[3]
- It usually presents in adults in second to fourth decade and show a female predilection.
- Hearing loss can be conductive, sensorineural, or mixed types and often bilateral in 80–85% of cases.[4] Progressive CHL with normal tympanic membrane and no middle ear infection is a typical presentation. "*Schwartze sign*" representing a pink tinge on promontory on otoscopic examination is also described. Clinically, superior SCC bone dehiscence may mimic otosclerosis.

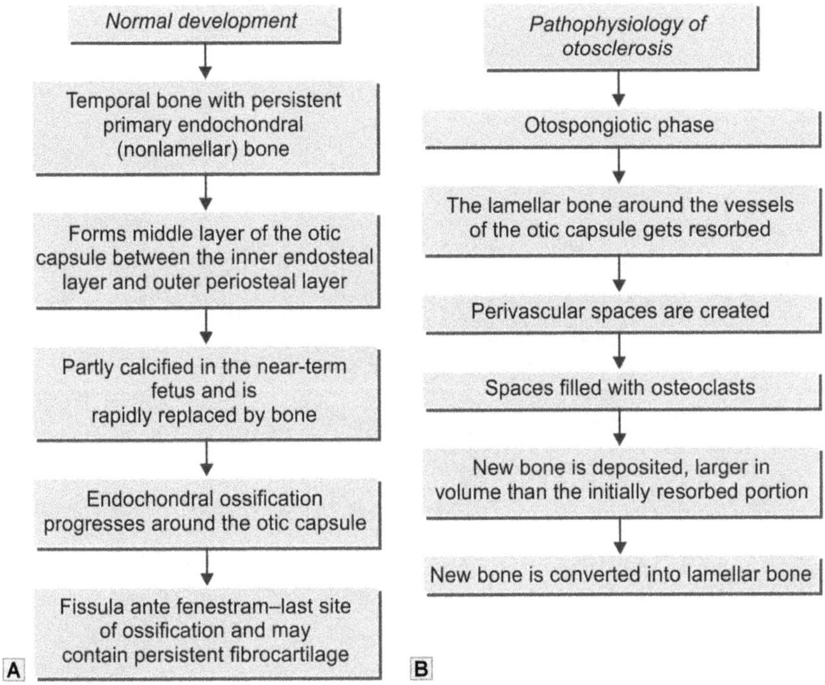

FLOWCHART 1: (A) Normal development and (B) pathophysiology of cochlear otosclerosis.

- The condition is slowly progressive and has a remitting-relapsing course.
- High-resolution CT is the investigation of choice (**Figs. 7A** to **F**).
- Magnetic resonance imaging is useful to assess the membranous labyrinth prior to cochlear implant. MRI also has a role to evaluate vascularity hence activity of the disease and cranial nerve involvement.

Types/Sites of Involvement

Fenestral Otosclerosis (Majority of Cases)

Involves oval window—

- *Sites of involvement*:
  - *Fissula ante fenestram*: It is located anteromedial to the oval window, and represents a cleft of fibrocartilaginous tissue that runs from the oval window to the cochleariform process. It is the most frequently affected site (95%).[5]
  - Rest of the otic capsule (49–60%)[4]
  - Round window niche (30%)
  - Stapes footplate (12–15%)
- *Phases*:
  - *Active phase*: Demineralization first anterior to oval window, then extends to foot plate of stapes causing its thickening and fixation. Facial

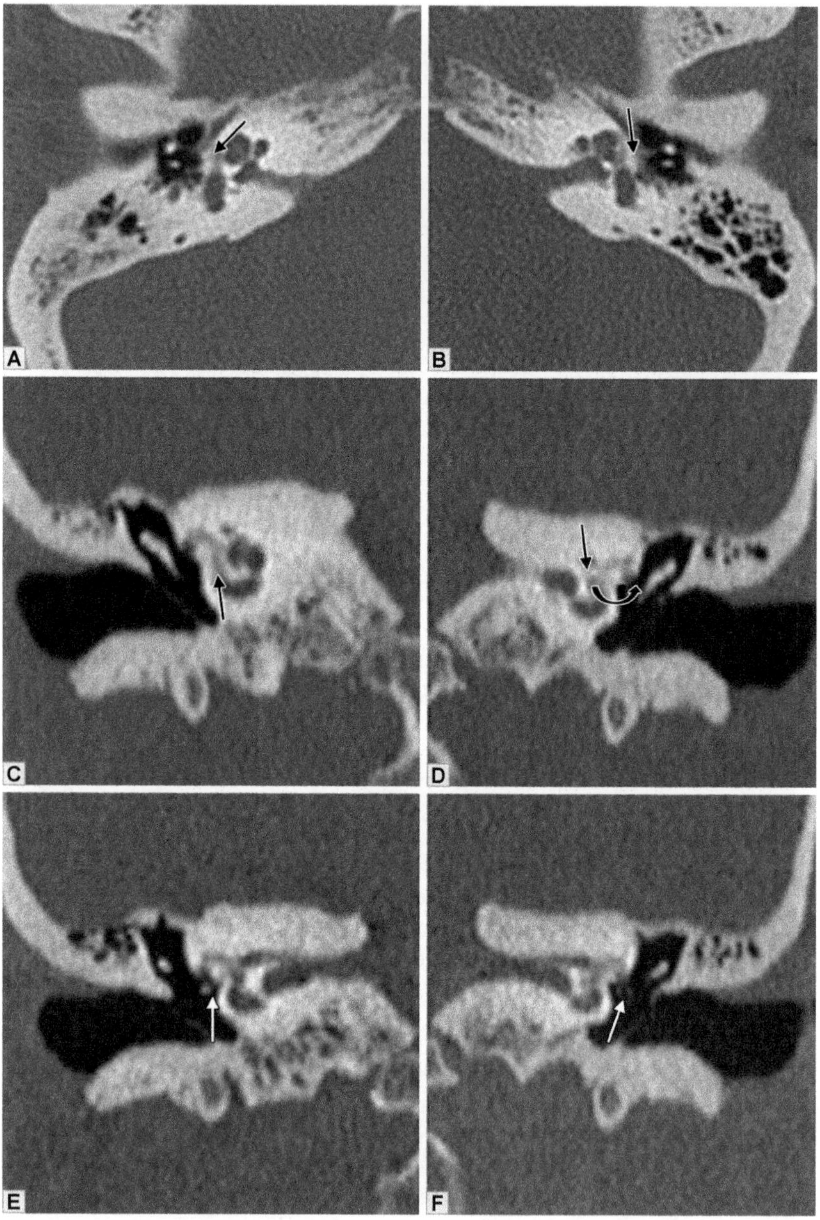

FIGS. 7A TO F: Otosclerosis: A 58-year-old male. (A and B) Axial HRCT sections showing sclerosis in the characteristic location of the fissula ante fenestram (anterior to oval window). The changes are more marked on the left side with cochlear involvement also; (C and D) Coronal HRCT sections reveal bilateral sclerosis just anterior to the oval window (curved arrow) with extension into basal turn of cochlea (arrows); (E and F) More posterior coronal sections show stapedial thickening and sclerosis. Bilateral fenestral and retrofenestral sclerosis: Stage: 2A.

Courtesy: Dr Barun Bagga.

nerve canal, cochlear promontory, and round window niche may also be involved, in which cases stapes surgery may not significantly improve hearing impairment.
  - During remission there is sclerosis and results in CHL.
  - Obliterative fenestral otosclerosis: It is seen when there is complete obliteration of the oval window. It is classified as three types:
    - Type 1: Thickening of entire footplate filling the oval window niche
    - Type 2: Bony overgrowth at the margins of oval window
    - Type 3: Footplate thickening and marginal overgrowth

Retrofenestral or Cochlear Otosclerosis

- It represents demineralization of cochlear capsule and is often seen in combination with fenestral otosclerosis and results in mixed type of HL and tinnitus.
- CT: *"Double ring effect"* due to confluence of spongiotic foci/extensive demineralization within the cochlear capsule in a ring-like fashion is seen on CT (**Fig. 8**). Lucent foci are seen disrupting the normally uniform border of the otic capsule. A lucent cavity may be seen anterior to IAC. Sclerosis develops later.
- On MRI, T1 and T2 intermediate signal in pericochlear and perilabyrinthine regions may be seen, and contrast enhancement in the active phase (**Fig. 9**). Loss of T2 hyperintense signal in membranous labyrinth due to fibrosis or bone deposition may also be noted.

Grading System

Symons and Fanning CT-based grading system is the most commonly followed system.[3,6]

- *Grade 1*: Only fenestral involvement
  - Spongiotic/sclerotic
  - CT findings: Thickened stapes footplate
  - Round window/oval window decalcified, narrowed/enlarged

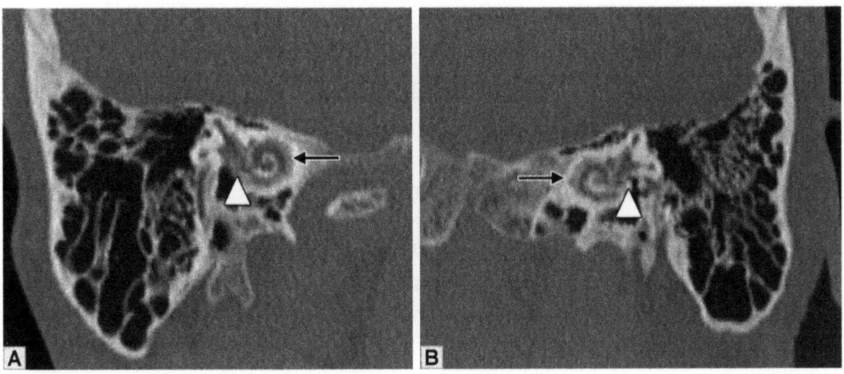

FIGS. 8A AND B: *Double-ring/Halo sign* in cochlea (arrows) with vestibular involvement (arrowheads) in a case of **cochlear otosclerosis**.

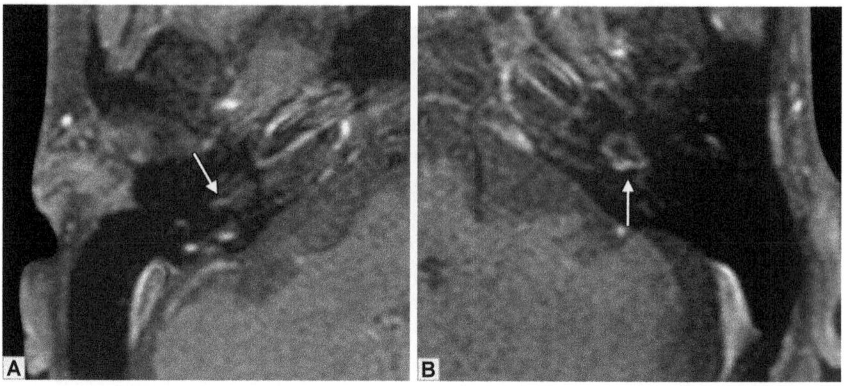

FIGS. 9A AND B: *Perilabyrinthine enhancement* along the cochlea bilaterally (arrows) in a case of **cochlear otosclerosis**.

- *Grade 2*: Localized cochlear disease (with or without fenestral involvement)
  - Basal turn of cochlea
  - Middle/apical turns
  - Both sites involved
- *Grade 3*: Entire cochlea involved: (Differentiation from grade 2C: In grade 2 the involvement is patchy, whereas it is diffuse in grade 3). As CT severity increases, the severity of SNHL increases.

Management

- *Medical management*: Fluorides and bisphosphonates
- Surgical:
  - *Fenestral otosclerosis*: Stapedectomy with stapes prosthesis is performed.
  - Cochlear implantation: Best treatment option in cases with severe to profound SNHL with diffuse cochlear involvement.
- Complication of stapedial surgery seen on CT (also see Chapter 21)
  - Displacement of the prosthesis
  - Perilymphatic fistula
  - Ossicular necrosis, or resorption
  - Air in the vestibule

Differential Diagnosis of Cochlear Otosclerosis

- *Cochlear cleft*: Commonly seen in children as a small space in the otic capsule, mimics fenestral otosclerosis
- *Osteogenesis imperfecta*: More extensive demineralization along the otic capsule
- *Tympanosclerosis*: Chronic otitis media resulting in fixation of stapes footplate
- Labyrinthitis ossificans, rheumatoid arthritis, otosyphilis, Paget disease, and ankylosing spondylitis could also mimic otosclerosis.

CONGENITAL HEARING LOSS

- Most causes of congenital CHL are due to bony anomalies within the middle or inner ear. HRCT of the temporal bones is the imaging study of choice for evaluation.
- Congenital SNHL is a common birth defect.[7]
- High-resolution CT reveals many types of bony inner ear malformations and takes less time to perform, requiring a shorter period of sedation.
- Magnetic resonance imaging provides better visualization of the membranous labyrinth and the ability to evaluate for cochlear nerve hypoplasia or aplasia (**Table 7**).

TABLE 7 **Imaging findings in congenital hearing loss.**

Diseases causing hearing loss	Imaging findings	Role of imaging
Conductive:		
Congenital aural atresia	• Atretic EAC • Ossicular chain anomalies • Inner ear abnormalities • Middle ear space abnormality • Abnormal course of the facial nerve • Pneumatization of mastoid	• Prognosis • Patient selection for surgery • Decrease risk for vascular/neural injury during reconstructive surgery
Congenital ossicular abnormalities	• Disconnection between the incus and stapes • Malformed malleus/incus complex • Bony bridge connecting the ossicles to the surrounding bone • Congenital stapes fixation—thickening of the footplate	• Critical for diagnosis and surgical planning
Sensorineural hearing loss:		
Inner ear dysplasia	• Labyrinthine aplasia (Michel's anomaly) • Cochlear aplasia • Common cavity • Cochlear hypoplasia • Incomplete partition I and II (classic Mondini) • IAC narrowing	• High-resolution CT successfully identifies bony abnormalities • MRI is needed for hypoplasia or aplasia of the cochlear nerve (important for cochlear implantation)

ACKNOWLEDGMENT

Dr Barun Bagga, Senior Resident, Department of Radiodiagnosis, AIIMS, New Delhi.

REFERENCES

1. Shekdar KV, Bilaniuk LT. Imaging of Pediatric Hearing Loss. Neuroimaging Clin N Am. 2019;29(1): 103-15.
2. Huang BY, Zdanski C, Castillo M. Pediatric sensorineural hearing loss, part 2: syndromic and acquired causes. AJNR Am J Neuroradiol. 2012;33(3):399-406.
3. Andreu-Arasa VC, Sung EK, Fujita A, Saito N, Sakai O. Otosclerosis and Dysplasias of the Temporal Bone. Neuroimaging Clin N Am. 2019;29(1):29-47.
4. Quesnel AM, Ishai R, McKenna MJ. Otosclerosis: Temporal Bone Pathology. Otolaryngol Clin North Am. 2018;51(2):291-303.
5. Maraghy AE, Aboelwafa W, Monem MA, Ghany AA, Sheref H, Mahmoud A. Role of high resolution multislice CT scan in otosclerosis. Egypt J Ear Nose Throat Allied Sci. 2015;16(3):247-54.
6. Marshall AH, Fanning N, Symons S, Shipp D, Chen JM, Nedzelski JM. Cochlear implantation in cochlear otosclerosis. Laryngoscope. 2005;115(10):1728-33.
7. van Beeck Calkoen EA, Engel MSD, van de Kamp JM, Yntema HG, Goverts ST, Mulder MF, et al. The etiological evaluation of sensorineural hearing loss in children. Eur J Pediatr. 2019;178(8):1195-205.

26

Approach to Vertigo

Shuchita Singh, Devasenathipathy Kandasamy

- Relevant Imaging Anatomy
- Clinical Presentation
- Diagnostic Approach
- Classification of Vertigo
- Imaging in Peripheral Causes
- Management

Vertigo is a commonly encountered symptom, with diverse etiologies.

RELEVANT IMAGING ANATOMY

- The utricle and saccule are the static labyrinth which detects the position of the head; and semicircular canals are the kinetic labyrinth which senses the rotational or angular motion of acceleration.
- Membranous labyrinths contain endolymphatic fluid and they are encapsulated in a bony labyrinth in the temporal bone. Perilymphatic fluid is seen in between the two labyrinths (see Chapter 20).
- Vestibule and the semicircular canals are innervated by the vestibular part of the vestibulocochlear nerve (8th cranial nerve) and the nerve courses through the internal auditory canal and reaches the vestibular nucleus in the brain stem. The central vestibular pathways extend to oculomotor nucleus, cerebellum, thalamus, and cortex.

CLINICAL PRESENTATION

- Vertigo can be associated with nausea or vomiting, unsteadiness (postural instability), falls, difficulty in walking, and motion sickness.
- Blurred vision, difficulty in speaking, altered level of consciousness, and hearing difficulty are the associated symptoms.
- Nystagmus may accompany.
- Symptoms may be persistent or episodic (lasting for seconds to minutes).
- Benign paroxysmal positional vertigo (BPPV) presents as repeated episodes of vertigo with head movement. It is episodic with periods of normalcy in between episodes. Each episode lasts <1 minute.
- Ménière's disease consists of a triad of tinnitus, vertigo, and hearing loss which may last for >20 minutes.
- *Labyrinthitis:* Sudden onset and the nystagmus occurs even without head movement.

DIAGNOSTIC APPROACH

- Differentiation from other causes of dizziness such as presyncope, hyperventilation syndrome, disequilibrium, or psychosomatic can be done by eliciting nystagmus.[1] This has been summarized in **Flowchart 1**.
- Vestibular system function can be evaluated by:
    - Electronystagmography (ENG)
    - Dix–Hallpike maneuver
    - Rotation tests
    - Head-thrust test
    - Caloric reflex test
- Auditory system function can be evaluated by:
    - Pure tone audiometry
    - Speech audiometry
    - Acoustic reflex
    - Electrocochleography (ECOG)
    - Auditory brainstem response test
    - Computerized dynamic posturography (CDP)
- CT scans or MRI are used only in selected few patients who present with atypical or refractory symptoms.

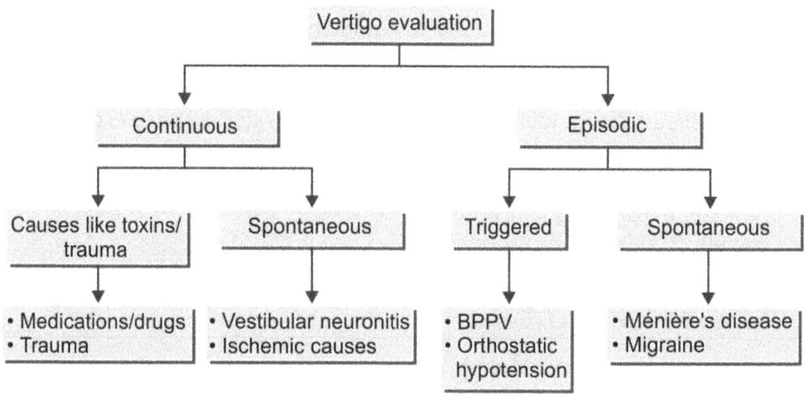

FLOWCHART 1: Algorithm for evaluation of vertigo.

CLASSIFICATION OF VERTIGO

- Depending on the site of involvement vertigo can be classified as peripheral or central (**Fig. 1**).[2]
- Vertigo can also be classified into objective, subjective, and pseudovertigo.

Peripheral

- Pathology within the inner ear or vestibular system is called "peripheral," "otologic," or "vestibular" vertigo.

- Imbalance, nausea, vomiting, hearing loss, tinnitus, fullness, and pain in the ear are the presenting features.
- Rapid compensation occurs and symptoms resolve in days to weeks.

Central

- Any abnormality in the balance centers in the brain can cause central vertigo and the symptoms are usually less severe than that of peripheral vertigo.
- It can be associated with difficulty in speech or nystagmus.

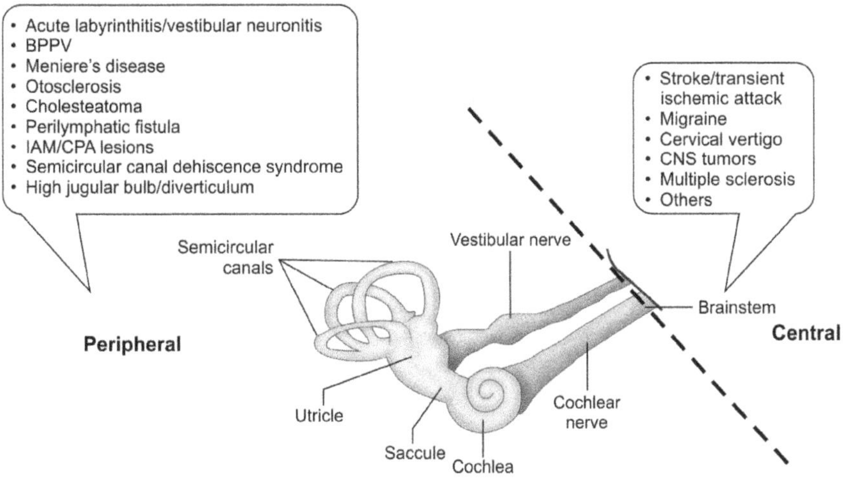

(BPPV: benign positional paroxysmal vertigo; IAM/CPA: internal acoustic meatus/cerebellopontine angle lesion)

FIG. 1: Line diagram for approach to vertigo: The causes mentioned to the left of interrupted line are the common causes of peripheral type of vertigo and the causes mentioned to the right of the line are the common causes of central type of vertigo.

IMAGING

- Computed tomography is the imaging modality of choice for abnormalities in bony labyrinth in which thin collimation with high-resolution reconstruction is mandatory.
- Magnetic resonance imaging is the preferred modality for the imaging of membranous labyrinth, conducting nerves, and the brain. Heavily T2-weighted sequences such as constructive interference in steady state (CISS)/sampling perfection with application-optimized contrasts by using different flip angle evolutions (SPACE) with thin sections and high-resolution are recommended for membranous labyrinth and the nerves.
- Whole brain imaging with diffusion-weighted imaging with or without postcontrast sequences is recommended for evaluating the central cause of dizziness.
- All peripheral causes are detailed in respective chapters; briefly listed in **Table 1**. Central causes of vertigo are discussed in **Table 2**.

TABLE 1 **Peripheral causes of vertigo.**

Causes	Imaging features and role of imaging
Acute labyrinthitis/ vestibular neuronitis	• Imaging is usually not necessary unless complicated or atypical • Contrast-enhanced MRI may show enhancement of labyrinth
Benign positional paroxysmal vertigo	• Diagnosis is by clinical examination, there is no role of imaging except in patients with no response to treatment
Ménière's disease	• Imaging is not necessary if the patient has typical clinical features • CT may show either narrowing or nonvisualization of vestibular aqueduct which contains the endolymphatic duct and sac • On 3T MRI, it may be possible to differentiate endolymphatic and perilymphatic spaces • Endolymphatic sac may be narrowed or may not be seen (see Chapter 20)
Otosclerosis	• CT is the imaging modality of choice and features depend on the phase of disease • Two types: (1) Fenestral and (2) Retrofenestral type • MRI is not a sensitive modality
Cholesteatoma[3]	• CT scan is the imaging of choice to evaluate the extent of involvement • Labyrinthine erosion is usually seen in the anterior limb of lateral semicircular canal (SCC) • MRI with diffusion-weighted imaging is also accurate in the characterization and also in recurrent disease
Perilymphatic fistula[4]	• Abnormal communication between the inner ear and middle ear • Fluctuating sensorineural hearing loss, tinnitus, and vertigo • Related to trauma, erosion or surgery • Oval window and round window are the common sites
	• *CT findings*: Unexplained fluid collection in middle ear or mastoid cavity and air in the inner ear (pneumolabyrinth) • In a post stapedectomy situation CT may reveal the displacement of prosthesis, bony fragment compressing the membranous labyrinth and may be the site of fistula
Internal acoustic meatus/ cerebellopontine angle lesions	• Imaging feature will depend on the lesion in these locations

Continued

Continued

Causes	Imaging features and role of imaging
SCC dehiscence syndrome (**Figs. 2A** and **B**)[5]	• Noise or static pressure triggers vestibular symptoms • Usually associated with a bony defect in the superior SCC and less commonly in the posterior SCC • A potentially treatable condition • CT scan in the coronal plane is accurate in demonstrating the defect and the size of the defect correlated with the severity of symptoms • MRI—not a sensitive modality to demonstrate the defect
High jugular bulb/ diverticulum	• Common radiological variant in which the jugular bulb is placed higher than the level of posterior SCC—best seen on CT scan

TABLE 2 **Central causes of vertigo.**

Causes	Imaging features and role of imaging
Stroke/transient ischemic attack	• Ischemia or hemorrhage involving the cerebellum and brainstem are important central causes of vertigo presenting acutely (**Figs. 3A** to **C**) • Chronic ischemia can also present with vertigo which can be longstanding and recurrent • Cerebellar infarction as a result of involvement of medial branch of posterior inferior cerebellar artery often lead to vertigo • Involvement of anterior inferior cerebellar artery and less commonly superior cerebellar artery can also lead to vertigo • CT is sensitive in detecting hemorrhages whereas posterior fossa infarcts can be missed on CT scans because of beam hardening artifacts • MRI with DWI is very sensitive in detecting posterior fossa infarcts
Migraine	• Imaging in these patients is unlikely to show any significant abnormality
Cervical vertigo	• Controversial entity • Radiographs may show the features of cervical spondylosis • Doppler USG may show decrease in flow in the vertebral artery during head rotation
CNS tumors	• Although CT can detect most of the intra-axial tumors, characterization and extent of spread are best evaluated using MRI
Multiple sclerosis (MS)	• MRI is the modality of choice for evaluating the demyelinating lesions of MS • Plaques in medial vestibular nucleus and superior cerebellar peduncles are usually associated with vertigo

(CNS: central nervous system; DWI: diffusion-weighted imaging)

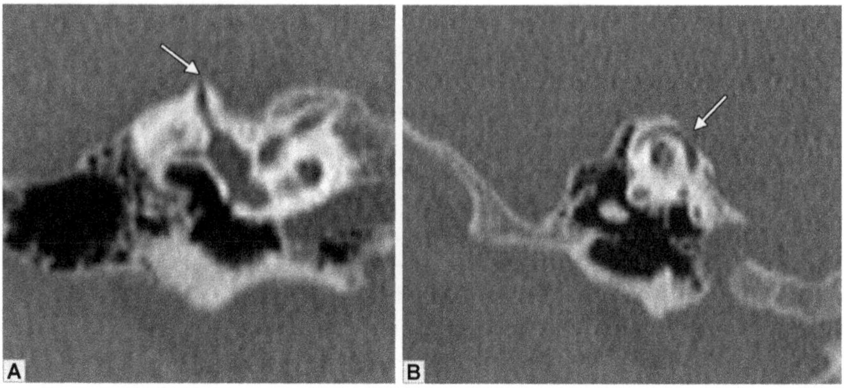

FIGS. 2A AND B: Example of peripheral cause: Superior semicircular canal dehiscence. HRCT scan of right temporal bone of a 12-year-old child shown in (A) coronal oblique and (B) sagittal oblique planes reveals a focal bony dehiscence of superior semicircular canal (arrow). The defect is too subtle that it may not be apparent on routine orthogonal reformatting planes. This highlights the importance of oblique reformatting planes.

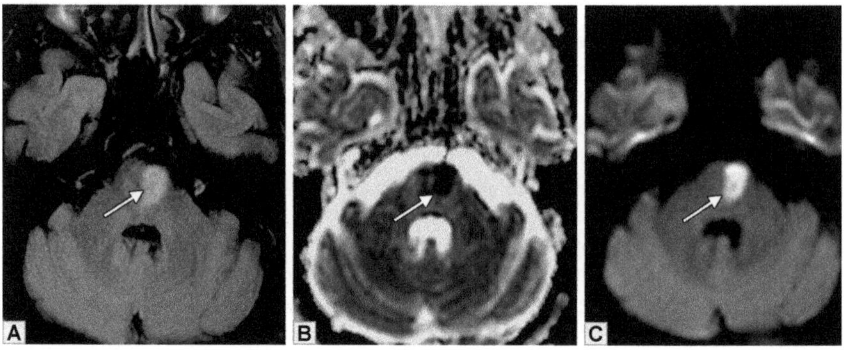

FIGS. 3A TO C: Example of central cause: Pontine infarct. Acute infarct in left half of pons (arrows), appearing (A) hyperintense on FLAIR, (B) hypointense on ADC map image, and (C) bright on diffusion-weighted image.
Courtesy: Professor Ajay Garg.

MANAGEMENT

- The aim is to treat the underlying cause of vertigo.
- *Medical therapy includes:*
  - Anticholinergics
  - Anticonvulsants and beta blockers for vestibular migraines
  - Antihistamines
  - Corticosteroids for inflammatory lesions
- *Vestibular rehabilitation*: This is a type of physical therapy aimed at strengthening the vestibular system. It is recommended for recurrent bouts of vertigo. It helps to train other senses to compensate for vertigo.

- *Canalith repositioning maneuvers.* There are guidelines about specific head and body movements for BPPV for repositioning of the otoliths.
- *Surgery*: In a few cases, surgery may be needed in specific situations.
- *Ménière's disease*: Conservative low-salt diet and intratympanic injections of antibiotics and steroids are employed. Surgical management is undertaken in refractory cases—shunt or ablation of the labyrinth.

CONCLUSION

- Vertigo is a complex clinical problem with diverse etiology which can purely be a clinical diagnosis if typical features are present.
- Imaging plays a key role when the presentation is atypical imaging and most of the times the role of imaging is to rule out the disorders which can closely mimic each other.
- In specific clinical situations such as peripheral type vertigo with associated asymmetrical or unilateral sensorineural hearing loss, vertigo in a patient with high risk of cerebrovascular disease or in patients with suspected central cause of vertigo should undergo some form of imaging to ascertain the cause.

REFERENCES

1. Herbert L, Muncie J, Sirmans SM, James E. Dizziness: Approach to Evaluation and Management. Am Fam Physician. 2017;95(3):154-62.
2. Thompson TL, Amedee R. Vertigo: A Review of Common Peripheral and Central Vestibular Disorders. Ochsner J. 2009;9(1):20-6.
3. Henninger B, Kremser C. Diffusion weighted imaging for the detection and evaluation of cholesteatoma. World J Radiol. 2017;9(5):217-22.
4. Venkatasamy A, Al Ohraini Z, Karol A, Karch-Georges A, Riehm S, Rohmer D, et al. CT and MRI for the diagnosis of perilymphatic fistula: a study of 17 surgically confirmed patients. Eur Arch Otorhinolaryngol. 2020;277(4):1045-51.
5. Gartrell BC, Gentry LR, Kennedy TA, Gubbels SP. Radiographic Features of Superior Semicircular Canal Dehiscence in the Setting of Chronic Ear Disease. Otol Neurotol. 2014;35(1):91-6.

27

Approach to Tinnitus

Devasenathipathy Kandasamay, Shuchita Singh

- ❑ Pathophysiology
- ❑ Clinical Presentation
- ❑ Types of Tinnitus
- ❑ Causes
- ❑ Diagnosis
- ❑ Imaging Features
- ❑ Management
- ❑ Prognosis

- The word "tinnītus" is derived from the Latin word "tinnīre" meaning "to ring".
- It is defined as the abnormality in which the affected person hears sound in the absence of any external sound stimulus.
- Ringing, clicking, hiss, or roaring sound are the most common presenting complaints.
- It is a common problem, which can be seen in around 10–15% of people however it is severe enough to be significant only in 3%.[1]
- The sound can be unilateral or bilateral, soft or loud, low- or high-pitched.
- Occasionally, the tinnitus could be objective, where the sound is audible to the examiner also through a stethoscope.
- It can cause depression, anxiety, or may interfere with concentration.
- A comprehensive audiological and neurological examination is mandatory for diagnosis.
- If the tinnitus is synchronous with the heartbeat, a thorough cardiological evaluation is a must.
- In case of an underlying cause, treating it may lead to improvements.
- Management involves counseling of the patient.
- Hearing aids may also be helpful for some.
- As of now, there are no effective medications.

PATHOPHYSIOLOGY

- Otoacoustic emissions is widely accepted mechanism and is shown in **Flowchart 1**.
- Damage to hair cells activates different sets of neurons giving the sense of hearing sound.
- Damage to receptor cells can also result in tinnitus.
- Although birds, reptiles and amphibians have the regenerative power to repair the damaged receptor cells, they can be formed only during embryogenesis in mammals.
- The mechanism of subjective tinnitus is not fully understood.
- Traumatic injury to the inner ear may also result in tinnitus.

Inner hair cells vibrate to sound waves

↓

Outer hair cells convert neural signals into basement membrane tension

↓

Sensor cells are linked with vibratory cells, which is regulated by brain

↓

This gives excellent sensitivity and selectivity to sound

↓

Any disturbance in the above system results in tinnitus

FLOWCHART 1: Pathophysiology of tinnitus.

CLINICAL PRESENTATION

- Tinnitus can be unilateral or bilateral.
- It is usually a ringing noise but, in many patients, it can take the form of a high-pitched whining, electric buzzing, hissing, humming, ringing or whistling sound or as ticking, clicking, roaring, "crickets" or "tree frogs" or "locusts (cicadas)," tunes, songs, beeping, sizzling, sounds that slightly resemble human voices or even a pure steady tone like that heard during a hearing test.
- It has also been described as a "whooshing" sound because of acute muscle spasms, as of wind or waves.
- Tinnitus can be intermittent or it can be continuous.
- Majority of people with tinnitus have some degree of hearing loss.
- The sound sensed by the patient may be as quiet as background noise or louder.
- In pulsatile tinnitus, patients perceive their own pulse or muscular contractions.

TYPES

There are several ways by which tinnitus can be classified: Subjective or objective, pulsatile or nonpulsatile, and primary or secondary tinnitus.[2]

- *Subjective tinnitus* is heard only by the patient and objective tinnitus is heard by patient and clinician.
- *Subjective tinnitus* is also known as "tinnitus aurium" "nonauditory," and "nonvibratory" tinnitus.
- *Objective tinnitus* is also known as "pseudo-tinnitus" or "vibratory" tinnitus.
- *Pulsatile tinnitus* is periodic and usually in sync with a patient's heartbeat whereas *nonpulsatile tinnitus* can be continuous.
- When a tinnitus does not have any known cause it is known as *primary tinnitus* and if there is a known cause such as otospongiosis then it is known as *secondary tinnitus.*

CAUSES

There are numerous causes of tinnitus. Some of them are intrinsic to the auditory apparatus and some of them are extrinsic causes. The common causes of tinnitus are listed in the schematic diagram (**Fig. 1**).

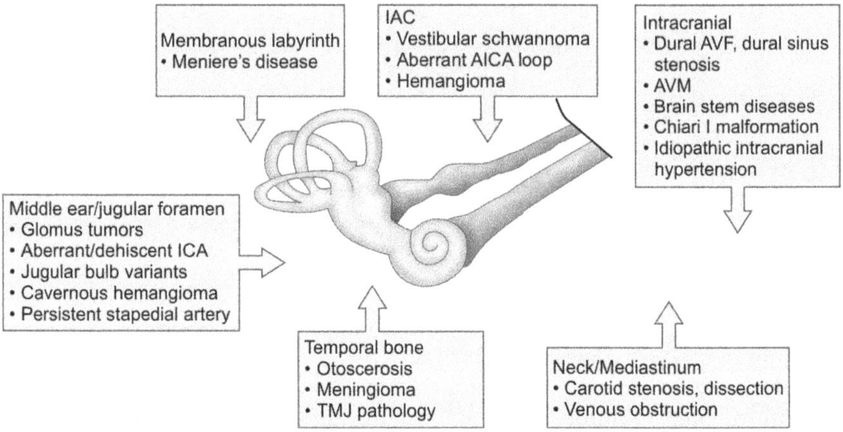

(AICA: anterior inferior cerebellar artery; AVF: arteriovenous fistula; AVM: arteriovenous malformations; IAC: internal auditory canal; ICA: internal carotid artery; TMJ: temporomandibular joint)

FIG. 1: Causes of tinnitus.

DIAGNOSIS

- The tinnitus measurement depends on the brain's tendency to select out only the loudest sounds heard.
- Tinnitus can be measured by playing various sounds with known amplitude.
- Subjective tinnitus, unlike the objective form, cannot be tested by comparative methods.

IMAGING

According to American Academy of Otolaryngology guidelines, imaging is indicated in patients with unilateral, pulsatile tinnitus which is associated with asymmetrical hearing impairment.[3,4] Imaging is also indicated if there are associated neurological symptoms. Diagnostic evaluation for tinnitus is illustrated in **Flowchart 2**. Common and important causes of tinnitus, and their imaging findings are described in **Tables 1** and **2**.

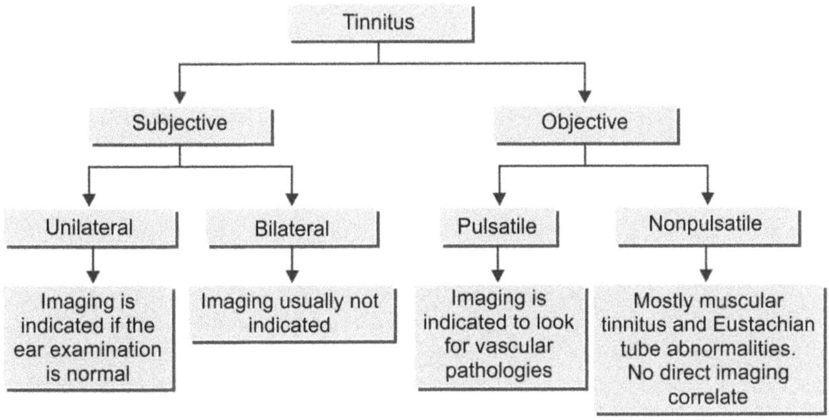

FLOWCHART 2: Diagnostic evaluation for tinnitus.

TABLE 1 **Pulsatile tinnitus.**

Causes	Imaging features and role of imaging
Glomus tumors (tympanicum, jugulare and jugulotympanicum) (**Figs. 2A** to **C**)	See Chapter 16
Cavernous hemangioma of middle ear (ME)	• Rare tumor, mimics glomus tumors on both clinical examination and imaging studies • Diagnosis usually made after surgery • *DD*: Low flow vascular malformations (**Figs. 3A** to **C**)
Cavernous hemangioma of FN	• Rare tumor, uncommonly causes tinnitus • Occurs in two locations: Geniculate ganglion, present with FN palsy and IAC, present with SNHL • *DD*: Glomus tumors, schwannoma, and meningioma
Meningioma	• Can cause pulsatile and nonpulsatile tinnitus • CT—may show sclerosis of the adjacent bone • *MRI*: Iso- to hyperintense on T2-weighted imaging, intense enhancement on CEMRI; presence of dural tail
Arteriovenous malformations (AVM)	• Can be extracranial, dural, or parenchymal • Most of them are clinically diagnosed • Imaging to delineate the extent of the lesion • Usually has a nidus with tuft of abnormal vessels • CT or MR can show the vascular lesion and parenchymal changes • *MRI*: Evidence of old bleed, arterial feeders, flow voids within the lesion and engorgement of veins and dural sinuses • DSA is the modality of choice for evaluating the AVM

Continued

Continued

Causes	Imaging features and role of imaging
Dural AVF	• Important cause of objective pulsatile tinnitus with normal clinical otoscopic examination • Direct communication of artery with the vein without any intervening nidus • Sigmoid, transverse, and cavernous sinuses are the most common locations • Supplied by the branches of ECA and the site of communication can be extracranial, intracranial, or both • *CECT/MR*: May or may not show the fistula itself, but can show the associated features, e.g., engorged cortical veins and dural sinuses and parenchymal changes • If high clinical suspicion, CT and MR negative; DSA is the modality of choice
Dural sinus stenosis	• Narrowing of dural sinuses such as transverse or sigmoid can cause turbulence in flow • May be associated with other features of intracranial hypertension • CT or MRV is usually sufficient
Venous compression/ obstruction	• Venous hum can be present in patients with hyperdynamic flow (thyrotoxicosis, severe anemia, etc.) which can cause tinnitus in few patients • Occasionally, the turbulent flow in jugular veins secondary to obstruction/compression in neck or mediastinum can cause tinnitus • CT/MRI can help to search for a cause of obstruction anywhere along the course of IJV
Aberrant ICA (**Fig. 4A**)	• Due to failure of development of cervical carotid artery • Compensatory enlargement of inferior tympanic artery which anastomoses with the caroticotympanic artery in the ME and continues as ICA from petrous part • On CT, the aberrant ICA is seen as a tubular horizontal structure coursing through the ME from posterior to anterior • The inferior tympanic canaliculus is markedly enlarged, which is otherwise a miniscule foramen • The vertical part of petrous ICA is absent • *DSA*: 7 or reversed 7 sign (abnormal lateral course) • The lateral wall of the aberrant vessel can be dehiscent: Seen on both otoscopy and CT
Persistent stapedial artery	• Rare congenital anomaly which can be associated with aberrant ICA or normal ICA • Persistent of a fetal artery which failed to regress before birth

Continued

Continued

Causes	Imaging features and role of imaging
	• It courses across the ME through the obturator foramen and enters the canal of tympanic part of FN, and eventually continues as middle meningeal artery • *CT*: Abnormal enlargement of the canal of the tympanic part of FN with absent foramen spinosum • DSA is the modality of choice • Can be missed on MRI due to its small size
Jugular bulb variants (**Fig. 4B**)	See Chapter 14
Carotid artery dissection/stenosis/ aneurysm	• Turbulence in the ICA caused by any lesion causing narrowing of lumen, e.g., dissection, atherosclerotic plaque can cause tinnitus • ICA aneurysm in relation to the petrous part can be the cause of tinnitus in a few patients • Fibromuscular dysplasia involving ICA: Beaded appearance of artery with multiple stenotic areas • CTA is a good tool in depicting them • MRA and vessel wall imaging can show the dissection and plaque better than CT scan
Aberrant anterior inferior cerebellar artery loops	See Chapter 12
Otosclerosis (see Chapters 20 and 21)	• It is an idiopathic infiltrative disorder involving the inner ear which can cause tinnitus • HRCT scan is the modality of choice to diagnose, classify, and characterize the lesions • MRI can also show changes of otosclerosis, however, it is less sensitive than CT scan
Idiopathic intracranial hypertension	• These patients can present with headache, visual disturbances +/– pulsatile tinnitus • MRI is better than CT in diagnosing this entity • *MRI*: Posterior globe flattening, optic nerve (ON) sheath distension, ON tortuosity, and empty sella

(AVF: arteriovenous fistula; CEMRI: contrast-enhanced magnetic resonance imaging; CTA: computed tomography angiography; DD: differential diagnosis; DSA: digital subtraction angiography; ECA: external carotid artery; FN: facial nerve; IAC: internal auditory canal; ICA: internal carotid artery; IJV: internal jugular vein; MRA: magnetic resonance angiography; MRI: magnetic resonance imaging; MRV: magnetic resonance venography; SNHL: sensorineural hearing loss)

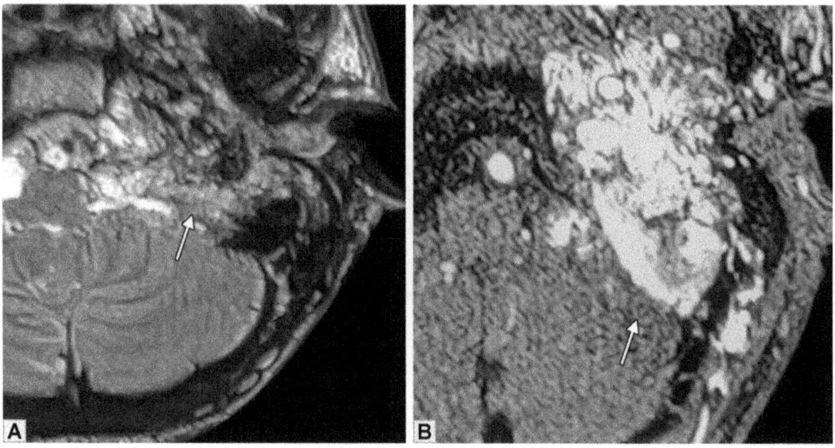

FIGS. 2A AND B: Glomus jugulare causing pulsatile tinnitus: T2-weighted image (A) showing a mass lesion causing destruction of the petrous temporal bone (thin arrow); (B) The mass showed characteristic intense enhancement after contrast with multiple vessels in the vicinity.

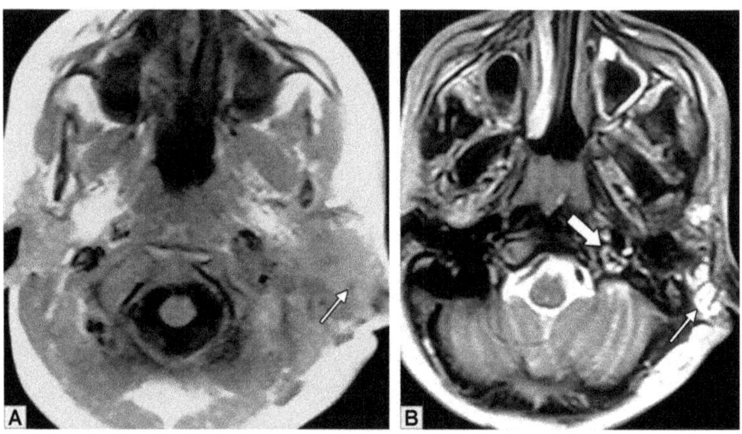

FIGS. 3A AND B: Slow flow vascular malformation: MRI image showing an ill-defined soft tissue and tubular channels which are isointense on T1W (A) image and hyperintense on T2W (B) image seen involving and the left side external ear (thin arrow) and petrous apex (thick arrow). On USG (not shown) the lesion showed slow flow suggestive of slow flow vascular malformation.

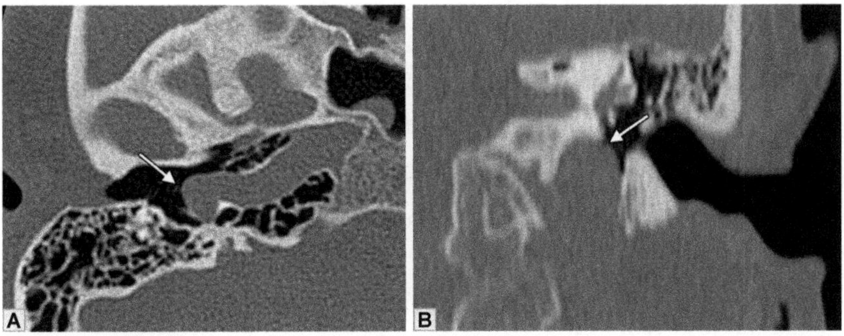

FIGS. 4A AND B: Variant vascular anatomy. Aberrant carotid artery (arrow in A). High riding dehiscent jugular bulb (arrow in B).

TABLE 2 Nonpulsatile tinnitus.

Causes	Imaging features and role of imaging
Cerebellopontine (CP) angle tumors (see Chapters 16 and 22)	• Most important consideration in nonpulsatile tinnitus • Vestibular schwannoma is the most common lesion in CP angle to cause tinnitus • CEMRI is the modality of choice
Palatal/ME myoclonus (muscular tinnitus)	• Palatal myoclonus involves tensor and levator palati, tensor tympani, salpingopharyngeus, and superior constrictor muscles • ME myoclonus is caused by abnormal contractions of stapedius and tensor tympani muscles • None of them have a direct imaging correlate • Occasionally, multiple sclerosis itself can cause tinnitus with fluctuating SNHL and vertigo • MRI: To look for brain stem and cerebellar lesions
Chiari I malformation	• Rarely associated with tinnitus • The stretching of 8th nerve secondary to herniation of posterior fossa structures is considered as cause • MRI is the modality of choice
Temporomandibular joint (TMJ)	• Degeneration involving the TMJ can cause continuous tinnitus • Tensor tympani and pterygoid muscles have a common innervation and the increased tension in the pterygoid muscle can lead to abnormal tension in tensor tympani muscle which can cause tinnitus • *CT and MRI*: Both can show degenerative changes
Ménière's disease	See Chapter 20
Miscellaneous	• Drugs such as NSAID, aminoglycosides • Noise-induced hearing loss and presbycusis can also be associated with tinnitus • After trauma and temporal bone surgery • Diagnosis is usually clinical and there may or may not be a imaging correlate in these entities

(ME: middle ear; NSAID: nonsteroidal anti-inflammatory drugs; SNHL: sensorineural hearing loss)

MANAGEMENT

- If a specific cause is found then treating the cause may improve symptoms. If no cause is found then treatment approaches like talk therapy and sound therapy may help.

Psychological:
- The most effective treatment for tinnitus is cognitive behavioral therapy (CBT). Reassurance is the key. Relaxation techniques may also be useful.

Physical:
- Ear wax to be removed
- Another approach is by using the "Finger Drumming" technique in which a patient is asked to snap the fingers by keeping the palm over the ears.

Medications:
- There are no effective medications for tinnitus. There is a doubtful role of antidepressants and benzodiazepines.
- Botulinum toxin has been used to treat muscular tinnitus.

Others:
- Hearing aids or tinnitus maskers can be used, however, there is no concrete evidence.
- Retraining therapy and transcranial magnetic stimulation are being used with limited success.

Alternative medicine:
- Ginkgo biloba and zinc supplementation are used.
- Melatonin can help in patients with sleep problems.

PROGNOSIS

Most people with tinnitus get used to it after a period of time, however, in few patients it remains a chronic problem.

REFERENCES

1. Shargorodsky J, Curhan GC, Farwell WR. Prevalence and Characteristics of Tinnitus among US Adults. Am J Med. 2010;123(8):711-8.
2. Cunnane MB. Imaging of Tinnitus. Neuroimaging Clin. 2019;29(1):49-56.
3. Tunkel DE, Bauer CA, Sun GH, Rosenfeld RM, Chandrasekhar SS, Cunningham Jr ER, et al. (2014). Clinical Practice Guideline: Tinnitus. [online] Available from https://journals.sagepub.com/doi/10.1177/0194599814545325 [Last accessed October, 2020].
4. Yew KS. Diagnostic Approach to Patients with Tinnitus. Am Fam Physician. 2014;89(2):106-13.

28

Approach to Facial Nerve Palsy

Arvind Kumar Kairo, Chandrashekhara SH

- Anatomy
- Causes
- Diagnosis
- Role of Imaging
  - CT
  - MRI
- Treatment

ANATOMY

- Facial nerve anatomy is illustrated in **Figure 1**.
- The intracranial part is formed by the motor and sensory roots.[1]
  - The cisternal and intracanalicular part of the nerve is surrounded by cerebrospinal fluid (CSF), and best visualized on magnetic resonance imaging (MRI).

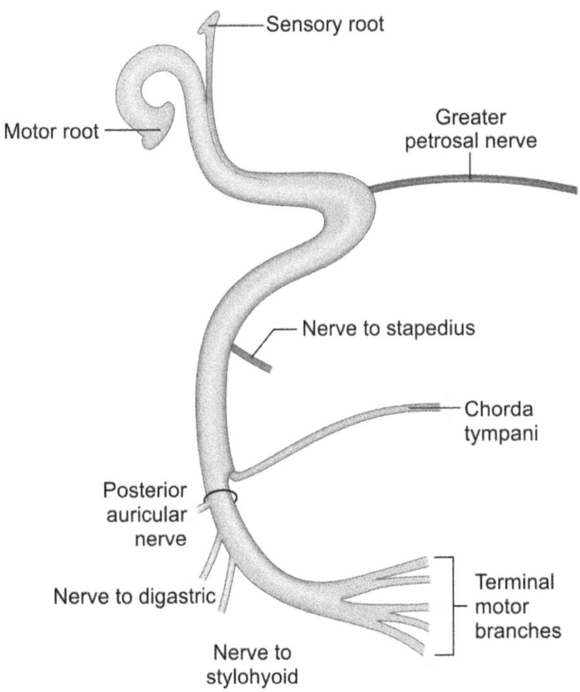

FIG. 1: Diagram showing the course and branches of facial nerve.

- Intratemporal part is best visualized on computed tomography (CT).
  - After exiting through the internal auditory canal (IAC), the first part of the nerve (labyrinthine segment) takes an acute bend at the first genu, where it joins the greater petrosal nerve.
  - The second (tympanic) part runs in the petrous temporal bone, closely related to the medial wall of the middle ear cavity. The only branch of FN in the ear is the nerve to stapedius.
  - The descending (mastoid) part of FN lies in the posterior wall of middle ear cavity and exits through stylomastoid foramen.
  - The branches related to it are chorda tympani nerve and posterior auricular nerve. Subsequently, the FN runs within the substance of the parotid gland and divides into five terminal branches. The branches of the FN are described in **Figures 1** and **2**.

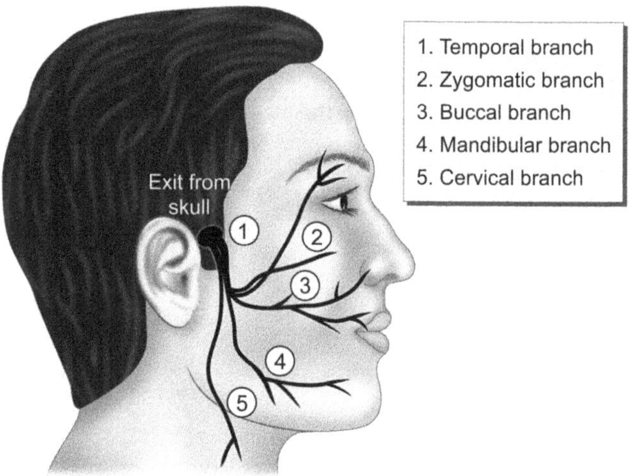

FIG. 2: Diagram showing the terminal branches of facial nerve.

CAUSES

- Facial nerve nucleus is located in the lateral midpons. FN paralysis can be subtyped into in upper motor neuron (UMN or supranuclear) lesion and lower motor neuron (LMN or infranuclear) paralysis. Causes according to level are described in **Figure 3**.
- In a LMN lesion, the patient cannot wrinkle their forehead but in UMN lesion patient can which can be easily tested during examination.
- Causes of UMN include multiple sclerosis, stroke (lacunar infract in internal capsule, infarcts involving pontine arteries), and intracranial tumors.
- Majority of the causes for FN paralysis are infranuclear type.
- Causes according to etiology are listed in **Table 1**.

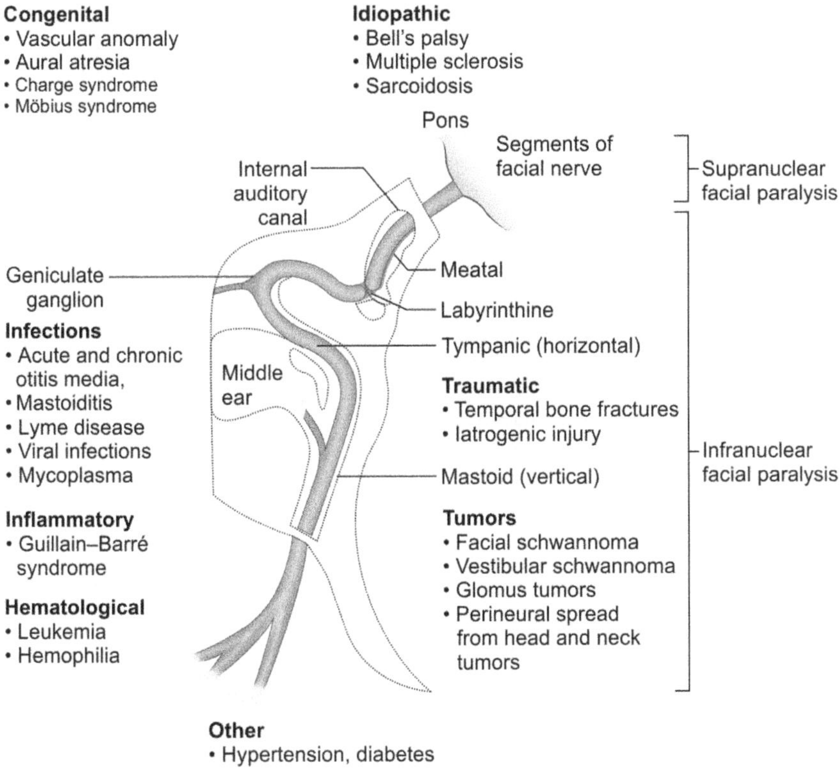

FIG. 3: Diagram showing the causes of facial nerve palsy, based on the site of involvement.

TABLE 1 **Causes of facial nerve paralysis.**

Causes	Conditions	Imaging
Congenital	Vascular anomaly, aural atresia, CHARGE syndrome, dehiscence of facial nerve canal, Möbius syndrome	CT and MRI are helpful in assessing the congenital anomalies of bone and soft tissue structures
Birth related	Traumatic or difficult delivery	MRI brain may demonstrate the hypoxic injuries in the brain
Idiopathic	• Bell's palsy • Multiple sclerosis • Sarcoidosis	MRI reveals abnormal and asymmetric enhancement of the intratemporal (the horizontal/tympanic; and the vertical/mastoid) parts of the facial nerve on MRI
Traumatic	• Temporal bone fracture • Iatrogenic injury • Brainstem injury • Penetrating trauma	CT demonstrates fracture line crossing through the facial canal, bony fragments which might cause impingement facial canal. MRI for associated soft tissue abnormality/hematoma

Continued

Continued

Causes	Conditions	Imaging
Infections	Viral infections (varicella-zoster virus, Ramsay Hunt syndrome, herpes simplex virus, Epstein–Barr virus, SARS-COV-2 infections), mycoplasma, lyme disease, acute and chronic otitis media (cholesteatoma), mastoiditis	Facial nerve involvement is seen as abnormal enhancement of the facial nerve on MRI
Tumors	Facial nerve schwannoma, vestibular nerve schwannoma, hemangioma, lipoma, glomus tumors, perineural spread of head and neck tumors	MRI is helpful in the evaluation of the tumors (also see Chapter 16)
Vascular	• MCA infarct • Pontine artery infarct • Lacunar infarct	MRI brain is helpful in the demonstration of infracts
Inflammatory	Guillain–Barré syndrome	Abnormal enhancement of the facial nerve on MRI
Hematologic	Leukemia and hemophilia	MRI is helpful in evaluating the facial nerve; CT for bony facial nerve canal
Other causes	Hypertension and diabetes mellitus	Imaging has limited role

DIAGNOSIS

- In examination, evaluation of any vesicular lesions on face, hematoma or other sign of skull base trauma, neck nodes, hearing evaluation, other lower cranial palsies, and corneal and ear examination should be done.
- Grade of palsy should be documented. The most commonly used staging system for categorizing and documenting is *House-Brackmann grading system* (**Table 2**).
- Localization of infranuclear lesion can be done by evaluating different functions of FN which have topological correlation along the length of FN (**Table 3**).
- *Electrodiagnostic testing*: It is used to differentiate neurapraxia from neural degeneration and to prognosticate.
  - *Nerve excitability test (NET)*: Electrode is applied over the stylomastoid foramen area. Lowest current eliciting a visible twitch of facial muscle is the threshold of excitation. Difference in thresholds between the two sides is calculated and compared. In cases of incomplete paralysis, this test is not contributory.
  - *Maximum stimulation test (MST)*: Levels of maximal current to elicit maximum facial twitch.
  - *Electroneuronography (ENoG) (also called electroneurography)*: This is done almost like the MST but bipolar electrodes are used to evoked

compound muscle action potential (CMAP). Peak-to-peak amplitude is measured in millivolts (mV).

- *Electromyography (EMG)*: Recording of spontaneous and voluntary muscle potentials using needles.

TABLE 2 House–Brackmann grading system.[3]

Grade I	Normal symmetrical function
Grade II	• Mild weakness, noticeable only on close inspection • Complete eye closure • Slight asymmetric smile with maximal effort • Synkinesis* absent
Grade III	• Obvious weakness, but not disfiguring • Inability to lift eyebrow • Complete eye closure • Strong but asymmetrical mouth movement • Obvious synkinesis*
Grade IV	• Obvious disfiguring weakness • Inability to lift brow • Incomplete eye closure • Asymmetry of mouth with maximal effort • Severe synkinesis*
Grade V	• Motion barely perceptible • Incomplete eye closure • Slight movement of the corner of mouth • Synkinesis*, contracture, and spasm usually absent
Grade VI	• No movement, loss of tone, no synkinesis*, contracture, or spasm

*Involuntary movements accompanying voluntary movements because of wrong connections of axons inside the nerve of nerves after healing of a damaged nerve.

TABLE 3 Branches of the facial nerve and the relevant clinical/laboratory tests.

Components of facial nerve	Functions	Clinical/Laboratory test
Nerve of Wrisberg/nervus intermedius/GSPN	Secretomotor fiber to lacrimal glands and nasal mucosa	Schirmer's test
Nerve to stapedius	To stapedius muscle	Checked by stapedial reflex (tympanometry)
Chorda tympani nerve*	Taste of anterior 2/3rd tongue	Electrogustometry
Muscular branches	Muscles of facial expression, occipitofrontalis, stylohyoid and posterior belly of digastric	Electrophysiologic tests
Cutaneous sensation	Skin of the external canal	Sensory testing seldom reveals hypoesthesia because of overlapping dermatomes

*Chorda tympani nerve also carries parasympathetic supply (general visceral efferent) to sublingual and submandibular gland which can be assessed by salivary flow test and salivary pH.

ROLE OF IMAGING

- The FN is often overlooked during interpretation.
- Both CT and MRI offer complimentary information in the evaluation of FN lesions.
- Detailed clinical history enables us to tailor imaging acquisition for optimal interpretation.

Computed Tomography

- Helpful for evaluation bony abnormalities of FN canal which may be seen in congenital anomalies of internal or middle ear; as well as in inflammatory pathology like cholesteatoma. CT is also ideal imaging modality in trauma and iatrogenic injuries.
- Technique- high-resolution temporal bone CT.

Magnetic Resonance Imaging

- In contrast to CT, MRI is helpful for evaluation of soft tissue abnormalities involving the FN canal, and hence, is the ideal imaging modality for suspected inflammation or neoplastic diseases.[2]
- Supranuclear lesions can be assessed in routine brain MRI; however, nuclear and infranuclear lesions may require additional dedicated sequences through the brainstem and temporal bone.
- *MRI sequences:*
    - Precontrast axial T2-weighted (T2W) sequence of brain
    - About 3 mm axial T1W of the IAC
    - Constructive interference in steady state (CISS) sequence
    - Postcontrast axial T1W brain
    - About 4 mm postcontrast coronal T1W of IAC
    - About 3 mm axial T1W fat-saturated sequence of IAC
- Diffusion tensor MR tractography helps in demonstrating the FN fibers in three-dimensional volumetric manner and in multiple planes.
- The evaluation of extracranial segments and branches of FN requires extra coverage of the parotid glands during MRI examination.
- The role of MRI in demonstrating the various segments of FN is illustrated in **Figures 4** to **6**.
- Several MR techniques have been tried for demonstration of nerve in the intratemporal part. The readers are referred to Chapter 1.

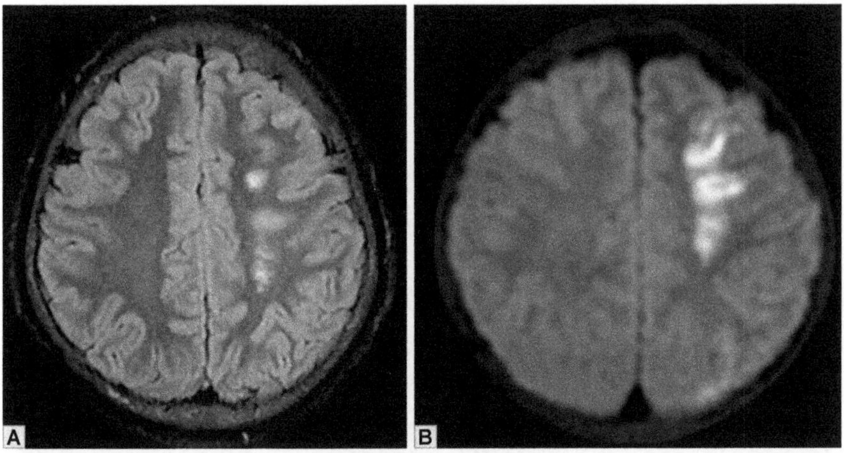

FIGS. 4A AND B: MRI in case right UMN facial palsy: MRI (A and B) showing areas of FLAIR hyperintensity (A) and restricted diffusion on DWI (B) in left external watershed area of MCA-ACA and MCA-PCA territory (left middle frontal region, centrum semiovale, and left posterior parietal region) sign of acute infarct.
Courtesy: Dr Ajay Garg.

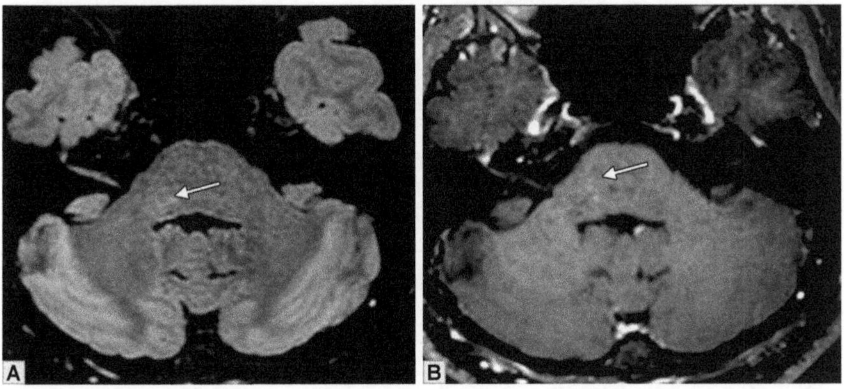

FIGS. 5A AND B: MRI in a case of mononeuritis multiplex with recent onset right 7th nerve palsy: MRI shows focal abnormal FLAIR hyperintensity in right lower hemipons in the expected location (A). Facial nerve motor nucleus showing enhancement on postcontrast study (B).
Courtesy: Dr Ajay Garg.

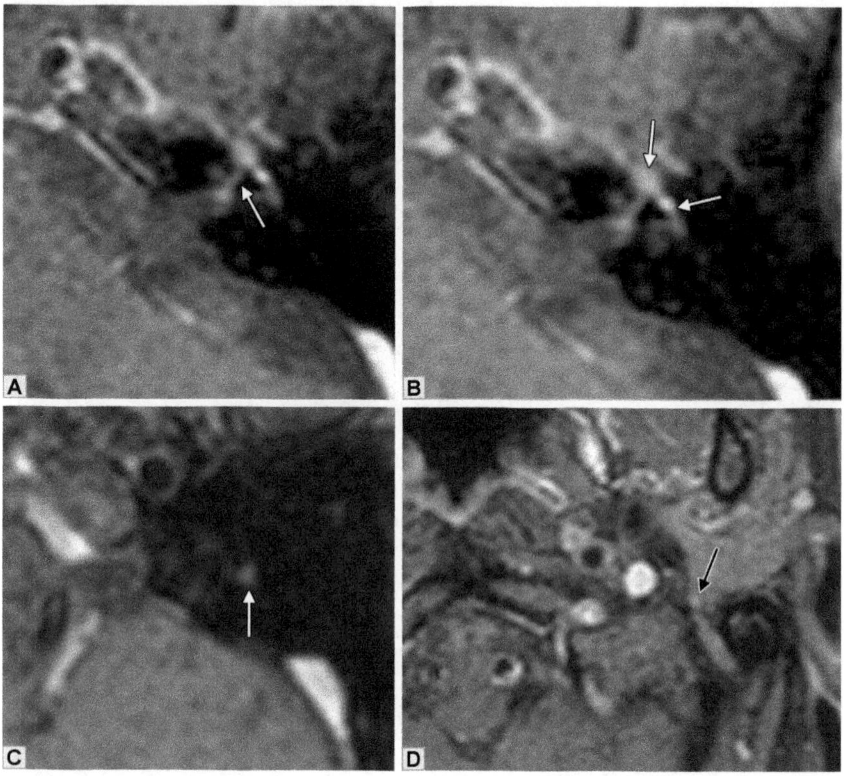

FIGS. 6A TO D: MRI in a case of facial neuritis: Postcontrast T1-weighted imaging showing thickening and enhancement of entire facial nerve involving (A) labyrinthine segment, (B) first genu and tympanic segment, (C) mastoid segment, and (D) extra-temporal segments.

TREATMENT

- *Medical:*
    - *Steroids*: Steroids are used in Bell's palsy (idiopathic), infections along with antimicrobial coverage, trauma, iatrogenic causes, inflammatory, and autoimmune condition (virtually in every case).
    - *Antiviral therapy (acyclovir/valacyclovir)*: When clinical suspicion of Ramsay Hunt syndrome, Bell's palsy is present.
- *General conservative:*
    - Observation—for spontaneous recover
    - Care of the eye:
        - Day time—eye drops and eye glasses
        - Night time—eye ointment with eye patching
        - Care of muscles of facial expression—physiotherapy
        - Tarsorrhaphy

- *Surgical*: Intraoperative FN monitoring is an important adjunct in surgery. Different surgical routes or approaches are required to reach different parts of FN as it has long intracranial and intratemporal course.
  - Retrolabyrinthine approach—from brainstem to IAC porus.
  - Middle cranial fossa approach—from IAC porus to tympanic segment.
  - Transmastoid approach—for intratemporal part of FN (first genu to stylomastoid foramen).

  Anatomic landmarks used during surgery to locate FN are described in ***Box 1****.*

Various types of surgical procedures are as follows:
- *Facial nerve decompression*: Bony canal (fallopian canal) of FN is removed around the site of nerve compression.
  - Criteria to consider FN decompression:[4-6]
    - Nerve excitability test: More than 3.5-mA threshold difference between sides
    - Maximal stimulation test: No response on injured side at maximal stimulation
    - Electroneurography: More than 90% degeneration within 14 days
- *Facial nerve neurorrhaphy*: Cut ends of FN are sutured surgically.
- *Facial nerve cable graft*: Cut ends of FN are joined surgically with an interpositioned nerve graft (either from greater auricular or from sural nerve).
- *Nerve transposition*: Distal ends of FN are connected to other nerves (other than FN as it is not always possible to anastomoses with proximal FN end), nerves which can be used are ipsilateral hypoglossal or ansa hypoglossi nerve (spinal accessory nerve are not used now a days).
- Muscle transposition innervated other muscles are used to function like facial muscle by transpositioning their attachments. Muscles in such surgeries are temporalis and masseter muscle.
- Microneurovascular transfer
- Static procedures—static facial sling

BOX 1 Anatomic landmarks used during surgery for facial nerve localization.

Middle ear and mastoid surgery	Parotid surgery
• Cog* • Processus cochleariformis • Oval window • Lateral semicircular canal dome • Short process of the incus • Pyramid • Posterior semicircular canal ampullary end • Digastric ridge	• Tragal pointer# *(of Conley)* • Tympanomastoid suture • Posterior belly of digastric muscle • Retrograde tracing of distal facial nerve branches

*Bony crest arising from tegmen tympani separating epitympanum from epitympanic sinus or recess.
#Medial most part of tragus (part of pinna).

- Surgical procedures to treat paralysis of the upper lid (lagophthalmos):
  - Gold weight insertion
  - Palpebral springs
  - Silicone (silastic) slings
  - Titanium chain link implants
- Botulinum toxin for management of synkinesis

REFERENCES

1. Ho ML, Juliano A, Eisenberg RL, Moonis G. Anatomy and pathology of the facial nerve. AJR Am J Roentgenol. 2015;204(6):W612-9.
2. Gupta S, Mends F, Hagiwara M, Fatterpekar G, Roehm PC. Imaging the facial nerve: a contemporary review. Radiol Res Pract. 2013;2013:248039.
3. House JW, Brackmann DE: Facial nerve grading system. Otolaryngol Head Neck Surg. 1985;93:146.
4. Wu Sh, Chen X, Wang J, Liu H, Qian Xz, Pan Xl. Subtotal facial nerve decompression in preventing further recurrence and promoting facial nerve recovery of severe idiopathic recurrent facial palsy. Eur Arch Otorhinolaryngol. 2015;272(11):3295-8.
5. Kim SH, Jung J, Lee JH, Byun JY, Park MS, Yeo SG. Delayed facial nerve decompression for Bell's palsy. Eur Arch Otorhinolaryngol. 2016;273(7):1755-60.
6. Kong K, Sevy A. Temporal bone fracture requiring facial nerve decompression or repair. Oper Techniques Otolaryngol. 2017;28:277-83.

9
SECTION

Examination Section

29

Subjective Assessment and MCQs

Anuradha Singh

The examination section has been devised to facilitate examination preparation for MD or DNB exit examinations as well as for entrance examinations. Hence, long questions, short notes and multiple choice questions (MCQs) have been enlisted in this section. The chapter numbers which discuss the answer to specific questions are given in parentheses.

SECTION A: SUBJECTIVE ASSESSMENT

Long Questions

1. Discuss the role of imaging in cochlear implantation (Chapter 14).
2. Discuss the role of imaging in the evaluation of pulsatile tinnitus (Chapter 27).
3. Discuss the imaging approach to sensorineural hearing loss (Chapter 25).
4. Tumors of temporal bone: Enlist and briefly discuss (Chapter 16).
5. Discuss the imaging approach to facial nerve palsy (Chapter 28).

Short Notes

Write short notes on:

1. Malignant otitis externa (Chapter 8)
2. Cholesteatoma (Chapter 8)
3. Glomus tumors of the skull base (Chapter 16)
4. Schwannoma of 8th nerve (Chapters 12 and 16)
5. Temporal bone fractures (Chapter 23)
6. Otosclerosis (Chapters 20 and 25)
7. Magnetic resonance imaging of internal auditory canal (Chapter 12)
8. High-resolution computed tomography (HRCT) temporal bone techniques (Chapters 1 and 2)
9. Endolymphatic sac tumor (Chapter 16)
10. Labyrinthitis ossificans (Chapters 14 and 20)

SECTION B: MCQS

Questions

1. **A 5-year-old child presented to the emergency department with fever and otalgia. Clinical examination revealed postauricular erythema and tenderness. Otoscopy revealed bulging and erythematous tympanic membrane. Which of the following statements is FALSE about this condition?**
   a. Primarily a disease of infancy and young children
   b. Cross-sectional imaging is indicated in all the cases
   c. HRCT may reveal opacities with air-fluid level in middle ear and mastoid cavity
   d. Ossicular resorption not a common feature
2. **Regarding complicated otomastoiditis which of the following statements is FALSE?**
   a. Outer mastoid cortex is first to be destroyed in complicated mastoiditis leading to the formation of coalescent mastoiditis
   b. Pneumatized petrous apex increases the risk of petrous apicitis
   c. Bezold abscess is commonly seen in children
   d. Otogenic brain abscess is most commonly located in temporal lobe or anteriorly in the lateral cerebellar hemispheres
3. **A 50-year-old diabetic male presented with fever, otalgia, and otorrhea. Clinical and otoscopic examination was suggestive of acute otomastoiditis for which he was instituted antibiotics and supportive management. However, he continued to have persistent otorrhea and 4 days later developed deep facial and retro-orbital pain. Which of the following statements is not true?**
   a. HRCT followed by contrast-enhanced CT (CECT)/CEMRI are the next step in evaluation
   b. Pneumatized bone increases the risk of this condition
   c. Vernet's syndrome is a known complication
   d. Common complication of acute otomastoiditis
4. **Regarding sequelae of chronic otitis media, which of the following statements is TRUE?**
   a. Petrous apex effusion (entrapped effusion) may cause expansion and erosion of the petrous apex
   b. Cholesterol granuloma can be reliably differentiated from an entrapped effusion on the basis of MR signal
   c. Granulation tissue encases middle ear structures without any erosion and shows intense enhancement
   d. On MRI, cholesteatoma is predominantly T1 hyperintense, T2 hypointense, and shows intense enhancement
5. **A 35-year-old female presented with right-sided facial nerve palsy, vertigo, and dizziness. HRCT revealed an expansile lesion at the petrous apex. MRI revealed hyperintense on T1- and T2-weighted imaging (T2WI) with hypointense rim without any enhancement. Which of the following is the correct diagnosis?**

a. Cholesteatoma
b. Glomus tumor
c. Petrous internal carotid artery (ICA) aneurysm
d. Cholesterol granuloma

6. **Regarding cholesteatoma, which of the following statements is FALSE?**
   a. Acquired pars flaccida cholesteatoma most commonly arises in Prussak's space and causes medial displacement and erosion of ossicles
   b. Acquired pars tensa cholesteatoma tends to arise lateral to the ossicles
   c. Most common site of occurrence of congenital cholesteatoma is hypotympanum
   d. Petrous apex cholesteatomas may be congenital or acquired
7. **Which of the following statements is FALSE regarding MRI imaging in cholesteatoma?**
   a. It is usually hypointense on T1WI, and mildly hyperintense on T2WI
   b. Echo-planar diffusion-weighted imaging (DWI) is better than nonechoplanar DWI
   c. In the postoperative setting, sensitivity of detection of cholesteatoma decreases on DWI
   d. Cholesteatoma may show delayed postcontrast enhancement
8. **A 25-year-old male presented with acute onset otalgia and conductive hearing loss bilaterally, with no otorrhea. HRCT revealed an expansile soft tissue in bilateral external auditory canals which was expansile and was causing smooth widening of the bony canal. There was no invasion of the adjacent structures. Which of the following is the diagnosis?**
   a. Wax
   b. Keratosis obturans
   c. EAC cholesteatoma
   d. Malignant otitis externa
9. **Which of the following statements is FALSE regarding keratosis obturans?**
   a. Affects older population with unilateral predisposition
   b. Frequently bilateral
   c. May have an association with sinusitis and bronchiectasis
   d. No bone erosion
10. **A 25-year-old male presented with headache, right-sided gradually progressive sensorineural hearing loss (SNHL), pulsatile tinnitus, aural fullness, and vertigo. HRCT temporal bone revealed an ill-defined infiltrative lesion with lytic-permeative bone destruction in the retrolabyrinthine petrous bone involving the vestibular aqueduct. Which of the following statements is FALSE regarding the lesion?**
    a. Mild enhancement on gadolinium-enhanced MRI
    b. Bony spicules may be present within the lesion
    c. May invade adjacent structures
    d. Genetic testing to be done
11. **A 45-year-old female presented with pulsatile tinnitus, SNHL, and hoarseness of voice. CT showed lytic permeative destruction at the petrous apex which was centered at jugular fossa and contiguously extending to**

the retrolabyrinthine petrous apex, middle ear, inner ear, and mastoid cavity. There was no matrix mineralization or internal calcification. On MRI, the lesion was hypointense on T1WI with foci of hyperintensity and intralesional flow voids. On T2WI, it was heterogeneously hyperintense and showed intense strong enhancement. Two other similar lesions were present in the soft tissue of neck. For the imaging appearance, differential consideration of paraganglioma versus endolymphatic sac tumor was kept. All of the following imaging findings differentiate paraganglioma from endolymphatic sac tumor over, EXCEPT:

a. Epicenter at jugular fossa
b. Lack of calcification
c. Presence of signal voids
d. Similar lesions in neck

12. **Most common lesion at petrous apex:**
    a. Trapped effusion
    b. Cholesterol granuloma
    c. Cholesteatoma
    d. Chondrosarcoma
13. **A noncontrast CT (NCCT) head in a trauma patient incidentally revealed an expansile soft tissue at the petrous apex with thinning of the cortical margins. Which of the following cannot be the diagnosis?**
    a. Cholesteatoma
    b. Cholesterol granuloma
    c. Petrous apex aneurysm
    d. Trapped effusion
14. **Which of the following statements is FALSE regarding petrous apex ICA aneurysms?**
    a. Calcification may be present
    b. Expansion of bony carotid canal may be present
    c. CT angiography is the noninvasive diagnostic modality of choice
    d. "Zipper artifact" on MRI suggestive of intralesional flow differentiates it from other expansile lesion at the petrous apex
15. **Regarding petrous apex cephaloceles, which of the following statements is TRUE?**
    a. Herniation of mesial temporal lobe
    b. CT cisternography highly sensitive in detecting the communication
    c. Coronal T2W sequence is the best sequence to demonstrate communication with the Meckel's cave
    d. Surgical correction of the defect is the treatment of choice
16. **Which of the following statements is FALSE regarding petrous apex tumors?**
    a. Most common tumor to metastasize at petrous apex is breast carcinoma
    b. Chondrosarcoma is the most common primary tumor of the petrous apex
    c. Chondrosarcoma arises from spheno-occipital synchondrosis
    d. Absence of chondroid matrix does not exclude the diagnosis of chondrosarcoma

17. A 32-year-old female underwent NCCT for evaluation of headache which revealed a cystic lesion of fluid attenuation in right cerebellopontine angle (CPA) which was extending into the ipsilateral internal auditory canal (IAC) with mass effect on the brainstem and cerebellar hemisphere. No calcification or fat density within. MRI was done for further evaluation which revealed the lesion to be T1 hypo- and T2 hyperintense (although the signal intensity was slightly higher than the CSF). There was no appreciable enhancement within the lesion. Which of the following MRI sequence is most helpful in ascertaining the diagnosis?

a. FLAIR
b. Heavily T2-WI
c. DWI
d. SWI

18. Regarding MR anatomy of IAC, which of the following statements is FALSE?

a. IAC lesions tend to present more likely with symptoms of SNHL than facial nerve palsy as the latter is more resistant to compression
b. In sagittal plane, volume of vestibulocochlear nerve is twice that of facial nerve
c. Cochlear branch runs anteroinferior to superior vestibular nerve
d. Gadolinium-enhanced MRI is imperative in the evaluation of adults with SNHL

19. All of the following determine hearing preservation in a case of vestibular schwannoma (VS) postoperatively, EXCEPT:

a. Volume of tumor occupancy in CPA cistern
b. Fluid signal intensity at the fundus of IAC on heavily T2-weighted sequence
c. Fluid signal intensity in the membranous labyrinth
d. Surgical approach—retrosigmoid versus translabyrinthine

20. For the differentiation of VS from a meningioma at IAC/CPA, which of the following statements is FALSE?

a. VS is centered at IAC whereas meningioma is usually centered at CPA
b. The cisternal component of the lesion makes obtuse angle with the petrous temporal bone in VS whereas it is acute in meningioma
c. IAC/porus acoustic widening is a feature specific to VS
d. Presence of calcification favors the diagnosis of meningioma

21. A 5-year-old child developed acute onset left-sided deafness and ipsilateral facial nerve palsy. MRI revealed enhancing lesion in left IAC with extension of the lesion to the geniculate ganglion and tympanic segment of the facial nerve. Also, there was enhancement of cochlea and lateral semicircular canal. Petrous apex on the ipsilateral side was hypointense on precontrast routine nonfat-suppressed T1WI and it also showed enhancement. There were no neurocutaneous stigmata. Which is most likely diagnosis?

a. Plexiform neurofibroma of the facial nerve
b. Vestibular schwannoma
c. Meningioma
d. High grade malignancy

22. **Which of the following is the most common congenital malformation of the inner ear?**
 a. Michel aplasia
 b. Mondini deformity
 c. Cystic cochleovestibular malformation
 d. Cochlear hypoplasia
23. **Which of the following statements is FALSE pertaining to type I and type II incomplete partition?**

		Type I	Type II
a.	Modiolus and internal scalar septum	Completely absent	Partially present
b.	Cochlea	Completely cystic	Cystic apex
c.	Size of vestibular aqueduct	Normal	Enlarged
d.	Diameter of internal auditory canal	Normal	Enlarged

24. **A 4-year-old girl presented with right SNHL. MRI demonstrated IAC to be of normal caliber; however, with an abrupt termination. Cochlea was not seen and vestibule was slightly dilated. Posterior semicircular canal was also dilated and stunted. HRCT done showed sclerotic focus anterior to IAC. Which of the following imaging findings is the best diagnostic clue to the correct diagnosis?**
 a. Flat medial wall of middle ear cavity
 b. Absence of cochlear nerve
 c. Size of the vestibular aqueduct
 d. Presence of similar findings contralaterally
25. **In a case of congenital SNHL planned for cochlear implant, HRCT demonstrates normal external, middle, and inner ear structures. Size of the IAC is also normal. Amongst the following, which is the most important structure to be evaluated on MRI before surgery?**
 a. Perilymphatic fluid in cochlea and vestibule
 b. Cochlear nerve
 c. Size of vestibular aqueduct
 d. Associated malformations in brain
26. **All of the following are contraindications (absolute or relative) for cochlear implant, EXCEPT:**
 a. Complete labyrinthine aplasia
 b. Cochlear aplasia
 c. Cochlear hypoplasia
 d. Deficient cochlear nerve
27. **Which is the most common inner ear malformation present in SNHL?**
 a. Cochlear hypoplasia
 b. Cystic vestibule
 c. Cochlear nerve agenesis
 d. Enlarged vestibular aqueduct
28. **Which of the following is an indication for emergency surgery in case of temporal bone trauma?**
 a. Complete facial nerve palsy
 b. CSF otorrhea

c. Perilymphatic fistula
d. Ossicular dislocation

29. As per the traditional system for temporal bone fracture classification, which of the following statements is a mismatch?

Injury	More common in
a. Tympanic membrane injury	Longitudinal fracture
b. Ossicular injury	Longitudinal fracture
c. Peripheral facial nerve palsy	Transverse fracture
d. Labyrinthine injury	Longitudinal fracture

30. Regarding ossicular injury, which of the following statements is FALSE?
a. More commonly seen in longitudinal than transverse fracture
b. Most common cause of conductive hearing loss following trauma
c. Ossicular dislocation is more common than ossicular fracture
d. Incudostapedial joint separation is the most common ossicular injury

31. A 35-year-old female presented with chronic progressive right-sided hearing loss from past 5 years. She also had otalgia and nonpulsatile tinnitus. Her symptoms had exacerbated during pregnancy; however, at times she used to feel better, relatively symptoms-free days during her course of illness. There was no other significant medical history. On otoscopy, tympanic membrane was intact and middle ear was normal. Audiology evaluation revealed mixed conductive–SNHL. HRCT showed mottled lucency along the basal turn of cochlea and in the region of oval window. Similar lesion was also noted incidentally adjacent to oval window. What is the diagnosis?
a. Cholesteatoma
b. Otosclerosis
c. Osteogenesis imperfecta
d. Paget's disease

32. A 40-year-old male had a long-standing history of vertigo, dizziness, feeling of moving of stationary objects, hearing loss, and pulsatile tinnitus. These symptoms were exacerbated while coughing, sneezing, or with loud sounds. What is the most likely finding on HRCT?
a. Dehiscent superior semicircular canal
b. Dehiscent jugular bulb
c. Retrofenestral otosclerosis
d. Cochlear malformation

33. A 25-year-old patient presented with complaints of fullness in right ear which was associated with tinnitus. He also used to feel dizzy as if he was about to fall, although he never had true vertigo. No significant medical or past history; however, socio-personal revealed him to be an adventure-loving person engaged in SCUBA diving and mountaineering which he had left now as there was worsening of symptoms with such activities. Which of the following is not an expected finding on cross-sectional (CT/MRI) imaging?
a. Enhancement of vestibulocochlear nerve
b. Presence of fluid in window (round/oval) niches
c. Pneumolabyrinth
d. Disorientation of stapes footplate

34. All of the following statements are true regarding exostoses of external ear, EXCEPT:
   a. Mostly is seen in swimmers
   b. Usually multiple
   c. Pedunculated
   d. Bilateral

35. Most common temporal bone tumor is:
   a. Vestibular schwannoma
   b. Glomus complex tumors
   c. Meningioma
   d. Facial nerve schwannoma

36. Which of the following is FALSE regarding cone beam CT (CBCT) as compared to multidetector computed tomography (MDCT) in temporal bone imaging?
   a. High spatial resolution
   b. Less sensitive to beam hardening and metallic artifacts
   c. Low radiation dose
   d. Less sensitive to motion artifacts

37. Which of the following is FALSE about microtia?
   a. Inner ear anomaly is usually not associated
   b. May be associated with congenital cholesteatoma
   c. Reconstructive surgery of EAC and ossicles remain equally difficult in atresia as well as stenosis of EAC
   d. Facial nerve may have anomalous anterolateral course

38. A 20-year-old male presented with history of chronic suppurative otitis media (CSOM) in right ear from past 5 years which was being managed conservatively. From past 1 year, he complained of progressive hearing loss (conductive); however, but there was no aural discharge this time. He underwent HRCT which showed soft tissue in the middle ear which was encasing the ear ossicles. There was no bone or ossicular erosion. On the contrary, stapes suprastructure was better delineated than contralateral normal ear. All of the following may be a finding in this entity, EXCEPT:
   a. Small calcific foci may be present in the tympanic cavity
   b. New bone formation may be seen in epitympanum
   c. Focus of demineralization in the region of oval window
   d. Thickened tympanic membrane which may have calcific foci

39. On HRCT, narrowed or nonvisualized vestibular aqueduct is seen in which of the following condition?
   a. Otosclerosis
   b. Méniére's disease
   c. Postinflammatory ossicular fixation (PIOF)
   d. Labyrinthine fibrosis

40. Regarding radiological reporting in surgical planning in chronic otomastoiditis which of the following statements is FALSE?
   a. Small, sclerotic opacified mastoid—canal wall down (CWD) mastoidectomy
   b. Large, well-aerated mastoid—canal wall up (CWU) mastoidectomy

c. Aeration of middle ear cavity prognosticates hearing outcome post ossicular reconstruction
d. Associated erosion of EAC—CWU mastoidectomy

41. Which of the following is a mismatch for initial imaging modality?
a. Conductive hearing loss in children—HRCT temporal bone
b. Conductive hearing loss in adults—CECT
c. Sensorineural hearing loss in children—noncontrast MRI
d. Sensorineural hearing loss in adults—CEMRI

42. Regarding glomus tumor and schwannoma in jugular foramen, which of the following statements is FALSE?
a. Lytic permeative bone destruction in glomus, scalloping/bone remodeling in schwannoma
b. Predominant direction of growth superomedially in glomus to involve the brainstem whereas it is superolaterally to involve hypotympanum in schwannoma
c. Schwannoma is less likely to infiltrate surrounding structures
d. Glomus is more responsive to radiotherapy

43. All of the following statements are true regarding imaging evaluation of pulsatile tinnitus (PT), EXCEPT:
a. PT with conductive hearing loss and/or vascular tympanic membrane—HRCT followed by MRI if needed
b. MRI including MRA is the modality of choice for evaluation of PT
c. PT with negative MRI and CT—psychiatric referral
d. Carotid Doppler, CT or MR angiography of neck vessels if risk of atherosclerosis

44. Which of the following statements is FALSE regarding labyrinthitis ossificans?
a. Enhancement on inner ear structures on MRI earliest imaging finding
b. Loss of fluid signal intensity on T2WI may precede the CT findings
c. Replacement of inner ear structures with bone in later stages
d. Narrowing of IAC and obliteration of cochlear promontory in end stage

45. Which of the following statements is FALSE regarding glomus tumors?
a. Ossicular destruction is common in both glomus tympanicum and glomus jugulotympanic tumors
b. "Salt and pepper appearance" on T1WI are usually seen in tumors >1 cm in size
c. Expansion and lytic permeative bone destruction in tumors arising from jugular foramen
d. Glomus tumor originates at cochlear promontory

46. All of the following is true regarding vascular anatomical variant pertaining to temporal bone on HRCT, EXCEPT:
a. Aberrant ICA—hypoplasia of vertical segment of carotid canal with a more lateral course
b. Persistent stapedial artery—tubular structure traveling against cochlear promontory
c. High-riding jugular bulb—if superior margin of bulb reaches epitympanum
d. Dehiscent jugular bulb—absent bone between jugular bulb and middle ear cavity

47. All of the following are true regarding imaging in suspected recurrence of paraganglioma, EXCEPT:
   a. Gadolinium-enhanced fat-saturated MRI differentiates recurrence from postoperative changes
   b. Slight progression of bone destruction is an expected finding postsurgery
   c. Octreotide scan may be helpful in some cases
   d. DSA is indicated if findings on other imaging modalities are inconclusive or indeterminate

48. Amongst the following, cholesteatoma is least likely to involve:
   a. Lateral epitympanic wall
   b. Lateral semicircular canal
   c. Long process of incus
   d. Cochlear promontory

49. Regarding imaging evaluation of facial nerve, which of the following statements is TRUE?
   a. Contrast-enhanced MRI is modality of choice in infective, inflammatory, or neoplastic involvement irrespective of the site of involvement along the course of nerve
   b. No enhancement in normal facial nerve
   c. All cases of post-traumatic facial palsy should be evaluated with MRI
   d. Certain benign tumors like lipoma and hemangioma of facial nerve should not be operated if not compromising the function of facial nerve

50. Which of the following statements is FALSE regarding HRCT anatomy of temporal bone?
   a. Mesotympanum has two recesses—facial recess and sinus tympani
   b. "Ice-cream cone" appearance is formed by head of malleus and body of incus
   c. Diameter of IAC <2 mm suggests hypoplasia
   d. Tympanic segment of facial nerve courses underneath posterior semicircular canal

Answers

Q1. Answer: b

The child herein is suffering from acute otitis media and the fact that he is additionally having postauricular erythema and tenderness points to complicated mastoiditis. Imaging is not indicated in uncomplicated acute otitis media. In complicated otomastoiditis as there is erosion of mastoid cortex and trabecula, cross-sectional imaging is mandated to rule out intratemporal/intracranial complications. Acute otomastoiditis may reveal an air-fluid level on imaging.

Q2. Answer: c

Bezold abscess is consequential to the tracking of the mastoid abscess/empyema through the tip of the mastoid cortex into the digastric fossa. It is seen usually in adults. In children, since the mastoid tip is not pneumatized, the abscess does not track there.

Q3. Answer: d

The clinical presentation in this case is classical of *Gradenigo's syndrome or petrous apex syndrome secondary to petrous apicitis.* It is a clinical triad comprising of otitis media, abducens nerve palsy, and deep facio-orbital pain; although all patients do not present with this classical triad. Petrous apex may be pneumatized in nearly 30% of the population which increases the risk of petrous apicitis in cases of acute otitis media and mastoiditis. The condition should be suspected if otorrhea is persistent despite adequate antibiotic coverage or even after surgery, with increased risk in diabetic and immunosuppressed/immunocompromised people. Facial and retro-orbital pain is due to the involvement of maxillary and ophthalmic division of trigeminal nerve. Horizontal diplopia is secondary to the involvement of the abducent nerve in the Dorello's canal under petrosphenoid ligament at petrous apex. Both CT and MRI are complimentary imaging modality in such cases. CT scan evaluates extent of pneumatization of petrous apex. CEMRI demonstrates hyperintensity at petrous apex with adjacent meningeal enhancement. Further, it helps to distinguish other differentials at this location like osteomyelitis, cholesteatoma, or tumors and hence, guide further management. It may further extend to the skull base leading to multiple cranial nerve palsies (Vernet's syndrome, 9th to 11th nerve palsies).

Q4. Answer: c

All of these entities on HRCT present as soft tissue opacification in middle ear and mastoid cavity or in the petrous apex and hence, remain differentials on imaging.

Entrapped effusion at petrous apex may mimic cholesterol granuloma on CT scan. Further, retained secretion may parallel the signal intensity of cholesterol granuloma on noncontrast MRI. However, bone expansion and ossicular erosion are not features of entrapped simple effusion whereas it is seen in cholesterol granuloma; thus, distinguishing the two. Granulation tissue is highly vascular and shows intense enhancement on gadolinium-enhanced MRI. In cholesteatoma, ossicular/bone erosion is a feature. On MRI, diffusion restriction and delayed gadolinium enhancement are other features.

Q5. Answer: d

For the location of the lesion at the petrous apex, excluding glomus tumor, rest other options are possible. Expansile lesions at petrous apex include mucocele, cholesterol granuloma, aneurysm, and cholesteatoma. Petrous apex aneurysm may have variable signal intensity depending upon the extent of thrombosis, size, and flow dynamics. Cholesteatoma is hypo on T1WI and hyper on T2WI. Expansion of the underlying bone without any enhancement with the presence of hypointense rim (due to hemosiderin deposition) suggests the diagnosis of cholesterol granuloma.

Q6. Answer: c

Most common location of the congenital cholesteatoma is anterosuperior part of the middle ear cavity just cranial to the opening of Eustachian tube.

Q7. Answer: b

Nonecho-planar turbo spin-echo DWI is more sensitive in detection of the cholesteatoma, as acquisition of even 2 mm thin slices is possible with this technique, with less susceptibility artifacts at the air-bone interface. In postoperative ear, specificity of detection of cholesteatoma on DWI remains high; however, sensitivity decreases especially in small lesions (<3 mm).

Q8. Answer: b

Q9. Answer: a

Keratosis obturans (KO) as well as external ear cholesteatoma occurs due to accretion of desquamated keratin debris in the external auditory canal (EAC). KO tends to occur in younger population, is frequently bilateral, acute in onset, and is usually a painful condition. On the contrary, EAC cholesteatoma affects older age groups, is unilateral, and is more chronic in onset, with otorrhea being more common than otalgia. On HRCT both may present as expansile soft tissue masses. However, expansion or smooth widening of the bony canal suggests diagnosis of KO. EAC cholesteatoma frequently erodes the inferior and posterior walls of the EAC, and extends into the mastoid cavity.

Q10. Answer: a

Patient is having symptoms classical of endolymphatic hydrops. The diagnosis is endolymphatic sac tumor. It is characterized by moth-eaten bone destruction of the retrolabyrinthine petrous segment which may extend to the adjacent structures. The tumor usually shows internal amorphous and posterior rim calcification on CT which are spicules of the residual bone. It is a highly vascular tumor and shows intense solid enhancement. For its hypervascularity, lesions >2 cm may show flow voids. It may be seen in 10–15% of cases of Von Hippel-Lindau syndrome in which case they may be bilateral.

Q11. Answer: c

Endolymphatic sac tumor and paraganglioma are differentials on imaging. Both cause aggressive lytic-permeative or moth-eaten bone destruction at the petrous apex which may extend contiguously to other segments. They share similar imaging features on MRI and remain indistinguishable. However, they may be distinguished by the predominant site of involvement—paraganglioma is epicentered at jugular fossa, whereas endolymphatic sac tumor is epicentered at the retrolabyrinthine petrous segment in the region of vestibular aqueduct. Moreover, presence of amorphous calcification or bony spicules on CT also favors the diagnosis of endolymphatic sac tumors over paraganglioma. These bony spicules may be seen as signal void on MRI in endolymphatic sac tumors.

Q12. Answer: b

Q13. Answer: d

Differential diagnosis of expansile lesion with smooth cortical margins at petrous apex includes cholesteatoma, cholesterol granuloma, petrous apex aneurysm, cephaloceles, and mucocele.

Q14. Answer: d

Petrous apex aneurysm is usually consequential to the congenital weakness in the wall of the artery at the site of origin of embryonic vessels. Unlike aneurysms elsewhere, it remains asymptomatic and grows insidiously for a considerable time before becoming symptomatic due to mass effect. As a result, nonuniform calcification may develop within its wall or within the thrombus, if present. Signal intensity on MRI may be variable depending on the size of aneurysm, luminal patency, and presence of thrombus. In a pulsatile aneurysm, intralesional flow may be suggested by motion artifact on MRI, most commonly on contrast-enhanced T1WI sequence. This artifact occurs in phase-encoding direction. Zipper artifact on the other hand occurs in frequency-encoding direction and is due to the release of electromagnetic energy.

Q15. Answer: c

Petrous apex cephaloceles, unlike cephaloceles elsewhere, do not contain any brain tissue but may have some prolapsed fibers of trigeminal nerve lined by dura and arachnoid mater. It is postulated to occur secondary to chronic cerebrospinal fluid (CSF) pulsations against an area of congenital bony weakness leading to its dehiscence which develops communication with the Meckel's cave. It may be bilateral in some cases. On CT, it appears as an expansile lobulated cystic lesion at the petrous apex which follows the CSF signal intensity on all the MRI sequence. However, its communication superomedially with the Meckel's cave is best demonstrated on coronal T2WI. CT cisternography may be used in doubtful cases. It is usually an incidental finding and requiring no intervention.

Q16. Answer: c

Most common cause of metastasis at the petrous apex is breast carcinoma followed by lung and prostate in that order. Chordoma and chondrosarcoma can be differentiated from the fact that chordoma is usually a midline lesion which arises from spheno-occipital synchondrosis. On the contrary, chondrosarcoma arises from petro-occipital synchondrosis. Chondroid matrix, if present, is diagnostic of chondrosarcoma; however, it is present in only 50% of the cases.

Q17. Answer: c

Differential diagnosis for a cystic lesion in CPA includes epidermoid cyst, arachnoid cyst, neurenteric cyst, and dermoid cyst, although, latter is more commonly in the midline. At times, cystic component of a tumor arising in the adjoining regions (e.g., cystic schwannoma) may extend into the CPA. Amongst these, epidermoid is most common in this location with this pseudocystic appearance and it can be differentiated from other lesions by characteristic restriction on DWI.

Q18. Answer: c

Vestibulocochlear nerve is almost twice in thickness to facial nerve. In fact, if they are of equal thickness, then agenesis of any component of vestibulocochlear nerve should be sought. Further, a normal cochlear nerve is approximately the same diameter as that of the facial nerve. In all the cases with SNHL, imaging evaluation should include thin T1WI (2 mm thickness) postcontrast sequence as some lesions, like infection/inflammation or metastasis may present only with enhancement of these nerves without any discernible lesion on heavily T2-weighted sequence.

Q19. Answer: a

Positive predictors for postoperative hearing preservation in a case of VS are presence of fluid signal intensity in the membranous labyrinth and the residual fluid signal in the fundus of IAC on heavily T2-weighted sequence. The latter is decided by volume of intracanalicular component of tumor and not cisternal. Retrosigmoid approach is more favorable for hearing preservation and is particularly suited for small lesions; however, it suffers from drawback of inadequate exposure to the canalicular segments of nerves. Translabyrinthine approach is reserved for large tumors or cases with complete deafness/profound SNHL.

Q20. Answer: b

Vestibular schwannoma (VS) is the most common IAC/CPA tumor followed by meningioma. These tumors may have similar imaging features on cross-sectional imaging. For their classical imaging appearance, neither "ice-cream cone sign" or "dural tail sign" are specific to VS and meningioma, respectively (**Table 1**). However, these may be distinguished by combination of findings as mentioned vide infra. Their preoperative distinction is imperative as preoperative embolization is done in meningioma for their high vascularity.

TABLE 1 **Differences between vestibular schwannoma and meningioma.**

Feature	Vestibular schwannoma	Meningioma
1. Location (with respect to IAC/porus acoustic)	Centered at porus acoustic	Often eccentric. Centered at CPA
2. Cisternal/CPA component of the lesion		
a. Shape	Spherical	Oval/hemispherical/plaque like obtuse
b. Its angle with petrous bone	Acute	
3. Calcification on CT	Not a feature unless treated	May be present in ~20% of cases
4. IAC widening	Present in large, long-standing tumor	Not a feature (even with canalicular extension)
5. Bony hyperostosis	Not a feature	May be present depending on location
6. MR perfusion	Low relative cerebral blood volume	High relative cerebral blood volume
7. MR spectroscopy	Myoinositol peak may be present	Alanine peak may be present

(CPA: cerebellopontine angle; IAC: Internal auditory canal)

Q21. Answer: d

Unlike adults, nerve sheath tumors are uncommon in children especially in the absence of stigmata of neurocutaneous syndrome. In this case, acute presentation with presence of solid lesion hints toward an aggressive pathology. Imaging description, otherwise, is fitting into plexiform neurofibroma of nerve sheath except for loss of marrow signal intensity at petrous apex in conjunction with its enhancement which hints toward its infiltration. Hence, the spectrum of IAC/CPA lesions in children is different than adults and a malignancy like rhabdomyosarcoma should be a concern in such age group in the absence of known neurocutaneous syndromes and aggressive findings on imaging.

Q22. Answer: b

Most common congenital malformation of the inner ear is type II incomplete partition a.k.a Mondini deformity (50%), followed by common cavity (~25%) and cochlear hypoplasia (~15%) in that order. Type I incomplete partition is also called cystic cochleovestibular malformation and accounts for ~6% of cases. Michel aplasia or complete labyrinthine aplasia is least common (1%).

Q23. Answer: d

Type I incomplete partition: Complete absence of modiolus and interscalar septum in cochlea, cochlea and vestibule cystic with partition between them (figure of 8 or snowman appearance on axial imaging), *IAC enlarged due to defective cribriform plate between IAC and cochlea predisposing to increased risk of meningitis*, and vestibular aqueduct normal sized.

Type II incomplete partition: Absence of modiolus and interscalar septum in middle turn and apex of cochlea (cystic cochlear apex), normal basal turn of cochlea, IAC normal sized, and *vestibular aqueduct enlarged.*

Q24. Answer: a

Sclerotic focus of bone anterior to IAC with no cochlea visible raises the possibilities of cochlear aplasia and labyrinthitis ossificans (LO). These two may be distinguished by the flat medial wall of the middle ear which is characteristically present in cochlear aplasia. Normally, bulge in medial wall is due to cochlear promontory which is because of the basal turn of cochlea which is preserved in LO. In long-standing LO, there may be atrophy of cochlear nerve. Cochlear aplasia may have associated malformations like in this case.

Q25. Answer: b

Size and morphology of IAC and normal anatomy of inner structures do not rule out cochlear nerve deficiency.

Q26. Answer: c

Q27. Answer: d

On CT, width of vestibular aqueduct is normally <1.5 mm and it is almost parallel and similar in width to the adjacent posterior semicircular canal. Its diameter is measured in midway when it exits vestibule and enters posterior fossa. This diameter is best measured in paracoronal plane reformatted perpendicular to the long axis of petrous bone. This abnormality may be isolated or seen along with other malformations like Type II incomplete partition, dysplasia of vestibule, or semicircular canals.

Q28. Answer: a

Complete facial nerve palsy may be due to bony fragment impinging on the nerve which requires immediate surgical correction. In rest other options, interval surgery is recommended.

Q29. Answer: d

Longitudinal fracture is more common (~70–80%), followed by transverse and mixed fractures. Longitudinal fracture more commonly involves middle ear structures as compared to greater involved of inner ear structures in transverse fracture. Facial nerve is most commonly injured around geniculate ganglion due to traction from greater superficial petrosal nerve. Such injury is most commonly seen in lateral subtype of transverse fracture.

Q30. Answer: b

Most common cause of conductive hearing loss following trauma is hemotympanum or tympanic membrane perforation. Ossicular injury may be missed on initial CT due to associated hemotympanum, but if conductive hearing loss persists beyond 1 month following injury, then associated ossicular injury should be sought. Ossicular disruption is more common than ossicular fracture. Incus is most commonly injured ossicle owing to its large size and lack of ligamentous and muscular support.

Q31. Answer: b

Otosclerosis is diagnosed on the basis of classical history with characteristic findings on audiology and HRCT. It usually presents in females in their 4–5th decade with progressive hearing loss with bilateral involvement in most of the cases (~85%). It may have episodes of remission. HRCT demonstrates foci of demineralization or resorption which is earliest seen anterior to stapes footplate or oval window a.k.a fissula ante fenestram. Depending upon the stage of disease, it may have involvement of other labyrinthine structures.

Q32. Answer: a

Symptomatology of this patient is classical for "third-window abnormalities" which include hearing loss, pressure (Valsalva, loud noise, shear forces, etc.) induced vestibular, and visual symptoms (Tullio and Hennebert signs). It includes defect in the bony integrity of the inner ear structures creating additional window apart from the two physiologic round and oval window. As a result, there is shunting of the acoustic energy from the oval window with further decrease in transmission to round window. Further, the third window can induce motion in endolymph in addition to the round and oval windows. Conditions which can produce this symptomatology include semicircular canal dehiscence (most commonly superior), enlarged vestibular aqueduct, perilabyrinthine fistula, cochlear dehiscence involving scala vestibuli, bone dyscrasias, etc. It is to be noted that the bony dehiscence of semicircular canal may sometimes be noted incidentally on HRCT.

Q33. Answer: a

Symptomatology here points to labyrinthine abnormality with "pressure sensitivity," meaning, replication/worsening of symptoms with change in atmospheric pressure (barotrauma) like SCUBA diving/mountaineering. Such pressure sensitivity may be present in many conditions including perilymphatic fistula (PLF), vestibular fibrosis, Méniére's disease, etc. Most common cause of PLF is head trauma, barotrauma, certain otological surgeries, (mastoidectomy, stapedectomy, and fenestration), as a complication of chronic otomastoiditis, and certain anatomic abnormalities (facial canal dehiscence and jugular bulb dehiscence). In this condition, there is development of abnormal communication between air-containing middle ear and fluid-containing inner ear. Such communication commonly develops at round window, oval window, otic capsule, and mastoid. A combination of CT and MRI findings helps to arrive at diagnosis. Most common findings include middle ear effusion and pneumolabyrinth. Additional findings can be replacement of normally air-containing window niches (round/oval) with effusion and disorientation of stapes footplate (normally oriented parallel to the long axis of vestibule and medial vestibular wall).

Q34. Answer: c

Exostoses are usually seen in swimmers due to contact with cold water. Its imaging differential is osteoma which is unilateral and pedunculated whereas exostoses are sessile.

Q35. Answer: a

Vestibular schwannoma is the most common tumor of temporal bone. Glomus complex (paraganglioma and nonchromaffin chemodectomas) tumors are the most common neoplasm of middle ear cavity.

Q36. Answer: d

CBCT is less sensitive to beam hardening artifact because image acquisition is based on conventional radiographic images. In it, a cone-shaped X-ray beam is directed through the center of temporal bone on a two-dimensional X-ray detector. Apart from the above-mentioned advantages, it also has shorter imaging time compared to MDCT. However, it is extremely sensitive to motion artifacts as head is to remain perfectly straight during the scanning time of nearly 40 seconds.

Q37. Answer: c

Microtia is usually associated with external and middle ear abnormality. Inner ear is usually normal or there may mild labyrinthine abnormality due to separate embryonic origin. Reconstructive surgery is usually facilitated in the presence of EAC, even if it is dysplastic or stenosed as it serves as landmark for safe accessibility to middle ear. There may be associated anatomical variations like anomalous course of facial nerve or aberrant ICA, which further increases the operative risk.

Q38. Answer: c

The diagnosis in this case is postinflammatory ossicular fixation (PIOF). Most important clinical clue to the diagnosis is "dry ear with conductive hearing loss." Differential diagnosis on this basis include: PIOF, otosclerosis, ossicular dysplasia, abnormalities in labyrinthine windows, etc. Causes of soft tissue in case of CSOM may be—fluid, cholesteatoma, and PIOF. HRCT shows findings characteristic of tympanosclerosis of stapes crura, i.e., increased visibility of stapes suprastructure which is "too well seen." In tympanosclerosis, there is uni- or multifocal calcific foci, calcification of tendons and ligaments in the middle ear are characteristic. Option c is characteristically seen in otosclerosis.

Q39. Answer: b

Correspondingly on high-resolution MRI, endolymphatic sac and duct may similarly be narrowed or nonvisualized.

Q40. Answer: d

Various surgical processes and surgical relevance of radiological findings are described in **Table 2**.

TABLE 2 Surgical relevance of radiological findings in cholesteatoma.

Radiological findings	Surgery/Surgical relevance
Cholesteatoma confined to Prussak's space—lateral attic and mastoid not involved	Atticotomy
Cholesteatoma extending beyond attic—mastoid and EAC not involved	CWU
Cholesteatoma extending beyond attic—small sclerotic mastoid and/or EAC erosion	CWD
Status of ossicular chain	For choice of ossicular reconstruction
Aeration of middle ear cavity	Prognosticates hearing outcome after ossicular reconstruction
• Position of jugular bulb • Position of sigmoid sinus with respect to posterior wall of EAC in sagittal plane • Position of tegmen tympani with respect to roof of middle ear cavity	Surgical landmarks in CSOM surgery (CWD/CWU)
• Dehiscent facial nerve canal • Aberrant carotid artery • Lateral semicircular canal fistula	Other surgical hazards

(CSOM: chronic suppurative otitis media; CWD: canal wall down; CWU: canal wall up; EAC: external auditory canal)

Q41. Answer: b

Conductive hearing loss in children or adults—HRCT temporal bone. SNHL in children is usually due to congenital inner ear anomalies in which noncontrast MRI is sufficient. On the other hand, in adults, SNHL is usually due to infection, inflammation, or tumor, hence CEMRI is recommended.

Q42. Answer: b

For jugular foramen tumors, paraganglioma predominantly grows superolaterally to involve medial hypotympanum whereas schwannoma grows superomedially to involve lateral brainstem. Glomus tumors are more infiltrative compared to schwannoma making surgical resection easier for latter. Lytic permeative pattern of bone destruction on CT and flow voids on MRI signifying their hypervascularity are characteristic feature of glomus tumors on imaging. On the other hand, schwannoma has slower growth rate and malignant potential as compared to glomus tumors.

Q43. Answer: c

Objective pulsatile tinnitus with apparently normal CT and MRI requires further confirmation with DSA (digital subtraction angiography) to rule out occult dural arteriovenous malformation (DAVF). Option A is typical presentation of glomus tumor.

Q44. Answer: d

Labyrinthitis ossificans (LO) has three stages with following imaging findings (**Table 3**):

TABLE 3 Imaging findings in various stages of LO.

Stage	CT	MRI
Acute	Normal	Enhancement of inner ear structures
Fibrous	Normal/slightly increased density	Loss of fluid signal intensity in membranous labyrinth
Ossifying	Replacement of inner ear structures with new bone depending upon severity of involvement	Obliteration of membranous labyrinth

- In suspected labyrinthitis, imaging modality of choice depends on stage
- Acute and fibrous—CEMRI
- Osseous stage—HRCT temporal bone
- In long-standing cases, there may be atrophy of cochlear nerve, but IAC dimensions and shape of cochlear promontory are maintained; hence, distinguishing it from cochlear or labyrinthine aplasia.

Q45. Answer: a

Bone and ossicular destruction are more common in jugulotympanic tumors as compared to tumors originating in middle ear cavity even if they are large enough.

Q46. Answer: c

If the highest level of jugular bulb is at or above the level of floor of IAC or above the basal turn of cochlea, then it is labeled as high-riding jugular bulb. Persistent stapedial artery arises at the junction of petrous and horizontal segment of ICA, enters hypotympanum, and travels along cochlear promontory.

Q47. Answer: b

Increase in bone destruction may be one of the earliest hints which should be carefully sought if recurrence is suspected.

Q48. Answer: d

Q49. Answer: d

Choice of imaging modality for evaluation of facial nerve depends on clinical localization of the segment of nerve involved. CT—for lateral segment if nerve: Beyond IAC to stylomastoid foramen (intratemporal course). MRI—for medial segment of nerve: From origin at brainstem to IAC, also for perineural spread of parotid malignancy (intracranial and extratemporal course)

If not localized, then CEMRI is indicated. Faint enhancement on MRI may be seen in geniculate, tympanic, and mastoid segments of nerve. Rest all enhancement along the course of nerve is abnormal. All facial nerve lesions need not be excised, especially, if there is no significant compromise of facial function and risk of progression, except cholesteatoma which should always be excised.

Q50. Answer: d

Tympanic segment of facial nerve courses underneath lateral semicircular canal.

30

Spotters

Ashu Seith Bhalla, Manisha Jana

- This chapter contains 50 imaging spotters with the answer key.
- Figure parts bearing same number belong to the same patient.
- Abnormal findings are marked with proper annotations, wherever required.
- Some spots have specific questions related to them, appropriately marked.

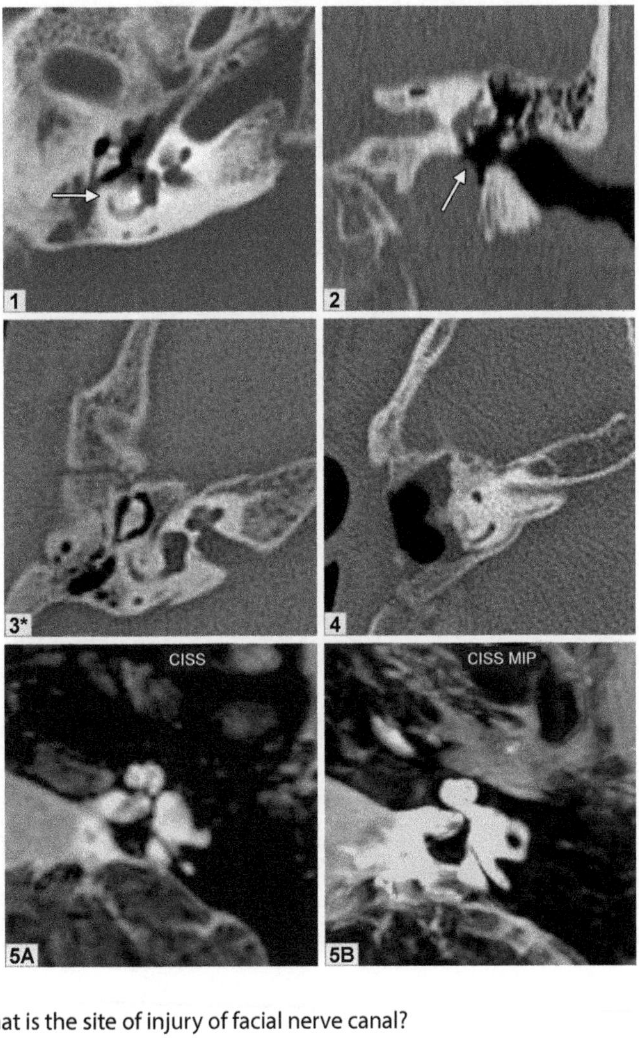

QUESTION

***Spot 3:** What is the site of injury of facial nerve canal?

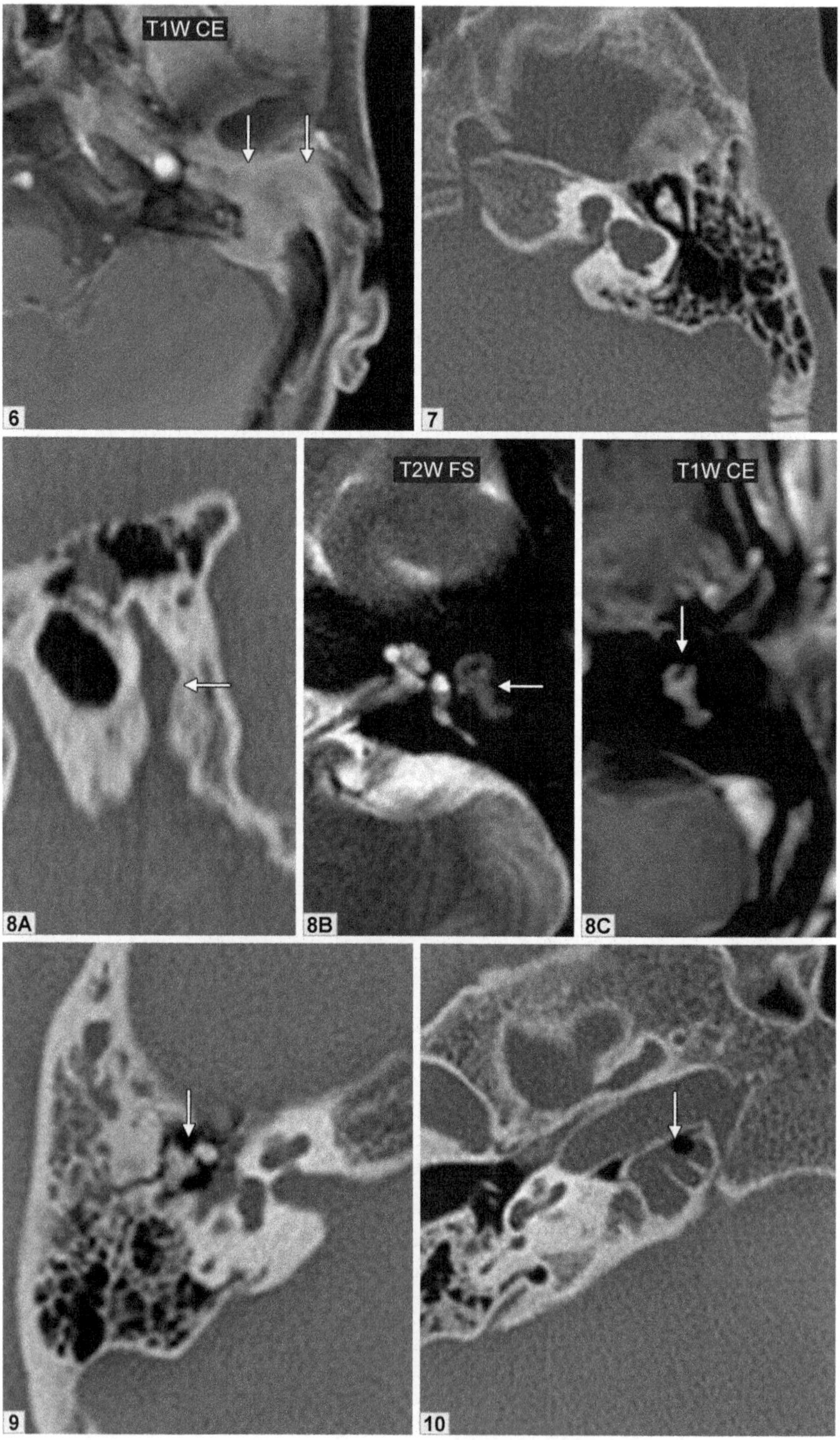
T1W CE
6
7
8A
T2W FS
8B
T1W CE
8C
9
10

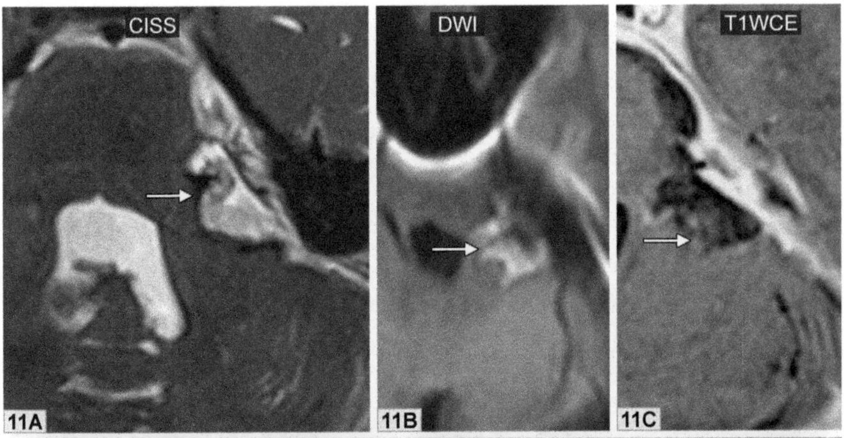
CISS
DWI
T1WCE
11A
11B
11C

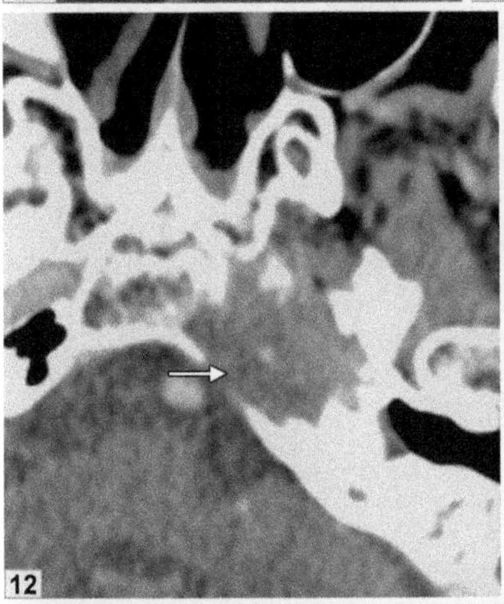
12

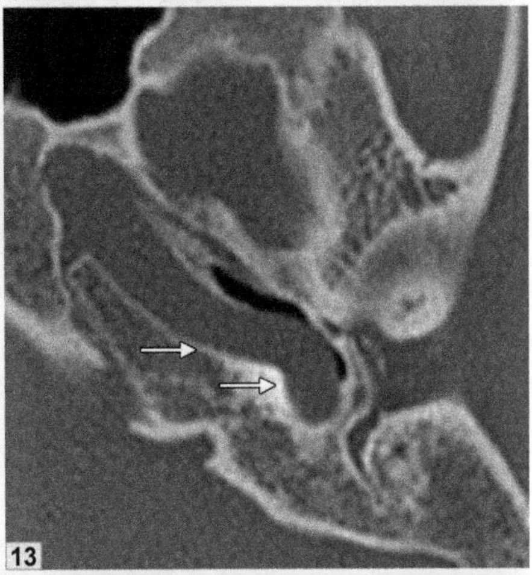
13

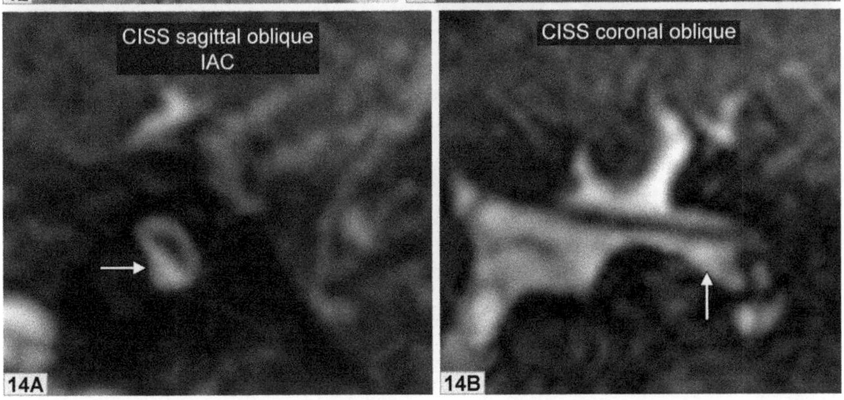
CISS sagittal oblique
IAC
CISS coronal oblique
14A
14B

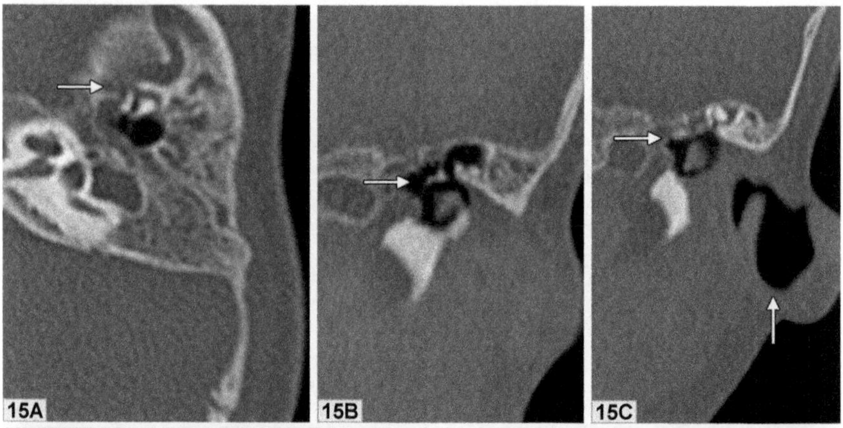
15A
15B
15C

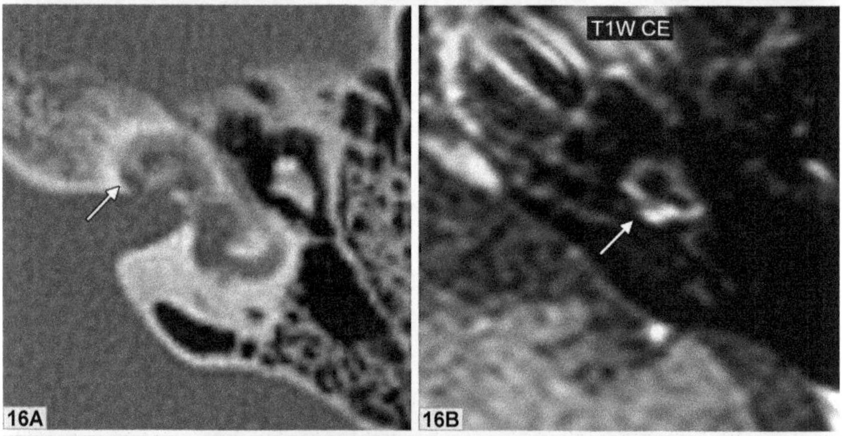
T1W CE
16A
16B

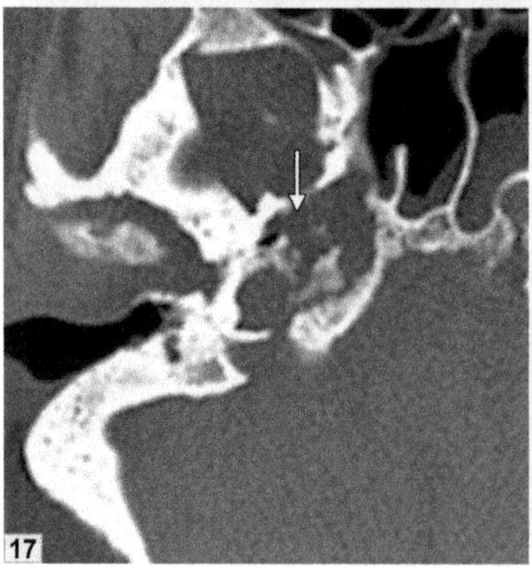
17

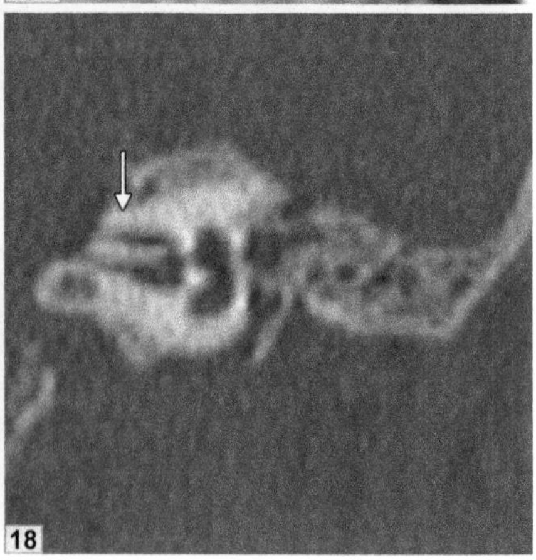
18

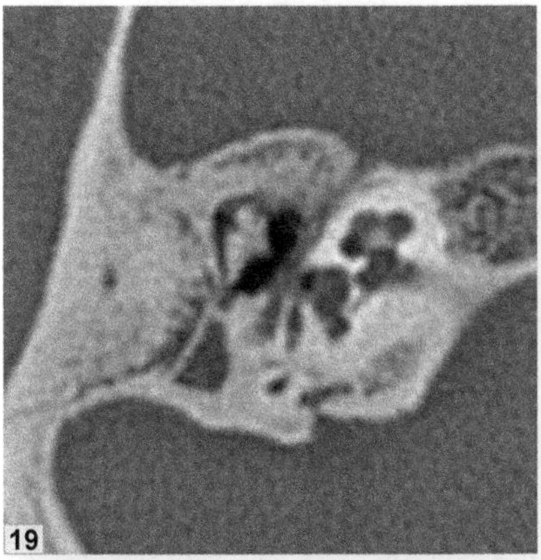
19

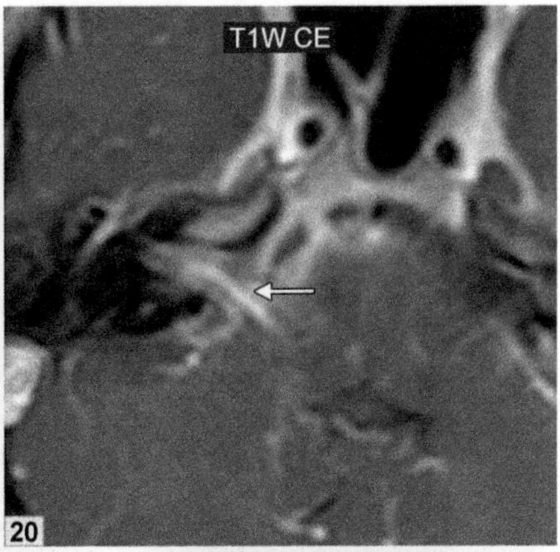
T1W CE
20

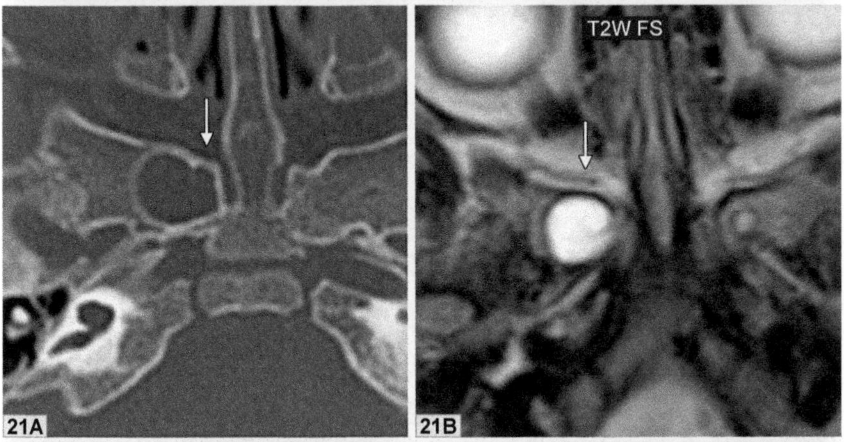
T2W FS
21A
21B

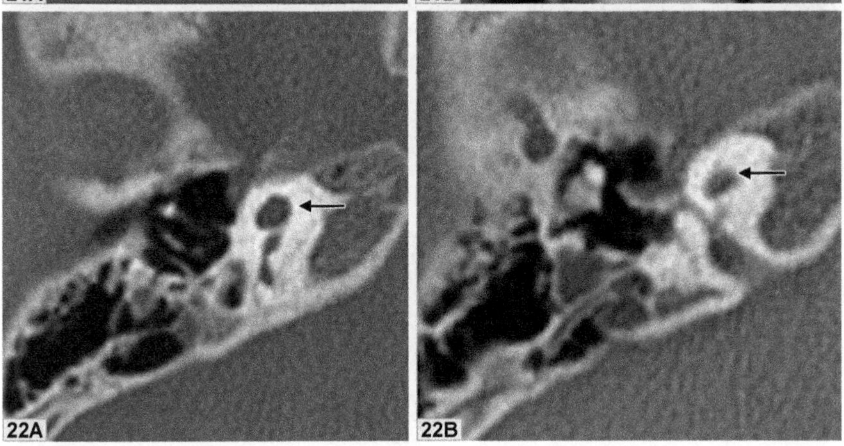
22A
22B

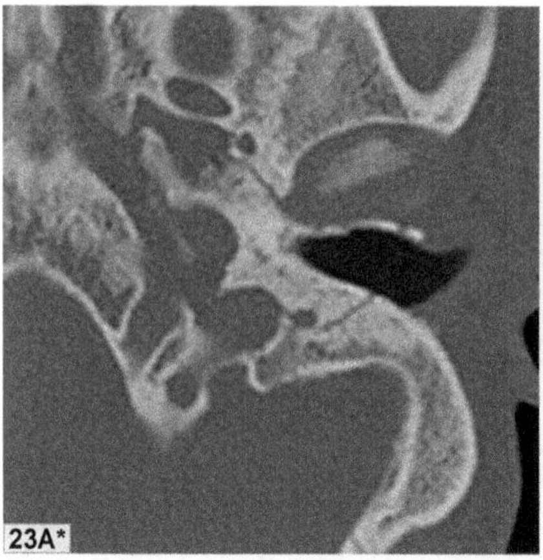

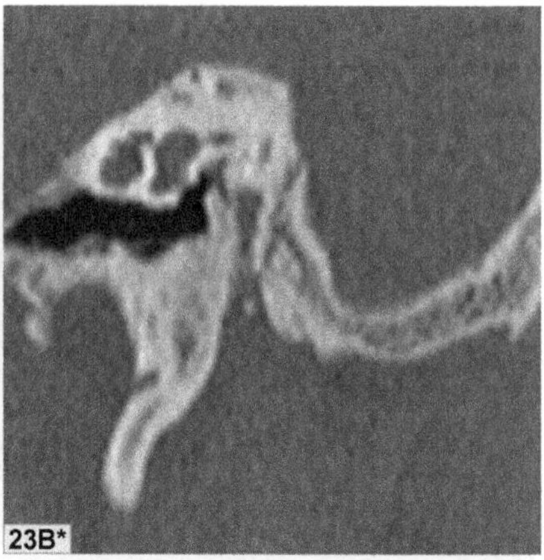

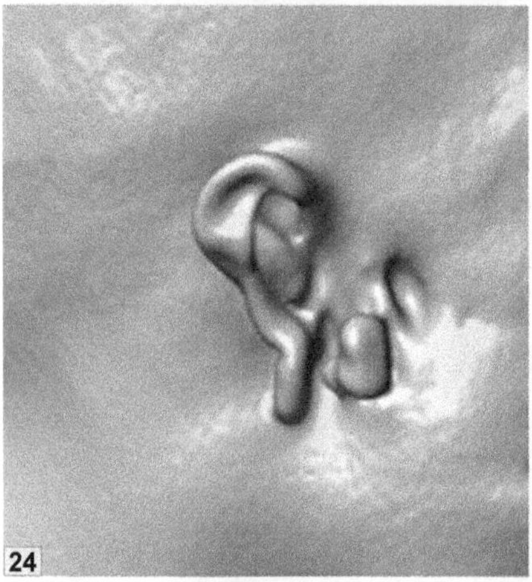

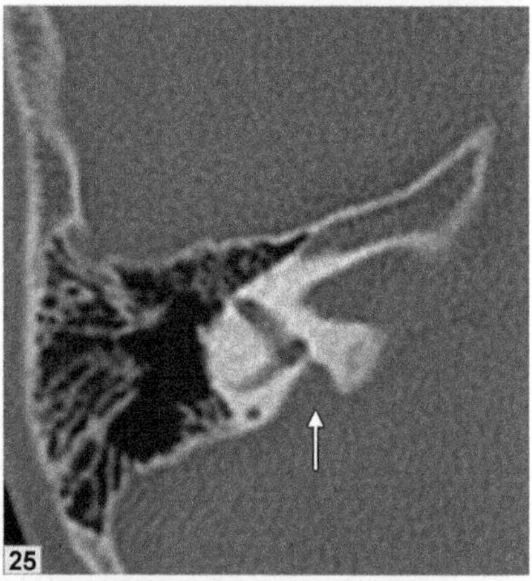

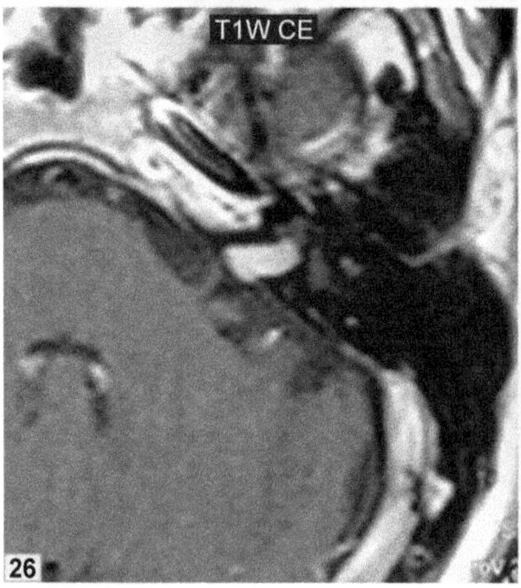

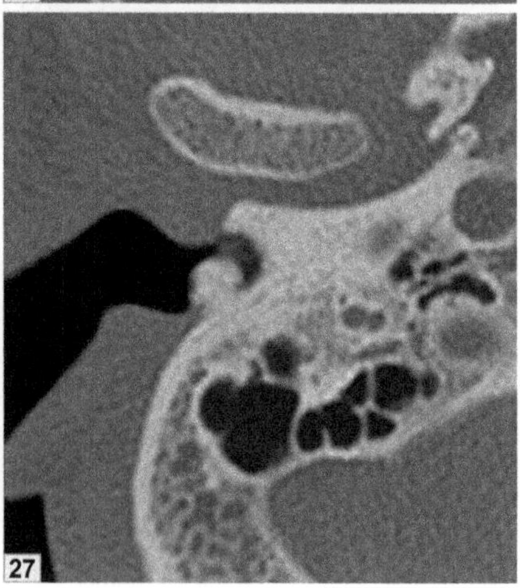

QUESTION

***Spot 23A AND B:** What is the site of injury of facial nerve canal?

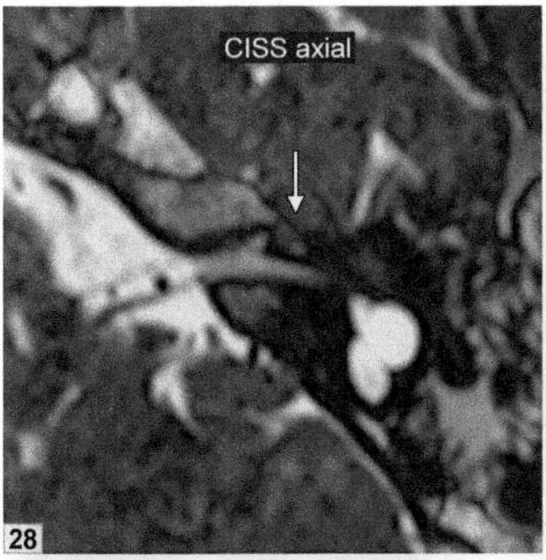

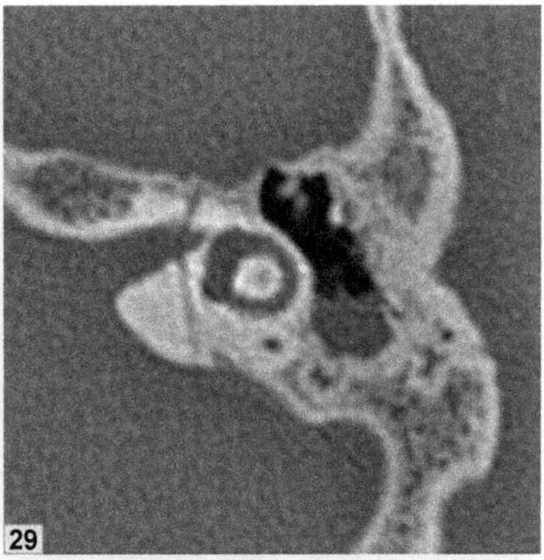

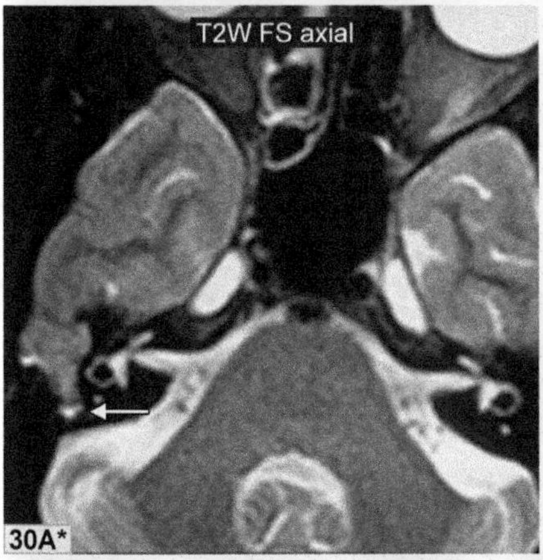

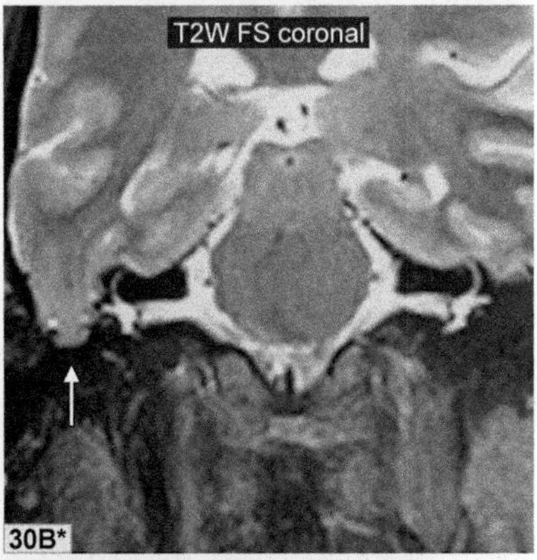

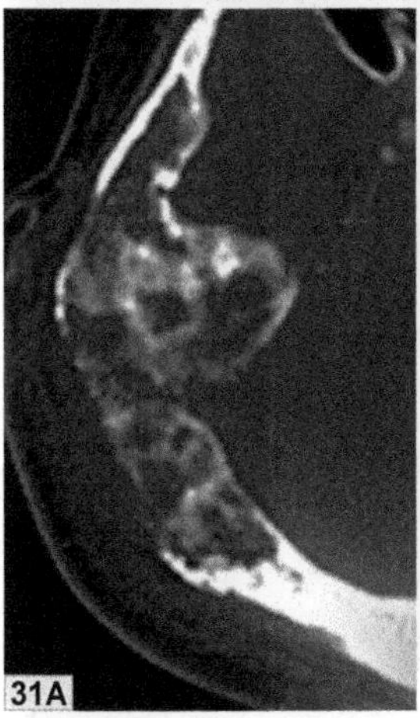

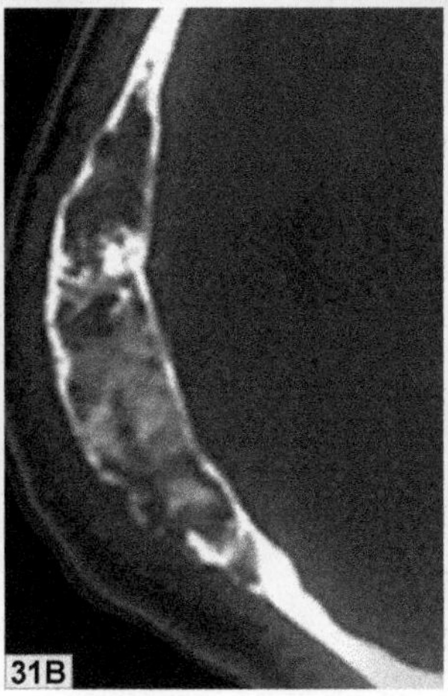

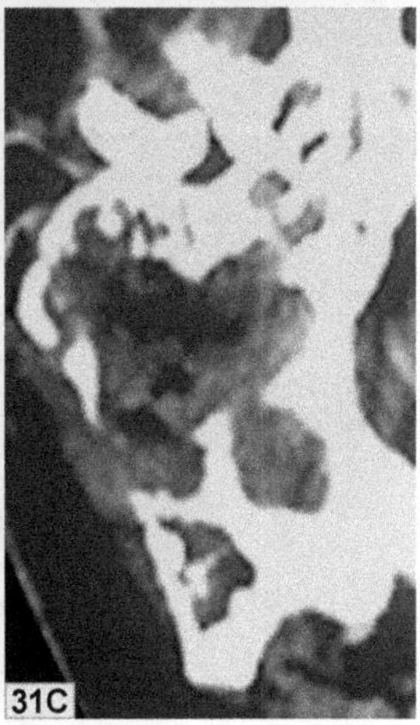

QUESTION

***Spot 30A AND B:** What postoperative complication is shown?

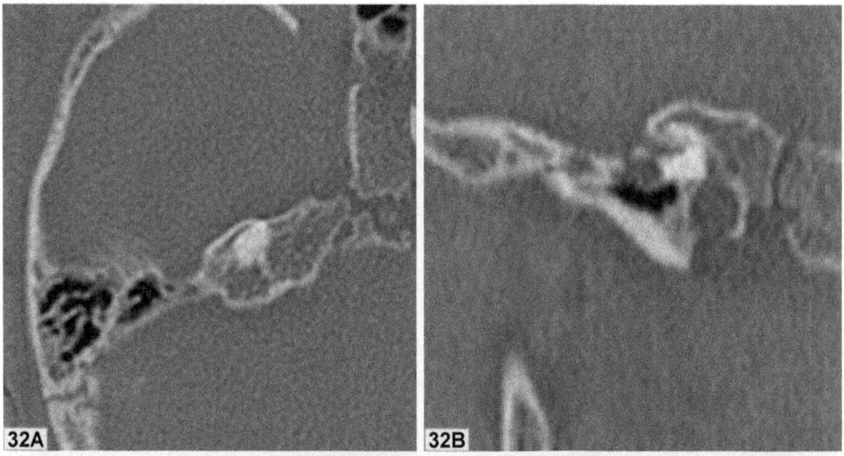

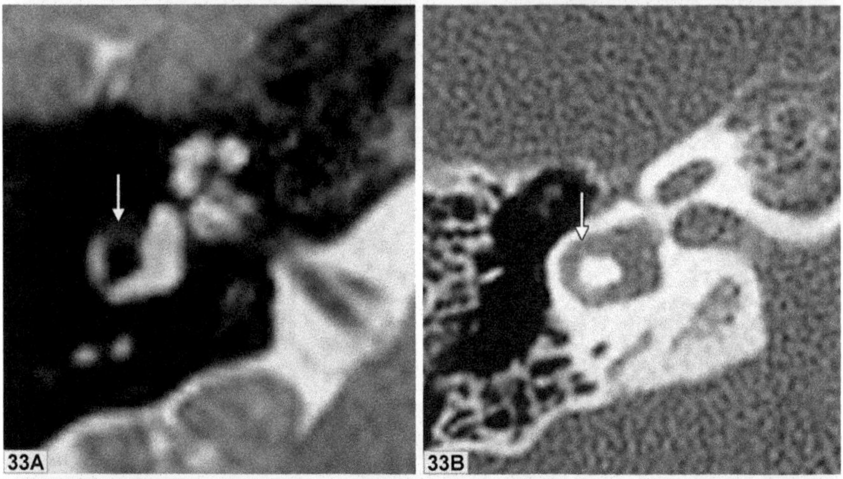

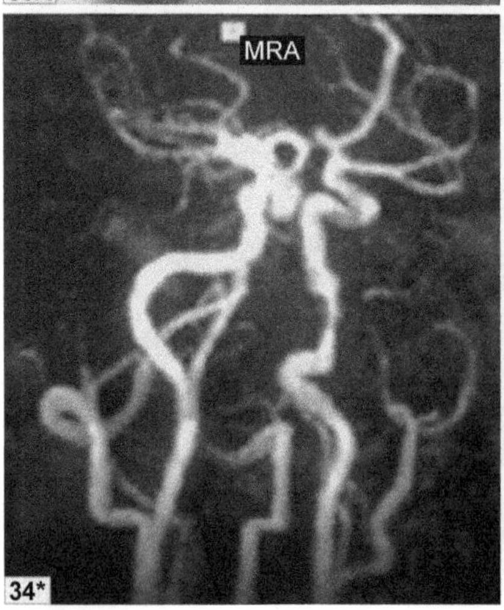

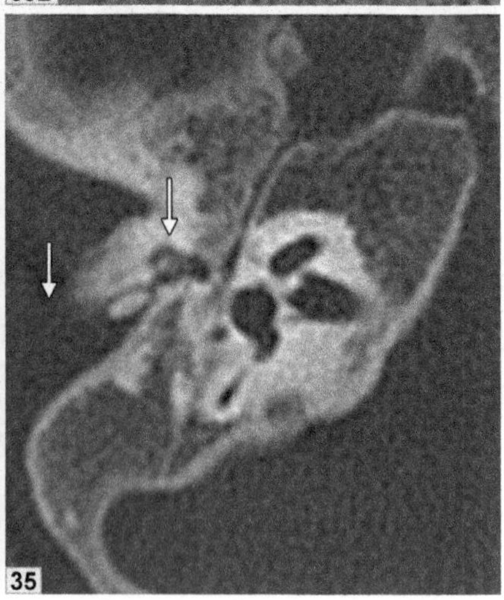

QUESTION

***Spot 34:** What complication of chronic suppurative otitis media (CSOM) is seen?

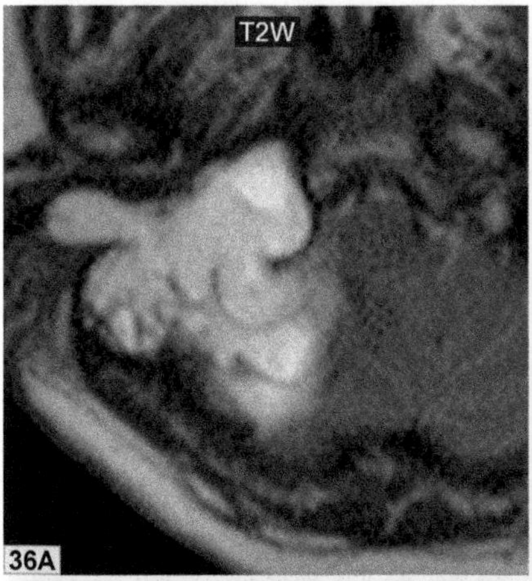
T2W
36A

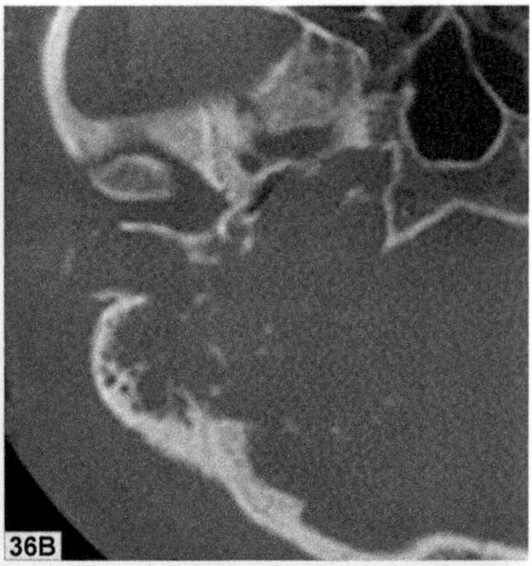
36B

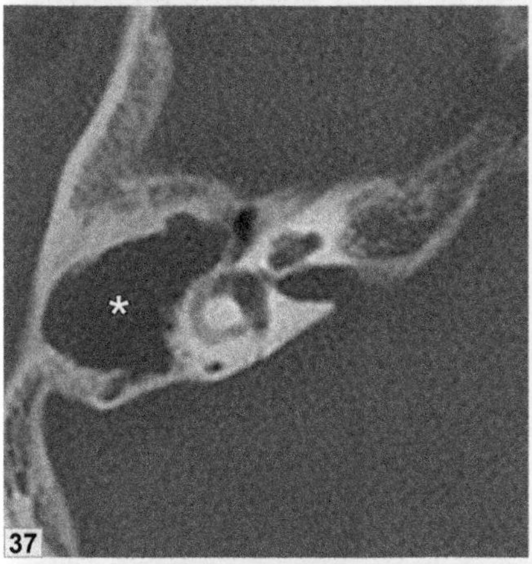
*
37

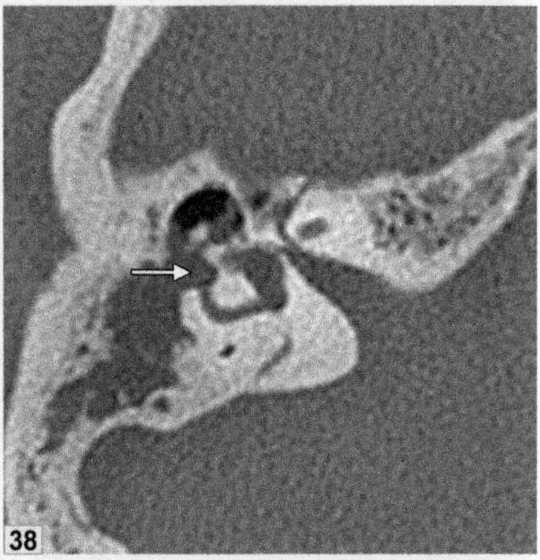
38

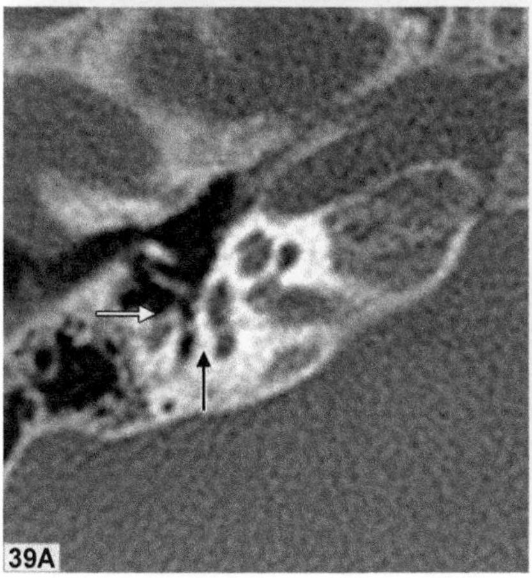
39A

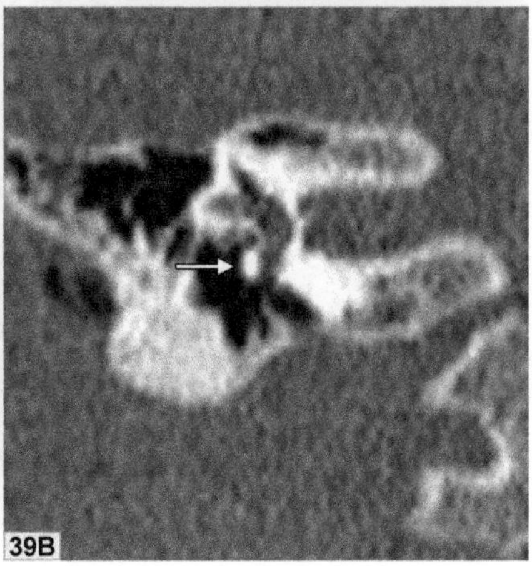
39B

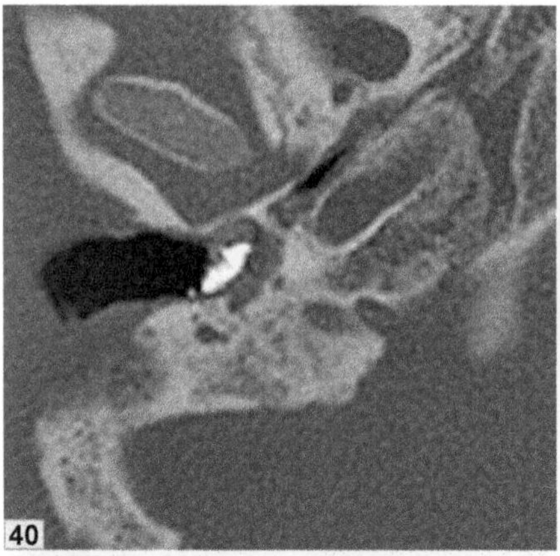

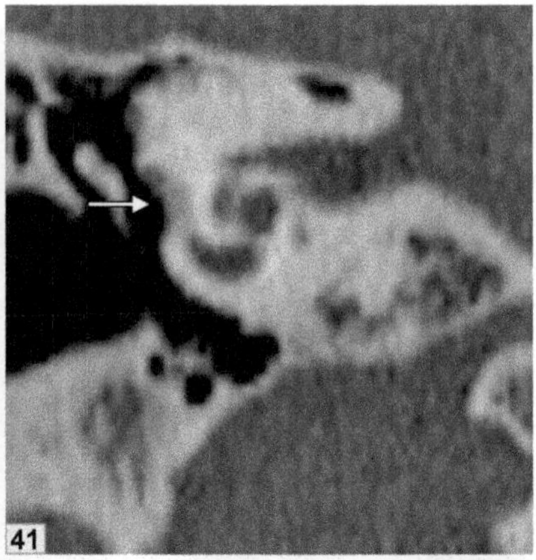

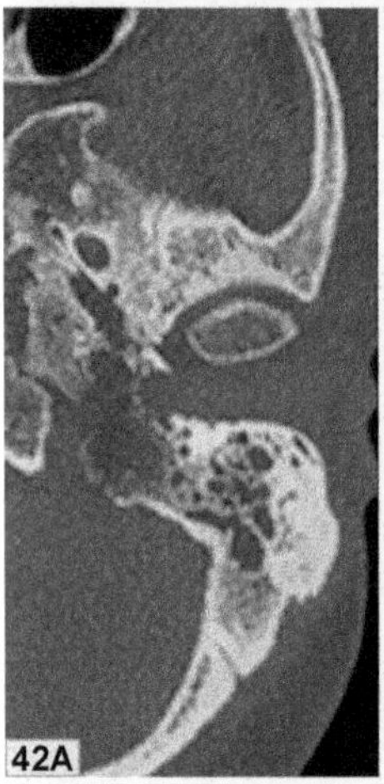

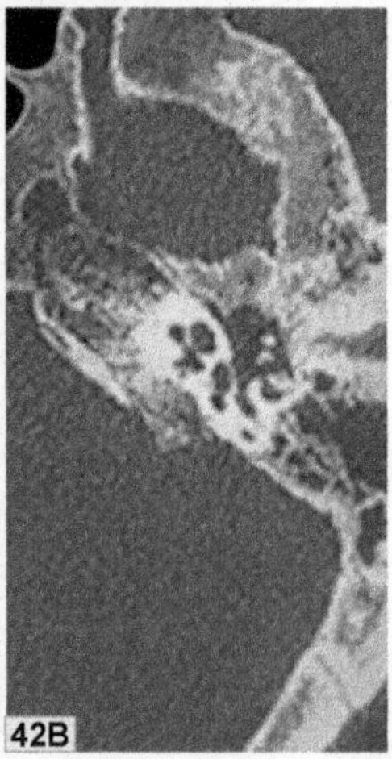

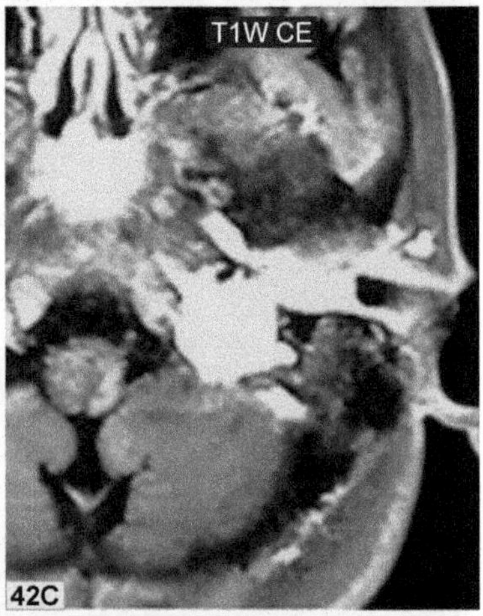

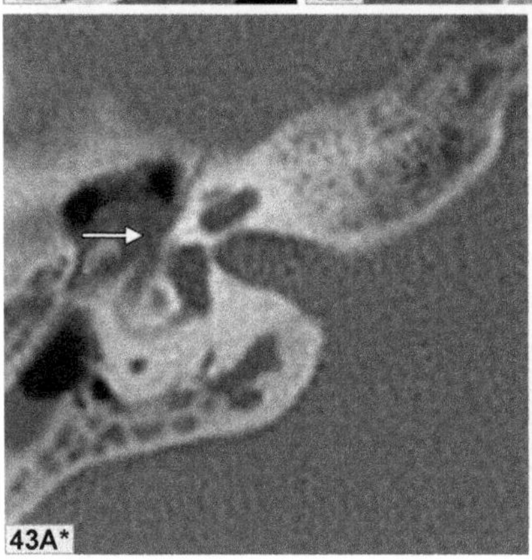

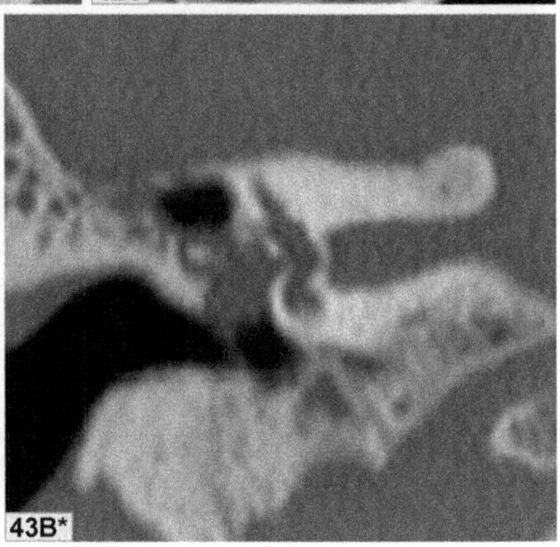

QUESTION

***Spot 43A AND B:** What complication of CSOM is shown?

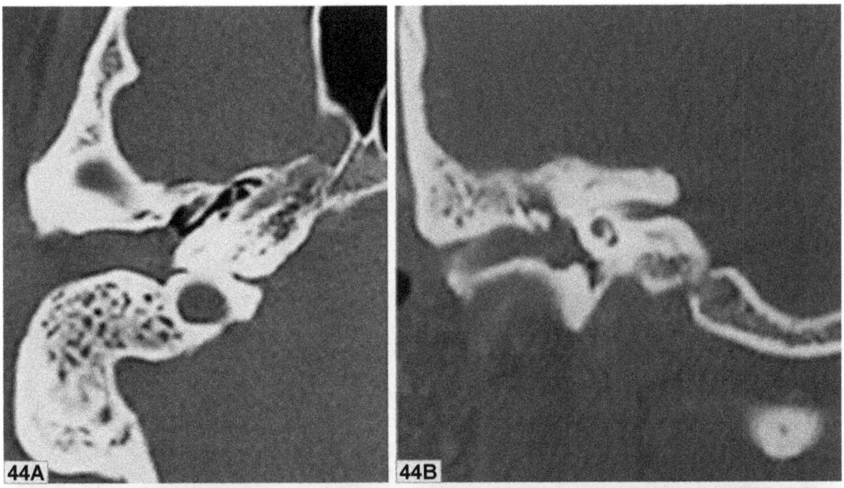

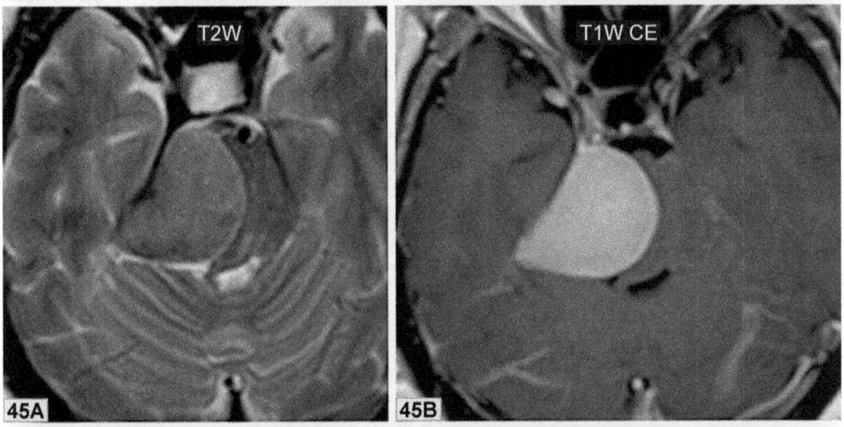

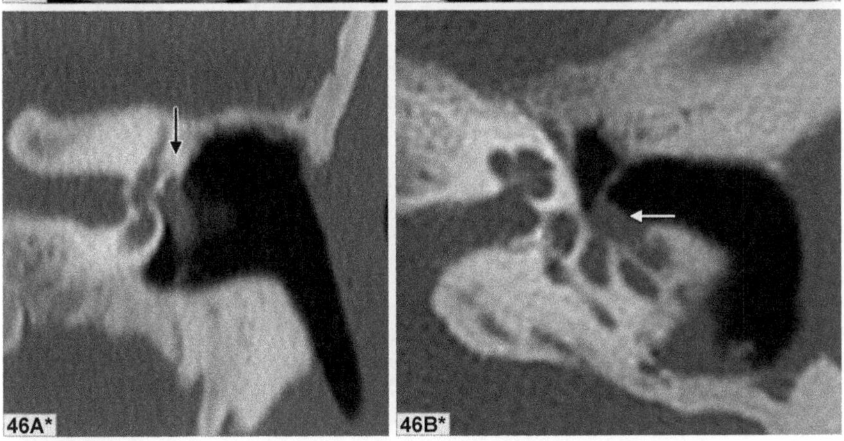

QUESTION

***Spot 46A AND B:** Which facial nerve abnormality is shown?

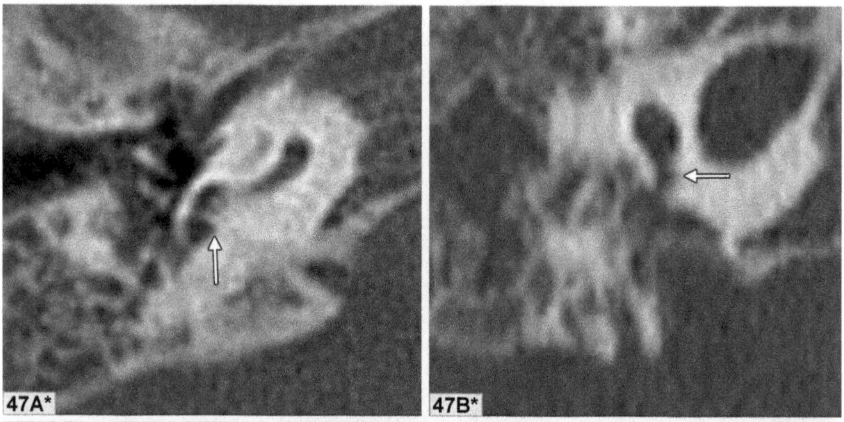

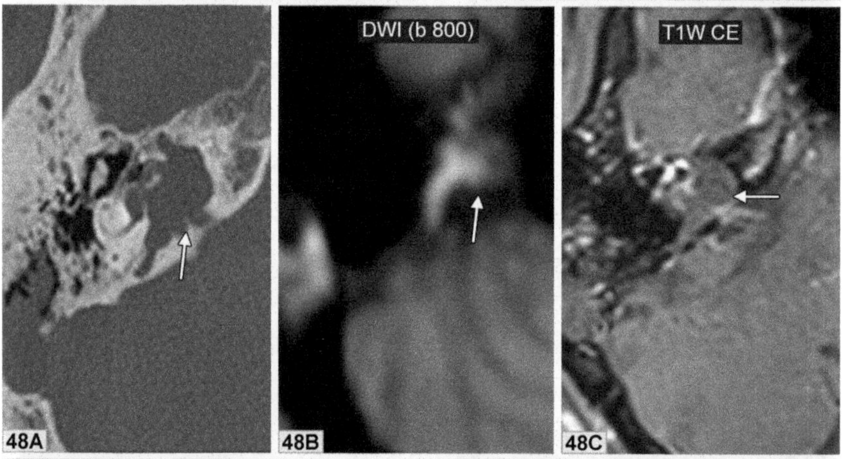

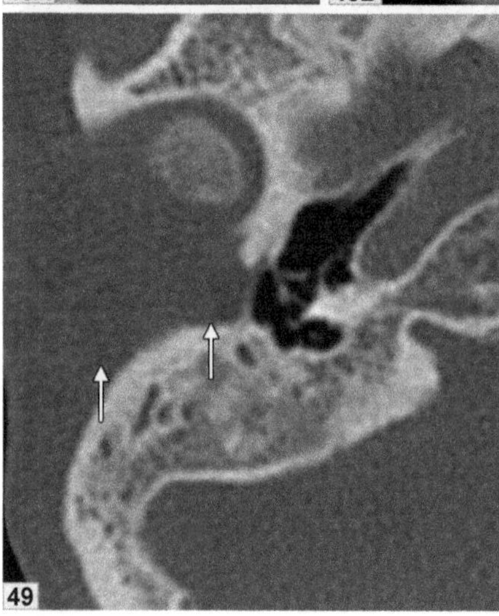

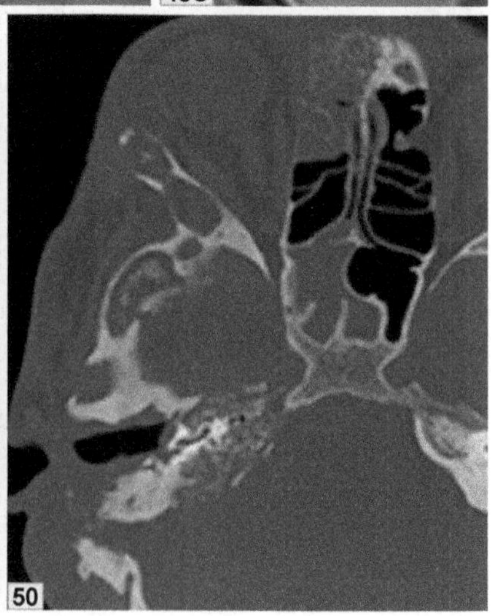

QUESTION

***Spot 47A AND B:** Which complication of labyrinthitis ossificans is shown?

KEY

Image Spot No.	Answer
1	Postinfective labyrinthitis ossificans
2	Dehiscent jugular bulb
3	Tympanic segment
4	Postmastoidectomy status
5 (A and B)	Incomplete partition type II
6	EAC carcinoma
7	Incomplete partition type I
8 (A to C)	Facial nerve schwannoma
9	Incudomalleal separation
10	Petrous apex mucocele
11 (A to C)	Cerebellopontine angle cistern epidermoid
12	Petrous apex metastasis
13	Aberrant course of ICA
14 (A and B)	Cochlear nerve aplasia
15 (A to C)	Microtia with ossicular dysplasia
16 (A to B)	Cochlear otosclerosis
17	Skull base osteomyelitis
18	Duplication of IAC
19	Longitudinal fracture of petrous temporal
20	Vestibular neuritis and meningitis
21 (A and B)	Lateral recess mucocele
22 (A and B)	Cochlear hypoplasia type 1 (CH1)
23 (A and B)	Mastoid segment
24	Grade 1 microtia with preauricular tag
25	Enlarged vestibular aqueduct
26	Acoustic schwannoma
27	EAC osteoma
28	Cochlear aplasia
29	Transverse fracture of temporal bone
30 (A and B)	Postmastoidectomy brain herniation
31 (A to C)	Fibrous dysplasia with mastoid abscess
32 (A and B)	Complete labyrinthine aplasia
33 (A and B)	Early labyrinthitis ossificans
34	Left IJV thrombosis and ICA stenosis

Continued

Continued

Image Spot No.	Answer
35	EAC atresia, reduced middle ear volume, and ossicular dysplasia
36 (A and B)	Petrous temporal chondrosarcoma
37	Postmastoidectomy recurrent CSOM
38	Lateral SCC fistula
39 (A and B)	RW stenosis due to bony bar; prominent pyramidal eminence
40	Ossicular implant
41	Fenestral otosclerosis
42 (A to C)	Glomus jugulotympanicum
43 (A and B)	Tympanic part of facial nerve canal erosion
44 (A and B)	Keratosis obturans
45 (A and B)	Meningioma
46 (A and B)	Overhanging tympanic segment of facial nerve
47 (A and B)	RW stenosis
48 (A to C)	Petrous apex cholesteatoma
49	Bony and cartilaginous EAC atresia
50	Tubercular otomastoiditis and osteomyelitis

(EAC: external auditory canal; CSOM: chronic suppurative otitis media; IAC: internal auditory canal; ICA: internal carotid artery; IJV: internal jugular vein; RW: round window; SCC: semicircular canal)

Index

Page numbers followed by *b* refer to box, *f* refer to figure, *fc* refer to flowchart, and *t* refer to table.

B

C

N

O

P

Q

R

T

EU GSPR Authorised Reprsentative
Logos Europe, 9 rue Nicolas Poussin
1700, La Rochelle, France
Phone: +33 (0) 6 67 93 73 78
E-mail: contact@logoseurope.eu

www.ingramcontent.com/pod-product-compliance
Ingram Content Group UK Ltd.
Pitfield, Milton Keynes, MK11 3LW, UK
UKHW060715180726
473396UK00005B/182
* 9 7 8 9 3 9 0 0 2 0 7 3 7 *